Women's Issues in
Thrombosis and Hemostasis

In Memory of

AMIRAM ELDOR, MD

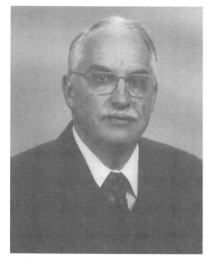

Amiram Eldor grew up in Tel Aviv. He graduated from the Hebrew University Hadassah Medical School in 1970. Following internship in hematology at Hadassah University Hospital and a two-year fellowship (1978–1980) at Cornell University Hospital, NY, he joined the senior staff of the Hematology Department at Hadassah University Hospital. In 1993 Professor Eldor was appointed as Director of the Hematology Institute at Tel Aviv Medical Center.

Professor Eldor was an outstanding hematologist, brilliant researcher, remarkable lecturer and an excellent mentor. His most meaningful studies were in the field of thrombosis, hemostasis and vascular biology. Among his remarkable contributions are insights into the understanding of prostacyclin secretion from endothelial cells, interactions between megakaryocytes and endothelial cells and description of hypercoagulability in patients with thalassemia. Professor Eldor was a leading investigator in the field of thrombophilia and gestational vascular complications, and he pioneered studies aimed at improvement of pregnancy results in women with these complications by using low molecular weight heparin.

Professor Amiram Eldor accomplished this work with extraordinary prominence until his untimely and tragic death in an airplane crash at the age of 59. Amiram is survived by his wife Sofia and his sons Roy and Eran. We extend our deepest sympathy to his family.

SHMUEL GILLIS, MD

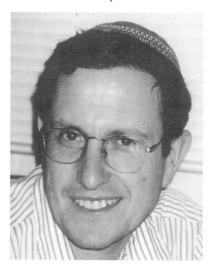

Shmuel Gillis was born in Sunderland, England in 1959. His family moved to Israel when he was aged eleven. He graduated from the Hebrew University Hadassah Medical School in 1982. Dr Gillis completed his training in internal medicine and hematology at Hadassah University Hospital in Jerusalem.

During his research fellowship with Dr Barbara and Bruce Furie at the New England Medical Center in Boston in 1994–1996 he focused on biochemical and functional aspects of factor IX. Since 1996 Dr Gillis served as senior hematologist supervising the field of thrombosis and hemostasis at Hadassah University Hospital. Clotting problems in women were a major interest for Dr Gillis, who was one of the pioneer users of LMWH in pregnancy and an active participant in trials of LMWH in women with gestational vascular complications.

Dr Shmuel Gillis was killed by Palestinian gunmen on his way home from Hadassah University Hospital. His chapter on 'DIC in pregnancy' was sent to the editor just two days before his untimely death in 2001. Shmuel Gillis was a dedicated physician, thoughtful colleague and a close friend and he is greatly missed.

Shmuel is survived by his wife Ruti and his children Reut, Amichai, Neta, Noam and Shai. We extend our deepest sympathy to his family.

Women's Issues in Thrombosis and Hemostasis

Edited by

Benjamin Brenner, MD
Director, Thrombosis and Hemostasis Unit,
Rambam Medical Center,
Haifa, Israel

Victor J Marder, MD
Director, Vascular Medicine Program,
Orthopaedic Hospital, UCLA,
Los Angeles, USA

Jacqueline Conard, PhD
Hemostasis and Thrombosis Unit,
Department of Biological Hematology,
Hôtel-Dieu, Paris, France

MARTIN DUNITZ

First published in the United Kingdom in 2002 by
Martin Dunitz Ltd
The Livery House
7–9 Pratt Street
London NW1 0AE

Tel: +44(0) 20-7482-2202
Tel: +44(0) 20-7267-0159
E-mail: info@dunitz.co.uk
Website: http://www.dunitz.co.uk

A CIP catalogue record for this book is available from the British Library

ISBN 1-84184-003-3

Distributed in the USA by
Fulfilment Center
Taylor & Francis
7625 Empire Drive
Florence, KY 41042, USA
Toll Free Tel.: +1 800 634 7064
E-mail: cserve@routledge_ny.com

Distributed in Canada by
Taylor & Francis
74 Rolark Drive
Scarborough, Ontario M1R 4G2, Canada
Toll Free Tel.: +1 877 226 2237
E-mail: tal_fran@istar.ca

Distributed in the rest of the world by
Thomson Publishing Services
Cheriton House
North Way
Andover, Hampshire SP10 5BE, UK
Tel.: +44 (0) 1264 332424
E-mail: salesorder.tandf@thomsonpublishingservices.co.uk

Composition by Scribe, Gillingham, Kent, UK
Printed and bound in Great Britain by Biddles Ltd, Guildford and King's Lynn

Contents

Preface

Women are affected by unique aspects of thrombosis and hemostasis throughout a large part of their life, starting at menarche and puberty, followed by issues of contraception, fertility and assisted reproductive techniques. During pregnancy, physiological changes are common and gestational vascular complications are a major cause of maternal and fetal morbidity and mortality. The role of inherited and acquired thrombophilia in these settings is rapidly emerging as a focus of attention and highlights issues of maternal and fetal health. At the menopause, hormone replacement therapy variably affects the coagulation system in both positive and negative ways.

The rapidly emerging spectrum of coagulation abnormalities in women is the foundation for this book, which is intended to serve as a comprehensive source of information for basic principles and clinical issues of thrombosis and hemostasis in women.

We hope that hematologists, gynecologists, obstetricians, neonatologists and other researchers in the field will find the book valuable for both clinical practice and research work.

Benjamin Brenner
Victor J Marder
Jacqueline Conard

Contributors

Regine Ahner, MD
Department of Obstetrics and Gynecology
The New York Hospital-Cornell Medical Center
525 East 68th Street
New York, NY 10021
USA

Ivan Bank, MD
Department of Vascular Medicine
Academic Medical Center
The University of Amsterdam
F4-277, Meibergdreef 9
1105 AZ Amsterdam
The Netherlands

Tiziano Barbui, MD
Divisione di Ematologia
Ospedali Riuniti di Bergamo
Largo Barozzi 1
24128 Bergamo
Italy

Katarina Bremme, MD, PhD
Department of Women & Child Health
Karolinska Hospital
Div Ob/Gyn, Kl
PO Box 140
Stockholm S-17176
Sweden

Benjamin Brenner, MD
Thrombosis and Hemostasis Unit
Department of Hematology
Rambam Medical Center
Technion–Israel Institute of Technology
Haifa 31096
Israel

James B Bussel, MD
Department of Obstetrics and Gynecology
The New York Hospital-Cornell Medical Center
525 East 68th Street
New York, NY 10021
USA

Jacqueline Conard, PhD
Hemostasis and Thrombosis Unit
Department of Biological Hematology
Hôtel-Dieu Hospital
1 Place du Parvis Notre-Dame
75181 Paris, Cedex 04
France

* Amiram Eldor, MD
Institute of Hematology
Tel-Aviv Sourasky Medical Center
6 Weizman Street
Tel-Aviv 64239
Israel

Yossef Ezra, MD
Department of Obstetrics and Gynecology
Hadassah Medical Center
Jerusalem 91120
Israel

Guido Finazzi, MD
Divisione di Ematologia
Ospedali Riuniti di Bergamo
Largo Barozzi, 1
24128 Bergamo
Italy

Monica Galli, PhD
Divisione di Ematologia
Ospedali Riuniti di Bergamo
Largo Barozzi, 1
24128 Bergamo
Italy

Grigoris T Gerotziafas, MD
Department of Biological Hematology
Hôtel-Dieu Hospital
1 Place du Parvis Notre Dame
75181 Paris, Cedex 04
France

Paul Giangrande, MD, FRCP, FRCPath
Oxford Haemophilia Centre and
Thrombosis Unit
Churchill Hospital
Oxford, OX3 7LJ
UK

* Shmuel Gillis, MD
Department of Hematology
Hadassah University Hospital
Ein Kerem
Jerusalem 91120
Israel

Ann Gompel, MD, PhD
UF de Gynecologie
Assistance Hôpitaux Publique de Paris
Hôtel-Dieu
1 Place du Parvis Notre-Dame
75181 Paris, Cedex 04
France

**Ian A Greer, MD, FRCP (Glas), FRCP (Ed),
FRCP (Lond), FRCOG**
Department of Obstetrics & Gynaecology
University of Glasgow
Glasgow Royal Infirmary
10 Alexandra Parade
Glasgow G31 2ER
UK

Marie-Hélène Horellou, MD
Hemostasis and Thrombosis Unit
Department of Biological Hematology
Hôtel-Dieu Hospital
1 Place du Parvis Notre-Dame
75181 Paris, Cedex 04
France

Berend Isermann, MD
Blood Research Institute
The Blood Center of Southeastern Wisconsin
8727 Watertown Plamk Road
Milwaukee, WI 53226
USA

Rezan A Kadir, MD, MRCOG, FRCS
Haemophilia Centre and Haemostasis Unit
Royal Free Hospital
Pond Street
London, NW3 2QG
UK

Cécile Kaplan, MD
Institut National de la Transfusion Sanguine
Laboratoire d'Immunologie Plaquettaire
6, rue Alexandre-Cabanel
75739 Paris, Cedex 15
France

Gili Kenet, MD
Pediatric Coagulation Service
The National Hemophilia Center
Sheba Medical Center
Tel-Hashomer, 52621
Israel

Andrea Kosch, MD
Klinik und Poliklinik für Kinderheilkunde -
Pädiatrische Hämatologie/Onkologie
Westfälische Wilhelms-Universität Münster
Albert-Schweitser-Straße 33
48149 Münster
Germany

Michael Kupfermincz, MD
Department of Obstetrics & Gynecology
Lis Maternity Hospital
Tel Aviv Sourasky Medical Center
6 Weizman Street
Tel Aviv, 64239
Israel

Christine Lee, MA, MD, DSc(Med), FRCP, FRCPath
Haemophilia Centre and Haemostasis Unit
Royal Free Hospital
Pond Street
London, NW3 2QG
UK

Delphine Levy, MD
UF de Gynecologie
Assistance Hopitaux Publique de Paris
Hôtel-Dieu
1 Place du parvis Notre-Dame
75181 Paris, Cedex 04
France

Marilyn J Manco-Johnson, MD
Department of Pediatrics and Pathology
The Children's Hospital
University of Colorado Health Sciences Center
1056 East 19th Avenue
Denver, CO 80218
USA

Victor J Marder, MD
Vascular Medicine Program
Orthopaedic Hospital
University of California Los Angeles
2400 South Flower Street
Los Angeles, CA 90007
USA

Saskia Middeldorp, MD, PhD
Department of Vascular Medicine
Academic Medical Center
The University of Amsterdam
F4-277, Meibergdreef 9
1105 AZ Amsterdam
The Netherlands

Dena M Minning, MD, PhD
Corporate Consultant
MEDACorp
60 State Street
Boston, MA 02109
USA

Ulrike Nowak-Göttl, MD
Klinik und Poliklinik für Kinderheilkunde -
Pädiatrische Hämatologie/Onkologie
Westfälische Wilhelms-Universität Münster
Albert-Schweitser-Straße 33
48149 Münster
Germany

Genevieve Plu-Bureau, MD
Hemostasis and Thrombosis Unit
Department of Biological Hematology
Hôtel-Dieu Hospital
1 Place du Parvis Notre-Dame
75181 Paris, Cedex 04
France

Martin H Prins, PhD
Department of Clinical Epidemiology and
Medical Technology Assessment
Academic Hospital Maastricht
The University of Maastricht
P. Debyelaan 25
6202 AZ Maastricht
The Netherlands

Meyer Samama, MD
Department of Biological Hematology
Hôtel-Dieu Hospital
1 Place du Parvis Notre Dame
75181 Paris, Cedex 04
France

Arnon Samueloff, MD
Feto-Maternal Medicine Unit
Department of Obstetrics and Gynecology
Shaare Zedek Medical Center
Jerusalem 91031
Israel

Sam Schulman, MD
Department of Internal Medicine
Karolinska Hospital
Stockholm S 171 76
Sweden

Ori Shen, MD
Feto-Maternal Medicine Unit
Department of Obstetrics and Gynecology
Shaare Zedek Medical Center
Jerusalem 91031
Israel

Isobel D Walker, MD
Department of Haematology
Glasgow Royal Infirmary and
Glasgow Royal Maternity Hospital
3rd Floor, Macewen Building
Castle Street
Glasgow G4 0SF
UK

Hartmut Weiler, PhD
Blood Research Institute
The Blood Center of Southeastern Wisconsin
8727 Watertown Plamk Road
Milwaukee, WI 53226
USA

Johnny S Younis, MD
Bruce Rappaport Faculty of Medicine
Technion, Haifa, and
Reproductive Medicine Unit
Department of Obstetrics and Gynecology
Poriya Medical Center
Tiberias 15208
Israel

1

Overview of hemostasis

Dena M Minning, Benjamin Brenner and Victor J Marder

INTRODUCTION

Humans have evolved an intricate hemostatic system that is designed to maintain blood in a fluid state under physiologic conditions but is primed to react to vascular injury in an explosive manner in order to stem blood loss by sealing the defect in the vessel wall. Hemostasis is a normal process that leads to cessation of blood flow from a damaged vessel. Thrombosis, however, is a pathological process, which may occur if the hemostatic stimulus is unregulated, either because the capacity of the inhibitory pathways is impaired or (more commonly) because the capacity of the natural anticoagulant mechanism is overwhelmed by the intensity of the procoagulant stimulus. Thrombosis may be regarded as an 'accident of nature' that has not had time to adapt through the lengthy process of evolution to the advances of modern medicine, which allow patients to survive the hemostatic challenge of major surgery and trauma but leave them vulnerable to thrombosis.

The entire hemostatic process – involving platelets, clotting factors, and endothelium, as well as inhibitory mechanisms of platelet aggregation, clotting, and fibrinolysis – serves to promote the perfect balance and location of hemostasis and recovery. This highly developed system of checks and balances allows a rapid and efficient hemostatic response to bleeding, but avoids a thrombogenic response away from the site of injury or persisting beyond the time of its physiologic need. Derangement of any portion of this intricate process can produce an imbalance, sometimes only slight, with a resultant hemorrhagic or thrombotic clinical disorder. A further complicating feature of this delicate balance is therapeutic intervention, which must be carefully regulated to correct a hemostatic defect without upsetting the balance too far, thus leading to thrombosis.

PLATELETS

The participation of platelets in hemostasis is a fundamental component of this physiologic process. Initially, platelets adhere to the compromised portion of a blood vessel. This is followed by the spreading of adherent platelets on the exposed subendothelial surface, secretion of stored platelet constituents (including molecules involved in hemostasis and wound healing), and formation of large platelet aggregates.[1] In addition, platelet membrane sites become available for binding and concentration of clotting factors, thereby accelerating plasma coagulation, resulting in the formation of a fibrin network that reinforces the otherwise friable platelet plug. The firm platelet–fibrin clot subsequently retracts into a smaller volume, a process that is also platelet-dependent.

Platelets do not adhere to normal vascular endothelial cells (Figure 1.1), but rather to an

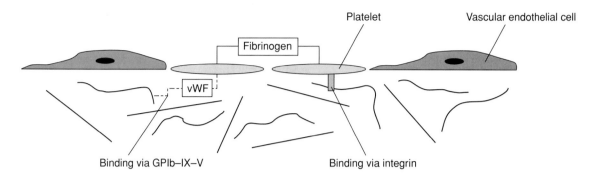

Figure 1.1 Platelet interactions. Platelets do not adhere to normal vascular endothelial cells. Via GPIb–IX–V, platelets bind vWF, which binds to subendothelium matrix proteins such as collagen. Platelets also bind to subendothelial components directly via integrins. Additionally, platelets are linked to one another by fibrinogen, which binds platelet GPIIb/IIIa.

area of endothelial disruption (e.g. the cut end of a divided blood vessel), which exposes subendothelial binding sites for an adhesive protein, von Willebrand factor (vWF), via the platelet glycoprotein (GP)Ib–IX–V complex, as well as fibrinogen and fibronectin through other integrin receptors.[2] These adhesive proteins are hypothesized to participate in the formation of a 'bridge' between platelets and subendothelial connective tissue, although this may be an oversimplification.

The importance of platelet adhesion to the subendothelium is illustrated by the occurrence of hemorrhage in Bernard–Soulier disease, in which patients lack GPIb–IX, or in von Willebrand's disease, in which von Willebrand factor (vWF) is decreased or defective. At high shear rates comparable to those found in arteries in the microvasculature (i.e. >800 per second), plasma vWF is required for normal adhesion of platelets to subendothelium, perhaps as a bridge between platelets and the fibrillar surface.[3] At low shear rates, adhesion of platelets to subendothelium is normal in patients with these disorders, suggesting that other proteins can substitute for the action of vWF, at least to some extent.

Other adhesive events probably include interactions of collagen with the platelet GPIa–IIa receptor,[4] followed by activation of intracellular signaling pathways by platelet GPVI.[5]

Abnormalities in either of these platelet receptors for collagen result in bleeding defects.

Once adherent to the subendothelium, platelets spread out on the surface, and additional platelets, delivered by the flowing blood, adhere first to the basal layer of adherent platelets and eventually to one another, forming a mass of aggregated platelets. A critical event in platelet aggregation and subsequent activation is induction of a change in the disposition of surface membrane GPIIb–IIIa,[6] which then acquires the capacity to bind fibrinogen, as well as vWF, fibronectin, and vitronectin.[7] Fibrinogen appears to be the most important protein in aggregation by virtue of its divalent structure, possibly allowing it to form a bridge from platelet to platelet, thereby mediating aggregation.

Several other integrins in the platelet membrane act as receptors for adhesive plasma proteins. These heterodimers, such as the vitronectin receptor, are present on the surface both of blood cells and of endothelial cells.[8] Whereas vWF and collagen can interact with resting platelets, fibrinogen forms a high-affinity bond only with the integrin GPIIb–IIIa on activated platelets.[9] In Glanzmann's thrombasthenia, a congenital disorder, the GPIIb–IIIa complex is deficient, and the associated defect in fibrinogen binding results in a bleeding tendency.[10] Likewise, the bleeding in congenital afibrinogenemia is caused, in part, by an abnormality of platelet aggregation.

Of the many platelet agonists with the ability to induce aggregation and granule secretion *in vitro*, those having the greatest physiological relevance are the proteolytic enzyme thrombin, adenosine diphosphate (ADP), collagen, arachidonic acid, and epinephrine. One major effect of these agonists is the unmasking of functional fibrinogen-binding sites via modulation of GPIIIb–IIIa. However, many of the major effects on platelets are actually visible, such as the disappearance of the equatorial band of microtubules that normally maintain the platelet's discoid shape, centralization of storage granules, and formation of pseudopodia. Epinephrine is unique since, unlike typical platelet agonists, it does not result in a detectable change in platelet shape.

Specific receptors exist on the platelet surface for these agonists.[11] Many of the receptor–agonist complexes interact in the platelet membrane with G proteins, which hydrolyze guanosine triphosphate (GTP). Evidently, some agonists interact with receptors that are coupled to ion-permeable channels in the platelet membrane, modulating ion flux – most importantly, the inward movement of calcium ions. Other agonist receptors are linked to protein tyrosine kinases (TK) that phosphorylate other sites on the receptor protein itself. Stimulatory agonists lead to activation of phospholipase C, which cleaves phosphatidylinositol bisphosphate (PIP_2) to form inositol trisphosphate (IP_3) and diacylglycerol. IP_3 reacts with receptors on calcium storage organelles known as the dense tubular system, analogous to the sarcoplasmic reticulum of muscle, leading to mobilization of calcium ions and increasing the cytoplasmic concentration of calcium.[12] Familial abnormalities in a G protein[13] and a phospholipase C[14] lead to mild hemorrhagic disorders.

Many processes involved in platelet activation are calcium-dependent. High concentrations of intracellular calcium (occurring, for example, after thrombin stimulation) lead to activation of a calcium-dependent neutral cysteine protease (calpain), which may participate in remodeling of cytoskeletal proteins, cleavage of receptor proteins[15] and thrombin-induced activation of platelets. Most importantly, calcium induces the enzyme, phospholipase A_2, to liberate arachidonic acid from membrane phospholipids.[16,17] Arachidonic acid is a substrate for the enzyme cyclo-oxygenase, ultimately forming the potent platelet agonist, thromboxane A_2, as well as stable prostaglandins such as prostaglandin D_2. Aspirin alkylates a reactive serine in glyco-oxygenase, thus permanently inactivating the enzyme; this accounts for the major pharmacological action on platelets of this widely used drug.

Diacylglycerol – like IP_3, a product of the action of phospholipase C – activates a ubiquitous enzyme, protein kinase C, in platelets.[18] Protein kinase C phosphorylates (among other substrates) pleckstrin, a 47 kDa protein that is a marker for activation of the kinase. Phosphatases provide a negative feedback, reducing the elevation of calcium ions by IP_3.[19] Diacylglycerol may be responsible for the alleged 'calcium-independent' reactions that occur during platelet activation, or it may act together with ionized calcium to activate protein kinase C, and thereby stimulate granule secretion.[20]

Platelets contain several classes of granules in which intracellular constituents are sequestered, including 'dense bodies' (containing serotonin, ATP, ADP, pyrophosphate, and calcium), α-granules (containing fibrinogen, vWF, factor V, high molecular weight kininogen (HMWK)), fibronectin, $α_1$-antitrypsin, (A5)b-thromboglobulin, platelet factor 4, and platelet-derived growth factor, and lysosomes (containing a variety of acid hydrolases).[21] Platelet stimulation results in centralization of these granules via activation of the platelet cytoskeletal contractile apparatus; polymerization of filamentous actin and phosphorylation of myosin are prominent reactions in platelets responding to receptor-mediated stimulation. In the presence of elevated cytoplasmic calcium, this leads to fusion of the granular envelope with the lining membranes of intracellular canaliculi and to external secretion of the granule contents.

During activation, platelets expose receptors for specific plasma clotting factors, particularly activated factor V (Va), which may be either secreted and expressed by the platelet or bound from plasma. This 'acquired' receptor, in conjunction with anionic phospholipids exposed on activated platelets, also functions as a binding site for factor Xa and thus provides an efficient catalytic environment for the conversion of prothrombin to thrombin by factor Xa.[22] An analogous system appears to exist for the binding of factor Ixa and subsequent conversion of factor X to Xa on platelets.

Platelet activation and its effects are modulated by several regulatory substances, of which the most potent inhibitor is cyclic 3',5'-adenosine monophosphate (cAMP).[23] In sufficient concentration, cAMP not only inhibits platelet aggregation, secretion, and shape change, but also platelet adhesion to surfaces. Like virtually all other animal cells except human red cells, platelets contain adenylate cyclase, the enzyme that converts ATP to cAMP. Adenylate cyclase is powerfully stimulated by the arachidonic acid products, prostaglandin D_2 in platelets and PGI_2 or prostacyclin (produced by endothelial cells). cAMP stimulates a protein kinase that mediates phosphorylation of an ATP-dependent calcium-pumping system that removes calcium from the cytosol.

Platelets also contain cyclic nucleotide phosphodiesterases that cleave cAMP to AMP, modulating intracellular cAMP concentration.[24] The major cAMP phosphodiesterase in platelets, PDE3A, is inhibited by cyclic 3',5'-guanosine monophosphate (cGMP). Thus, compounds that increase cGMP also inhibit platelet activation by indirectly increasing cAMP levels.

Other checks on unbridled platelet activation exist on the surface of endothelial cells, including an ADP-destroying ectoenzyme (ADPase), and thrombomodulin, a powerful thrombin inhibitor. Endothelial cells, when stimulated by agonists such as ATP, produce nitric oxide (NO), a potent vasodilator that also inhibits platelet function by raising platelet cGMP.[25] There is evidence to indicate that platelets themselves have the capacity to form NO from L-arginine, leading to a rise in the concentration of cGMP.[26]

COAGULATION

Blood coagulation is a cascade of steps in which plasma zymogens of serine proteases are transformed into active enzymes. These enzymes act to convert their procofactor substrates into active cofactors, which then assemble the proteases on cell surfaces. The assembly of cofactor, enzyme, and substrate on a phospholipid-containing surface, such as a cell membrane, is a recurrent theme in blood coagulation, resulting in maximal efficiency and velocity of the molecular reactions. This assembly increases the local concentrations of the reactants. The sequential nature of the reactions in which the product serves as the next enzyme amplifies the overall velocity of the reaction. The final event in coagulation is the formation of thrombin, which converts a soluble protein (fibrinogen) into an insoluble polymer (fibrin) that forms the clot.

Traditionally, the coagulation system is divided into 'intrinsic' and 'extrinsic' pathways, which converge on the 'common' pathway to produce thrombin (Figure 1.2). Although useful for *in vitro* laboratory testing, such a distinction does not occur physiologically, since the extrinsic pathway is capable of activating the intrinsic pathway *in vivo*.

Extrinsic pathway

Normally, no coagulation takes place in the bloodstream, owing to the properties of the endothelium and the inactive form of the proteins, which are either zymogens or procofactors. Initiation of this cascade depends on exposure of the blood to components that are not present physiologically in the bloodstream. These activators of coagulation are revealed as a result of mechanical injury (i.e. after a vessel is severed), endothelium damage or denudation (i.e. during coronary angioplasty), or biochemical alteration, such as the release of cytokines, which in turn induce biosynthesis of activators. Each of these events is capable of initiating coagulation via exposure of blood to a single critical component, tissue factor (TF). TF is a single-chain membrane receptor for coagulation

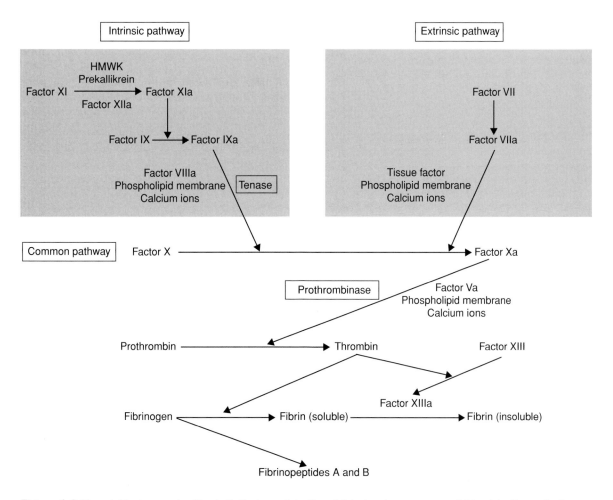

Figure 1.2 The clotting cascade. The initiating event is thought to involve exposure of blood to tissue factor, which binds factor VIIa. In the presence of a phospholipid membrane, the TF–VIIa complex activates both factor IX and factor X. The intrinsic pathway is activated *in vitro* by the 'contact' system, factor XIIa, high molecular weight kininogen (HMWK), and prekallikrein, which activate factor XI. Factor XI activates factor IX to IXa. Factor IXa, in concert with factor VIIIa, the phospholipid membrane, and calcium ions, forms the 'tenase' complex, which activates factor X. Factor Xa interacts with factor Va, the phospholipid membrane, and calcium ions to form the 'prothrombinase' complex, which activates prothrombin to thrombin. In turn, thrombin cleaves fibrinopeptides A and B from fibrinogen to form soluble fibrin. Fibrin is covalently crosslinked by factor XIIIa, which is activated by thrombin.

factor VII.[27] TF is expressed constitutively on most cells (other than hepatocytes) that do not normally contact the blood, such as fibroblasts. Alternatively, endotoxin can stimulate monocytes and endothelial cells to biosynthesize two cytokines, tumor necrosis factor and interleukin-1, which, in turn, induce the biosynthesis of TF.[28,29]

The major plasma component of the extrinsic pathway is factor VII, one of a group of vitamin K-dependent proteins (including factors IX and X, prothrombin, and protein C), synthesized as zymogens and activated to serine proteases by a limited number of proteolytic cleavages. Protein S, another a vitamin K-dependent protein, is a cofactor rather than a zymogen. Common to these proteins are unique γ-glutamyl carboxyl acid (Gla) residues at the *N*-terminal end of the molecule that require vitamin K for proper synthesis by hepatocytes. This postribosomal modification of the protein is required for calcium binding; one calcium binds the two carboxyl groups of a Gla residue, thereby serving as a bridge for protein binding to the phospholipid surface. Gla-less factors are essentially non-functional, which is the basis for warfarin, a pharmacological anticoagulant that indirectly inhibits Gla modification of coagulation proteins.

Factor VII binds to constitutive and induced TF on fibroblasts and monocytes, respectively. In all normal people, trace levels of active factor VII (factor VIIa) are present in the circulation, accounting for approximately 1% of the total factor VII concentration.[30] Therefore, exposure of TF to plasma results in binding of both factor VII and factor VIIa; however, only the TF–VIIa complexes are enzymatically active. Factor VII bound to TE is then activated by TF–VIIa, termed autoactivation.[31]

The factor VIIa–tissue factor enzyme complex, which assembles on the fibroblast, activated monocyte, or perturbed endothelial cell, has two principal substrates – factor IX and factor X, both of which are vitamin K-dependent proteins. Cleavage of either protein results in an active serine protease, factor IXa or Xa, that remains membrane-bound via its Gla residues, which facilitate further reactions if appropriate cofactors are present. The cofactor, factor VIII, is required for factor IXa to catalyze the conversion of factor X to factor Xa, whereas another cofactor, factor V, is required for Xa conversion of prothrombin to thrombin.

Measurement of the ability of the extrinsic pathway to produce fibrin effectively is accomplished *in vitro* using the prothrombin time. Any deficiency of factor in this pathway, whether absolute or functional (as occurs with warfarin therapy), results in a prolongation of the prothrombin time. A congenital deficiency of factor VII or factor X produces a similar hemorrhagic condition, and distinguishing one from the other requires the determination of specific coagulation factor activities. A clinically defin-

able decrease in tissue factor has not been described.

Intrinsic pathway

Parallel with the extrinsic system is the intrinsic system, which can be defined as coagulation initiated by components contained entirely within the vascular system. This pathway results in the activation of factor IX by a novel dimeric serine protease, factor XIa (Figure 1.2), providing a pathway that is independent of factor VII for blood coagulation. However, an important difference exists between these two pathways in the clotting cascade. Whereas the activation of factor IX by VIIa requires both calcium and the protein cofactor, tissue factor, which is embedded in the lipid bilayer of a cell membrane, the activation of factor IX by Xia requires only the presence of ionized calcium.

Initiation of the intrinsic system *in vitro* is mediated by a group of proteins, factor XII, HMWK, and prekallikrein. This group of proteins is called the 'contact' system, since activation occurs via binding to negatively charged surfaces, such as kaolin, dextran sulfate, and sulfatides. The net effect of the contact system is the activation of factor XI. Once activated, factor XIa then activates the vitamin K-dependent zymogen, factor IX. Factor IXa and its cofactor, factor VIII, assemble on a phospholipid-containing surface and together form the 'tenase' complex, which activates factor X.

Measurement of the ability of the intrinsic pathway to produce fibrin effectively *in vitro* is accomplished using the partial thromboplastin time. Analogous to prothrombin time assessment of extrinsic pathway function, any factor deficiency in the intrinsic pathway results in slow generation of thrombin and, thus, a prolonged partial thromboplastin time.

The role of the contact system proteins in initiation of the intrinsic pathway of coagulation in hemostasis is questionable, as deficiency of factor XII, HMWK, or prekallikrein does not lead to a bleeding disorder, despite marked prolongation of the partial thromboplastin time. In fact, factor XII deficiency has been implicated as a risk factor in venous (and perhaps arterial) thrombosis,[32] so it may serve as a natural anti-coagulant. Additionally, the contact proteins participate in the initiation of the inflammatory response, complement activation, fibrinolysis, angiogenesis, and kinin formation.

In plasma, factor VIII is primarily found in a non-covalent complex with vWF, which protects factor VIII from undesirable proteolytic attack. After dissociation from vWF, factor VIII is converted to the active cofactor, factor VIIIa, by factor Xa or thrombin. Factor VIIIa functions as a cofactor to accelerate the factor IXa-mediated conversion of factor X to Xa. The absence of factor VIII or IX underlies the hemophilia syndromes (classic hemophilia A and hemophilia B, respectively), which produce identical hemorrhagic states. Probably the similarity of these hemorrhagic conditions, secondary to deficiency of either factor VIII or IX, is due to the functional lack of a proper 'tenase' complex, which is critical for factor X activation (see Figure 1.2). The severity of the clinical disorder directly reflects the concentration of factor VIII or IX. The most severe clinical disease, manifested by spontaneous joint hemorrhage (hemarthroses), occurs with factor VIII or factor IX levels of 0–1%. At factor levels of 5–30%, symptoms may be mild or even non-existent, except in serious trauma such as surgery, and activity above 30% usually suffices for normal hemostasis. The presence of more than twice as much factor VIII or IX in normal persons as is present in hemophilia carriers (mean 50%) indicates that clotting proteins are typically present in excess, and thus, deficiencies must be relatively severe to produce clinically significant effects.

Interestingly, factor XI deficiency, even when biochemically severe (<1% of normal), is clinically mild. The major manifestation is post-traumatic bleeding, and only one-half of affected patients have some excessive bleeding. Moreover, the mechanism of activation of factor XI remains controversial. As previously mentioned, deficiency of the contact factors (XII, HMWK, and prekallikrein) does not lead to a hemorrhagic disorder, only to a prolongation of the *in vitro* partial thromboplastin time. Thus, *in vivo*, it is likely that blood coagulation is initiated not by the contact system of the intrinsic system, but rather via factor VIIa–TF of the extrinsic system.

Common pathway

Once factor Xa is formed by either the extrinsic or intrinsic pathway, it catalyzes the conversion of prothrombin to thrombin, but the reaction is slow. Efficient activation of prothrombin requires four components, factor Xa, factor Va, phospholipid, and calcium. Factor V that participates in this 'prothrombinase complex' is probably supplied by either fusion of plasma-derived factor V with the platelet plasma membrane or via secretion from platelet α-granules. The procofactor, factor V, is activated to factor Va by either factor Xa or thrombin. Factor Va then functions as a cofactor in the prothrombinase complex by serving as a receptor for factor Xa on the activated platelet surface. Once assembled, this 'prothrombinase complex' has a markedly increased rate of prothrombin activation – more than 300,00-fold faster than that with enzyme (factor Xa) and substrate (prothrombin) alone. Owing to a mutation in the 3' untranslated region, G20120A, elevated prothrombin levels result in a common genetic cause of the hypercoagulable state.[33] Additionally, elevated plasma levels of factor VIII, as well as factor XI, are also associated with venous thromboembolic disease.[34,35]

Owing to the involvement of platelets, factor V deficiency typically manifests itself with bleeding that resembles qualitative platelet disorders (ecchymoses, epistaxis, menorrhagia, and bleeding from the gingiva, gastrointestinal tract, umbilicus, and central nervous system). Interestingly, the severity of bleeding in factor V-deficient patients may be more closely related to levels of platelet-associated factor V than to plasma factor V.

Regulation of coagulation

Regulation of blood coagulation is achieved by several mechanisms, including factor dilution and the rate of blood flow, fibrinolysis, proteolytic inhibitors, and thrombin itself. The hemostatic plug is exposed to the disruptive pull of blood flow, and small clumps of platelets that are inadequately attached to the main body of platelets or to the vessel wall can be washed free into the circulation. Additionally, soluble activated coagulant proteins such as factor Xa or thrombin may diffuse away from the clot, to be bound to inhibitory plasma proteins that destroy or at least markedly decrease their coagulant potential.

Antithrombin III (AT-III) is a serpin (serine protease inhibitor) that primarily inhibits thrombin and factor Xa and, to a lesser extent, factor IXa. The catalytic-site serine of thrombin reacts with an arginine in the active center of AT-III to form a covalent inactive complex. The inhibition produced by AT-III is potentiated by heparin, a sulfated polysaccharide with the highest negative charge of any naturally occurring polymer and a close relation of the heparan sulfate that exists on the endothelial surface. Heparin binds to a basic group in AT-III to increase its rate of inactivation of thrombin. However, once thrombin is bound to fibrin, it is resistant to AT-III and even more so to the AT-III–heparin complex.[36,37] This phenomenon may explain the limitation of heparin both in preventing the propagation of venous thrombi and in inhibiting rethrombosis after successful coronary thrombolysis. Although enough AT-III is present to neutralize three times the total amount of thrombin that could form in the blood, a decrease to 40–50% predisposes to thrombotic disorders. The fact that congenital AT-III deficiency is associated with a strikingly increased risk of venous thromboembolism indicates that inhibitors play a major regulatory role and that a delicate balance exists between procoagulant and anticoagulant forces.

Heparin cofactor II is a serpin that selectively inactivates thrombin (not factor Xa) in the presence of heparin or dermatan sulfate.[38] α_2-macroglobulin is a secondary or back-up inhibitor for many plasma coagulant and fibrinolytic enzymes, including kallikrein, thrombin, and plasmin. Because enzymes trapped in the cage structure of this inhibitor exhibit some activity, α_2-macroglobulin–enzyme complexes may serve as a repository of enzymatic activity

that is protected against other inhibitors. No clinical disorder of severe α_2-macroglobulin deficiency has been described.

The fibrin clot itself is an important reservoir of active thrombin, which is protected from inhibition by AT-III. Hirudin, argatroban, inogatran, and melagatran directly bind to thrombin and inhibit the enzyme in a heparin-independent manner.[39] Inogatran is particularly effective at inhibiting clot-bound thrombin, probably because of its relatively small molecular size.[40] Currently, the direct thrombin inhibitors that are available in the USA include lepirudin, argatroban, and bivalirudin, which are administered parenterally. Melagatran, the active form of the oral agent, ximelagatran,[41] is currently being developed and has been shown to inhibit fibrin-bound thrombin.[42] In addition, there are direct factor Xa inhibitors, such as tick anticoagulant peptide, antistatin, and DX-9065a, which bind to the active site of the enzyme.[39,43] Also, an indirect factor Xa inhibitor, SR 90107/ORG 31540 binds AT-III, which subsequently inhibits soluble factor Xa.[44]

One important consideration in the pharmacological manipulation of hemostasis is that venous and arterial thrombi have subtle differences. Venous thrombi primarily consist of fibrin, whereas platelets comprise the major component of arterial thrombi. Thus, traditionally, warfarin and inhibitors of thrombin have been used in the primary treatment and prevention of venous thrombi. Unfractionated and low molecular weight heparins have been used as adjunct therapies for arterial thrombi, in concert with fibrinolytic agents or angioplasty. However, direct thrombin inhibitors are also capable of inhibiting thrombin-mediated platelet activation,[45] suggesting a role for such agents in the treatment and prevention of arterial thrombotic conditions. Additionally, unlike warfarin, direct thrombin inhibitors, owing to their 1:1 stoichiometric binding of thrombin, may have the advantage of relatively wide therapeutic windows, reducing the risk of bleeding or insufficient anticoagulation.

The extrinsic pathway results in activation of factor IX (intrinsic pathway) and factor X (common pathway). Cleavage of either protein results in a cell-bound serine protease, factor IXa or factor Xa. However, the TF–VIIa complex is tightly regulated by tissue factor pathway inhibitor (TFPI),[46] a protein consisting of three Kunitz domains that is produced by the endothelial cell.[47] The first domain binds to and inhibits factor VIIa–TF and the second, factor Xa. Ligation of factor Xa is required for TFPI to inhibit TF–VIIa.[46] Thus, the direct activation of factor Xa is rapidly down-regulated.

The contribution of the contact system (factor XII, HMWK, prekallikrein) to activation of the intrinsic pathway *in vivo* is questionable, given the lack of bleeding tendency in patients deficient in these factors. Therefore, coagulation is probably initiated by the extrinsic pathway on exposure of the blood to tissue factor found in the subendothelium or on perturbed endothelial cells. However, in the presence of TFPI, which readily inhibits the extrinsic pathway, the major pathway for the propagation of coagulation is probably the intrinsic pathway, which can be activated by TF–VIIa mediated conversion of factor IX to IXa. Additionally, different cell

surfaces have markedly different abilities to facilitate enzymatic reactions in the coagulation cascade.[48] This could potentially provide yet another level of regulation whereby TF-expressing cells, such as a fibroblast in the subendothelium, would initiate coagulation via the extrinsic pathway, and propagation of coagulation would occur on the platelet surface via specific receptors for coagulation proteins.

Thrombin plays a central role in hemostasis, serving not only procoagulant functions, but also key inhibitory roles (Figure 1.3). Thrombomodulin is expressed on normal endothelium and inhibits the ability of thrombin to cleave fibrinogen and activate platelets and factors V and VIII. Thrombomodulin also markedly enhances the ability of thrombin to activate protein C, a natural anticoagulant enzyme. Protein C binds to endothelial cell protein C receptor, which enhances its activation.[49] Protein C, in turn, inactivates the clotting cofactors, factors Va and VIIIa, and enhances fibrinolysis, probably by binding an inhibitor of plasminogen activators.[50] Thrombin, once

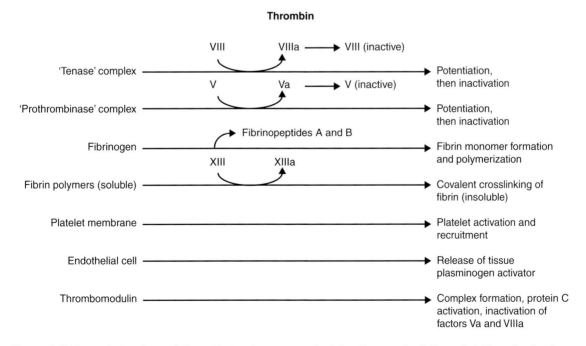

Figure 1.3 The varied actions of thrombin involve procoagulant functions, potentiation of clotting, feedback inhibition, and limitation of clotting.

bound to thrombomodulin, is also activated by circulating AT-III, a step accelerated by heparan sulfate. Protein C activity is stimulated by its cofactor, protein S, and is controlled by protein C inhibitor (PAI-3) as well as α_1-proteinase inhibitor.[51,52] Protein S is controlled by C4b, which complexes it, thus preventing its cofactor action.[53] The enhancement of fibrinolysis by protein C also may be dependent on protein S.[54] Thus, the net effect of thrombin binding to thrombomodulin is the loss of the procoagulant functions of thrombin and the enhancement of its ability to activate protein C and therefore to inhibit thrombogenesis. The fact that thrombomodulin is expressed on normal endothelial cells serves to localize the procoagulant stimulus to sites of endothelial disruption, thereby limiting clot extension. Patients deficient in either protein C or its cofactor, protein S, have a lifelong tendency for pathologic thromboembolic disease. Furthermore, mutation of arginine 506 to glutamine in factor V (factor V Leiden) results in a factor V that is resistant to inactivation by protein C.[55] Protein C resistance (factor V Leiden) is the single most common genetic risk factor for venous thromboembolism, further highlighting the physiological importance of this natural anticoagulant pathway.

FIBRIN FORMATION AND FIBRINOLYSIS

The formation of fibrin strands represents the second phase in hemostasis (the first being the primary platelet aggregate). The precursor of fibrin is fibrinogen, a large glycoprotein of molecular weight 340 kDa that is present in high concentration in plasma and in platelet granules. Fibrinogen interacts with other proteins, including factor XIII, fibronectin, α_2-plasmin inhibitor, plasminogen, and plasminogen activator.[56] The location and surface concentration of these modifying proteins influence the orderly process of fibrin formation, cross-linking, and lysis. Thrombin binds to the fibrinogen central domain and liberates fibrinopeptides A and B, resulting in fibrin monomer and polymer formation.[57] Progressive lengthening of the polymer chain occurs by a half-overlap, side-to-side approximation of fibrin monomer molecules

(Figure 1.4), and the two-stranded protofibrils interact laterally to form long, thin fibrin strands or short, broad sheets of fibrin.[58,59]

Although the degree of lateral fibrin strand association probably contributes to the tensile strength of the clot, its resistance to degradation by plasmin is influenced mainly by factor XIIIa-mediated crosslinking.[60] In addition, factor XIIIa, by linking α_2-plasmin inhibitor to fibrin, may protect the clot against fibrinolysis. Factor XIII exists in plasma as a four-chain precursor molecule of molecular weight 320 kDa, and after activation by thrombin, factor XIIIa (with calcium) induces cross-linking of the fibrin polymer.[61] Covalent isopeptide bonds form between lysine donors and glutamine receptors, with two γ-chains cross-linked rapidly to form γ–γ-dimers; α-chains are crosslinked more slowly, each with two other such chains to form a polymer network.[62,63] In mature forms, the fibrin fiber contains approximately 100 protofibrils, with a somewhat random pattern of branching that links the fibers together.

The fibrin mesh binds platelets together and contributes to their attachment to the vessel wall, mediated by binding to platelet receptor glycoproteins and by interactions with other adhesive proteins such as thrombospondin, fibronectin, and platelet fibrinogen (released from platelet granules but probably otherwise equivalent to plasma fibrinogen).[64] After attachment to platelet binding sites, these proteins may serve as molecular bridges between plasma proteins and the platelet interior, between platelets and the vessel wall, and between plasma fibrin fibers and the subendothelial matrix. For instance, fibronectin is cross-linked by factor XIIIa to fibrin, and its separate binding site for collagen could serve to bridge fibrin to the vessel wall.[65,66] vWF also could serve as a bridge between platelet membrane GPIb–X (or IIb–IIIa) and a subendothelial matrix component.[67] Additionally, the platelet membrane GPIIb–IIIa could join plasma or α-granule fibrinogen to platelet intracellular actin, thereby mediating clot retraction and vessel wall constriction.[68]

The potential for hemorrhagic or thrombotic disease resulting from derangements in fibrino-

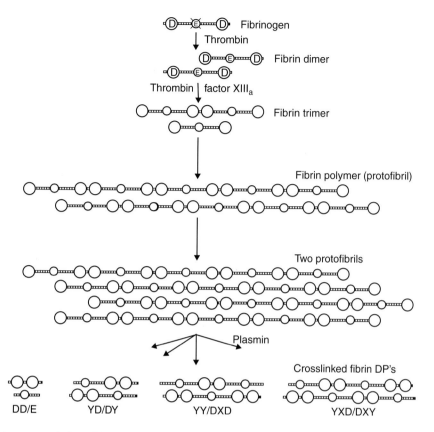

Figure 1.4 Fibrinogen and thrombin-induced fibrin monomer and polymer formation, factor XIIIa-induced fibrin crosslinking, and plasmin-induced crosslinked fibrin degradation. The curly lines represent coiled coils between central and terminal domains, and the double horizontal lines represent cross-link sites induced by factor XIIIa between γ-chains of two contiguous fragment D domains. The central and two terminal domains of fibrinogen are included in the frgament E and D domains, respectively. The fibrinopeptides are indicated as small vertical lines connected to the central (E) domain of fibrinogen and are absent from the fibrin monomer molecules after thrombin action. Plasmin action is depicted here as limited to cleavage of the coiled coils between center (E) and terminal (D) domains, to yield the complexes noted at the bottom. These complexes consist of two noncovalently bound fragments (for instance, fragments DD and E in the DD–E complex).

gen structure, concentration, or interaction with thrombin or factor XIII, is great and varied. It could, for instance, manifest as a poorly polymerizing protein, by slow or absent liberation of a fibrinopeptide, or as an inadequately cross-linked fibrin.[69] The latter situation similarly could be produced by an absent or faulty factor XIII molecule, which could contribute both to a hemorrhagic condition and to inadequate wound healing. The most common acquired disorders of fibrinogen are those of consumption (the disseminated

intravascular coagulation (DIC) syndromes), which may reflect excessive or inappropriate coagulation or proteolytic degradation of plasma fibrinogen and can result in a variety of hemorrhagic and thrombotic manifestations, depending to a great extent on the underlying pathological process.[70]

A major mechanism for limiting clot formation is fibrinolysis (Figure 1.5), which, along with endothelial cell regrowth and vessel recanalization, constitutes a repair mechanism. Fibrinolysis resembles the cascade mechanism

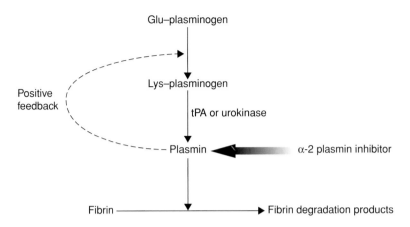

Figure 1.5 Fibrinolysis. Plasminogen is activated to plasmin by t-PA and urokinase. Plasmin cleaves fibrin to fibrin degradation products. Plasmin is inhibited by α2 plasmin inhibitor. Plasmin exerts positive feedback by converting glu–plasminogen to lys–plasminogen.

of clotting factor activation in that it involves zymogen-to-enzyme conversions, feedback potentiation and inhibition, and a finely tuned balance with inhibitors. The inactive precursor protein is plasminogen, present in plasma at twice the molar concentration of its inhibitor, α_2-plasmin inhibitor. During the initial period of hemostatic plug formation, platelets and endothelial cells release plasminogen activator inhibitors that serve to facilitate fibrin formation.[71] However, in response to a poorly understood but precisely timed and orchestrated sequence of stimuli, endothelial cells liberate tissue plasminogen activator.[72] Both tissue plasminogen activators (tPA) and prourokinase have the capacity to convert plasminogen (especially plasminogen bound to fibrin) to the serine protease-active form, plasmin, which effectively degrades fibrin.[73] Pharmacologically, different forms of tPA, such as alteplase, as well as the bacterial plasminogen activator, streptokinase, are used to induce fibrinolysis.

Plasmin exerts positive feedback by cleavage of an activation peptide from plasminogen (converting Glu–plasminogen to Lys–plasminogen), rendering it more susceptible to surface binding and subsequent activation by plasminogen activators. Perhaps more critical is the markedly heightened reactivity of plasminogen after it is bound to fibrin by lysine binding sites located on its kringle structures. Lipoprotein A with multiple kringles and histidine-rich glycoprotein also modulates fibrin-plasminogen interactions by inhibiting plasminogen binding to fibrin.[73,74]

Once plasmin is produced locally on the hemostatic plug, the potential for fibrin degradation exists. Although only a small proportion of plasma plasminogen is bound to fibrin during particulate clot formation, this is sufficient to influence subsequent physiological fibrinolysis.[75] The process is a balanced one, however, because α_2-plasmin inhibitor also is bound to the fibrin, covalently attached by factor XIIIa action.[76] Active plasmin molecules may be released into the circulation during fibrinolysis, but in solution, plasmin is extremely susceptible to inhibition by α_2-plasmin inhibitor, whereas, when bound to fibrin, plasmin is resistant to inhibition.[77] The relative proportions and positions of profibrinolytic plasminogen and plasminogen activator molecules and antifibrinolytic α_2-plasmin inhibitor molecules on the fibrin strand influence the timing and degree of clot dissolution.

By an intricate balance of the simultaneous forces of coagulation and platelet aggregation, inhibition of coagulation, profibrinolytic and antifibrinolytic reactions, and cellular mechanisms for both coagulation and lysis (in leukocytes as well as in platelets and endothelial cells), the clot is gradually reduced. The neutral serine protease (elastase) released from the primary granules of neutrophils also contributes to the local fibrinolytic potential.[78] The surface of the clot may be removed first, revealing fresh surfaces that are progressively attacked until the process is completed.[79] Clinical derangements of the fibrinolytic system include hemorrhagic disorders caused by deficient or defective α_2-plasmin inhibitor or plasminogen activator-1 (PAI-1).[80]

During hemostatic plug or thrombus dissolution, solubilized fibrin degradation products are liberated into the circulation; some of these products represent unique cross-linked derivatives, such as D-dimer, that can be distinguished from fibrinogen degradation products.[81] The circulating degradation products serve as diagnostic markers of thrombin or factor XIIIa, or both, plus plasmin action that reflects prior clot formation and ongoing fibrinolysis. The surface of a clot and circulating fibrin derivatives may possess a small but significant amount of active thrombin that could serve to propagate the coagulant process elsewhere in the circulation.[82]

Studies have elucidated an important connection between the coagulation and fibrinolytic pathways by virtue of thrombin–thrombomodulin-mediated activation of both protein C and thrombin-activated fibrinolytic inhibitor (TAFI), a carboxypeptidase B proenzyme. The mode of action of TAFI is to cleave C-terminal lysine residues from fibrin, thereby preventing plasminogen, plasmin, or tPA from binding to fibrin and thus, secondarily, inhibiting fibrinolysis. Whereas activation of protein C leads to inactivation of factors Va and VIIIa and curtailment of further clot formation, TAFI activation promotes stabilization of fibrin and therefore persistence of formed fibrin clots. Clinical conditions of decreased coagulation, such as classic hemophilia, are not only deficient in thrombin and fibrin formation but, by virtue of low levels of activated TAFI, also allow fibrinolysis to proceed relatively unimpeded. The combination of less fibrin and more lysis together contributes to the bleeding seen in patients with factor VIII deficiency. Similarly, patients with deficiency of 'intrinsic' coagulation factors also appear to have decreased TAFI activation, perhaps by inadequate completion of clotting after initial fibrin formation. On the other hand, patients with deficiency of protein C manifest a thrombotic tendency by virtue of a failure of 'feedback inhibition' of factors Va and VIIIa by thrombin. The predilection to thrombosis may also receive a contribution from excessive TAFI formation caused by continuously high production of thrombin. In this case, not only are thrombin and fibrin formed, but such fibrin is rendered resistant to plasmin-mediated lysis by excessive TAFI. Thrombin inhibitors may not only impair clot-formation, but also promote fibrinolysis by inhibiting thrombomodulin-thrombin mediated activation of TAFI.[83]

ENDOTHELIUM

Normal vascular endothelium (Figure 1.6) maintains blood fluidity by producing inhibitors of blood coagulation and platelet aggregation, modulating vascular tone and permeability, and providing a protective envelope that separates hemostatic blood components from procoagulant subendothelial structures. Endothelial cells synthesize and secrete basement membrane and extracellular matrix, which contains adhesive proteins, such as collagen, fibronectin, laminin, vitronectin, and vWF. The endothelium has several actions; it inhibits blood coagulation by synthesizing and expressing thrombomodulin and heparan sulfate on its surface; it modulates fibrinolysis by synthesizing and secreting tPA, urokinase plasminogen activator (uPA), and plasminogen activator inhibitors; it inhibits platelet aggregation by releasing PGI_2 and NO; and it regulates vessel wall tone by synthesizing endothelins (which induce vasoconstriction) and PGI_2 and NO (which produce vasodilation).

Defective vascular function can lead to abnormal bleeding if the endothelium becomes more permeable to blood cells, if the vasoconstrictive response is impaired because of structural abnormalities of the vessel wall or extravascular supporting tissues, or if physiological fibrinoly-

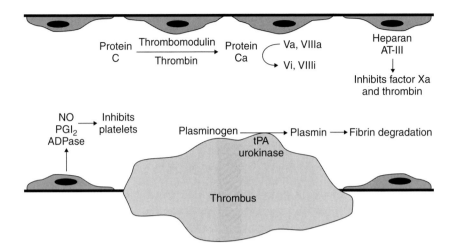

Figure 1.6 Thromboresistant properties of endothelium. Endothelial cells produce nitric oxide (NO), prostacyclin (PGI$_2$), and adenosine diphosphatase (ADPase), which inhibit platelets. Normal vascular endothelial cells express thrombomodulin and heparan proteoglycans on their surfaces. Thrombomodulin binds thrombin, which then cleaves and inactivates the clotting cofactors, factors Va and VIIIa, to factors Vi and VIIIi. Heparan proteoglycans bind and activate AT-III, which inhibits soluble factor Xa and thrombin. Additionally, endothelial cells secrete plasminogen activators, tPA, and urokinase, resulting in the activation of plasmin, which degrades fibrin.

sis is not controlled by the normal production of plasminogen activator inhibitors. Bleeding associated with endothelial injury may be mediated by immune complexes and viruses.[84,85] Proteolytic enzymes released from leukocytes in inflammatory states perturb endothelial cells and alter connective tissue proteins and could also contribute to petechial hemorrhage in vasculitic disorders.[86,87] Attenuation and fenestration of the vascular endothelium may contribute to the hemorrhagic manifestations of idiopathic thrombocytopenia purpura, which may respond to prednisone therapy promptly, even before a detectable rise in platelet count.[88]

Endothelial cells lose their non-thrombogenic protective properties after they are stimulated by enzymes (such as thrombin), by hypoxia, by fluid shear stress, by oxidants, by cytokines (such as interleukin-1, tumor necrosis factor, and γ-interferon), by synthetic hormones (such as desmopressin acetate), and by endotoxin. Synthesis of tissue factor and PAI-1 is induced, and the concentration of surface-bound thrombomodulin is reduced by cytokines and endotoxin; whereas desmopressin acetate

results in the release of high molecular weight vWF multimers from Weibel–Palade bodies[89] that may augment platelet adhesion to the injured vessel wall. Endothelial cells contain integrins of the very late antigen (VLA) type, which allow binding of fibronectin (α_1-β_1), collagen (α_v-β_1), and laminin (α_3-β_1, α_6-β_1), and of the cytoadhesive type, notably the vitronectin receptor (α_2-β_3).[90] The stimulated endothelial cell synthesizes chemokines such as monocyte chemoattractant protein, interleukin-8, RANTES, and gro. Endothelial cells also contain intercellular adhesion molecules, such as ICAM-1 and ICAM-2, and VCAM-1, which act as counter-receptors for leukocyte integrins.[91,92] Before tight adhesion to the endothelium, platelets and leukocytes roll, an interaction mediated by E-selectin and P-selectin (which is stored in Weibel–Palade bodies).

Endothelium is heterogeneous, both metabolically and structurally.[93] For instance, converting enzyme is synthesized by most endothelial cells but principally by aortic endothelium, not by cardiac microvessel endothelium; on the other hand, thromboxane A$_2$ is not synthesized by most endothelial cells but is synthesized by pulmonary arterial endothelium. Additionally, shear stresses caused by blood flow modulate endothelial gene expression, as well as the activity of certain endothelial enzymes.[94] For example, endothelial cell turnover is low under resting conditions but varies with location; however, at sites of hemodynamic stress and injury, proliferation is especially increased. Endothelial cells contain a full array of contractile proteins, but of special importance are the stress fibers involved in cell attachment and maintenance of endothelial junctional apposition by vascular endothelial (VE) cadherin and platelet-endothelial cell adhesion molecule (PECAM). Endothelial cells also contain caveolae that concentrate glycosyl–phosphatidyl-linked proteins such as the urokinase receptor.

Endothelial cell permeability is influenced by the functional adaptations that join the cells to their neighbors. Macromolecules pass across the endothelium into the vessel wall through patent intercellular junctions, by endocytosis, and via transendothelial pores. Vessel permeability is increased by vasodilatation, by induction of severe thrombocytopenia, and by high doses of heparin. Spontaneous bleeding observed with a low platelet count or after heparin infusion may actually be induced by increased vascular permeability.

Increased fenestration and attenuation of endothelium may account for the loss of barrier function associated with experimental thrombocytopenia. The thrombocytopenia-induced extravasation of erythrocytes, which manifest clinically as petechiae, occurs principally through postcapillary venular interendothelial channels. The loss of endothelial barrier function, associated with extreme platelet depletion, may be related to a loss of serotonin and norepinephrine delivered by platelets to the microvascular milieu. Exogenous sources of either amine prevent both petechial formation in severely thrombocytopenic animals, as well as failure of platelets to plug gaps at intercellular junctions between retracted endothelial cells.

Endothelial cells are highly negatively charged, a feature that may repel the negatively charged platelets. This anionic surface as well as other antithrombotic properties of endothelium could be important in limiting the intravascular extension of the hemostatic reaction induced by vessel injury.[95] Thus, PGI_2, synthesized and released from endothelial cells close to the site of hemostatic plug formation, could inhibit intravascular platelet aggregation.[96–99] Thrombomodulin and heparan sulfate, the two endothelial surface-bound thrombin inhibitors, could limit the intravascular spread of fibrin beyond the confines of the hemostatic plug.[100–104] Heparan sulfate, a glycosaminoglycan, activates AT-III and thus catalyzes the inhibition of thrombin and factor Xa. Endothelial cell-associated ADPase (CD39) cleaves ADP to AMP, thus modulating this stimulatory platelet agonist.[105]

Thrombin and other stimuli, including epinephrine and trauma, stimulate PGI_2 synthesis by endothelial cells.[106] Other agonists, including histamine, ATP, bradykinin, and acetylcholine, stimulate endothelial cell guanylate cyclase, raising the levels of intracellular cGMP, which results in the synthesis of NO. Thus, endothelial cells exposed to appropriate stimuli synthesize and release two distinct mediators of vasodilatation and inhibition of platelet function.[107] Endothelial-mediated platelet inhibition serves as yet another mechanism to limit clot formation to the site of endothelial perturbation, similar to thrombomodulin–thrombin inhibition of coagulation. Stimulated endothelial cells also synthesize a group of peptides known as endothelins, which have counter-regulatory properties, including vasoconstriction.[108]

Endothelial cells elaborate plasminogen activators, which, in the presence of fibrin, promote fibrinolysis and can aggravate a bleeding tendency in susceptible patients. Synthetic and natural fibrinolytic inhibitors can control this bleeding tendency. PAI-1 is also elaborated with a different time course and in response to different stimuli.[109] Deficiency of PAI-1 causes a bleeding tendency, indicating that unopposed physiological fibrinolysis disrupts the hemostatic balance.

Endothelial cells are stimulated by cytokines and other mediators to mount a procoagulant response, which is characterized by an increased synthesis and release of PAI-1, release of vWF, synthesis and availability of tissue factor, and reduction of cell membrane-associated thrombomodulin. The postoperative and post-traumatic fibrinolytic shutdown is associated with increased synthesis of PAI-1 and could be mediated by cytokines elaborated as a response to tissue damage.[109] Thrombin bound to thrombomodulin not only activates protein C but also more efficiently activates the thrombin-activated fibrinolytic inhibitor (TAFI).[83] This response not only protects the newly formed hemostatic plug from premature dissolution but may also contribute to the increased risk of postoperative venous thrombosis.

The complex interplay between mediators and countermediators derived from the vessel wall, the endothelial lining, and even the vasomotor regulation of arteries and veins affects hemostasis and wound healing. All of these vascular processes act in concert with similarly complex processes in the platelet, plasma coagulation, and fibrinolytic and inhibitory pathways to maintain normal hemostasis. Occasionally, however, the hemostatic response is excessive and leads to intravascular thrombosis.

REFERENCES

1. Ruggeri ZM, Dent JA, Saldivar E. Contribution of distinct adhesive interactions to platelet aggregation in flowing blood. *Blood* 1999;**94**:172–8.
2. Pytela R, Pierschbacher MD, Ginsberg MH et al. Platelet membrane glycoprotein Iib/IIIa: member of a family of Arg–Gly–Asp-specific adhesion receptors. *Science* 1986;**231**:1559–62.
3. Weiss HJ, Turitto VT, Baumgartner HR. Effect of shear rate on platelet interaction with subendothelium in citrated and native blood. I. Shear rate-dependent decrease of adhesion in von Willebrand's disease and the Bernard–Soulier syndrome. *J Lab Clin Med* 1978;**92**:750–64.
4. Staatz WD, Rajpara SM, Wayner EA et al. The membrane glycoprotein Ia–IIa (VLA-2) complex mediates the Mg++-dependent adhesion of platelets to collagen. *J Cell Biol* 1989;**108**:1917–24.
5. Howard JB. Methylamine reaction and denaturation-dependent fragmentation of complement component 3: comparison with alpha-2-macroglobulin. *J Biol Chem* 1980;**255**:7082–4.
6. Shattil SJ, Kashiwagi H, Pampori N. Integrin signaling: the platelet paradigm. *Blood* 1998;**91**:2645–57.
7. Shattil SJ, Hoxie JA, Cunningham M et al. Changes in the platelet membrane glycoprotein IIb/IIIa complex during platelet activation. *J Biol Chem* 1985;**260**:11107–14.
8. Lam SC, Plow EF, D'Souza SE et al. Isolation and characterization of a platelet membrane protein related to the vitronectin receptor. *J Biol Chem* 1989;**264**:3742–9.
9. Bennett JS, Vilaire G. Exposure of platelet fibrinogen receptors by ADP and epinephrine. *J Clin Invest* 1979;**64**:1393–401.
10. Nurden AT, Caen JP. The different glycoprotein abnormalities in thrombasthenic and Bernard–Soulier platelets. *Semin Hematol* 1979;**16**:234–50.
11. Colman RW. Platelet receptors. *Hematol Oncol Clin North Am* 1990;**4**:27–42.
12. Feinstein MB. The role of calcium in blood platelet function. In: Weiss GB, ed. *Calcium in Drug Action*. New York: Plenum; 1978:197–239.
13. Gabbeta J, Yang X, Kowalska MA et al. Platelet signal transduction defect with G-alpha subunit dysfunction and diminished G-alpha-q in a patient with abnormal platelet responses. *Proc Natl Acad Sci USA* 1997;**94**:8750–5.
14. Lee SB, Rao AK, Lee KH et al. Decreased expression of phospholipase C-beta 2 isozyme in human platelets with impaired function. *Blood* 1996;**88**:1684–91.
15. Colman RW, Hoffman I. Calpains and hemostasis. In: Mellgren R, Murachi T, eds. *Intracellular Calcium-Dependent Proteolysis*. Florida: CRC Press; 1990;211–14.
16. Adelstein RS, Conti MA. Phosphorylation of platelet myosin increases actin-activated myosin ATPase activity. *Nature* 1975;**256**:597–8.
17. Pickett WC, Jesse RL, Cohen P. Initiation of phospholipase A2 activity in human platelets by the calcium ion ionophore A23187. *Biochim Biophys Acta* 1976;**486**:209–13.
18. Nishizuka Y. The role of protein kinase C in cell surface signal transduction and tumour promotion. *Nature* 1984;**308**:693–8.
19. Berridge NJ. Inositol triphosphate and diacylglycerol as second messengers. *Biochem J* 1984;**220**:345–60.

20. Rink TJ, Sanchez A, Hallam TJ. Diacylglycerol and phorbol ester stimulate secretion without raising cytoplasmic free calcium in human platelets. *Nature* 1983;**305**:317–19.

21. Holmsen H. Platelet secretion and energy metabolism. In: Colman RW, Hirsh J, Marder VJ *et al.*, eds. *Hemostasis and Thrombosis: Basic Principles and Clinical Practice*, 3rd ed. Philadelphia: JB Lippincott; 1993;524–45.

22. Hoyer LW, Colman RW, Wyshock EG. Coagulation cofactors: factors VIII and V. In: Colman RW, Hirsh J, Marder VJ *et al.*, eds. *Hemostasis and Thrombosis: Basic Principles and Clinical Practice*, 3rd ed. Philadelphia: JB Lippincott; 1993;109–33.

23. Haslam RJ, Davidson MM, Fox JE *et al.* Cyclic nucleotides in platelet function. *Thromb Haemost* 1978;**40**:232–40.

24. Colman RW. Platelet cyclic nucleotide phospho-diesterases. In: Rao GHR, ed. *Handbook of Platelet Physiology and Pharmacology*. Boston: Kluwer Academic; 1999;251–67.

25. Rapoport RM, Murad F. Endothelium-dependent and nitrovasodilator-induced relaxation of vascular smooth muscle: role of cyclic GMP. *J Cyclic Nucleotide Protein Phosphor Res* 1983;**9**:281–96.

26. Radomski MW, Palmer RM, Moncada S. An L-arginine/nitric oxide pathway present in human platelets regulates aggregation. *Proc Natl Acad Sci USA* 1990;**87**:5193–7.

27. Rao LV, Williams T, Rapaport SI. Studies of the activation of factor VII bound to tissue factor. *Blood* 1996;**87**:3738–48.

28. Geczy CL. Cellular mechanisms for the activation of blood coagulation. *Int Rev Cytol* 1994;**152**:49–108.

29. Camerer E, Kolsto AB, Prydz H. Cell biology of tissue factor, the principal initiator of blood coagulation. *Thromb Res* 1996;**81**:1–41.

30. Morrissey JH, Macik BG, Neuenschwander PF, Comp PC. Quantitation of activated factor VII levels in plasma using a tissue factor mutant selectively deficient in promoting factor VII activation. *Blood* 1993;**81**:734–44.

31. Neuenschwander PF, Fiore MM, Morrissey JH. Factor VII autoactivation proceeds via interaction of distinct protease-cofactor and zymogen–cofactor complexes. Implications of a two-dimensional enzyme kinetic mechanism. *J Biol Chem* 1993;**268**:1489–92.

32. Halbmayer WM, Mannhalter C, Feichtinger C *et al.* The prevalence of factor XII deficiency in 103

orally anticoagulated outpatients suffering from recurrent venous and/or arterial thromboembolism. *Thromb Haemost* 1992;**68**:285–90.

33. Poort SR, Rosendaal FR, Reitsma PH *et al.* A common genetic variation in the 3'-untranslated region of the prothrombin gene is associated with elevated plasma prothrombin levels and an increase in venous thrombosis. *Blood* 1996;**88**:3698–703.

34. Koster T, Blann AD, Briet E *et al.* Role of clotting factor VIII in effect of von Willebrand factor on occurrence of deep-vein thrombosis. *Lancet* 1995;**345**:152–5.

35. Meijers JCM, Tekelenburg WLH, Bouma BN *et al.* High levels of coagulation factor XI as a risk factor for venous thrombosis. *N Engl J Med* 2000;**342**: 696–701.

36. Hogg PJ, Jackson CM. Fibrin monomer protects thrombin from inactivation by heparin–antithrombin III: implications for heparin efficacy. *Proc Natl Acad Sci USA* 1989;**86**:3619–23.

37. Weitz JI, Huboda M, Massel D *et al.* Clot-bound thrombin is protected from inhibition by heparin–antithrombin III but is susceptible to inactivation by antithrombin III-independent inhibitors. *J Clin Invest* 1990;**86**:385–91.

38. Tollefsen DM, Majerus DW, Blank MK. Heparin cofactor II. Purification and properties of a heparin-dependent inhibitor of thrombin in human plasma. *J Biol Chem* 1982;**257**:2162–9.

39. Weitz JI, Hirsh J. New antithrombotic agents. *Chest* 1998;**114**(suppl):715S–27S.

40. Berry CN, Girardot C, Lecoffre C *et al.* Effects of the synthetic thrombin inhibitor argatroban on fibrin- or clot-incorporated thrombin: comparison with heparin and recombinant hirudin. *Thromb Haemost* 1994;**72**:381–6.

41. Heit JA, Colwell CW, Francis CW *et al.* A comparison of the oral direct thrombin inhibitor H 376/96 with enoxaparin sodium as prophylaxis against venous thromboembolism after total knee replacement surgery: a phase II dose-finding study. *Arch Intern Med* 2001;**161**:2215–21.

42. Elg M, Gustafsson D, Deinum J. The importance of enzyme inhibition kinetics for the effect of thrombin inhibitors in a rat model of arterial thrombosis. *Thromb Haemost* 1997;**78**:1286–92.

43. Hauptmann J, Sturzebecher J. Synthetic inhibitors of thrombin and factor Xa: from bench to bedside. *Thromb Res* 1999;**93**:203–41.

44. Samama MM, Kher A. The old and the new. *Heamostaseologie* 1998;**18**:S27–S32.

45. Gandossi E, Lunven C, Gauffeny C *et al.* Platelet

aggregation induced in vitro by rabbit plasma clot-associated thrombin, and its inhibition by thrombin inhibitors. *Thromb Haemost* 1998;**80**:840–4.

46. Rao LV, Rapaport SI. Studies of a mechanism inhibiting the initiation of the extrinsic pathway of coagulation. *Blood* 1987;**69**:645–51.

47. Broze GJ, Warren LA, Novotny WF *et al.* The lipoprotein-associated coagulation inhibitor that inhibits the factor VII–tissue factor complex also inhibits factor Xa: insight into its possible mechanism of action. *Blood* 1988;**71**:335–43.

48. Hoffman M, Monroe DM III. A cell-based model of hemostasis. *Thromb Haemost* 2001;**85**:958–65.

49. Fukudome K, Esmon CT. Identification, cloning, and regulation of a novel endothelial cell protein C/activated protein C receptor. *J Biol Chem* 1994;**269**:26486–91.

50. Esmon NL, Owen WG, Esmon CT. Isolation of a membrane-bound cofactor for thrombin-catalyzed activation of protein C. *J Biol Chem* 1982;**257**:859–64.

51. Heeb MJ, Espana F, Geiger M *et al.* Immunological identity of heparin-dependent plasma and urinary protein C inhibitor and plasminogen activator inhibitor-3. *J Biol Chem* 1987;**262**:15813–16.

52. Walker FJ. Regulation of activated protein C by protein S. The role of phospholipid in factor Va inactivation. *J Biol Chem* 1981;**256**:11128–31.

53. Dahlback B. Inhibition of protein Ca cofactor function of human and bovine protein S by C4b-binding protein. *J Biol Chem* 1986;**261**:12022–7.

54. de Fouw NJ, Haverkate F, Bertina RM *et al.* The cofactor role of protein S in the acceleration of whole blood clot lysis by activated protein C *in vitro*. *Blood* 1986;**67**:1189–92.

55. Bertina RM, Koeleman BPC, Koster T *et al.* Mutation in blood coagulation factor V associated with resistance to activated protein C. *Nature* 1994;**369**:64–7.

56. Doolittle RF, Goldbaum DM, Doolittle LR. Designation of sequences involved in the 'coiled-coil' interdomainal connections in fibrinogen: constructions of an atomic scale model. *J Mol Biol* 1978;**120**:311–25.

57. Blomback BBM. The molecular structure of fibrinogen. *Ann NY Acad Sci* 1972;**202**:77–97.

58. Ferry JD. The mechanism of polymerization of fibrin. *Proc Natl Acad Sci USA* 1952;**38**:566.

59. Hermans J, McDonagh J. Fibrin: structure and interactions. *Semin Thromb Hemost* 1982;**8**:11–24.

60. Robbins KD. A study on the conversion of fibrinogen to fibrin. *Am J Physiol* 1994;**142**:581–90.

61. Schwartz ML, Pizzo SV, Hill RL *et al.* Human factor XIII from plasma to platelets. Molecular weights, subunit structures, proteolytic activation, and cross-linkings of fibrinogen and fibrin. *J Biol Chem* 1973;**248**:1395–407.

62. Folk JE, Finlayson JS. The epsilon-(gamma-glutamyl)lysine crosslink and the catalytic role of transglutaminases. *Adv Protein Chem* 1977;**31**:1–133.

63. McKee PA, Mattock P, Hill RL. Subunit structure of human fibrinogen, soluble fibrin, and cross-linked insoluble fibrin. *Proc Natl Acad Sci USA* 1970;**66**:738–44.

64. Kaplan KL, Broekman MJ, Chernoff A *et al.* Platelet alpha-granule proteins: studies on release and subcellular localization. *Blood* 1979;**53**:604–18.

65. Mosher DF. Action of fibrin-stabilizing factor on cold-insoluble globulin and alpha 2-macroglobulin in clotting plasma. *J Biol Chem* 1976;**251**:1639–45.

66. Ruoslahti E, Pekkala A, Engvall E. Effect of dextran sulfate on fibronectin-collagen interaction. *FEBS Lett* 1979;**107**:51–4.

67. Wagner DD, Urban Pickering M, Marder VJ. von Willebrand protein binds to extracellular matrices independently of collagen. *Proc Natl Acad Sci USA* 1984;**81**:471–5.

68. Nachmias V, Sullender J, Asch A. Shape and cytoplasmic filaments in control and lidocaine-treated human platelets. *Blood* 1977;**50**:39–53.

69. McDonagh J, Carrell N. Dysfibrinogens and other disorders of fibrinogen structure and function. In: Colman RW, Hirsh J, Marder VJ *et al.*, eds. *Hemostasis and Thrombosis: Basic Principles and Clinical Practice*, 3rd ed. Philadelphia: JB Lippincott; 1993;314–34.

70. Marder VJ, Colman RW, Francis CW *et al.* Consumptive thrombohemorrhagic disorders. In: Colman RW, Hirsh J, Marder VJ *et al.*, eds. *Hemostasis and Thrombosis: Basic Principles and Clinical Practice*, 3rd ed. Philadelphia: JB Lippincott; 1993;1023–63.

71. Plow EF, Collen D. The presence and release of alpha 2-antiplasmin from human platelets. *Blood* 1981;**58**:1069–74.

72. Levin EG, Marzec U, Anderson J *et al.* Thrombin stimulates tissue plasminogen activator release from cultured human endothelial cells. *J Clin Invest* 1984;**74**:1988–95.

73. Lijnen HR, Collen D. Interaction of plasminogen activators and inhibitors with plasminogen and fibrin. *Semin Thromb Hemost* 1982;**8**:2–10.

74. Mao SJ, Tucci MA. Lipoprotein(a) enhances plasma clot lysis *in vitro*. *FEBS Lett* 1990;**267**:131–4.

75. Alkjaersig N, Fletcher NP, Sherry S. The mechanism of clot dissolution by plasmin. *J Clin Invest* 1959;**38**:1086–90.

76. Sakata Y, Aoki N. Cross-linking of alpha 2-plasmin inhibitor to fibrin by fibrin-stabilizing factor. *J Clin Invest* 1980;**65**:290–7.

77. Collen D. On the regulation and control of fibrinolysis. Edward Kowalski Memorial Lecture. *Thromb Haemost* 1980;**43**:77–89.

78. Plow EF. Leukocyte elastase release during blood coagulation: a potential mechanism for activation of the alternative fibrinolytic pathway. *J Clin Invest* 1982;**69**:564–72.

79. Francis CW, Marder VJ, Martin SE. Plasmic degradation of crosslinked fibrin. I. Structural analysis of the particulate clot and identification of new macromolecular-soluble complexes. *Blood* 1980;**56**:456–64.

80. Aoki N, Moroi M, Sakata Y *et al.* Abnormal plasminogen. A hereditary molecular abnormality found in a patient with recurrent thrombosis. *J Clin Invest* 1978;**61**:1186–95.

81. Kopec M, Teisseyre E, Dudek-Wojciechowska G. Studies on 'Double D' fragment from stabilized bovine fibrin. *Thromb Res* 1973;**2**:283.

82. Francis CW, Markham RE Jr, Barlow GH *et al.* Thrombin activity of fibrin thrombi and soluble plasmic derivatives. *J Lab Clin Med* 1983;**102**:220–30.

83. Nesheim ME, Wang W, Boffa M *et al.* Thrombin, thrombomodulin and TAFI in the molecular link between coagulation and fibrinolysis. *Thromb Haemost* 1997;**78**:386–91.

84. Cines DB, Tomaski A, Tannenbaum S. Immune endothelial-cell injury in heparin-associated thrombocytopenia. *N Engl J Med* 1987;**316**:581–9.

85. MacGregor RR, Friedman HM, Macarak EJ *et al.* Virus infection of endothelial cells increases granulocyte adherence. *J Clin Invest* 1980;**65**:1469–77.

86. LeRoy EC, Ager A, Gordon JL. Effects of neutrophil elastase and other proteases on porcine aortic endothelial prostaglandin I2 production, adenine nucleotide release, and responses to vasoactive agents. *J Clin Invest* 1984;**74**:1003–10.

87. Janoff A, Sloan B, Weinbaum G *et al.* Experimental emphysema induced with purified human neutrophil elastase: tissue localization of the instilled protease. *Am Rev Respir Dis* 1977;**115**:461–78.

88. Kitchens CS. The anatomic basis of purpura. *Prog Hemost* 1982;**5**:211–44.

89. Wagner DD, Olmsted JB, Marder VJ. Immunolocalization of von Willebrand protein in Weibel–Palade bodies of human endothelial cells. *J Cell Biol* 1982;**95**:355–60.

90. Hynes RO. Integrins: a family of cell surface receptors. *Cell* 1987;**48**:549–54.

91. Dustin ML, Garcia Aguilar J, Hibbs ML *et al.* Structure and regulation of the leukocyte adhesion receptor LFA-1 and its counterreceptors, ICAM-1 and ICAM-2. *Cold Spring Harb Symp Quant Biol* 1989;**54**:753–65.

92. Hession C, Osborn L, Goff D *et al.* Endothelial leukocyte adhesion molecule 1: direct expression cloning and functional interactions. *Proc Natl Acad Sci USA* 1990;**87**:1673–7.

93. Rosenberg RD, Aird WC. Vascular-bed-specific hemostasis and hypercoagulable states. *N Engl J Med* 1999;**340**:1555–64.

94. Topper JN. Blood flow and vascular gene expression: fluid shear stress as a modulator of endothelial phenotype. *Mol Med Today* 1999;**5**:40–6.

95. Ofosu FA, Buchanan MR, Anvari N *et al.* Heparin, heparan sulfate and dermatan sulfate. *Ann NY Acad Sci* 1989;**556**:123.

96. Marcus AJ, Weksler BB, Jaffe EA. Enzymatic conversion of prostaglandin endoperoxide H2 and arachidonic acid to prostacyclin by cultured human endothelial cells. *J Biol Chem* 1978;**253**:7138–41.

97. Moncada S, Vane JR. The role of prostacyclin in vascular tissue. *Fed Proc* 1979;**38**:66–71.

98. Weiss HJ, Turitto VT. Prostacyclin (prostaglandin I2, PGI2) inhibits platelet adhesion and thrombus formation on subendothelium. *Blood* 1979;**53**:244–50.

99. Weksler BB, Marcus AJ, Jaffe EA. Synthesis of prostaglandin I2 (prostacyclin) by cultured human and bovine endothelial cells. *Proc Natl Acad Sci USA* 1977;**74**:3922–6.

100. Esmon CT, Owen WG. Identification of an endothelial cell cofactor for thrombin-catalyzed activation of protein C. *Proc Natl Acad Sci USA* 1981;**78**:2249–52.

101. Lollar P, Owen WG. Clearance of thrombin from circulation in rabbits by high-affinity binding sites on endothelium. Possible role in the inactivation of thrombin by antithrombin III. *J Clin Invest* 1980;**66**:1222–30.

102. Hatton MW, Berry LR, Regoeczi E. Inhibition of thrombin by antithrombin III in the presence of

certain glycosaminoglycans found in the mammalian aorta. *Thromb Res* 1978;**13**:655–70.

103. Busch C, Owen WG. Identification in vitro of an endothelial cell surface cofactor for antithrombin III. Parallel studies with isolated perfused rat hearts and microcarrier cultures of bovine endothelium. *J Clin Invest* 1982;**69**:726–9.

104. Teien AN, Abildgaard U, Hook M. The anticoagulant effect of heparan sulfate and dermatan sulfate. *Thromb Res* 1976;**8**:859–67.

105. Marcus AJ, Safier LB, Hajjar KA *et al.* Inhibition of platelet function by an aspirin-insensitive endothelial cell ADPase. Thromboregulation by endothelial cells. *J Clin Invest* 1991;**88**:1690–6.

106. MacIntyre DE, Pearson JD, Gordon JL. Localisation and stimulation of prostacyclin production in vascular cells. *Nature* 1978;**271**:549–51.

107. Warner TD, Mitchell JA, de Nucci G *et al.* Endothelin-1 and endothelin-3 release EDRF from isolated perfused arterial vessels of the rate rabbit. *J Cardiovasc Pharmacol* 1989;**13**:S85–S88.

108. MacCumber MW, Ross CA, Glaser BM *et al.* Endothelin: visualization of mRNAs by in situ hybridization provides evidence for local action. *Proc Natl Acad Sci USA* 1989;**86**:7285–9.

109. Wiman B, Chmielewska J, Ranby M. Inactivation of tissue plasminogen activator in plasma. Demonstration of a complex with a new rapid inhibitor. *J Biol Chem* 1984;**259**:3644–7.

2

Introduction to the reproductive tract in women

Johnny S Younis, Ori Shen and Arnon Samueloff

INTRODUCTION

Obstetrics and gynecology is a medical and surgical specialty involving many situations that require frequent consultations with a hematologist with a special interest in thrombosis and hemostasis. Emergency situations include postpartum hemorrhagic shock, disseminated intravascular coagulopathy, and thromboembolic phenomena. Common non-urgent medical conditions include hemoglobinopathies, thrombocytopenias, and inherited coagulopathies.

In the past decade great progress has been made, with new evidence of several prevalent mutant genes that may increase susceptibility to thrombosis. This is especially true in obstetrics and gynecology, in which several situations (Table 2.1) defined in the past to be idiopathic are now coming to be associated with inherited or acquired thrombophilia. It is anticipated that this ongoing co-operation between obstetricians and gynecologists and hematologists will provide opportunities for successful prevention or treatment of these disorders.

This chapter presents a short introduction to the female pelvic vasculature and reproductive endocrinology. In addition, it discusses ovarian hyperstimulation syndrome (OHSS) and recurrent pregnancy loss. In Chapter 3, a short introduction to placental physiology is presented and an overview of the main vascular pregnancy complications, including pre-eclampsia,

Table 2.1 Gynecological and obstetrical situations associated with thrombophilia

Gynecological disorders
Venous thrombosis associated with oral contraception
Venous thrombosis associated with hormone replacement therapy
Thromboembolic phenomena associated with OHSS
Recurrent pregnancy loss

Obstetrical disorders
Thromboembolic phenomena associated with pregnancy or puerperium
Postpartum ovarian vein thrombosis
Pre-eclampsia
Placental abruption
Intrauterine growth restriction
Intrauterine fetal death

intrauterine growth restriction, placental abruption and intrauterine fetal death is given.

PELVIC VASCULATURE

The organs of the female reproductive tract are traditionally divided into the external and internal genitalia. The external genital organs are located in the vulvar region. The internal genital organs are placed in the true pelvis and include the vagina, cervix, uterus, fallopian tubes, ovaries, and surrounding supporting structures.[1–4]

The vascular supply to the internal pelvic organs is derived from three main sources; the internal iliac (hypogastric) artery, the middle sacral artery, and the superior rectal (hemorrhoidal) artery.[4] As a rule, the arterial supply to the pelvis is paired and bilateral and has multiple collaterals. The arteries enter their organs laterally and then unite with anastomotic vessels from the other side of the pelvis near the midline. The pelvic reproductive viscera lie within a loosely woven basket of large veins with numerous interconnecting venous plexuses. The arteries pass through this interwoven mesh of veins, giving off numerous branching vessels to provide a rich blood supply.[1–4]

The uterus receives its blood supply from two major sources: the uterine and ovarian arteries. The uterine artery is the major blood supplier in the non-pregnant state. However, during pregnancy both arteries have an important role in vascular supply.[4]

The ovary receives a dual blood supply derived from two major vessels, the internal iliac through the ovarian branch of the uterine artery and the aorta through the ovarian artery. These two arteries anastomose in the meso-ovarium. The ovarian artery becomes markedly enlarged during pregnancy and is capable of providing a major proportion of blood supply to the fundus of the gravid uterus. It may also significantly contribute to the placental blood flow during pregnancy.[4]

The vascular architecture of the endometrium is of special importance in the physiology of menstruation, implantation and pregnancy development. The uterine artery arises from the anterior division of the hypogastric artery and courses medially toward the isthmus of the uterus. The ascending branch of the uterine artery passes through the broad ligament and anastomoses with the ovarian artery in the meso-ovarium. Through its tortuous route in the parametrium the uterine artery gives off numerous branches that unite with arcuate arteries

from the contralateral side. This series of arcuate arteries gives off radial branches (the basal or straight arteries) that supply the myometrium and the basalis layer of the endometrium. The arcuate arteries also supply the spiral arteries (or coiled arteries) of the functional layer of the endometrium.[1,2] It has been shown that, unlike the basal arteries, the coiled arteries are hormone-dependent and thus may serve an important role in the mechanism of menstruation as well as implantation.[2]

The venous drainage of the pelvis begins in small sinusoids that drain to profuse venous plexuses contained within or immediately adjacent to the pelvic organs. Invariably there are numerous anastomoses between the parietal and visceral branches of the venous system. In general, the veins of the female pelvis and peritoneum are thin-walled and have few valves.[1] Veins that drain the pelvic plexuses follow the course of the arterial supply and their names are similar to those of the accompanying arteries. Often multiple veins run alongside a single artery. Venous systems are paired and mirror each other in their drainage, with the notable exception of the ovarian veins.[2] The left ovarian vein empties into the left renal vein, whereas the right ovarian vein connects directly with the inferior vena cava.[1]

The pelvic vasculature is a high-volume, high-flow system with substantial expansive capabilities throughout reproductive life.[3] Blood flow through the uterine arteries increases to approximately 500 ml/minute in late pregnancy. In non-pregnant women, certain conditions such as uterine leiomyomas, OHSS, and malignant neoplasm may be associated with new vascularization and hypertrophy of existing vessels and a corresponding increase in pelvic blood flow.[3]

Clinical impact of pelvic vascular anatomy

Pelvic hemorrhage

A degree of vascular redundancy in the pelvis is important to ensure adequate supply of oxygen and nutrients in the event of major pelvic damage or other vascular compromise. In certain emergency clinical situations associated with profound hemorrhage from the female pelvis, drastic operative measures may be called for. These clinical situations are usually encountered during pregnancy or after delivery (either vaginal or Caeserean delivery), usually as a result of uterine atony, placental accreta, uterine rupture, or another obstetrical complication. In rare cases, extensive bleeding occurs during surgery for an advanced female pelvic malignancy.

In these situations, lifesaving ligations of the uterine, ovarian, or internal iliac arteries are sometimes warranted. Uterine artery ligation reduces blood loss associated with uterine atony or lacerations. In addition it may, in certain circumstances, permit uterine conservation. The complication rate for this procedure has been reported to be low.[5,6]

Internal iliac artery ligation is performed when other measures have failed. Unilateral internal iliac artery ligation reduces distal ipsilateral blood flow by half. An even more important clinical effect is an 85% reduction in pulse pressure distal to the ligation. This reduction changes the hemodynamics of the distal arterial tree to a situation that more resembles that of a venous system and so is amenable to hemostasis via simple clot formation.[6] Branches of the anterior division of the internal iliac artery provide the major blood supply to organs of the female pelvis. Fortunately, none of these procedures results in hypoxia of the pelvic viscera. Reports of successful full-term pregnancies after bilateral ligation of internal iliac, uterine, and ovarian arteries attest to the abundant collateral blood supply of the female reproductive tract.[1,3,6]

Iliac vein compression syndrome (May–Thurner syndrome or Cockett's syndrome)

Deep vein thrombosis (DVT) is one of the most prevalent disorders in women during the reproductive years, especially during pregnancy. Its major complication, pulmonary embolism, is still a leading cause of maternal death. Based on studies using objective radiographic testing, it is estimated that DVT affects 0.5–3.0 per 1000 women during pregnancy.[7] Using objective criteria, antepartum DVT has been found to be as least as common as postpartum thrombosis, and it occurs with equal frequency in all three trimesters.[8] However, pulmonary embolism has been found to be more common in the postpartum period.

It has long been noticed that DVT occurs predominantly in the left leg. This predisposition to the left side has been first perceived and reported by May and Thurner[9] and by Cockett and Thomas[10] more than 30 years ago. Later studies have confirmed the left leg predominance.[11–13] In a cohort study of 60 consecutive pregnant women with a first episode of DVT, 58 women had an isolated left leg thrombosis and two patients had bilateral vein thrombosis.[11] In a recent meta-analysis of all published studies of DVT during pregnancy and the puerperium between 1966 and 1998, 14 studies were found using objective testing for diagnosis.[12] A cumulative rate of 82% was found for left-sided or bilateral vein thrombosis.

Several anatomical–mechanical explanations have been presented to explain the left-sided predominance of DVT. The outstanding anatomical feature is the peculiar anatomical relationship of the pelvic vessels, specifically compression of the left common iliac vein at its origin against the pelvic rim by the overlying right common iliac artery.[13] Pressure by the gravid uterus and the lumbosacral hyperlordosis developing in normal pregnancy could accentuate compression on the left iliac veins, thus promoting venous stasis.

Primary endovenous structures mainly 'spur' outgrowths in the left common iliac vein was also suggested as an alternative pathogenic factor for the left sided dominance of DVT. It was implied that such endovenous outgrowths may alter blood flow within the vessel and predispose to stasis or injury.[12] However, this 'spur' phenomenon is debated, and the present-day view tends to consider it as secondary to compression of the left iliac vein by the overlying artery.[13] However, this does not preclude that part of this phenomenon could have a congenital basis.

Factors other than pregnancy may also predispose to the development of iliac vein thrombosis and compression. These factors include confinement to bed, trauma, surgery, oral contraception, pelvic or other malignancy, and acquired or inherited thrombophilia (see Chapters 12 and 13).

REPRODUCTIVE ENDOCRINOLOGY

The hypothalamic–pituitary–ovarian axis (Figure 2.1) is one of the fundamental cornerstones of reproductive endocrinology in the female. The hypothalamic gonadotropin-releasing hormone (GnRH) is the hormone that controls release of the pituitary gonadotropin (follicular stimulating hormone (FSH) and luteinizing hormone (LH)). The GnRH molecule is a decapeptide with a very short half-life of only 2–5 minutes. The hypothalamus has many cerebral connections that may affect GnRH production and secretion. The greatest concentration of GnRH-producing neurons is located in the arcuate nucleus. From here the GnRH is transported along the axons of these neurons, which terminate in the median eminence, around the capillaries of the primary portal plexus.[14–16]

There is no direct nervous connection between the hypothalamus and the anterior pituitary. There is also no direct arterial blood supply to the anterior pituitary. Its major source of blood flow is also its source of hypothalamic input, the portal vessels.[16] Gonadotropin-releasing hormone molecules are secreted into the portal vessel system. The direction of the blood flow is from the median eminence to the anterior pituitary.[15]

Normal gonadotropin secretion requires pulsatile GnRH discharge with a frequency and amplitude that is within a critical range. The amplitude and frequency of the pulse vary throughout the menstrual cycle.[14,15] The control of GnRH pulsatility is complex and is regulated by several negative and positive feedback mechanisms, including the ovarian sex steroids estradiol (E_2) and progesterone, the pituitary gonadotropins LH and FSH, and central neurotransmitters and neuromodulators.[14]

LH and FSH are glycoproteins of high molecular weight (28,000 Da and 37,000 Da, respectively). They each have the same α-subunit (molecular weight 14,000 Da) of about 90 amino acids, which is similar in structure to the α-subunit of thyroid-stimulating hormone and human chorionic gonadotropin (hCG). The β-subunits of all these hormones have different amino acids and carbohydrates and provide the specific biological activity. The α- and β-subunits are joined by disulfide bonds. The half-life of LH is shorter (30 minutes) than that of FSH (3.9 hours).

Although the two gonadotropins act synergistically, FSH acts primarily on the granulosa cells

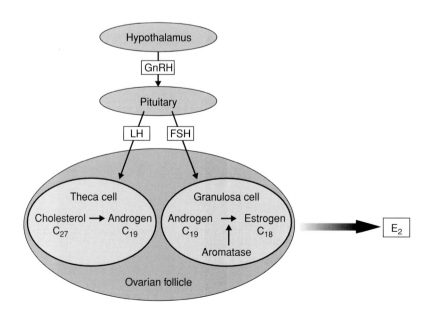

Figure 2.1 The endocrine hypothalamic–pituitary–ovarian axis.

to stimulate follicular growth and E_2 synthesis, whereas LH acts primarily on the theca cells in the ovary to induce steroidogenesis.[14,15] *In vitro* studies support the two-cell theory of E_2 production in the ovary. This theory proposes that LH acts on the theca to produce androgens (androstenedione and testosterone), which are then transported to the granulosa cells, where they are transformed into estrogens (estrone and E_2) by the action of FSH. The aromatase enzyme catalyzes this conversion.[14,15]

LH receptors exist on the theca cells at all stages of the cycle. They also appear on granulosa cells after follicular maturation. In addition, they exist on the corpus luteum. The main action of LH is to stimulate androgen synthesis by the theca cells and progesterone synthesis by the corpus luteum.[15]

FSH receptors exist primarily on the granulosa cells. FSH also stimulates follicular growth by increasing both the FSH and LH receptor content in granulosa cells. This action is enhanced by E_2. In addition, FSH activates the aromatase enzyme. After a sufficient number of LH receptors have been produced by the action of FSH and E_2, LH acts directly on the granulosa cells to cause luteinization and production of progesterone. The mid-cycle LH peak initiates the ovulatory process. Ovulation occurs about 32 hours after the initial rise in LH and about 12–16 hours after the LH peak. LH also stimulates synthesis of prostaglandin and proteolytic enzymes. Prostaglandins are also involved in luteinization, progesterone production, and follicle rupture.[15] Moreover, the mid-cycle LH surge initiates germinal vesicle disruption and resumption of meiosis in the oocyte.

The ovarian hormones E_2 and progesterone are steroids with a low molecular weight (220–387 Da). In women of reproductive age these steroids must be produced and secreted in an orderly, cyclic fashion in order to stimulate endometrial proliferation and secretion in preparation for normal implantation of the embryo. The average length in humans, of each of the proliferative and secretory phases in the endometrium is 14 days.[16] Failure of implantation causes corpus luteum demise and resumption of menstrual bleeding. As the corpus luteum of the previous cycle fades, luteal production of progesterone and E_2 decreases, allowing FSH level to rise again and to start a new cycle.

If pregnancy does occur, placental hCG will mimic LH action and continuously stimulate the corpus luteum to produce progesterone. Continued corpus luteum function is essential for implantation and pregnancy maintenance until the developing placenta is capable to produce sufficient progesterone.[16] This luteal–placental shift usually occurs between the 7th and 10th week of gestation.[15]

Disorders of the hypothalamic–pituitary–ovarian–endometrial physiology may lead to many pathological states, including menstrual disturbances, anovulation, infertility, recurrent pregnancy loss, and malignancy. These disorders are some of the most frequent reasons for women to seek medical care.

OVARIAN HYPERSTIMULATION SYNDROME

Infertility

Infertility is defined as inability to conceive after 1 year of unprotected sexual intercourse. This condition may be further classified as primary infertility, in which no previous pregnancies have occurred, and secondary infertility, in which a previous pregnancy, although not necessarily a live birth, has occurred. Fecundability is the probability of achieving pregnancy within a single menstrual cycle, and fecundity is the probability, within a single menstrual cycle, of achieving pregnancy that results in a live birth. The fecundability of a normal couple has been anticipated at 20–25%. On the basis of this assessment, about 85–90% of couples restraining from contraception should conceive after 12 months.[17,18]

About 10–15% of couples in the reproductive age group will have difficulties in achieving pregnancy. Infertility may be the result of several etiologic factors. The distribution rate of each of these etiologies is summarized in Table 2.2. Other issues such as age, ovarian reserve, lifestyle factors (including smoking, exercise,

Table 2.2 Etiological factors of infertility in couples	
Factor	**Distribution rate (%)**
Tubal and/or pelvic pathology (including endometriosis)	35
Male factor infertility	35
Ovulatory dysfunction	15
Unexplained infertility	10
Other factors	5

and diet), and environmental and occupational circumstances may also affect incidence of infertility and success of treatment.[17]

Most long-term infertility problems are managed today with one of three treatment modalities. Ovulatory dysfunction is usually treated with ovulation-induction drugs. Mild male factor infertility and unexplained infertility are treated with superovulation and intrauterine insemination. Mechanical infertility, severe male factor infertility, and other conditions are treated with assisted reproductive technologies, mainly *in vitro* fertilization and embryo transfer. In all of these treatment modalities, ovulation-induction drugs are used in order to stimulate the ovaries to ovulate or alternately to produce numerous follicles and multiple fertilizable oocytes for *in vivo* or *in vitro* fertilization.[18] This supraphysiological pharmacological intervention is termed 'controlled ovarian hyperstimulation'.

Ovulation-induction drugs include, mainly, clomiphene citrate, urinary gonadotropins (human menopausal gonadotropins and human chorionic gonadotropins), recombinant gonadotropins and gonadotropin releasing hormone analogs (GnRH agonists and GnRH antagonists). A combination of these drugs is usually given in accordance with the specific protocol used.

Several complications may result from the use of ovulation-induction medications, the main two being OHSS and multiple pregnancy. In some cases, the abortion rate and the ectopic pregnancy rate are increased. Some protocols of treatment may also adversely affect corpus luteum function.

The clinical syndrome

OHSS is usually defined as an iatrogenic complication caused in the course of pharmacological ovarian stimulation. Marked ovarian enlargement, high E_2 levels and extravascular exudate accumulation occur in this clinical syndrome. The pathophysiological hallmarks are increased vascular permeability and a significant shift of fluid and protein from the intravascular space into the third space, primarily the peritoneal cavity. Depletion of the intravascular space results in electrolyte imbalances, hemoconcentration, and diminished organ perfusion. Consequently, renal, hepatic, or respiratory dysfunction can result. This may be followed, in severe cases, by potentially lethal thromboembolic phenomena.

Because of the ovarian enlargement, torsion of the adnexa is a relatively common complication of this syndrome. The possibility of an ovarian rupture and intraperitoneal bleeding should also be considered, especially if there is an unexplained fall in the patient's hematocrit.[18]

The incidence of clinically important OHSS is remarkable. The mild type is relatively common. The incidence of severe OHSS ranges from 1% to 2% following ovulation induction and controlled ovarian stimulation. The incidence of OHSS is no greater in assisted reproduction as compared to conventional ovulation-induction treatment. However, the incidence of hyperstimulation following GnRH-agonist therapy seems to be higher. About two-thirds of cases of OHSS occur early in the conception cycle, the remainder occur in non-conception cycles. The risk

Table 2.3 Risk factors for OHSS
Young age
Polycystic ovary syndrome
Asthenic habitus
High serum estradiol in the late follicular phase
Multiple follicles on transvaginal scan
A conception cycle
Human chorionic gonadotropin supplementation in the luteal phase
Gonadotropin releasing hormone agonist treatment

factors for the development of OHSS, especially the severe form, are listed in Table 2.3.

Critical cases of OHSS are complicated by multiple system failure. The most severe consequences of these cases are renal failure, adult respiratory distress syndrome, and thromboembolic phenomena.[18,19]

Several factors have been implicated in the pathophysiology of OHSS. It is now clear that the OHSS is associated with the process of ovulation induced by either LH or hCG. Following ovulation, one or more substances produced by the ovary are secreted in excess, increasing capillary permeability and resulting in the clinical syndrome. Histamines, prostaglandins, cytokines (mainly interleukin-1), the ovarian renin–angiotensin system, vascular endothelial growth factor, and nitric oxide have all been suggested to be involved in the pathogenesis of OHSS.[18,19] Research in this field is still ongoing and final conclusions have yet to be drawn.

The vast majority of thrombotic complications that affect women with OHSS are venous thrombosis in the lower limbs, the pelvis, the upper limbs, the neck, or the cerebrum. A complete list of the venous sites published in the literature is presented in Table 2.4. Rare cases of acute arterial thrombosis associated with OHSS have also been published.[20,21]

Recently, several reports have been published describing the development of severe thrombotic vein events in mild to moderate cases of the OHSS with no evidence of hemoconcentration.[22–24] Interestingly, another unique report of spontaneous OHSS complicated by a deep vein thrombosis in a pregnant woman carrying the factor V Leiden mutation has also been presented.[25] Thromboses developed during the second trimester of gestation and affected the left subclavian, axillary, humeral, and internal jugular veins.

Taken together, these case reports[22–25] emphasize that thrombophilic pleomorphisms may be a significant pathogenic risk factor for thromboembolic phenomena in women who develop OHSS. A detailed review on this topic is presented in Chapter 10.

RECURRENT PREGNANCY LOSS

About 15–20% of all human pregnancies are clinically aborted. However, the actual total human embryo loss is estimated to be much higher. Early morphological data have estimated that about 40% of embryos do not implant or are ejected from the uterus before the next menstrual cycle. Later prospective studies using sensitive β-hCG levels have shown that the rate of pregnancy loss in a normal population could be as high as 30–50%.[26,27] In most cases pregnancy loss occurs without the woman's

Table 2.4 Sites of vein thrombosis in ovarian hyperstimulation syndrome
Internal jugular vein
External jugular vein
Superior vena cava
Cortical vein
Deep cerebral vein
Subclavian vein
Femoral vein
Iliac vein
Upper limbs
Lower limbs

knowledge. However, since not all fertilized oocytes are implanted, some have no opportunity to secrete β-hCG. Therefore, it is anticipated that the actual pregnancy loss in humans is even higher, perhaps as high as 60–70%.

About 80% of clinical pregnancy loss occurs in the first trimester of gestation. As pregnancy progresses, the risk of abortion diminishes. The vast majority of early abortions are the result of a chromosomal or genetic defect of the conceptus itself.[27] The risk of a recurrent abortion in a woman who has already aborted once is of the same magnitude as the abortion rate in the general population. However, if a woman has already aborted three times, her chances of losing her next pregnancy increases significantly.

Recurrent pregnancy loss in women is a distinct and serious clinical disorder that should be evaluated and treated. As many as 5% of all couples attempting to conceive have two successive pregnancy losses, and 1% have three or more consecutive losses. Uncertainties about the etiology and the controversies surrounding management of repeat fetal demise are two reasons why this issue remains a particularly frustrating challenge for physicians and patients.

There is general agreement today that recurrent pregnancy loss is associated with genetic, uterine, endocrine, and autoimmune factors, as well as with multiple pregnancies. However, there is still considerable disagreement about other potential conditions associated with consecutive losses, such as infectious, environmental (teratogenic), and alloimmune factors. Until several years ago, as many as 50% of all cases of recurrent pregnancy loss were considered 'unexplained'. Recently, new developments have brought this topic back into the focus of the medical community. Table 2.5 summarizes these etiologies and lists new factors under current investigation.

Genetic factors

Genetically balanced structural chromosome rearrangements are present in approximately 2–3% of couples with recurrent spontaneous

Table 2.5 Etiologies of recurrent pregnancy loss
Non-controversial factors
Genetic factors
Uterine factors (congenital)
Uterine malformations
Diethylstilbestrol exposure *in utero*
Uterine factors (acquired)
Intrauterine adhesions (Asherman's syndrome)
Cervical incompetence
Myoma uteri
Endocrinological factors
Corpus luteum dysfunction
Uncontrolled diabetes mellitus
Uncontrolled hypothyroidism
Autoimmune factors
Systemic lupus erythematosus (and other autoimmune disorders)
Antiphospholipid syndrome
Multiple pregnancies
Controversial factors
Infectious etiologies
Environmental (teratogenic) factors
Alloimmune factors
New developments
Low ovarian reserve
Polycystic ovary syndrome
Congenital thrombophilia

abortions. Balanced translocation account for the largest proportion of karyotypic abnormalities in couples with recurrent pregnancy loss. The most common type of structural abnormality involves the exchange of chromatin between two non-homologous chromosomes (reciprocal translocation) or the addition of part of one chromosome to another non-homologous chromosome (simple translocation).[27]

Uterine factors

About 10–15% of women with recurrent pregnancy loss have congenital uterine anomalies. The most common anomalies are unicornuate, bicornuate, septate, and didelphic uteri. Acquired uterine abnormalities, such as severe endometrial synechiae, submucous leiomyomata, and cervical incompetence, may also be associated with recurrent pregnancy loss. It is suggested that all of these abnormalities may be related to recurrent abortions because of limited potential for uterine volume expansion or because of inadequate placentation resulting from a poorly vascularized endometrium.

Endocrinological factors

Corpus luteum dysfunction (or luteal phase defect) is considered to be a cause of recurrent early pregnancy loss. Some uncontrolled studies indicate that such patients may benefit from progesterone or hCG supplementation.[28–30] Other endocrinological disorders, such as diabetes mellitus or hypothyroidism, have been implicated as causes of recurrent pregnancy loss, although only when associated with severe systemic metabolic derangement. There is no evidence from controlled studies that asymptomatic disorders cause pregnancy loss.[27]

Autoimmune factors

Systemic lupus erythematosus (SLE) is the leading autoimmune disease that causes recurrent pregnancy loss in humans. It is now apparent that most cases of recurrent pregnancy loss in women with SLE are associated with the presence of antiphospholipid antibodies (APLA).[31] About 7–30% of patients with SLE have APLA.[32] These antibodies are also associated with recurrent pregnancy loss in otherwise healthy women.[32] These antibodies have also been associated with venous and arterial thrombosis, autoimmune thrombocytopenia, and autoimmune hemolytic anemia. When one of these manifestations occurs in a person with significant serum levels of APLA, that person is considered to have the antiphospholipid syndrome. Since the 1980s antiphospholipid syndrome has been considered to be an etiology of recurrent pregnancy loss, and it has been found in 5–10% of patients.[27]

Multiple pregnancies

Abortion is more likely with multiple fetuses. Detailed pathological reviews of abortuses have identified three times as many twins among aborted pregnancies as among term pregnancies.[33] Monochorional twins greatly outnumber dichorial twins in abortuses (at a 18:1 ratio), implicating monozygosity as a major risk factor for spontaneous abortion.

In the past decade, as a result of ultrasound studies performed during the first trimester, there is evidence to suggest that the incidence of multiple pregnancies in humans is higher than previously estimated and that a significant proportion of early pregnancy loss takes place in these gestations. This has led to the concept of the 'vanishing twin'. The reported incidence of this phenomenon in the first trimester differs between series; it ranges between 13% and 78%.[34]

New developments

In the past few years, several novel factors have been implicated in the etiology of recurrent pregnancy loss. Table 2.6 shows the authors' work-up protocol for patients with recurrent pregnancy loss, including tests concerning the contemporary knowledge of our understanding in this field.

Table 2.6 Evaluation of recurrent pregnancy loss

Karyotype of husband and wife
Hysterosalpingography and/or hysteroscopy
Late luteal endometrial biopsy
Fasting glucose
TSH level
Antinuclear factor level
Lupus anticoagulants and anticardiolipin antibodies
Day 3 FSH, E_2 and LH serum levels
Congenital thrombophilia evaluation

Low ovarian reserve

During the past decade, several studies have been published that have investigated day 3 FSH and E_2 serum levels in infertile patients attempting assisted reproduction.[35] These studies have shown that high FSH or E_2 levels (or both) are correlated with low ovarian reserve and unfavorable results of infertility treatment. Some studies have also shown that day 3 FSH is a better predictor than age for success of infertility treatment by assisted reproduction.[36]

High day 3 FSH levels are estimated to be the result of poor-quality ovarian follicles and granulosa cells that secrete low quantities of inhibin. Low inhibin B levels preclude the hypothalamic negative feedback and therefore early follicular FSH and E_2 levels are higher. Low-quality follicles produce low quality oocytes and embryos that have a diminished potential for implantation.

Recently, two preliminary retrospective reports have concluded that low ovarian reserve may also be associated with recurrent pregnancy loss.[37,38] These studies suggested that ovarian reserve screening should be considered in the work-up of recurrent pregnancy loss before therapy is attempted. Although these preliminary reports seem to be promising, more prospective research in this field should be performed before final conclusions are drawn.

Polycystic ovary syndrome

Polycystic ovary syndrome (PCOS) is usually defined as a state of chronic anovulation coupled with signs of hyperandrogenism. The main characteristics of women with PCOS are oligoovulation or anovulation, oligomenorrhea, hirsutism, high serum LH levels, and a typical ovarian appearance on pelvic sonography. Several reports in the past decade have shown that pregnancies achieved in women with PCOS have a high rate of recurrent early fetal loss.[39] Other reports have shown that reducing follicular LH levels using GnRH-agonists in these women may reduce the abortion rate considerably.[40–42]

Several explanations have been proposed for the pathogenesis of this occurrence. The first explanation implicated the high follicular LH levels in premature oocyte maturation as causing the oocyte to ovulate prematurely. This would result in failure of the oocyte to be fertilized or, if fertilized, the embryo being miscarried. The second explanation concerned over-secretion of ovarian androgens that could adversely affect granulosa cell function and lead to follicular atresia. The third explanation involved endometrial abnormality secondary to premature luteinization developing in this setting.[39]

These reports are still preliminary and it is too early to draw final conclusions, especially since not all investigators agree on an association between recurrent pregnancy loss and PCOS. A recent report has concluded that polycystic ovarian morphology on ultrasound is not predictive of pregnancy loss among ovulatory women with recurrent miscarriage who conceive spontaneously. Neither an elevated LH level nor an increased serum testosterone level was associated with an increased rate of miscarriages.[43] The search for a specific endocrine (or other) abnormality that can separate women with PCOS into those with a good prognosis and those with a poor prognosis for a future successful gestation should be pursued.

Congenital thrombophilia

For several decades, clinicians have presumed that a significant proportion of patients with recurrent pregnancy loss have a hemostatic disturbance in the placental bed. The assumption was that microthrombi in the placental bed vessels could lead to multiple placental infarctions that adversely affect the fetomaternal circulation, leading eventually to fetal death.[44] Unfortunately, no evidence for the 'thrombosis theory' has been presented. Several empirical antithrombotic treatments have been advocated in the past but without any scientific validation or medical proof of efficacy.

The discovery of the antiphospholipid syndrome, in the early 1980s, as an etiology for recurrent pregnancy loss might be taken as evidence in favor of the 'thrombosis theory'. However, this syndrome has been found in no more than 5–10% of all patients with recurrent pregnancy loss. Moreover, at that time, as many as 50% of all cases of repeated fetal loss were still considered to be unexplained.

Until recently, primary hypercoagulable states were responsible for less than 10% of cases presenting with thrombotic phenomena. The discovery of activated protein C resistance caused by a single point mutation of factor V

gene (factor V Leiden) has changed this situation dramatically.[45]

Indeed, in the past few years, several investigators have shown an association between activated protein C resistance, factor V Leiden, and other new thrombophilic polymorphisms and recurrent pregnancy loss in humans.[46–49] A detailed description of this association and its treatment are presented in Chapter 16.

REFERENCES

1. Droegemueller W. Anatomy. In: Droegemueller W, Herbert AL, Mishel DR Jr, Stenchever MA (eds), *Comprehensive Gynecology*. St Louis: CV Mosby; 1987:42–75.

2. Anatomy of the reproductive tract. In: Cunningham FG, MacDonald PC, Gant NF *et al.* (eds), *Williams Obstetrics*, 20th ed. Stamford, USA: Appleton and Lange; 1997:37–67.

3. Anderson JR, Genadry R. Anatomy and embryology. In: Berek JS, Adashi EY, Hillard PA (eds), *Novak's Gynecology*, 12th ed. Baltimore: Williams and Wilkins; 1996:71–122.

4. Gould SF. Anatomy. In: Gabbe SG, Niebyl JR, Simpson JL (eds), *Obstetrics: Normal and Problem Pregnancies*. New York: Churchill Livingstone; 1986:3–38.

5. O'Leary JA. Stop of hemorrhage with uterine artery ligation. *Contemp Obstet Gynecol* 1986;**28**:13–19.

6. Hankins GDV, Clark SL, Cunningham FG, Gilstrap LC III. Management of postpartum hemorrhage. In: *Operative Obstetrics*. Norwalk: Appleton and Lange; 1995:475–92.

7. American College of Obstetricians and Gynecologists. Thromboembolism in pregnancy. *ACOG Practice Bulletin* No 19. August 2000.

8. Gherman RB, Goodwin TM, Leung B *et al.* Incidence, clinical characteristics, and timing of objectively diagnosed venous thromboembolism during pregnancy. *Obstet Gynecol* 1999;**94**:730–4.

9. May R, Thurner J. The cause of the predominantly sinistral occurrence of thrombosis of the pelvic veins. *Angiology* 1957;**8**:419–26.

10. Cockett FB, Thomas ML. The iliac compression syndrome. *Br J Surg* 1965;**52**:816–21.

11. Ginsberg JS, Brill-Edwards P, Burrows RF *et al.* Venous thrombosis during pregnancy: leg and trimester of presentation. *Thromb Haemost* 1992;**67**:519–20.

12. Ray JG, Chan WS. Deep vein thrombosis during pregnancy and the puerperium: a meta-analysis of the period of risk and the leg presentation. *Obstet Gynecol Survey* 1999;**54**:265–71.

13. Verhaeghe R. Iliac vein compression as an anatomical cause of thrombophilia: Cockett's syndrome revisited. *Thromb Haemost* 1995;**74**:1398–401.

14. Mishell DR Jr. Reproductive endocrinology. In: Droegemueller W, Herbert AL, Mishel DR Jr, Stenchever MA (eds), *Comprehensive Gynecology*. St Louis: CV Mosby; 1987:76–127.

15. Neuroendocrinology. In: Speroff L, Glass RH, Kase NG (eds), *Clinical Gynecology, Endocrinology and Infertility*, 6th ed. Baltimore: Lippincott Williams and Wilkins; 1999:159–99.

16. Palter SF, Olive DL. Reproductive physiology. In: Berek JS, Adashi EY, Hillard PA (eds), *Novak's Gynecology*, 12th ed. Baltimore: Williams and Wilkins; 1996:149–72.

17. Guzick DS. Human infertility: an introduction. In: Adashi EY, Rock JA, Rosenwaks Z (eds), *Reproductive Endocrinology, Surgery, and Technology*. Philadelphia: Lippincott–Raven; 1996:1897–913.

18. Female infertility. In: Speroff L, Glass RH, Kase NG (eds), *Clinical Gynecology, Endocrinology and Infertility*, 6th ed. Baltimore: Lippincott Williams and Wilkins; 1999:1013–42.

19. Navot D, Bergh PA, Laufer N. The ovarian hyperstimulation syndrome. In: Adashi EY, Rock JA, Rosenwaks Z (eds), *Reproductive Endocrinology, Surgery, and Technology*. Philadelphia: Lippincott–Raven; 1996:2215–32.

20. Choktanasiri W, Rojanasakul A. Acute arterial thrombosis after gamete intrafallopian transfer: a case report. *J Assist Reprod Genet* 1995;**12**:335–7.

21. Germond M, Wirthner D, Thorin D *et al.* Aortosubclavian thromboembolism: a rare complication associated with moderate ovarian

hyperstimulation syndrome. *Hum Reprod* 1996;**11**:1173–6.

22. Aboulghar MA, Mansour RT, Serour GI, Amin YM. Moderate ovarian hyperstimulation syndrome complicated by deep cerebrovascular thrombosis. *Hum Reprod* 1998;**13**:2088–91.

23. Loret de Mola JR, Kiwi R, Austin C, Goldfarb JM. Subclavian deep vein thrombosis associated with the use of recombinant follicle-stimulating hormone (gonal-F) complicating mild ovarian hyperstimulation syndrome. *Fertil Steril* 2000;**73**:1253–6.

24. Aurousseau MH, Samama MM, Belhassen A *et al.* Risk of thromboembolism in relation to an in-vitro fertilization programme: three case reports. *Hum Reprod* 1995;**10**:94–7.

25. Todros T, Carmazzi CM, Bontempo S *et al.* Spontaneous ovarian hyperstimulation syndrome and deep vein thrombosis in pregnancy: case report. *Hum Reprod* 1999;**14**:2245–8.

26. Wilcox AJ, Weinberg CR, O'Connor JF *et al.* Incidence of early loss of pregnancy. *N Engl J Med* 1988;**319**:189–94.

27. American College of Obstetricians and Gynecologists. Early pregnancy loss. *ACOG Technical Bulletin* No 212. September 1995.

28. Tho PT, Byrd JR, McDonough PG. Etiologies and subsequent reproductive performance of 100 couples with recurrent abortion. *Fertil Steril* 1979;**32**:389–95.

29. Jones GS. The luteal phase defect. *Fertil Steril* 1976;**27**:351–6.

30. Somuel S, Daya S, Collins J, Hughes EG. The role of luteal phase support in infertility treatment: a meta-analysis of randomized trials. *Fertil Steril* 1994;**61**:1068–76.

31. Lockshin MD, Druzin ML, Goei S *et al.* Antibody to cardiolipin as a predictor of fetal distress or death in pregnant patients with systemic lupus erythematosus. *N Engl J Med* 1985;**313**:152–6.

32. Silver RM, Branch DW. Recurrent miscarriage: autoimmune considerations. *Clin Obstet Gynecol* 1994;**37**:745–60.

33. Multifetal pregnancy. In: Cunningham FG, MacDonald PC, Grant NF *et al.* (eds), *Williams Obstetrics*, 20th ed. Stamford, USA: Appleton and Lange; 1997:861–94.

34. Landy HJ, Keith LG. The vanishing twin: a review. *Hum Reprod Update* 1998;**4**:177–83.

35. Scott RT, Hofmann GE. Prognostic assessment of ovarian reserve. *Fertil Steril* 1995;**63**:1–11.

36. Toner JP, Philput CB, Jones GS, Muasher SJ. Basal follicle-stimulating hormone level is a better predictor of in vitro fertilization performance than age. *Fertil Steril* 1991;**55**:784–91.

37. Trout SW, Seifer DB. Do women with unexplained recurrent pregnancy loss have higher day 3 serum FSH and estradiol values? *Fertil Steril* 2000;**74**:335–7.

38. Hofmann GE, Khoury J, Thie J. Recurrent pregnancy loss and diminished ovarian reserve. *Fertil Steril* 2000;**74**:1192–5.

39. Balen AH, Tan SL, Jacobs HS. Hypersecretion of luteinizing hormone: a significant cause of infertility and miscarriage. *Br J Obstet Gynecol* 1993;**100**:1082–9.

40. Johnson P, Pearce M. Recurrent spontaneous abortion and polycystic ovarian disease: comparison of two regimens to induce ovulation. *BMJ* 1990;**300**:154–6.

41. Regan L, Owen EJ, Jacobs HS. Hypersecretion of luteinizing hormone, infertility, and miscarriage. *Lancet* 1990;**336**:1141–4.

42. Homburg R, Levy T, Berkovitz D *et al.* Gonadotropin-releasing hormone agonist reduces the miscarriage rate for pregnancies achieved in women with polycystic ovarian syndrome. *Fertil Steril* 1993;**59**:527–31.

43. Rai R, Backos M, Rushworth F, Regan L. Polycystic ovaries and recurrent miscarriage: a reappraisal. *Hum Reprod* 2000;**15**:612–15.

44. Younis JS, Ohel G, Brenner B, Ben-Ami M. Familial thrombophilia: the scientific rationale for thrombophylaxis in recurrent pregnancy loss? *Hum Reprod* 1997;**12**:1389–90.

45. Dahlback B, Carlsson M, Svensoon PJ. Familial thrombophilia due to a previously unrecognized mechanism characterized by poor anticoagulant response to activated protein C: prediction of a cofactor to activated protein C. *Proc Natl Acad Sci USA* 1993;**90**:1004–8.

46. Preston FE, Rosendaal FR, Walker ID *et al.* Increased fetal loss in women with heritable thrombophilia. *Lancet* 1996;**348**:913–16.

47. Rai R, Regan L, Hadley E *et al.* Second-trimester pregnancy loss is associated with activated protein C resistance. *Br J Haematol* 1996;**92**:489–90.

48. Brenner B, Mandel H, Lanir N *et al.* Activated protein C resistance can be associated with recurrent fetal loss. *Br J Haematol* 1997;**97**:551–4.

49. Brenner B, Sarig G, Weiner Z *et al.* Thrombophilic polymorphisms are common in women with fetal loss without apparent cause. *Thromb Haemost* 1999;**82**:6–9.

3

Human gestation and pregnancy complications

Ori Shen, Johnny S Younis and Arnon Samueloff

The human placenta is the primary interface between mother and fetus. Through this organ nutrients and oxygen are delivered to the fetus and waste products are cleared. Apart from this metabolic function, the placenta performs vital endocrine and immunological functions.

ANATOMY

The origin of the term 'placenta' is from the Latin word *plac* meaning 'cake'.[1]

The gross anatomy of the placenta[2] can be clearly observed after it has been delivered. The uterine side of the (usually) disc-shaped placenta has a distinct lobular structure. This side of the placenta, which is in direct contact with the maternal decidua, is known as the 'basal plate'. The other side, known as the 'chorionic plate', is in direct contact with the fetal membranes. The fetus is linked to the placenta via the umbilical cord and its vessels, which insert into the placental chorionic plate.

Integral to the function of the placenta as the primary maternal–fetal interface is an intimate transport mechanism that exists between the maternal and fetal blood systems. The fetal arterial system branches out from the two umbilical arteries to the multiple truncal arteries, each supplying a single placental lobe (cotylelone). From there, the vessels diverge into the capillary network that circulates within a complex structure of chorionic villi – the end-unit for metabolic fetal–maternal blood exchange. The villi bathe in maternal blood circulating within the intervillous space. The outer layer of the villi is composed of trophoblast cells, which are extraembryonic cells that are in direct contact with the maternal blood system. This type of structure (termed 'hemochorioendothelial') is unique and essential to the immunological interaction of the maternal–conceptus diad.

A key event in the development of this intricate vascular interface is the trophoblastic invasion of maternal blood vessels. Initially, surface endometrial capillaries and, eventually, uterine spiral arteries are invaded by the growing trophoblast, which erodes the walls of these vessels. The end-point of this process is a maternal circulation in which blood flows from the spiral arteries into a lacunar system that surrounds the chorionic villi that contain the fetal capillaries.

Occasionally, the placental 'barrier' is breached by fetal or maternal cells. Allo-immunization disorders, in which the mother becomes sensitized to fetal tissue, is a notable example. Furthermore, fetal blood cells, in small numbers, have been directly identified in the maternal bloodstream.[3]

PLACENTAL FUNCTION

Transfer

The transplacental transfer of nutrients and waste products was suspected in ancient times, and its nature and mechanisms were speculated on centuries ago. Multiple transfer mechanisms are operative at the hemochorioendothelial interface.[4] These mechanisms include:

- diffusion – small molecules, such as oxygen, carbon dioxide and water, diffuse easily between maternal and fetal circulations, driven by molecular concentration or partial pressure;
- facilitated diffusion (which is also driven by the molecular concentration gradient via specific carrier proteins) – rapid uninhibited transport by which many molecules, notably glucose, are transported at the placental interface; and
- selective transfer – a mechanism operating at the placental interface for substances concentrated in the fetus (iron, iodine and probably certain amino acids).

Endocrine function

The placenta is a veritable hormone factory that is responsible for producing a variety of substances, some of them in large quantities. These have a profound effect on the physiology of maternal gestation and may have an effect on fetal physiology as well. Certain products produced by the trophoblast (e.g. estriol, progesterone, human placental lactogen) affect maternal carbohydrate and lipid metabolism, modulate the maternal immune response, and are possibly instrumental in maintaining uterine quiescence until the onset of labor. Current research focuses on decidual derived products such as insulin growth factor binding protein-1, which may play a regulatory role in fetal growth. The endocrinological changes induced by placental function have been frequently implicated in the pathophysiology of various pregnancy-related pathologies, most notably pregnancy-induced hypertension and gestational diabetes.

Immunological function

Fetal tissue is an allogenic graft and the fact that it is not rejected by the maternal immune system has been, and still remains, a major focus of research and speculation. It seems reasonable to assume that acceptance of the fetus is, to some degree at least, a responsibility of the trophoblast cells. These fetus-derived extra-embryonic cells are the only cells in direct contact with maternal blood and other immuno-competent cells. The process of trophoblastic invasion of the decidua and its arterial vessels, up to the level of the spiral arteries, is typically completed by the middle of the second trimester. This 'invasion' process requires some deviation from the standard recognition of 'self' and 'non-self' tissue.

Theories to explain this phenomena are still unsuccessful in providing a comprehensive model to account for the multiple facets of these issues. A fairly recent development is recognition of the role of human leukocyte antigen (HLA) class G in trophoblast cells.[5] This gene is monomorphic (i.e. it has a single known allele). It has been shown that HLA class G is the only major histocompatibility complex (MHC) class 1 antigen expressed by a trophoblast. It has been known for some time that MHC class 2 antigens are not expressed at all by trophoblasts, which would explain how a trophoblast is recognized as 'self' by material immune cells. Incompatibilities between trophoblast and maternal expression might lead to placental-related diseases such as pre-eclampsia. This is elaborated in reviews by Loke *et al.*[6] and Dekker and Sibai.[7]

PRE-ECLAMPSIA

Pre-eclampsia is pregnancy-induced or aggravated hypertension that may be associated with proteinuria or generalized edema (or both). If left untreated, convulsions and death may occur. This severe disease is responsible for 10–20% of maternal deaths. Pre-eclampsia typically affects nulliparous women and women over 40 years of age. Its incidence ranges between 5 and 10% and is affected by racial and familial predisposition.

The cure for pre-eclampsia is delivery of the fetus and of the placenta.

Etiology

The etiology of pre-eclampsia is unknown. Although many hypotheses have been explored[7] in recent years, none has been proven to be true. At the present time, at least three hypotheses provoke tremendous interest:

- the genetic hypothesis;
- the placental ischemia hypothesis; and
- the immune dysfunction hypothesis.

Although a specific gene for pre-eclampsia has yet to be discovered, there is a large body of circumstantial evidence supporting a genetic predisposition. In one study, daughters of women with pre-eclampsia had a 26% incidence of pre-eclampsia compared with an incidence of 8% in matched controls.[8] Fetal genotypes have been implied in determining susceptibility, since women who were born to an eclamptic mother have been observed to have a higher prevalence than their sisters born after a non-eclamptic pregnancy.[9] Some of the genes implied include HLA antigen-coding genes, angiotensin II receptor genes and altered tumor necrosis factor-α messenger RNA expression.

Haig[10] suggested that a 'genetic conflict' might exist between maternal and paternally imprinted fetal genes. According to this theory, fetal genes serve to increase nutrient transfer to the fetus by raising maternal blood pressure (and thus the placental perfusion pressure). Maternal factors act to check this by reducing blood pressure. An abnormality in the balance of forces might result in excessive vasoconstriction and pre-eclampsia.

According to placental ischemia hypothesis, placental perfusion is abnormal as a result of a process involving the radial arteries. Thus, relative placental ischemia may be associated with abnormally increased systemic deportation of placental tissue that brings about systemic endothelial dysfunction, a hallmark of severe pre-eclampsia.

The reader interested in theories on the etiology and pathogenesis of pre-eclampsia will find the review by Decker and Sibai[7] illuminating.

To date, none of these or other theories offer a comprehensive or coherent view of what the etiology might be for this enigmatic disease. It is likely that in order to explain all the clinical and experimental observations that have been made, a theory that combines elements from all the theories mentioned above, and probably from others as well, will be formulated in the future.

Pathophysiology

Vasospasm with generalized arteriolar constriction is a fundamental feature of the pathophysiology of pre-eclampsia. Eventually, these vascular changes manifest clinically as hypertension, owing to elevated total peripheral resistance. The vasospasm is ubiquitous and can be found in multiple organs, specifically in the kidneys, liver, brain and the placenta.

An associated phenomenon is increased sensitivity to endogenous pressor agents such as angiotensin II and vasopressin. Typically, pregnant women become refractory to infusion of these agents. In pre-eclampsia this refractoriness is lost.[11]

Diagnosis

Table 3.1 illustrates the current classification of hypertensive disorders in pregnancy. Pre-eclampsia is diagnosed when hypertension develops during pregnancy and is accompanied by proteinuria and/or pathological edema.[12] It is further classified as mild or severe according to Table 3.2. Mild pre-eclampsia may rapidly progress to severe pre-eclampsia. Unfortunately, the resolution or regression of severe pre-eclampsia seldom occurs before the fetus and placenta are delivered.

Manifestations

Pre-eclampsia is a disease with multiple-organ involvement; clinically, the disorder may affect one or more of these organs in any combination.

Table 3.1 Classification of hypertensive disorders complicating pregnancy

Pregnancy-induced hypertension

Hypertension that develops as a consequence of pregnancy and regresses postpartum

Hypertension without proteinuria or pathological edema

Pre-eclampsia (with proteinuria or pathological edema)

Mild

Severe

Eclampsia (proteinuria or pathological edema with convulsions)

Coincidental hypertension

Chronic underlying hypertension that antedates pregnancy or persists postpartum

Pregnancy-aggravated hypertension

Underlying hypertension exacerbated by pregnancy

Superimposed pre-eclampsia

Superimposed eclampsia

Transient hypertension

Hypertension that develops after the mid-trimester of pregnancy and is characterized by mild elevations of blood pressure that do not compromise the pregnancy; this form of hypertension regresses after delivery, but may return in subsequent gestations

From Cunningham[12]

Table 3.2 Clinical manifestations of severe disease in patients with pregnancy-induced hypertension

Blood pressure >160–180 mmHg systolic or >110 mmHg diastolic

Proteinuria >5 g/24 hours (normal <300 mg/24 hours)

Elevated serum creatinine

Grand mal seizures (eclampsia)

Pulmonary edema

Oliguria <500 ml/24 hours

Microangiopathic hemolysis

Thrombocytopenia

Hepatocellular dysfunction (elevated alanine aminotransferase or aspartase aminotransferase)

Intrauterine growth retardation or oligohydramnios

Symptoms that suggest significant end-organ involvement: headache, visual disturbances, or epigastric or right upper quadrant pain

Contracted plasma volume related to generalized vasoconstriction is a hallmark of the disease. It leads to relatively low tolerance to volume loss in pre-eclampsia.

The most frequent hematological change in pre-eclampsia is thrombocytopenia. This may be isolated or part of a broader microangiopathic disorder known as HELLP syndrome (Hemolysis, Elevated Liver enzymes and Low Platelet count).

Renal function is affected to varying degrees, with proteinuria ranging from excretion of minimal amounts of protein to massive loss of protein via 'leaking' capillaries. Glomerular filtration rate is typically slightly decreased. Rarely, there is severe dysfunction to the level of acute renal failure. Sodium retention and decreased clearance of uric acid are early manifestations of renal involvement.

Severe neurological manifestations include visual blurring, persistent severe headaches or eclamptic seizures. Eclamptic seizures have a relatively high mortality rate and are typically preceded by headaches or other neurological symptoms.

Hepatic involvement may be limited to mild transaminase elevation, or it may be as severe as a subcapsular hematoma or a frank hepatic rupture, with catastrophic consequences.

Not infrequently, the placental vasculature is affected as well. This may result in diminished transport capacity leading to intrauterine growth restriction and other forms of fetal compromise.

Management

Unfortunately, there are no measures or medications that have proven efficacy in the prevention of pre-eclampsia. Bed rest, aspirin and countless other modalities have been investigated, and no doubt the search will continue for an effective way to prevent this common and frequently severe disease.

Once the diagnosis has been made, the only way to reverse the process and cure the disease is by delivery. If the disease occurs at or near term, this seldom presents a problem and delivery should be carried out preferably by the vaginal route. When diagnosed far from term, the problem may prove difficult and the possibly beneficial effect on the fetus that might be gained from delaying delivery must be weighed against the dangers that progression of the disease pose both to mother and to fetus. Generally, in severe cases, there is little benefit in prolonging pregnancy beyond week 32–34. When a decision has been taken to delay delivery, intensive monitoring is essential, with cosideration given to administration of antihypertensive medication as well as to seizure prophylaxis. The universally accepted agent for preventing as well as treating eclampsia is magnesium sulfate.

INTRAUTERINE GROWTH RESTRICTION

Intrauterine growth restriction (IUGR) is diagnosed when the fetus is estimated to be small for its gestational age. The clinical issues involving such a fetus are dominated by the need for accurate knowledge of gestational age, by the inherent inaccuracies with all current weight estimation techniques, by the etiology of this condition (if one can be established), and by additional parameters of fetal well-being.

Unfortunately, there is a paucity of evidence-based data about the optimal management approach. Concerns revolve around both short-term and long-term somatic and neurological outcome parameters.

Definition

Clearly, many genetic and environmental factors influence the weight distribution of fetuses in any given population. It is therefore critical to have detailed knowledge of fetal growth curves pertaining to that specific population. The cut-off point used to define growth restriction has been put arbitrarily by numerous authors and institutions at points ranging from below the third percentile to the 10th percentile. The American College of Obstetrics and Gynecology has suggested the 10th percentile,[13] and this is used by many institutions. Most of these children will not be sick or suffer any measurable developmental delay. Yet unfortunately, we still lack efficient tools to identify those fetuses that might suffer ill effects and those that might benefit from intervention.

Etiology

Both prognosis and management vary and are dependent on the etiology as well as on the severity of growth restriction. The various etiologies might be divided between three groups: maternal, fetal and placental. This division might appear arbitrary at times, and overlap between categories is not uncommon.

Severe maternal systemic disease or pathology can bring about IUGR. Advanced pregestational diabetes with vascular pathology[14] and systemic lupus erythematosus are common examples of maternal systemic diseases that adversely affect the placental vasculature or blood flow, leading to metabolic deprivation and IUGR. Antiphospholipid antibodies and other autoimmune disorders are associated with IUGR, as are substance abuse, exposure to teratogenic agents such as radiation, drugs and viruses (typically cytomegalovirus or rubella). A growing interest in the relationship between various thrombophilic disorders and perinatal complications such as IUGR, pre-eclampsia, placental abruption and others has accelerated research efforts in this area,[15] which might generate an effective prevention plan for those at risk. 'Placental-related' etiologies include hypertensive disorders (specifically pre-eclampsia), multiple gestations, tumors, placental mosaicism and chronic placental abruption or placental 'insufficiency'. Fetal etiologies range from severe structural anomalies or aneuploidy to wrong dates or simply being constitutionally small.

Risk

Small-for-gestational-age infants are at risk of increased morbidity and mortality. This is especially true for those below the third percentile. One study found a ten-fold increase in neonatal mortality for these small infants as well as an increased risk of neonatal sepsis, an increased need for intubation and an increased risk of seizures and low cord pH.[16]

Long-term growth cannot be accurately predicted from neonatal anthropometric measurements, let alone from ultrasound measurements *in utero*. The same can be said about long-term neurological and intellectual performance. Some studies have found more learning disabilities and others an increased rate of cerebral palsy[17] in children who are born with IUGR. However, much of the research in this area is plagued by the lack of uniform entry criteria or short follow-up. Future studies are required to identify at-risk fetuses, since clearly most fetuses are not.

Management

The management of IUGR is dependent on its etiology. A diagnostic work-up to clarify this might include a karyotype, detailed fetal organ scan, anthropometric measurements, biophysical score and Doppler studies, viral antibody testing and a thrombophilia battery.

If a fetus is suspected of being constitutionally small or if there is doubt as to gestational age, no intervention is called for. If the etiology involves a fetal defect, either inherited or acquired, typically no intervention will be of benefit to the

affected fetus. When a so-called 'placental factor' is assumed or it is thought that a maternal condition is adversely affecting placental function or blood flow, it is implied that the supply of nutrients and oxygen to the fetus might be compromised. In such circumstances there might be an advantage in intervening in the form of an elective delivery. If fetal testing indicates fetal compromise, this can be done pre-term. The logic in this approach is that once the placenta fails to provide for adequate metabolic exchange, the fetus might benefit both in the short and in the long term from induced premature delivery. If, when and how to do so are determined by multiple factors, especially gestational age, ultrasonographic anthropometric measurements, tests of fetal well-being, and standard obstetrical parameters. When expectant management is offered, any of several fetal surveillance protocols are followed. These typically use maternal counting of fetal movements, frequent non-stress tests, sonographic biophysical score (including ultrasound measurements of amniotic fluid volume), fetal movements, tone and breathing movements, and Doppler flow studies of any number of fetal arterial or venous vessels. Serial ultrasounds to establish a growth curve are typically performed every 2 weeks.

At the present time, there is at least one prospective multicenter study under way that is attempting to clarify the issue of whether and when such an intervention might benefit the child, both in the short and in the long term. The Growth Restriction Intervention Trial (GRIT) is a trial designed to compare the effect of delivering growth restricted babies early to prevent damage from intrauterine hypoxia, with delaying delivery for as long as possible to minimize the risk of prematurity.

In some cases, treatment or prevention can be directed towards those factors that are thought to cause IUGR. Patients should be counseled to avoid or decrease smoking and other substance abuse. Adequate nutrition should be supplied and teratogenic exposure avoided or kept to a minimum.

With the proliferation of hematological testing, more patients are found to have various thrombophilia-related disorders. The treatment and prevention of IUGR and other perinatal complications by means of administering anticoagulants is a logical option but unfortunately is currently of unproven benefit. Sadly, prophylactic anticoagulant therapy with low molecular weight heparin has become accepted practice in many institutions as the standard of care for patients at risk. This creates a climate in which it will become more difficult to conduct controlled studies designed to establish or negate its effectiveness. The American College of Obstetrics and Gynecology states, as a level A recommendation that 'heparin and aspirin therapy have not been shown to be effective for prevention or treatment of IUGR'.[13]

Additional interventions such as nutritional or oxygen supplementation, various other medications, or volume expansion are of no proven benefit.

PLACENTAL ABRUPTION

Placental abruption (or abruptio placentae, a term borrowed from the Latin) is defined as premature separation of a normally located placenta.[1] 'Premature' in this situation refers to the fact that the placenta separates from the uterine wall before delivery of the fetus. The inevitable consequence is bleeding and this bleeding typically finds a path through the cervix to produce vaginal bleeding. It may happen that some – and, at times all – of the blood becomes trapped between the uterine wall and the separated placenta, producing a concealed hemorrhage.

The incidence of placental abruption varies between various studies but the rate is in the area of around 0.5% of deliveries. The recurrence rate in subsequent pregnancies is high, with a relative risk of up to 15:1.

The clinical appearance of abruption is highly variable, ranging from mild bleeding to severe and life-threatening hemorrhage. Bleeding is frequently accompanied by painful uterine contractions or hypertonicity (or both). Occasionally, concealed hemorrhage causes painful contractions with no evident external bleeding. To detect the abruption, it is important

to maintain a high level of vigilance when contractions are associated with hypertonicity and the uterus appears larger than expected. The fetus, too, may be affected to various degrees. Fetal compromise or death are not uncommon in severe cases.

Etiology

The etiology of placental abruption is unknown, but some clear associations have been described. Hypertension, both chronic and pregnancy-induced, smoking and cocaine abuse, pre-term premature rupture of membranes, multiple gestations and trauma are associated, if not instrumental, in the pathogenesis of placental abruption. Especially noteworthy in this last category is placental abruption secondary to external cephalic version. Uterine fibroids, especially when in a submucous location, may cause abnormal placentation and, if the placenta has implanted in proximity of the fibroid, an increased risk of placental abruption is to be expected.[18] Situations in which rapid decompression of the uterus occurs may predispose to placental abruption for purely mechanical reasons. This happens physiologically postpartum, but placental abruption may occur when the waters break from a polyhydramniotic sac or after delivery of a first twin.

Thrombophilic disorders have been implied and are being considered as a possible cause for placental abruption. Thrombophilia has generated considerable interest as a cause of various perinatal complications,[15,19] including placental abruption. It is unfortunate, however, that these studies tend to group together several complications, since this makes it difficult to obtain strong evidence to establish that coagulation disorders are a causative factor or a risk factor for placental abruption and other conditions.

Clinical presentation

Clinical evaluation of placental abruption must consider both maternal and fetal status. Maternal status is directly related to the amount of bleeding and to the existence and degree of associated consumptive coagulopathy. Bleeding, both overt and concealed, can easily result in hemorrhagic shock. Intensive crystalloid and blood component replacement, combined with prompt delivery to control hemorrhage, can be life-saving for both mother and fetus.

In mild cases, if the fetus is immature, supportive measures and adequate surveillance may suffice, provided that the option for immediate delivery in the event of deterioration is available.

Coagulopathy

Severe coagulation defects can occur within minutes after symptoms of placental abruption have appeared. Hypofibrinogenemia, prolonged prothrombin time and elevated fibrin split products are all to be expected, as is a degree of thrombocytopenia. It has been speculated that the mechanism involved in triggering this process is one of disseminated intravascular coagulation induced by various instigating factors forced into the maternal circulation. Support for this comes from two observations:

- coagulopathy is rarely observed in cases of hemorrhage from a prematurely separated placenta previa when all the blood escapes into the vagina;
- coagulopathy is more common with concealed hemorrhage.

Many cases require massive transfusion therapy, and this may serve to compound any coagulation disorder. In cases of severe abruption, therefore, it is critical to timely administer blood products in a balanced way in order to replace the various components lost in this dangerous situation.

Chronic placental abruption

Placental abruption can assume a relatively mild form; when this happens far from term, it is prudent to allow expectant management to allow fetal maturation. The natural progression when this occurs is variable and depends on existing risk factors. It can develop into the severe, full-blown clinical syndrome or remain as a low-grade abruption, or the bleeding may cease altogether, possibly recurring later in the pregnancy. Whatever the course of events, the patient is at risk of developing severe placental abruption with its potentially catastrophic outcome for both mother and fetus.

Fetal to maternal hemorrhage

Fetal to maternal hemorrhage occasionally occurs with placental abruption, particularly when the abruption is associated with trauma; in these cases, anti-D immunoglobulin administration should be considered. Since the size of the breach of the fetal barrier is unpredictable, variable amounts of fetal blood have been detected in the maternal circulation during and after placental abruption. The amount of bleeding in cases not associated with trauma is typically small and does not pose a threat to fetal well-being.

Management

In acute cases, expedient delivery is the rule. The mode of delivery is a clinical decision that must be made with regard to the severity of the condition for both mother and fetus, any associated coagulopathy, and the standard obstetric parameters. In general, the vaginal route is preferred if expedient delivery can be anticipated. Labor may be augmented or induced by amniotomy or oxytocin. Aggressive replacement of fluid and blood products are lifesaving for both patients.

In cases where expectant management is selected, coagulation functions must be monitored, as must the quantity of blood loss and the fetal status. When contractions or hypertonicity dominate, consideration might be given to tocolytic treatment. Theoretically, this might decrease the shearing forces applied to the placental surface during contractions. However, in practice the clinical value of this is uncertain and it should be used only in selected mild cases in which prematurity is a major issue and the patient is hemodynamically stable.

INTRAUTERINE FETAL DEATH

The World Health Organization defines intrauterine fetal death (IUFD) as death before complete expulsion or extraction from the mother, regardless of the duration of pregnancy. This chapter focuses on fetal death after 20 gestational weeks. Most states in the USA require cases of fetal death after this time to be reported. The fetal death rate in the USA (after 20 gestational weeks and per 1000 live and stillbirths) decreased from 18.8 in 1950 to 7.3 in 1991.[20] The etiologies involved in producing this grim outcome are many. In some cases the connection is obvious and evident (Rh isoimmunization, hydrops fetalis and eventual fetal death), while in others the links can only be suspected.

Fetal death may be diagnosed when maternal perception of fetal movement has ceased. The diagnosis is confirmed on ultrasound by a failure to visualize fetal heart activity.

Etiology and diagnostic work-up

It is important to identify the cause of IUFD for both future treatment and psychological considerations. A proportion of fetal deaths are attributed to factors that may recur in a subsequent pregnancy. A clear-cut diagnosis of such a condition would significantly affect counseling and future treatment. Psychologically, guilt feelings may prevail, and isolating an identifiable cause for this frequently tragic event may facilitate a healthy grieving process.

Overt conditions associated with IUFD include severe hypertension (chronic or pregnancy-induced), uncontrolled diabetes, and a number of other severe systemic diseases. A typical diagnostic work-up includes a detailed autopsy,[21] for the purpose of detecting fetal anomalies as well as other pathologies that might explain the fetal death. Given that aneuploidy is more prevalent in stillbirths than in live births,[22] a genetic evaluation of the fetus to detect chromosomal anomalies should be considered, although this might prove at times to be technically challenging because of cell autolysis. Both parents should also have a karyotype study, as various cytogenetic imbalances might create a risk of recurrent aneuploidy in future pregnancies.

Infections are not an infrequent cause of fetal death. Occasionally this might be clinically obvious, as in cases of full-blown chorioamnionitis. At other times, however, the infection may have only a minimal direct effect on the mother and will be suspected as the cause of fetal demise only if actively sought by appropriate culture, immunological and histological testing. Some examples include listeriosis[23] and cytomegalovirus infection.

Cord entanglement is often blamed for IUFD. It should be remembered, however, that nuchal cords are very common[24] and have not been proven to cause fetal death. True knots in the cord are not so common. Six percent of cases of cord knots are associated with perinatal death.[25]

An etiology of declining incidence is red blood cell isoimmunization. Since the introduction of anti-D immunoglobulin, the incidence of this potentially lethal disease has dramatically declined in the developed world, to a degree that most cases of red blood cell isoimmunization are related to non-D antigens.

One area of growing interest that might be related in part to IUFD is thrombophilia. It has been known for some time that antiphospholipid antibodies and lupus anticoagulant are associated with IUFD. One of the proposed mechanisms is by means of the formation of multiple microthrombi within the placenta. In the past few years there has been evidence of an apparent association with antithrombin deficiency, protein S deficiency and protein C deficiency and other thrombophilias. This is an important finding, since these conditions may be treatable with anticoagulant therapy.

Finally, intrapartum fetal death is a rare and dramatic event. It might be the result of placental abruption or of a cord accident, and rigorous intrapartum fetal surveillance is essential to prevent this from occurring.

Management of fetal death

Once a diagnosis of fetal death has been made, a decision must be made whether to await the development of spontaneous labor or to induce labor. The considerations here[26] are the emotional burden of carrying a dead fetus and the danger of coagulopathy on one hand, and the risks of labor induction on the other.

In most cases spontaneous labor develops within 2 weeks of IUFD. The length of the latency period (i.e. the period between fetal death and the onset of spontaneous labor) is inversely related to the gestational week the fetal death occurred. Coagulopathy may develop after at least 1 month has elapsed since fetal demise. Unlike the disseminated intravascular coagulation that may accompany placental abruption, this coagulopathy is typically of gradual onset and is rapidly reversed with replacement therapy. If a non-interventional approach is selected, monitoring coagulation functions, especially fibrinogen, is recommended.

Finally, the emotional aspects of IUFD must be addressed in a sensitive manner so as to assist the patient in coping with this major emotional crisis.

REFERENCES

1. *Stedman's Medical Dictionary*, 24th ed. New York: Williams and Wilkins; 1988.
2. Panigel M. Anatomy and morphology in the human placenta. *Clin Obstet Gynecol* 1986;**13**: 421–45.
3. Bianchi DW, Flint AF, Pizzimenti MF *et al*. Isolation of fetal DNA from nucleated erythrocytes in maternal blood. *Proc Natl Acad Sci USA* 1990;**87**:3279–83.
4. Morriss FH Jr, Boyd RDH, Mahendren D. Placental transport. In: Knobil E, Neill E, eds. *The Physiology of Reproduction*, vol 2. New York: Raven Press; 1994:813–61.
5. McMaster MT, Librach CL, Zhou Y *et al*. Human placental HLA-G expression is restricted to differentiated trophoblasts. *J Immunol* 1995;**154**: 3771–8.
6. Loke YM, King A. Trophoblastic interaction with extracellular matrix. *Cell Biology and Immunology*. Cambridge: Cambridge University Press; 1995:151–79.
7. Dekker GA, Sibai BM. Etiology and pathogenesis of pre-eclampsia: current concepts. *Am J Obstet Gynecol* 1998;**179**:1359–75.
8. Chesley LC, Annitto JE, Cosgrove RA. The familial factor in toxemia of pregnancy. *Obstet Gynecol* 1968;**32**:303–11.
9. Cooper DW, Brennecke SP, Wilton AN. Genetics of pre-eclampsia. *Hypertens Pregn* 1993;**12**:1–23.
10. Haig D. General conflicts in human pregnancy. *Q Rev Biol* 1993;**68**:495–532.
11. Talledo OE, Chesley LC, Zuspan FP. Renin–angiotensin system in normal and toxemic pregnancies. III. Differential sensitivity to angiotensin II and norepinephrine in toxemia of pregnancy. *Am J Obstet Gynecol* 1968;**100**; 218–22.
12. Cunningham FG, MacDonald PC, Gant NF *et al*. Hypertensive disorders in pregnancy. In: *Williams Obstetrics*, 20th ed. Stanford, Connecticut: Appleton and Lange; 1997:694–5.
13. ACOG Practice Bulletin, Number 12, January 2000. *Intrauterine Growth Restriction*. Washington DC: ACOG.
14. Moore TR. Fetal growth in diabetic pregnancy. *Clin Obstet Gynecol* 1997;**40**:771–86.
15. Kupferminc MJ, Eldor A, Steinman N *et al*. Increased frequency of genetic thrombophilia in women with complications of pregnancy. *N Engl J Med* 1999;**340**:9–13.
16. McIntire DD, Bloom SL, Casey BM, Leveno KJ. Birth weight in relation to morbidity and mortality among newborn infants. *N Engl J Med* 1999;**340**:1234–8.
17. Spinillo A, Capuzzo E, Egbe TO *et al*. Pregnancies complicated by idiopathic intrauterine growth retardation: severity of growth failure, neonatal morbidity and two-year infant neurodevelopmental outcome. *J Reprod Med* 1995;**40**:209–15.
18. Rice JP, Kay HH, Mahoney BS. The clinical significance of uterine leiomyomas in pregnancy. *Am J Obstet Gynecol* 1989;**160**:1212–16.
19. Brenner B. Inherited thrombophilia and fetal loss. *Curr Opin Hematol* 2000;**7**:290–5.
20. National Center for Health Statistics. Vital statistics of the United States, 1988. Vol II, Mortality, Part A. DHSS Pub. No. (PHS) 91-1101. Washington, DC: US Government Printing Office; 1991.
21. Mueller RJ, Sybert VP, Johnson J *et al*. Evaluation of a protocol for post-mortem examination of stillbirths. *N Engl J Med* 1983;**309**:586–90.
22. Boué A, Boué J. Chromosomal abnormalities associated with fetal malformations. In: Schrimgeout J, ed. *Towards the Prevention of Fetal Malformation*. Edinburgh: Edinburgh University Press; 1978:49–65.

23. Linnan MJ, Mascola L, Lou XD *et al.* Epidemic listeriosis associated with Mexican-style cheese. *N Engl J Med* 1988;**319**:823–8.

24. Kan PS, Eastman NJ. Coiling of the umbilical cord around the fetal neck. *Obstet Gynaecol Br Commonw* 1957;**64**:227–8.

25. Spellacy WN, Gravem H, Fisch RO. The umbilical cord complications of true knots, nuchal coils and coils around the body. *Am J Obstet Gynecol* 1966;**94**:1136–42.

26. ACOG Technical Bulletin, No 176, January 1993. *Diagnosis and Management of Fetal Death.* Washington DC: ACOG.

4

Laboratory assessment of hemorrhagic diathesis

Grigoris T Gerotziafas and Meyer Michel Samama

INTRODUCTION

Life is associated with the experience of some blood loss. Women are much more familiar with bleeding than men since menses is a regular phenomenon in their life. Abnormal menstruation is frequently the first feature of bleeding disorder and there may be intractable bleeding in adolescence. It is noteworthy that the first patient described by Erik von Willebrand in 1926 died of uncontrollable menstrual bleeding at the age of 13. During pregnancy, the balanced function of blood coagulation allows the normal development of the fetus without maternal hemorrhage or thrombosis, and it restricts blood loss during delivery. Normal hemostasis ensures that all the bleeding episodes are limited to minimal blood loss that will not affect the homeostasis of the whole body. Since bleeding is a common experience, the line between 'physiological' blood loss and abnormal bleeding tendency or hemorrhage is sometimes ambiguous. On the other hand, bleeding tendency may reflect either primary alterations of some of the components of the hemostatic system or secondary alterations, induced by an underlying disease or by a treatment. Thus, the exploration of the hemorrhagic diathesis must be polyvalent and must combine classic differential diagnostic procedures such as patient's personal and family history and clinical examination with either simple or sophisticated laboratory assays

that explore all the aspects of the hemostatic system. It should be stressed that a detailed personal and family history and clinical examination is of paramount importance and must precede any laboratory investigation.

This chapter discusses the current concepts of the approach to the patient, the traditional and newer assays used for the laboratory exploration of blood coagulation, and the pathology of blood coagulation disorders.

APPROACH TO THE PATIENT

Complete medical history

It is important to stress the relevance of a good history, which will not only indicate which laboratory tests should be requested but also help to explain any abnormality found in the results. The history must be taken rigorously using standardized questionnaires (Table 4.1).

The history of any significant bleeding must be covered, particularly spontaneous episodes or bleeding or bruising following injury, dental extractions, or surgical procedures. Menorrhagia, heavy menses, frequently accompanied by the passage of clots, hematuria, or gastrointestinal bleeding must be asked about, as must poor healing of superficial lacerations, easy bruising, mucocutaneous bleeding, purpura, petechiae, ecchymoses, epistaxis, hemarthrosis, bleeding into muscles or other organs, and telangiectasies.

Table 4.1   Principal elements of a questionnaire designed for the exploration of a hemorrhagic syndrome

Research of personal or family history of bleeding diathesis	*Perioperative*	Significant bleeding during or after the operation disproportional to the type of intervention
		Need for blood transfusion
	Non-surgical	Hemorrhagic delivery
		Menorrhagia
		Ecchymoses (multiple, recessive, spontaneous or provoked)
		Prolonged bleeding after minor trauma, bruising or venepuncture
		Repeated epistaxis
		Hematomas after intramuscular injections
		Poor healing of superficial lesions
		Gingival bleedings
		Recessive macroscopic hematuria or gastrointestinal bleeding
		Spontaneous hemarthrosis
		Hemarthrosis after minor trauma
	Underlying disease	Multiple myeloma
		Autoimmune disease
		Liver disease
		Infections (localized or general)
		Cancer, liver metastasis
		Leukemia
		Myeloproliferative disorders
Drug-induced	*List of the treatment received during the previous 10 days*	Anticoagulant treatment
		Antibiotics
		Non-steroidal anti-inflammatory agents
		Antiplatelet agents
		Hepatotoxic drugs
		Chemotherapy

Bleeding that recurs hours to days after the original trauma is significant, as is an incidental finding of an abnormal hemostatic test.

The patient's drug history (including antiplatelet agents, oral anticoagulants, heparin, non-steroidal anti-inflammatory, and hepatotoxic drugs) is essential information. Information about underlying medical illnesses (specifically, there may be jaundice or symptoms of hepatic or renal failure, symptoms of localized or generalized infection, or symptoms or signs of cancer) must be covered. The age of the patient at the time of the first recurrent or significant bleeding episodes, especially if it has been present since childhood, is important, as is a positive family history.[1,2]

Physical examination

Physical examination is as important as the medical history. The following points should attract the attention of the physician who investigates patients suspected of having a disorder of hemostasis:

- localization of the bleeding – repeated bleeding in the same territory are suggestive of a local lesion whereas a disseminated distribution (as in purpura or petechiae) favors a hemorrhagic disease;
- severity of the bleeding, or the presence of symptoms of anemia;
- clinical signs of systemic disease (e.g. renal, hepatic or cardiac failure; cancer; hepatosplenomegaly; lymphadenopathy; recent surgery; abdominal mass; hematoma of psoitis – which must be distinguished from appendicitis; muscular or arterial swelling; joint abnormalities or deformed joints; jaundice; symptoms and signs of gastrointestinal bleeding; cough and bloody sputum);
- apparent cause of bleeding (e.g. signs of injury or surgical procedure) or spontaneous bleeding.

Laboratory evaluation

A complete blood cell count – including hemoglobin, white cell count and platelet count, erythrocyte sedimentation rate and blood smear – and serum biochemical evaluation should never be neglected.

Exploration of platelet function defects

Bleeding time

Bleeding time screens for primary hemostasis; it looks at the interaction between platelets in the presence of traces of fibrinogen (platelet aggregation) and vascular wall in the presence of von Willebrand factor (vWF) (adhesion). Thus, prolongation of bleeding time is seen in platelet function disorders (thrombocytopathies). It is also prolonged in von Willebrand's disease and in severe hypofibrinogenemia. Antiplatelet treatment (aspirin, ticlopidine or clopidogrel) results in an increase in bleeding time. Severe anemia (hemoglobin <7 g/l) induces a prolongation of bleeding time via a rheological mechanism. Bleeding time is also prolonged in thrombocytopenia (platelet count >100 × 10^6/l). Bleeding time is not significantly prolonged in most disorders that cause prolongation of prothrombin time (PT) or activated partial thromboplastin time (aPTT) (Figure 4.1).

There are two procedures for the assessment of bleeding time.[3] Duke bleeding time measures the time until the cessation of bleeding from a 5 mm horizontal incision on the ear lobe. It is not standardized since it largely depends on the operator's experience. The blood is collected with blotting paper every 30 seconds without contact with the incision. The diameter of the second drop should be 5–10 mm. The diameter and the intensity of the blood drops are progressively reduced. The normal value is 2–4 minutes.

Ivy bleeding time is a more standardized technique. It is performed using a template device that produces one or two standardized horizontal or vertical incisions on the volar aspect of the forearm. A sphygmomanometer around the arm is inflated to 40 mmHg to standardize venous pressure. The time required for bleeding to cease is determined by carefully blotting the blood that emerges from the wound with filter paper every 30 seconds. The normal values for Ivy bleeding time is 4–8 minutes. The three-point bleeding time is a variant of Ivy bleeding time where, instead of an incision, nips are made with a needle on the volar aspect of the forearm. The normal value is 3–5 minutes.

The depth, location and direction of the incision, as well as the skin thickness, temperature, vasoconstriction resulting from emotional factors, and the experience of the operator are major factors that influence the reproducibility of the bleeding time. The most reliable and reproducible results are obtained with the horizontal incision Ivy bleeding time, since this procedure is more standardized than the Duke bleeding time.

Occlusion time

Occlusion time is an *in vitro* assay that uses a new instrument (PFA-100 Dade Behring) that

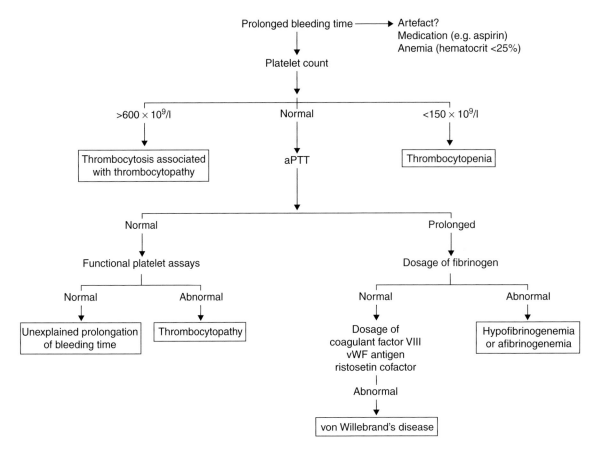

Figure 4.1 Diagnostic procedure for the investigation of prolonged bleeding time.

allows the global functional capacity of platelets to be measured. It is performed on citrated whole blood without any previous preparation of the blood samples. The test stimulates *in vitro* the conditions observed after a lesion of the arteriolar vascular wall. Aspirated blood passes into a cartridge composed of a microcapillary (of 200 μm diameter) and a nitrocellulose membrane (covered by collagen, epinephrine or adenosine diphosphate) that is perforated by a central micro-orifice (of 150 μm diameter). A pump keeps the blood flowing into the cartridge by simulating the arteriolar shear conditions. The micro-orifice simulates the vascular lesion. Platelets passing through the membrane are activated and adhere to and obstruct the micro-orifice. The PFA-100 measures the time that is necessary to complete obstruction of the micro-orifice; this time is defined as the occlusion time.

Occlusion time is sensitive to the most common alterations of primary hemostasis, such as the use of aspirin and vWF deficiency. It also detects major thrombocytopathies but it is insensitive to abnormalities of platelet secretion (i.e. in the context of a myelodysplastic syndrome). Occlusion time is significantly more sensitive than the Ivy bleeding time for the detection of vWF deficiency. Owing to rheological mechanisms, the occlusion time is affected by severe anemia (hemoglobin <6 g/dl) or thrombocytopenia (platelet count $<70 \times 10^9$/l).

Platelet aggregation assay
Platelet function is studied mainly by the platelet aggregation assay. The pattern of platelet aggregation in citrated, platelet-rich plasma (with a standardized platelet count) is studied after the addition of a standardized concentra-

Table 4.2	Factors which affect the main global tests of hemostasis			
Bleeding time	Platelets, vWF, vascular wall			
Occlusion time	Platelet function analyzer (PFA-100), vWF	Global exploration of platelet function		
aPTT	Prekallikrein, high molecular weight kininogen, factor XII, factor XI, factor IX, factor VIII, inhibitor	Factor V, factor X, factor II	Fibrinogen	
PT	Factor VII	Factor V, factor X, factor II	Fibrinogen	
Thrombin clotting time			Fibrinogen	

tion of a platelet agonist (e.g. arachidonic acid, adenosine diphosphate, epinephrine, thrombin, collagen). The platelet aggregation patterns can diagnose most thrombocytopathies and can estimate residual platelet activation during antiplatelet therapy (aspirin, ticlopidine, clopidogrel, or antiGPIIb–IIIa antibodies) and the influence of non-steroid anti-inflammatory treatment on platelet activability.[4–6]

Screening tests for hemostasis

When a bleeding problem emerges or is suspected, it is necessary to decide which laboratory tests should be performed. The patient's history and the clinical examination point to the most useful test (or combination of tests) to establish the diagnosis and determine the appropriate treatment.

The first step is to perform global clotting tests and blood cell count (Table 4.2). The next step is to perform analytical tests in order to explore platelet aggregation, or to measure the activity of clotting factors, or to search for a circulating anticoagulant or a specific inhibitor of a clotting factor. Which clotting factor should be measured usually depends on the results of the global clotting tests, the personal and family history of hemorrhagic diathesis and the presence of any underlying disease. Special attention must be given to systemic coagulation disorders, such as disseminated intravascular coagulation or

hyperfibrinolysis (Table 4.3). The rationale is similar for the performance of platelet aggregation tests. In the case of thrombocytopenia, it must be clarified whether the thrombocytopenia has a central origin or not, whether it is drug-induced or idiopathic, whether it is associated with a decrease in other blood cells, or whether it is associated with abnormal peripheral blood cells.[7]

Global clotting tests

The principal clotting times are the PT and the aPTT. Both tests measure the time to the formation of sufficient thrombin to initiate fibrinogen clotting and detectable fibrin clot formation to the extent that the optical density of the plasma is changed (clotting assay) or a detectable amount of color appears in assays using chromogenic substrate. Global clotting tests do not estimate the amount of generated thrombin.[8,9]

Prothrombin time or Quick clotting time
The PT explores the tissue factor pathway (or extrinsic pathway). It measures the lag-time of thrombin formation and fibrinogen clotting, after initiation of the coagulation by $CaCl_2$ addition in citrated platelet-poor plasma in the presence of an excess of thromboplastin (tissue extract that is the source of tissue factor and phospholipids). The PT is not correlated with the amount of

Table 4.3   Laboratory tests used for the etiological diagnosis of hemorrhagic syndrome

Global tests for diagnostic orientation	Full blood count Bleeding time PT, aPTT
Specific tests in case of abnormality or clinical indication	Clotting factor activities Circulating anticoagulant Fibrinogen level, search for dysfibrinogenemia Thrombin generation and endogenous thrombin potential Occlusion time (PFA-100)
Tests in case of normal results of the previous clinic profile	von Willebrand disease: Ivy bleeding time, occlusion time (PFA-100), vWF level, ristocetin cofactor, FvW antigen Alteration of fibrinolysis: shortened lysis time, deficiency of a_2-antiplasmin or PAI-1 Deficiency of factor XIII Thrombocytopathy: specific platelet aggregation tests

Table 4.4   Differential diagnosis of PT prolongation

Hereditary deficiency (rare) • Factor VII, factor V, factor X, factor II or fibrinogen Hereditary dysfibrinogenemia Acquired disorders: • liver disease • vitamin K deficiency • amyloidosis (deficiency of factor X, a_2-antiplasmin) Severe fibrinopenia: • reduction of hepatic synthesis • increased consumption (DIC) • destruction by plasmin (primary hyperfibrinolysis) Acquired dysfibrinogenemia (cirrhosis, hepatoma) Lupus type circulating anticoagulant (anti-prothrombinase) Treatment with unfractionated heparin Hirudin	Normal levels of factor V but decreased levels of factor VII, factor X, factor II

generated thrombin. Prothrombin time is affected by factor VII, the factors of the prothrombinase complex (factors V and X), prothrombin, and fibrinogen. The PT is prolonged in qualitative abnormalities of fibrinogen as well as in the presence of high concentrations of heparin and other antithrombin drugs (e.g. hirudin) (Figure 4.2, Table 4.4). The PT is the assay of choice for monitoring treatment with vitamin K antagonists (the coumarins).

The sensitivity of the PT depends mainly on the thromboplastin reagent used. Thrombo-

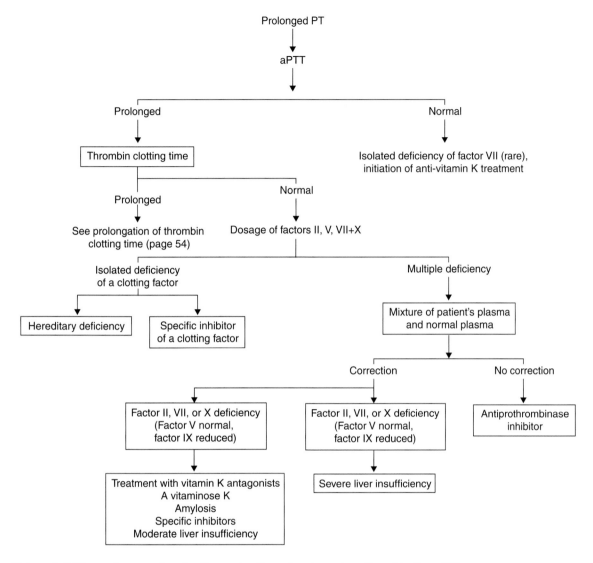

Figure 4.2 Diagnostic procedure for the exploration of prolonged prothrombin time (PT).

plastin preparations come from different origins (human brain, human placenta, rabbit, bovine sources, or recombinant tissue factor).

The PT is expressed in seconds (patient's PT versus a normal control), as a ratio (of the patient's PT to a control's PT), or as a percentage of prothrombin. However, there are important variations of PT ratio or percentage of prothrombin, depending on the thromboplastin used; for example, for a given patient receiving oral anticoagulant treatment with vitamin K antagonists, the prolongation of PT (expressed as PT ratio or percentage of prothrombin activation) is different when different thromboplastin reagents are used. The World Health Organization has established a reference thromboplastin derived from human brain that has been used to calibrate secondary standards, available to manufacturers and laboratories for the evaluation of thromboplastin reagents. The sensitivity of a thromboplastin is described by the International Sensitivity Index (ISI). Most commercial thromboplastins derived from animal sources are less sensitive than the reference standard (ISI = 1) and have ISIs of 1.2–1.8. Thus, in order to normalize the variations, PT results are expressed as an International Normalized Ratio (INR), especially for the patients under oral anticoagulant treatment with vitamin K antagonists. INR converts the ratio of the patient's PT to the control PT to the value expected if the test had been performed with the reference thromboplastin. It is given by the equation:

$$INR = (PT \text{ patient}/PT \text{ control})^{ISI}.$$

However, it has been recognized that the coagulation analyzer may influence the apparent ISI value for a given thromboplastin. Instrument-specific ISI values may be required to overcome this discrepancy.

Activated partial thromboplastin time (aPTT)
The aPTT explores the commonly named intrinsic clotting pathway. It essentially measures the lag-time of thrombin formation and fibrinogen clotting after initiation of the coagulation by addition of calcium chloride to citrated platelet-poor plasma in the presence of phospholipids and an activator (e.g. kaolin, silicon, ellagic acid) of the contact system. Cephaline is the source of phospholipids (substitute for platelets in a variable composition and concentration). The aPTT, like the PT, is not correlated with the amount of generated thrombin after coagulation has been triggered. The aPTT is affected by the factors that participate in the formation of the intrinsic tenase enzymatic complex (factors VIII and IX), the factors of the prothrombinase enzymatic complex (factors V and X), prothrombin (factor II), fibrinogen, factors XI and XII, and the factors of the contact system (prekallikrein and high-molecular-weight kininogen).

Isolated prolongation of aPTT usually reveals congenital hemophilia A or B, von Willebrand disease or the presence of specific inhibitors against factor VIII, factor IX or circulating anticoagulant (lupus anticoagulant). Moreover, the aPTT is the established test for monitoring treatment with unfractionated heparin, but it is not significantly affected by the treatment with low molecular weight heparins (Figure 4.3 and Table 4.5).

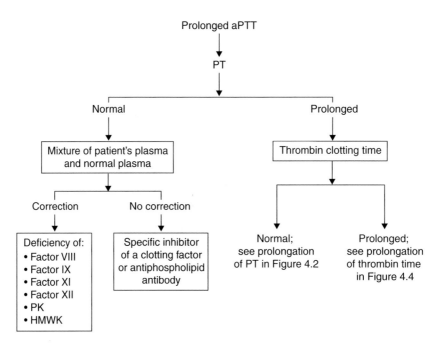

Figure 4.3 Diagnostic procedure for the exploration of prolonged activated partial thromboplastin time (aPTT). PK, prekallikrein; HMWK, high molecular weight kininogen.

Table 4.5 Differential diagnosis of aPTT prolongation	
Normal PT	**Prolonged PT**
Congenital deficiency of clotting factors	Congenital deficiency of
• factor VIII: hemophilia A	• factor X, factor V, factor II or fibrinogen
• factor IX: hemophilia B	Liver disease
• factor XI: Rosenthal disease	DIC
• factor XII, prekallikrein, high molecular weight kininogen: non-hemorrhagic diathesis	Circulating anticoagulant
	Treatment with oral anticoagulants anti-vitamin K
Treatment with heparin	Heparin
Circulating anticoagulants	

The sensitivity of the test depends on the phospholipids and the activator that are used. It is commonly accepted that a decrease in clotting factor activity of more than 30–40% induces significant prolongation of the aPTT. In reality, this depends on the reagents used. Thus, the reagents must be selected according to the differential diagnosis of the suspected disorder.

Thrombin clotting time
The thrombin clotting time explores the two steps of fibrin formation – the proteolytic activity of thrombin on fibrinogen and the polymerization of fibrin. However, it is independent of factor XIII (the factor that stabilizes the fibrin network). It is performed by the addition of a known concentration of thrombin (of human or animal origin) to platelet-poor plasma. The results are expressed in seconds compared with a normal control. Thrombin clotting time depends on fibrinogen. It is prolonged if fibrinogen level is less than 1 g/l or more than 6 g/l. In the latter case, a dilution of the plasma normalizes the clotting time. Thrombin clotting time is sensitive to the presence of a thrombin inhibitor (circulating anticoagulant, high levels of fibrin–fibrinogen degradating products, heparin, or hirudin). Since thrombin clotting time is very sensitive to the presence of heparin, the test is widely used to explore if heparin is present into the studied sample. Finally, thrombin clotting time is prolonged in the presence of a qualitative abnormality of fibrinogen (Figure 4.4).

Reptilase clotting time
The reptilase clotting time is based on the proteolytic action of reptilase, a snake venom from *Bothrops atrox*, which directly cleaves only the fibrinopeptide A of fibrinogen and forms end-to-end fibrin clot instead end-to-end plus the side-to-side fibrin polymerization resulting from the action of thrombin. In qualitative or quantitative fibrinogen abnormalities, the reptilase clotting time is correlated with the thrombin clotting time. However, the reptilase clotting time is not affected by the presence of heparin. Thus, in the case of prolonged thrombin clotting time, a normal reptilase clotting time suggests the possibility of heparin contamination of the sample (see Figure 4.4). Moreover, the reptilase clotting time is prolonged in the presence of fibrinogen and/or fibrin degradation products in disseminated intravascular coagulation (DIC).

Ecarine clotting time
The ecarine clotting time uses another snake venom (ecarin). It is more sensitive than the aPTT for monitoring treatment with hirudins and other thrombin inhibitors.

Transmittance waveform analysis
Transmittance waveform analysis is the optical profile generated on standard coagulation assays such as PT and aPTT that charts changes in light transmittance during the process of clot formation. Normal subjects and patients who have clotting factor deficiencies or are receiving

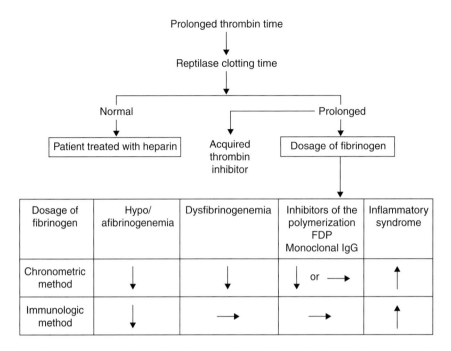

Figure 4.4 Diagnostic procedure for the exploration of prolonged thrombin clotting time. Thrombin clotting time may also be prolonged in patients treated with thrombin inhibitors such as hirudin, melargatran, or agatroban. ↑, increased; ↓, decreased; →, not modified.

heparin have a monophasic waveform on the aPTT assay. Critically ill patients suffering from overt DIC (diagnosed by clinical and laboratory evidence) have a biphasic waveform. Similarly, a biphasic transmittance waveform is observed in patients with pre-DIC or a hypercoagulable state. Changes in the transmittance waveform of the aPTT assay are currently under evaluation, and they could become useful for early diagnosis of hypercoagulable states and DIC.[10]

Other tests
A clotting time in tissue factor-initiated whole blood coagulation has been proposed by Rand *et al.*[11] This test is performed on whole blood loaded with corn trypsin inhibitor (which specifically inhibits intrinsic pathway activation). Coagulation is initiated by the addition of relipidated tissue factor and calcium chloride. This test measures the lag-time of thrombin generation and thrombus formation (without estimating the total amount of generated thrombin) in the presence of blood cells (simulating the natural conditions). It is currently under clinical evalua-

tion. A recent study shows that this clotting time is prolonged in severe thrombocytopenia.

Special tests to define the precise nature of the defect or the abnormality

Specific tests can establish the cause of a hemorrhagic syndrome by exploring the nature of the deficit and the precise part of the whole hemostatic system that is affected.

Thrombin generation test (thrombogram) and endogenous thrombin potential
The thrombin generation test is a sophisticated test that measures the total amount of generated thrombin after *in vitro* initiation of coagulation and, consequently, the global capacity of the hemostatic system to generate and inhibit thrombin. The general form of the thrombogram is shown in Figure 4.5. There may or there may not be a lag-time, then an explosive rise to a peak value is seen and a slow decline follows, caused by the inhibition of thrombin, mainly by antithrombin but also by a_2-macroglobulin. A

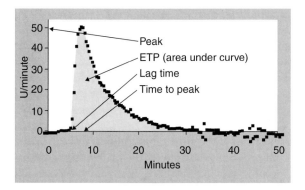

Figure 4.5 A typical pattern of thrombin generation curve (thrombogram). www.thrombin.com. ETP, endogenous thrombin potential.

clot forms at the end of the lag-time as soon as the first traces of measurable thrombin are formed. The lag-time, therefore, for practical purposes, equals the clotting time; depending on the trigger used, it may correspond to the classic global clotting times (i.e. PT or aPTT). During the lag-time, traces of thrombin are formed that, through feed-back activation, cause explosive thrombin formation (the ascending part of the curve). In addition to the lag-time, the 'endogenous thrombin potential' (ETP) is the most important information given by the thrombogram. The ETP has been defined by Hemker and Beguin[12] as 'the hemostatic activity that develops in a wound or thrombus [which is] essentially dependent upon the number of "man-hours" of thrombin that can develop in blood. That means that the amount of thrombin that generates as well as the length of time that it is active both count. The amount of work that can potentially be done by thrombin is reflected in the area under the curve that describes the concentration of thrombin in time during clotting'.

In a clotting time measurement, this thrombin goes unobserved but *in vivo* it may diffuse away from the site where blood has clotted and exert its hemostatic and thrombotic actions in the surrounding area. The thrombogram can be assayed with automated computerized instruments using platelet-rich or platelet-poor plasma (after activation of the tissue factor or the intrinsic clotting pathway) or amidolytic substrate that is specific to thrombin, or it can be assayed in whole blood using a fluorogenic substrate. The thrombogram provides precise information about the hemostatic balance in patients with hemorrhagic diathesis or hypercoagulable state and in patients undergoing antithrombotic treatment.[12]

Thromboelastography

Thromboelastography is a global test that explores the time to clot formation, the quality and the firmness of the clot, and the procedure of the clot lysis *in vitro*. The thromboelastograph is performed on native blood, or recalcified citrated whole blood or plasma. Despite more than 25 years of clinical experience, however, several basic questions relating thromboelastograph parameters to standard coagulation tests remain unanswered, and the value of the thromboelastograph is established only in the setting of orthotopic liver transplantation and cardiopulmonary bypass surgery. A new generation of computerized instruments allows assessment of thromboelastography at the bedside or in the operation room. Thromboelastography is a 'near patient' test of coagulation. It is easy to perform and can provide information on a patient's coagulation status within 30 minutes. This allows rapid estimation of blood coagulation or fibrinolysis alterations in an emergency.[13]

Dosage of coagulation factors (clotting activity and antigen levels)

Diluted citrated platelet-poor plasma from the patient is mixed with substrate-citrated platelet-poor plasma that is immunodepleted of the clotting factor that is going to be measured. Clotting is initiated by calcium chloride in the presence of either phospholipids or an activator if a clotting factor of the intrinsic pathway (factor XII, XI, IX, or VIII) is being measured or in the presence of thromboplastin if factor VII or a factor of the prothrombinase complex (factor V or X) is being measured. The results are expressed as a percentage of activity versus that obtained for the same clotting factor from normal pool plasma, which is used to construct a calibration curve. The protein concentration (antigen) of each clotting factor can also be measured with an immunologic assay (enzyme-linked immunosorbent assay (ELISA) or Lowrell electrophoresis). Important information on the nature of a clotting factor deficiency (qualitative deficiency, quantitative deficiency or both) can be derived when both dosages (clotting activity and antigen levels) are combined.

Prothrombin consumption
The prothrombin consumption test is performed with non-anticoagulated whole blood, which is collected in non-siliconized glass tubes incubated at 37°C for 1 hour. Serum prothrombin levels are then measured. The clot appears when about 1% of the thrombin is formed, whereas until a stable clot is formed in whole blood or plasma, about 5–10% of the prothrombin is activated to thrombin. Prothrombin consumption is abnormal in thrombocytopenia, thrombocytopathies, hemophilia A and B, and in the presence of a circulating anticoagulant antibody. Treatment with oral anticoagulants or unfractionated heparin, low molecular weight heparins, or synthetic pentasaccharide also render prothrombin consumption abnormal. Prothrombin consumption is an old test, which is not in use any more except in diagnosing Scott syndrome.

Exploration of a circulating anticoagulant or specific inhibitor
Usually the presence of a specific inhibitor against a clotting factor (most commonly immunoglobulin) is related to hemorrhagic manifestations, whereas the presence of a circulating anticoagulant against an enzymatic complex or phospholipids, although it causes prolongation of the clotting time, is clinically associated with thrombotic rather than hemorrhagic tendency. To reveal the presence of a circulating anticoagulant (a specific inhibitor against a clotting factor), an established approach is followed. The PT, aPTT, or both might be prolonged. The first step is the elimination of the possible interference of an antithrombotic drug. Then, the abnormal clotting test is performed by mixing equal volumes of the patient's plasma with normal plasma. The mixture is incubated for several time intervals until 2 hours with and without phospholipids in order to demonstrate any dependence of the

clotting time prolongation on phospholipids. With lupus-type circulating anticoagulant, the prolongation of the clotting time depends on the presence of phospholipids, whereas with a specific antibody against a clotting factor, the prolongation of the clotting time is independent of the presence of phospholipids. Then the PT or aPTT is performed on the plasma mixture. If the addition of the normal plasma normalizes the prolongation of the clotting time, the presence of an inhibitor is excluded. If the addition of the normal plasma does not affect the prolonged clotting time, this means that an antibody that is present in the patient's plasma neutralizes the clotting factor from the normal plasma that is added. The addition of phospholipids and the different incubation times allow the optimum conditions to be achieved so that the inhibitor reveals its effect. The next step is the investigation of the clotting factor that is inhibited, as well as the determination of the type of antibody.

An isolated clotting factor deficiency (most commonly factor VIII) is also mandatory for the diagnosis of a specific inhibitor. The procedure is based on the same principle – mixing patient's plasma with control plasma and measuring the specific clotting factor according to a standardized procedure of dilutions. Titration of the inhibitor is based on dilution of the patient's plasma that inhibits the clotting factor by 50% of the control plasma. This dilution is defined as 1 Bethesda unit. It must be stressed that the presence of an immunological inhibitor against a clotting factor is related to an increased hemorrhagic risk, whereas the presence of a lupus-type circulating anticoagulant is related to an increased thromboembolic risk.[14–16] In the latter case, a search for antiphospholipid antibody (using a specific ELISA) must be performed and an aPTT using sensible reagents should also be performed.

Investigation of hyperfibrinolysis
Global functional assays for the exploration of fibrinolysis (such as the clot lysis time) lack sensitivity, and they are not routinely used. Of these tests, the euglobulin lysis time (ELT) is the most frequently used. The ELT provides some evidence of circulating plasmin or a plasminogen activator. The ELT is performed by creating

a plasma-derived clot that is free of fibrinolytic inhibitors in a test tube and then observing it closely over the next 60 minutes for accelerated clot lysis. Fibrinolysis, however, is studied by analytic functional and antigenic assays, which measure the levels of PAI-1 (by amidolytic assay and ELISA), tissue plasminogen activator (tPA) activity in special acidic citrate solution and ELISA, plasminogen (by amidolytic assay), and plasmin–antiplasmin complex (by ELISA).

Global fibrinolytic capacity
Global fibrinolytic capacity is a new global test that measures the D-dimers generated after the addition of a standardized concentration of fibrin in the presence of a constant and limited concentration of tPA. It is a semiquantitative assay, which is currently being evaluated in clinical practice.

D-Dimers

D-dimers are generated after the proteolytic action of plasmin on the fibrin network that has been stabilized by factor XIIIa. During this proteolysis, plasmin releases fibrin fragments, which contain the domain D of fibrinogen. The dimeric structure is formed by the action of factor XIIIa. The molecular structure of D-dimers is heterogeneous, and several monoclonal antibodies specific to particular epitopes of the D-dimers have been produced. These monoclonal antibodies are used for the measurement of D-dimers, either by the quantitative ELISA method, by latex semiquantitative assay, or by turbidimetric assay. The measurement of D-dimers is principally used to exclude thromboembolic disease. However, increased levels of D-dimers are observed in hyperfibrinolytic syndromes and, especially, in disseminated intravascular coagulation (DIC). D-dimers are elevated in physiological conditions such as pregnancy and old age.

INVESTIGATION OF THE HEMORRHAGIC SYNDROME

Classification of hemorrhagic disorders is based on their pathogenic mechanisms. The medical history, the clinical examination, and the findings of laboratory tests leads to the choice of more specific tests that might allow a precise investigation of the different stages of hemostasis:

- primary hemostasis;
- coagulation; or
- fibrinolysis.

In addition, specific tests can also access the nature of the abnormality:

- quantitative or qualitative platelet disorder – disorders of platelet aggregation or adhesion (or both);
- coagulation deficit – acquired or inherited, quantitative or qualitative deficiency of a specific clotting factor;
- reduced synthesis, increased consumption, or increased clearance of a clotting factor;
- hyperfibrinolysis.

Pathology of primary hemostasis

'Primary hemostasis' refers to three principal elements: the vascular wall, the platelets themselves, and vWF. Traces of fibrinogen are also required to achieve primary hemostasis. Hemorrhagic syndromes or disorders of primary hemostasis may affect:

- the vascular component;
- the platelets (qualitative or quantitative disorders); or
- vWF (congenital or acquired von Willebrand's disease).

Alterations in the vascular wall
Abnormalities in capillary vessel wall are usually associated with the clinical characteristics of purpura, which may coexist with petechiae or ecchymoses. Purpura, petechiaes, or ecchymoses are frequently associated with vascular diseases that affect the capillary wall. Different forms of purpura have been described. The cause may be immunologic (autoimmune syndrome), infectious, metabolic, or (most commonly) undetermined or idiopathic.

Purpura associated with leukocytic vasculitis

which affects the lower limbs and is associated with myalgia, arthralgia, edema, and nephropathy or peripheral neuropathy. Purpura results from the deposition of circulating immune complexes in the cutaneous capillaries. The presence of cryoglobulins may be documented, which are usually mixed, rarely monoclonal. In the context of isolated capillary vessel wall involvement, platelet counts, platelet functional tests, and clotting times are normal and there is no qualitative or quantitative defect in the clotting factors.

PLATELET DISORDERS

Quantitative platelet disorders

Thrombocytopenia is commonly defined as a platelet count <150 × 10^9/l. It indicates an underlying disease process but does not constitute the diagnosis. Thrombocytopenic disorders have been classified into:

- disorders of production;
- disorders of distribution (with platelet sequestration into splenic pool);
- disorders of destruction (immune or consumptive); and
- hemodilution.

Thrombocytopenia due to decreased platelet production
The diagnosis of thrombocytopenia due to decreased platelet production is established by bone marrow examination, which assesses the quantity and the morphology of megacaryocytes. Non-invasive methods have been described (such as measurement of the serum concentration of the glycocalicin fragment of GPIb, the detection by flow cytometry with fluorogenic dyes of residual RNA in platelets, and the measurement of endogenous thrombopoetin (TPO) levels) but they are not in common use.

Acquired disorders of platelet production
Production disorders are commonly observed when the marrow is involved with metastatic cancer, lymphoma, acute or chronic leukemia,

myelodysplasia, myeloma, myelofibrosis, Gaucher's disease, osteopetrosis, histiocytosis, or infectious processes. The marrow shows a decrease or absence of megacaryocytes; any megacaryocytes present may have morphological abnormalities. Alterations of the other lines are also observed.

Administration of chemotherapeutic agents or irradiation induces destruction of megacaryocytes, their progenitors or both. Other causes of production platelet disorders associated with mild thrombocytopenia, are severe alcoholism and viral infection (mumps, rubella, measles, varicella, cytomegalovirus, infectious mononucleosis, dengue or other hemorrhagic fevers, hepatitis, parvovirus, or HIV). Many drugs and toxins have been implicated in the suppression of platelet production.

Varying degrees of thrombocytopenia may be observed with either folate or vitamin B12 deficiency; in some cases it may be severe. Rare patients with iron deficiency become thrombocytopenic. Aplastic anemia involves multiple lineages, although thrombocytopenia may be the presenting feature. Thrombocytopenia at the time of diagnosis of paroxysmal nocturnal hemoglobinuria is a poor prognostic indicator. Acquired pure amegakaryocytic purpura is a rare disorder. Refractory thrombocytopenia due to myelodysplasia (the usual laboratory findings include macrocytosis of platelets and red cells; clonal chromosomal abnormalities are required to confirm the diagnosis with chromosomes 3, 5, 8, or 20 being most commonly involved).

Hereditary platelet production disorders
Congenital aplastic anemia, Fanconi's anemia, and congenital amegacaryocytic thrombocytopenia are rare disorders of infancy and early childhood of unknown etiology. The inheritance pattern is mixed, with some cases being X-linked and others being autosomal recessive. There is isolated severe thrombocytopenia with normal marrow cellularity but scant megakaryocytes. Platelet survival is normal. Anemia and macrocytosis are commonly observed and occasionally hemoglobin F is elevated.

Thrombocytopenia with absent radius syndrome is an autosomal-recessive disorder manifested by hypomegakaryocytic thrombocytopenia and absent radii. Chromosomal abnormalities are absent. Other autosomal recessive thrombocytopenia include Bernard–Soulier syndrome, which is associated with moderate and occasionally severe thrombocytopenia and megakaryocytic abnormalities such as failure to express the GP Ib–IX complex. Although in most cases megakaryocytes are not enlarged despite the marked increase in platelet size, there is abnormal development of the membrane system.

Gray platelet syndrome (see below) is a disorder in which megakaryocytes are unable to package endogenously synthesized proteins into developing-granules; a production deficit may contribute to the thrombocytopenia.

Familial thrombocytopenia with micromegacaryocytes, marrow examination shows a decrease in mean megakaryocyte diameter and the presence of numerous micromegakaryocytes. The syndrome is characterized by modest thrombocytopenia accompanied by giant granules (15% of all platelets) and a mild hemorrhagic tendency. Platelet survival is normal. Although platelet function is globally normal, the abnormal platelets with giant granules fail to release their contents on stimulation.

Paris–Trousseau thrombocytopenia is a syndrome characterized by the presence of a deletion in the long arm of chromosome 23.[17,18]

May-Hegglin anomaly is an autosomal-dominant disorder characterized by giant platelets, moderate thrombocytopenia and leukocyte inclusion bodies, easy bruising, and menorrhagia. About 40% of patients are asymptomatic. The pathognomonic feature is the Dohle-body-like inclusion bodies found in neutrophils and eosinophils and occasionally in monocytes. The platelets are large but exhibit no intrinsic structural abnormalities. Marrow megakaryocytes appear normal.

Alport's syndrome (hereditary interstitial nephritis, cataracts and high frequency of sensorineural deafness) has been associated with thrombocytopenia and giant platelets in a number of families (when it is referred to as Epstein's syndrome). Ultrastructural abnormalities have been seen in megakaryocytes. This syndrome can occur in association with leukocyte inclusions (Fechtner's syndrome). The Sebastian platelet syndrome is a variant of Fechtner's syndrome without the other clinical defects seen in Alport's syndrome. The genetic defects in Alport's syndrome are deletions or rearrangements in the collagen IV gene on Xq22.

Other autosomal-dominant thrombocytopenias include Mediterranean macrothrombocytopenia and Wiskott–Aldrich syndrome (immunodeficiency, thrombocytopenia and eczema).

Thrombocytopenia due to disorders of distribution

Disorders of distribution are seen in the context of hypersplenism caused by infections, inflammation, congestive splenomegaly, red cell disorders, myeloproliferative disease, chronic leukemia, lymphoma, and benign neoplasia (e.g. hamartoma, hemangioma, lymphangioma).

Thrombocytopenia due to platelet destruction

Infection is a common cause of thrombocytopenia, which is generally mild to moderate. Thrombocytopenia occurs secondary to several viral or bacterial infections, including acute platelet reaction to auto-antibodies; recent infection from measles, mumps, or rubella; infectious mononucleosis; hepatitis; infection or seropositive diagnosis of cytomegalovirus or parvovirus; HIV infection; and parasitosis (e.g. malaria, toxoplasmosis, leishmaniasis).

Drugs are another common cause of thrombocytopenia. Thrombocytopenia-inducing drugs include quinine, quinidine, sulfonamides, rifampicin, cimetidin, digoxin, thiazides, chlorothiazides, penicillins, aspirin, and heparins.

Other causes of thrombocytopenia due to platelet destruction include immune thrombocytopenic purpura, idiopathic thrombocytopenic purpura, systemic lupus erythematosus, antiphospholipid syndrome, hemophagocytic syndrome, incidental thrombocytopenia of pregnancy, pre-eclampsia and eclampsia, thrombocytopenia associated with cardiovascular disease, heparin induced thrombocytopenia (although most frequently not associated with bleeding), immune thrombocytopenia after

Table 4.6 Summary of the most important congenital thrombocytopathies, the molecular defects, and the platelet function abnormalities

Thrombocytopathy	Functional defect	Molecular abnormality	Phenotype
Bernard–Soulier syndrome	Defect of adhesion	GPIb, GPV, GPIX	VWF binding to platelets platelet adhesion to microfibrils giant platelets
von Willebrand's disease	Defect of adhesion	GPIb	VWF binding to platelets Plasmatic vWF Platelet adhesion to subendothelium
Defect of reactivity to collagen		GPIa	Platelet adhesion to collagen
Abnormality in intracellular calcium ion fluxes	Defect of activation		Defect in enzymatic reactions and metabolic events responsible for activation Platelet release and aggregation
Abnormality in the prostaglandin pathway		Cyclo-oxygenase or thromboxane synthetase deficiency	Platelet release and aggregation
Defect of reactivity to adenosine diphosphate	Defect of aggregation	Defect of adenosine diphosphate receptors (P2Y1 and P2Y12)	Defect in activation and aggregation to adenosine diphosphate
Defect response to epinephrine	Defect of secretion or aggregation	Decrease in platelet α_2-adrenergic receptors	Defective activation induced by epinephrine
Montreal platelet syndrome	Decrease of calpain	Spontaneous aggregation by increased exposure of binding sites for adhesive proteins	Impaired platelet aggregation
Dense body deficiency in Hermansky–Pudlak syndrome	Quantitative and functional defect in dense bodies	α-granule content and	Impaired platelet secretion and aggregation induced by adenosine diphosphate, collagen, or epinephrine

Gray platelet syndrome	Defect of secretion of adhesive proteins	number	Release of adhesive proteins, adhesion, and aggregation
Paris–Trousseau syndrome	Defect of secretion	Giant α-granules	Defect of secretion after stimulation by thrombin
Quebec syndrome	Increased proteasic activity within platelet α-granules	Decrease of intraplatelet multimerin	Defect of release of factor V stored in α-granules
δ-storage pool disease	Defect of secretion of dense granules	Dense bodies number and function	Release of adenosine diphosphate and aggregation
Hermansky–Pudlak syndrome	Defects in vesicles of lysosomal lineage	Quantitative and functional dense-body deficiency	Absent or minimal second wave of aggregation following stimulation with epinephrine or adenosine diphosphate
Chediak–Higashi syndrome	Defects in vesicles of lysosomal lineage	Quantitative and functional dense-body deficiency	Absent or minimal second wave of aggregation following stimulation with epinephrine or adenosine diphosphate
Glanzmann disease	Defect of aggregation	GPIIb–IIIa	Fibrinogen binding, aggregation
Variant thrombasthenia	Defect of aggregation	Abnormal GPIIb–IIIa	Fibrinogen binding, aggregation
Ticlid like thrombocytopathy	Deficiency of adenosine diphosphate induced aggregation	Alterations of PY12 receptor	Reversible adenosine diphosphate induced aggregation
Platelet factor 3 deficiency	Defect of procoagulant activity	Abnormality in phospholipids involved in the binding of factors Va and Xa	Defect of activation in situ of plasmatic factors

platelet transfusions and cardiopulmonary bypass surgery.

The diagnostic procedure involves peripheral blood smear to exclude pseudothrombocytopenia; the morphology of the platelets helps in the differential diagnosis (e.g. giant platelets suggest a hereditary or myelodysplastic syndrome). Marrow examination is required to evaluate the megakaryocytes. A biopsy is more reliable than an aspirate to determine whether megakaryocytes are decreased in number. However, an aspirate showing abundant megakaryocytes in the presence of thrombocytopenia is sufficient to suggest platelet destruction or ineffective production. Megakaryocyte morphology is occasionally valuable.

The bleeding time, although not a useful measurement to predict the propensity of bleeding, may be helpful in distinguishing ineffective production of platelets from platelet destruction. In destructive processes such as immune thrombocytopenia, the bleeding time may be shorter than predicted on the basis of the platelet count alone.

Qualitative platelet disorders (thrombocytopathies)

Thrombocytopathies may be classified as defects of adhesion, or platelet activation, or secretion, of aggregation or of platelet procoagulant activity (Table 4.6). It must be mentioned that hereditary thrombocytopathies are very rare.

Hereditary thrombocytopathies

Defects of platelet adhesion
Bernard–Soulier syndrome is characterized by prolonged bleeding time, moderate thrombocytopenia with giant platelets and typical granulations clustered to the center of the cell leading a pseudolymphocytic appearance (12–15 fl), and normal clot retraction but abnormal prothrombin consumption. Mucocutaneous hemorrhage is the only consistent symptom, which may be moderate but is often severe and even fatal. The platelet membrane glycoprotein GP Ib–IX is affected. GPIb is linked to GPIX and GPV to form a complex. GPIb is the most important

platelet receptor for plasma vWF, which is involved to the reaction with a microfibrillar component of the subendothelium.

Functional assays show lack of agglutination in the presence of ristocetin or bothrocetin, delayed aggregation after stimulation by thrombin, and normal aggregation induced by adenosine diphosphatase, collagen or arachidonic acid.

Inheritance is autosomal. In clinical practice, accurate estimation of the amount of platelet GPIb is essential for establishing the diagnosis. This is possible immunologically by fluorocytometry, ELISA, or bidimensional immunoelectrophoresis. Detection of heterozygous subjects or antenatal diagnosis are now possible, though difficult; they are facilitated by and more reliable with molecular biology assays since GPIb, GPIX and GPV have been cloned. With molecular biology assays, variant forms of Bernard–Soulier syndrome can be diagnosed by revealing mutations related to qualitative abnormalities of GPIb or GPIb-IX complex.[18]

In the platelet type von Willebrand's disease, inheritance seems to be autosomal dominant. Hemorrhage is most often mucocutaneous and is of variable intensity; it is sometimes severe. Thrombocytopenia fluctuates with normal platelet survival. Platelets are of increased size and tend to agglutinate spontaneously. The bleeding time is usually prolonged independently of the platelet count. Platelet aggregation induced by physiological agonists is normal or slightly decreased, but the main abnormality is the increased reactivity to ristocetin, especially at low doses. Plasma levels of factor VII coagulant activity (factor VII:C) are slightly decreased; vWF is also decreased, and ristocetin cofactor activity is lower than that of vWF antigen. Immunoelectrophoresis and SDS page gel electrophoresis confirm the decrease in high multimeric forms of vWF. The platelet type of von Willebrand's disease is caused by structural abnormality within the GPIb–IX complex, and it must be distinguished from von Willebrand's disease type IIb, in which vWF is intrinsically abnormal with a high affinity for platelets.

Defects of reactivity to collagen in which collagen does not induce platelet activation, secretion, adhesion, or aggregation. The defect is related to a defect in GPIa/IIa or to a deficiency to GPIV.

Defects of platelet activation

Defect of calcium ion mobilization occurs rarely. Platelet aggregation to classical agonists is decreased, but the membrane glycoproteins are present. Synthesis of thromboxane B2 is normal, ruling out an abnormality in the prostaglandin metabolic pathway. The unique alteration is calcium ion mobilization, documented using the ionophore A23187, which normally permits mobilization of calcium outside its storage vesicles. This defect may be defined more precisely by measurement of changes of fluorescence employing Quin 2.

Defects in prostaglandin metabolic pathway (aspirin-like syndromes) occur in cases of cyclo-oxygenase or thromboxane synthetase deficiency. They too are rare. In these patients, hemorrhagic tendency is of variable severity and bleeding time is generally slightly prolonged. Aggregation induced by adenosine diphosphatase, thrombin, or collagen is decreased, whereas there is no response to arachidonic acid. In cyclo-oxygenase deficiency prostaglandin synthesis and aggregation are normal after stimulation by natural endoperoxide. In contrast, in thromboxane A_2 synthetase deficiency, natural endoperoxide-induced aggregation remains decreased and there is a reorientation of prostaglandin synthesis towards prostaglandins E_2 or D_2 at the expense of thromboxane A_2. A new thrombocytopathy marked by defective sensitivity of platelets to thromboxane A_2 has been reported, implicating an underlying abnormality of thromboxane A_2 receptors.

Defects of platelet response to adenosine diphosphate is a bleeding disorder characterized by severe impairment of platelet responses to adenosine diphosphate. It is similar to the thrombocytopathy induced by ticlopidine or clopidogrel. Platelet aggregation induced by adenosine diphosphate is impaired while platelet aggregation induced by other agonists (such as thrombin, collagen, and epinephrine) is either normal or only slightly decreased. Agglutination induced by ristocetin is normal.

The mobilization of calcium ions is also decreased when adenosine diphosphate is used as agonist. Adenosine diphosphate-induced platelet activation results from the stimulation of at least two P2 receptors – the P2Y 1 metabotropic receptor, which is responsible for the mobilization of ionized calcium from internal stores, which initiates aggregation, and the P2Y 12 receptor (previously called P2Y T receptor), which influences the size of the platelet aggregates and their stabilization in response to released adenosine diphosphate through adenylcyclate inhibition. The defect is probably associated either with a decreased number of adenosine diphosphate receptors on platelet membranes or with a defective interaction between adenosine diphosphate and its membrane receptors.[19–23]

Montreal platelet syndrome is transmitted in an autosomal-dominant manner. It is characterized by the appearance of giant platelets, by a reduced platelet count, and by impaired, spontaneous platelet aggregation. The bleeding time is prolonged but thrombin generation and clot retraction are normal. Aggregation induced by ristocetin is normal but the response to thrombin is impaired or completely absent.

Other rare anomalies of platelet activation concern defects in reactivity to epinephrine.

Defects of platelet secretion

In idiopathic dense body deficiency (storage pool disease), there is complete failure of aggregation after collagen stimulation and decreased response to adenosine diphosphate or epinephrine, with rapid disaggregation. Platelet aggregation induced by arachidonic acid is also impaired. These abnormalities are due to a decreased number of dense bodies. The inheritance of this disorder is autosomal dominant.

Dense-body deficiency in Hermansky-Pudlak syndrome (HPS) is an autosomal-recessive disorder characterized by the presence of tyrosine-positive oculocutaneous albinism, accumulation of ceroid-like pigment in macrophages, prolonged bleeding time, and mild hemorrhagic tendency associated with platelet storage pool deficiency. Functional platelet studies demonstrate a decrease in dense bodies and defective release of their components. Platelets show impaired response to adenosine diphosphate, collagen, or epinephrine (attenuated secondary aggregation), and they have a decreased number of dense granules. Two genes associated with HPS have been mapped, one to chromosome 10q23.1-23.3, the other being ADTB3A.[24]

Chediak-Higashi syndrome (CHS) is a very rare autosomal-recessive disorder that is characterized by infectious diathesis, variable degrees of oculocutaneous albinism, and a platelet storage pool deficiency associated with mild hemorrhagic diathesis and giant intracellular granules in platelets, megakaryocytes, polymorphonuclear leucocytes, neurons, conjunctival fibroblasts, and cultured lymphoblasts. CHS patients have reduced or irregular platelet-dense bodies. Aggregation studies reveal an absent or minimal second wave of aggregation following stimulation with epinephrine or adenosine diphosphate. No gene mutation associated with CHS has been discovered. Both HPS and CHS result from defects in vesicles of lysosomal lineage.[24]

Wiskott–Aldrich syndrome is another thrombocytopathy with recessive X-linked inheritance. It is characterized by the extensive eczema, recurrent infections due to severe lymphocyte T and B immunodeficiency, and severe thrombocytopenia with small platelets and serious bleeding tendency. Dense body deficiency is also present in thrombocytopenia with absent radii.

Thrombocytopathies with defect of granules
Gray platelet syndrome is characterized by thrombocytopenia, hemorrhagic diathesis, and morphological abnormalities of platelets and megakaryocytes. Platelets are slightly larger than normal and they lack granules. In Romanowsky-stained blood film the platelets have a peculiar gray color due to the absence of normal α granules. The platelet α-granule contents (factor V, vWF, P-selectin, PF4, platelet derived growth factor (PDGF), β-thromboglobulin, thrombospondin, fibronectin, and PAI-1) are also reduced. Functional studies show normal adhesion but impaired aggregation to collagen,

thrombin, epinephrine, and ionophore A2317, and slightly decreased aggregation after adenosine diphosphate. Prostaglandin metabolism is normal, but release of serotonin is decreased. Myelofibrosis is discovered in most cases.

The Paris–Trousseau syndrome is a thrombocytopathy with autosomal-dominant inheritance characterized by mild hemorrhagic diathesis, mild thrombocytopenia, giant granules in platelets, and dysmegacaryopoiesis (micromegakaryocytes with dystrophic maturation). Platelet survival is normal. Bleeding time is prolonged. Platelet aggregation studies indicate normal platelet function but platelets are unable to release their contents after stimulation with thrombin. Paris–Trousseau syndrome is associated with a deletion at the distal long arm of chromosome 11 extending from 11q23.3 to the 11q terminus.[25]

The Quebec syndrome was described in 1984. It is an autosomal-dominant disorder and is associated with mild thrombocytopenia and a moderate bleeding tendency. A decrease in multimerin and the constituents of platelet granules has been shown, probably due to increased proteasic activity within the granules. The abnormal multimerin induces a defect of factor V release *in situ*, and there is no platelet response to epinephrine.

Defects of platelet aggregation
In Glanzmann thrombasthenia, there is normal platelet count and morphology, absence of clot retraction, prolonged bleeding time, and a bleeding tendency with mucocutaneous bleedings. There is a great variability in the severity of bleeding, and the severity and frequency of bleeding episodes decrease with age. Molecular abnormalities affect the structural genes of GPIIb or GPIIIa (mutations, deletions, or even insertions), leading to a defect in the expression of the GPIIb–GPIIIa complex. In type 1 Glanzmann thrombasthenia, there is about 5% of residual GPIIb–IIIa complex on platelet membrane; in type 2 there is 20% residual GPIIb–IIIa complex. There is no fibrinogen binding in type 1 and it is significantly decreased in type 2. The defect of GPIIb–IIIa complex accounts for the lack of aggregation,

since binding of fibrinogen to GPIIb–IIIa is the critical step for platelet aggregation. Tyrosine phosphorylation of a number of platelet proteins that are dependent on GPIIb–IIIa and its role in platelet aggregation was found to be lacking or considerably decreased. Functional studies show normal shape change and secretion of adenosine triphosphate. Platelet adhesion and agglutination induced by collagen type III and ristocetin are normal. Platelet aggregation is completely absent to adenosine diphosphate, thrombin, epinephrine, collagen, and arachidonic acid. Several variant forms of Glanzmann thrombasthenia have been described.

Defects of platelet procoagulant activity

Some rare cases with severe hemorrhage and an isolated deficiency of platelet factor (PF)3 (phosphatidylserine) have been published. This phenotype has been named Scott syndrome. PF3 is an anionic phospholipid that is exposed outside the platelet membrane on platelet activation; it contributes to enzymatic complex formation on the platelet membrane (prothrombinase and intrinsic tenase). Scott syndrome is probably associated with either a deficiency of PF3 or impaired mobilization of anionic phospholipids at the platelet membrane. It is very difficult to document the deficiency in PF3. The prothrombin consumption test is abnormal. The thrombin generation test using platelet-rich plasma might be mandatory for these defects. This syndrome has been shown to be transmitted as an autosomal-recessive trait, and probably the causal mutation affects a phosphatidylserine translocase. Moreover, a defect in the generation of procoagulant microparticles has been described.

Acquired thrombocytopathies

Acquired thrombocytopathies are much more common than hereditary disorders and may affect all the platelet functions. Patients suffering from an acquired thrombocytopathy do not have a previous personal or family history of hemorrhagic diathesis. Medication is the most frequent cause; more specifically, drugs such as non-steroidal anti-inflammatory drugs are considered the major cause of impaired platelet

function. Known anti-aggregating agents such as aspirin, ticlopidine, and clopidogrel cause iatrogenic impairment of platelet aggregation. Thrombocytopathy is a side effect of several other drugs, including antibiotics (cephalosporins and penicillin), diuretics, calcium channel blockers, chemotherapeutic agents, anesthetic agents, tricyclic antidepressants, dextran, hypolipidemic agents, and alcohol. Several diseases may also induce impaired platelet function, including myeloproliferative syndromes, leukemias, myelodysplastic syndrome, renal insufficiency, extracorporeal circulation, cardiac valvulopathies, autoimmune diseases with autoantibodies directed against platelet membrane glycoproteins, and hepatic disorders.

HEREDITARY DISORDERS OF COAGULATION

Hereditary disorders of coagulation are relatively rare. The severity of the hemorrhagic tendency is related to the specific clotting factor deficiency and the degree of reduction in the clotting factor. The deficiency of a given clotting factor may be quantitative (reduced protein synthesis), qualitative (normal protein levels but reduced activity), or both. The symbolism nomenclature of hereditary deficiencies of a clotting factor (factor V for example) is as follows:

- FV$^+$ – qualitative deficiency of factor V;
- FV$^-$ – a quantitative deficiency of factor V; and
- FV^R – a combined qualitative and quantitative deficiency of factor V.

The incidence and the severity of bleeding of the hereditary clotting factor deficiencies are summarized in Table 4.7.

Hemophilia A

All the clinical features of hemophilia A are due directly or indirectly to a deficiency of factor VIII. The gene for factor VIII is located near the tip of the long arm of the factor X chromosome (Xq 2.8 ter), which accounts for the X-linked

Table 4.7	Incidence and bleeding severity of clotting factor deficiencies	
Clotting factor deficiency	**Estimated incidence**	**Bleeding severity**
I	Very rare	Mild to severe
II	Very rare	Mild to moderate
V	1/100,000	Moderate
VII	1/500,000	Mild to severe
VIII	1/100,000	Mild to severe
IX	1/300,000	Mild to severe
X	1/500,000	Mild to severe
XI	Rare (except in Ashkenazi Jewish)	Mild to moderate
XII	Unknown	No bleed
XIII	1/100,000	Moderate to severe
V/VIII	1/100,000	Mild to moderate

Modified from Roberts and Hoffman.[31]

pattern of inheritance. The deficiency of factor VIII is the result of several mutations in factor VIII locus.

Almost all patients are male. The joints most affected are the main load-bearing joints – ankles, knees, and elbows; however, any joint can be the site of bleeding. Muscle bleeding can be seen in any anatomical site but most often presents in the large load-bearing muscle groups of the thigh, calf, iliopsoas, posterior or abdominal wall, and buttocks. Hematuria is less common than joint or muscle bleeding, but most severely affected patients have one or two episodes per decade. Central nervous system bleeding, although less common, is clinically dangerous. Surgery and open trauma may lead to life-threatening hemorrhage.

Classification of the severity of hemophilia has been based on either clinical bleeding symptoms or plasma procoagulant levels. The most widely used classification is based on plasma procoagulant levels:

- <1% of normal factor VIII levels defined as severe;
- 1–5% (or 1–7%) of normal factor VIII levels defined as moderately severe; and
- >5% (or >7%) of normal factor VIII levels defined as mild.

At the same time, classification based on clinical symptoms has been used because occasional patients with a factor VIII or levels <1% of normal exhibit little or no spontaneous bleeding and appear to be clinically 'moderate' or 'mild'; conversely, occasional patients with procoagulant activities of 1–5% of normal may have frequent spontaneous bleeds and appear to be clinically severe. Accordingly, the Factor VIII and Factor IX Subcommittee recommends that plasma procoagulant levels, rather than clinical bleeding symptoms, should be used for the classification of hemophilia (Table 4.8).[26–28]

Screening tests show prolongation of aPTT but normal PT, thrombin clotting time, bleeding time, and platelet count. Specific functional assays show factor VIII clotting activity below 50 u/dl (50%), with all other factors normal and vWF antigen and ristocetin cofactor also normal. A test for antibodies to factor VIII should also be performed. The female carriers usually have 15–50% of normal factor VIII levels.

Hemophilia B

Hemophilia B is six times less common than hemophilia A. Clinically, hemophilia B resembles hemophilia A. It is also an X-linked disorder and the gene of factor IX is located at the tip of

Table 4.8 Classification of hemophilia A and hemophilia B	
Factor VIII or factor IX level	**Classification**
<0.01 IU/ml (<1% of normal)	Severe
0.01–0.05 IU/ml (1–5% of normal)	Moderate
>0.05–<0.40 IU/ml (>5–<40% of normal)	Mild

Normal is 1 IU/ml of factor VIII:C (100%), as defined by the current World Health Organization International Standard for Plasma Factor VIII:C (as distributed by The National Institute for Biological Standards and Control, Potters Bar, Hertfordshire, UK).

the long arm of the X chromosome. The phenotypic resemblance is to be expected since factor VIIIa is the cofactor of factor IXa when the enzymatic complex of intrinsic tenase is formed. However a decrease in factor IX must be distinguished from an acquired reduction in factor IX levels because factor IX is a vitamin K-dependent clotting factor and its levels are affected by hepatic function, vitamin K intake, and intestinal absorption as well as by the use of vitamin K antagonists. In hemophilia B, only factor IX clotting activity and protein levels are decreased, whereas all the other clotting factors are normal. The differential diagnosis is not difficult if the clinical context and the specific assays are taken into consideration. Bleeding time is normal but prothrombin consumption is impaired.

von Willebrand's disease

von Willebrand's disease is the most common hereditary hemorrhagic disorder, with a prevalence of 1–3%.[29] The classical picture is of an autosomal-dominant, mild to moderately severe bleeding tendency. Patients suffer from mucocutaneous bleeding, bruising, petechiae and ecchymoses, prolonged bleeding after minor cuts, menorrhagia and excessive but not life-threatening bleeding after trauma or surgery. The disease is classified in three types (Table 4.9). The majority of patients (80%) are found to have type 1 disease; types 2A and 2B together are found in about 15% of cases. Much less common

is the autosomal-recessive (type 3) von Willebrand's disease, in which the phenotype resembles that of hemophilia.[30]

For laboratory diagnosis, the following tests are necessary:

- platelet count, plasma activity of ristocetin cofactor, performed with a platelet aggregometric assay; ristocetin modifies certain glycoproteins of platelet membrane and provokes spontaneous agglutination by enhancing the binding of vWF to GPIb–IX. It is a quantitative test that is easy to perform;

Table 4.9 Variants of von Willebrand's disease		
Type 1		Partial quantitative deficiency of vWF
Type 2		Qualitative deficiency of vWF
	2A	Decreased platelet dependent function associated with absent high molecular weight multimers of vWF
	2B	Variants with increased affinity for platelet GPIb
	2M	As type 2A but high molecular weight multimers are present
	2N	Variants with decreased affinity for factor VIII
Type 3		Virtually complete deficiency of vWF (homozygous)

- vWF antigen levels, performed either with immunoelectrophoresis (Laurell method) or (more commonly) with immunoenzymatic assay using microlatex or ELISA;
- factor VIII coagulant activity, performed with the conventional clotting assay; and
- platelet–vessel wall interactions, investigated with the bleeding time.

Additional tests are required to establish the diagnosis of the subtype of von Willebrand's disease, principally vWF multimer size analysis at low and high resolution. This will demonstrate the distribution of vWF polymers and the pattern of flanking bands. The variant 2N ('N' because this variant of von Willebrand's disease was first described in a family from Normandy) may be misdiagnosed as mild hemophilia, because laboratory investigation reveals only reduced levels of factor VIII (15–30%), since the only disorder is the reduced affinity of vWF to factor VIII. To clarify the diagnosis, specific binding studies are required. A family history is very helpful.

Pseudo-von Willebrand's disease

Pseudo-von Willebrand's disease is a disorder that resembles type 2B von Willebrand's disease. It is a mild bleeding syndrome but the defect is situated in the platelets rather than in the plasma. Patients with pseudo-von Willebrand's disease have moderately reduced plasma vWF antigen, moderate thrombocytopenia, and enhanced response of their platelet-rich plasma to low concentrations of ristocetin. Structure of platelet membrane GPI is modified, resulting in increased and spontaneous binding to high multimers of vWF.

Prothrombin deficiency

Prothrombin (factor II) deficiency is the rarest cause of hereditary clotting factor deficiency. It is transmitted in an autosomal-recessive manner. Two types of prothrombin deficiency have been described:

- a qualitative deficiency (dysprothrombinemia), characterized by decreased factor II activity but normal levels of factor II antigen; and
- a quantitative deficiency (hypoprothrombinemia), characterized by decreased factor II activity and factor II antigen.

Heterozygotes are asymptomatic whereas the homozygotes suffer from mild hemorrhagic diathesis, which is manifested mainly as postoperative bleeding. The severity of the hemorrhagic manifestations is inversely proportional to the residual factor II activity.

Hereditary deficiency of factor II must be differentiated from an acquired deficiency, which is usually due to the inhibition of factor II by autoantibodies associated with lupus-like circulating anticoagulants or to the antiphospholipid syndrome. Hemostatic bandages with absorbed bovine thrombin has been shown to provoke the formation of antibodies, which cross-react and neutralize plasma prothrombin. Only one case with severe deficiency of prothrombin has been described. Liver disease, reduced vitamin K intake or anti-vitamin K oral anticoagulant treatment reduce factor II levels as well as the other vitamin K-dependent clotting factors.

The diagnosis may be suspected when the prothrombin time is slightly or moderately prolonged and factor II levels in functional assays are reduced while the other vitamin K-dependent clotting factors are normal.[31]

Factor VII deficiency

Factor VII deficiency is a rare autosomal-recessive disorder. Laboratory investigation shows prolonged PT and normal aPTT, thrombin time and bleeding time. The factor VII clotting activity is reduced. However, only patients with very low or absent factor VII levels (<1%) manifest severe bleeding. When factor VII levels are above 2% the bleeding tendency is mild or even absent.

Factor V deficiency

Factor V deficiency is another rare autosomal-recessive disorder. The plasma levels of factor V are not always correlated with the severity of the bleeding tendency. However, most usually the bleeding is severe and for this reason the deficiency of factor V was called 'para-hemophilia'. Probably the factor V originated from platelets and the platelet surface-associated factor V is the critical determinant for the severity of the bleeding. Both PT and aPTT are prolonged; thrombin time is normal but bleeding time may be prolonged in some patients.

Factor X deficiency

Factor X deficiency is a rare autosomal-recessive disorder. Bleeding is typically hemophilia-like. Bleeding tendency correlates with residual factor X levels. Experiments with different animal thromboplastins and dosage of factor X antigen concentration in patients' plasma, showed that the prolongation of PT and the levels of factor X coagulant activity depends on the factor X variant form.

Factor XI deficiency

Factor XI deficiency is more common in Ashkenazi Jews. Heterozygotes have factor XI levels between 15 and 65 u/dl. Homozygotes have levels below 4 u/dl. Bleeding is infrequent and occurs mainly after open trauma or surgery. Five percent of women with deficiency of factor XI suffer from menorrhagia.

Factor XIII deficiency

Factor XIII is a transamidase plasma protein that stabilizes the fibrin network. Hereditary disorders of factor XIII are extremely rare and are transmitted in an autosomal-recessive manner. Very low plasma concentration of factor XIII (about 5%) is required to achieve effective hemostasis thus, only the homozygous patients are suffering from bleedings which are manifested either after the apoptosis of the umbilical cord or after circumcision, or as profound hematomas. Diagnosis is based on the level of factor XIII in plasma. Autoantibodies against factor XIII have been described mainly after prolonged administration of isoniazid. Some patient's with rheumatoid purpura have

been described as having acquired deficiency of factor XIII. Very low plasma concentration of factor XIII (about 5%) are required to achieve effective hemostasis, and most cases have been diagnosed after circumcision.

Fibrinogen deficiency

Fibrinogen deficiencies are classified as either hypofibrinogenemias (characterized by quantitative deficiency of fibrinogen) or as dysfibrinogenemia (characterized by qualitative deficiency of fibrinogen). Some mixed cases have also been described.

Afibrinogenemia is an extremely rare disorder that is transmitted in an autosomal-recessive manner. It usually manifests itself during the perinatal period and is characterized by ecchymoses, mucocutaneous bleeding, and severe postoperative bleeding; paradoxical thrombosis has also been reported in some anecdotal cases. Global clotting times (PT, aPTT, and thrombin time) are prolonged and they are partially corrected by mixing the patient's plasma with normal plasma. Fibrinogen is unmeasurable, but the other clotting factors are normal. Platelet aggregation is defective to all agonists.

Hypofibrinogemia is transmitted in an autosomal-dominant or an autosomal-recessive manner. In some exceptional cases, paradoxical venous and arterial thrombosis have been observed. The severity of the clinical manifestations is related to the fibrinogen levels.

Dysfibrinogenemia is more common. It is transmitted in an autosomal-dominant manner. In the majority of published cases, it is asymptomatic (55%). Bleeding tendency is reported in 25% of patients and a tendency to thrombosis in 20%.[32] Structural abnormalities of the fibrin network result in the formation of porous clots which are resistant to fibrinolysis. Defective binding of thrombin to this clot may lead to hypercoagulability because free thrombin levels are increased. Moreover, a defective stimulatory function of abnormal fibrin in tPA-mediated fibrinolysis results in thrombosis. On the other hand, because the clots are made up of thick fibers and large pores with greatly reduced stiffness and increased slippage of protofibrils, fibrinolysis occurs more rapidly and this may predispose to bleeding.[33,34] Moreover, fibrin polymerization is impaired and the formation of fibrin network is delayed. Laboratory assessment shows prolonged PT, aPTT, thrombin clotting time, and reptilase time. Thrombin clotting time is the most sensitive of these tests. In some patients with dysfibrinogenemia predisposing to thrombosis, the thrombin clotting time may be significantly shorter than normal. Turbidity kinetics and light-scattering technology can also be used to detect abnormal fibrinogen molecules. The fibrinogen level varies. In some dysfibrinogenemias it is normal with immunological and gravimetric assays but it is reduced with the Clauss thrombin clotting time. In other dysfibrinogenemias there is a concordance between functional and immunological concentrations of fibrinogen. The gold standard for the diagnosis of dysfibrinogenemia is the identification of the molecular defect. The disorder is autosomal-dominant and detailed study may reveal two populations of fibrinogen – one normal and one abnormal. Molecular biology allows the causal mutations to be identified.

Combined deficiencies

Combined factors V and VIII deficiency is an autosomal-recessive bleeding disorder identified in at least 58 families from a number of different ethnic groups, mostly Mediterranean. Affected patients present with a moderate bleeding tendency and have factor V and factor VIII levels in the range of 5–30% of normal. The severity ranges from mild (factor V and VIII levels of 10–20 u/dl) to moderate (5–10 u/dl). Linkage of the combined factor V and factor VIII deficiency locus to human chromosome 18q was reported in nine non-Ashkenazi Jewish families by homozygosity mapping and in 19 families of Iranian, Pakistani, and Algerian origin by classical linkage analysis. The highest frequency of the mutant gene is found in Jews of Sephardic and Middle Eastern origin living in Israel, in whom there is an estimated disease frequency of one in 100,000. It was shown by mutation analysis that the gene responsible for combined factor V and factor VIII deficiency codes a 53 kDa transmembrane protein resident in the endoplasmic reticulum–Golgi intermediate compartment (ERGIC-53), a distinctive vesicular organelle in the secretory pathway. The importance of ERGIC-53 protein in the efficient secretion of the coagulation factors V and VIII has clearly been established by its causative role in combined factor V and factor VIII deficiency. Factor V and factor VIII are homologous proteins that share a conserved domain structure, being derived from a common ancestor molecule, with the A and C domains of the two factors showing 40% sequence identity. Both factor V and factor VIII are subject to extensive post-translational modification, which includes the addition of multiple oligosaccharide residues, predominantly in the B-domain. Therefore, ERGIC-53 probably interacts with the B-domains of factor V and factor VIII via a lectin-like linkage. Numerous mutations in the ERGIC-53 gene were found to be responsible for the disease. These mutations accounted for a total of 70 mutant alleles (74%). In addition, a number of polymorphisms have been identified, some of which result in amino acid changes. However, there is still some factor V and factor VIII activity in the plasma of the affected patients, suggesting that there may be several bypass mechanisms for the transport of factor V and factor VIII from the endoplasmic reticulum to the Golgi complex. The existence of further loci responsible for combined factor V and factor VIII deficiency is currently under investigation. Moreover, there are some cases with this combined deficiency who have no known mutation or polymorphism.[35–37]

Deficiency of factors II, VII, IX, and X results from an abnormality of the metabolism of vitamin K as a consequence of icterus, sprue, celiac disease, or intestinal resection. A mutation in the γ-carboxylase has been described in very rare patients. Any hepatocellular dysfunction and intestinal malabsorption must be managed, as must the intake of vitamin K antagonists.

SPECIAL ISSUES IN HEREDITARY HEMORRHAGIC DISORDERS IN WOMEN

Special attention must be given to early diagnosis of hereditary hemorrhagic disorders in women. Regular excessive blood loss during menses in women with underlying hemorrhagic disorders may cause anemia which affects the quality of life. Pregnancy and especially the delivery is another critical condition where diagnosis and close medical care are important. A recent study demonstrated that menorrhagia was confirmed in 74% of women with von Willebrand's disease, 57% of female carriers of hemophilia and 59% of women with factor XI deficiency, respectively, in comparison with 29% in age-matched controls.[38] Menorrhagia has been reported in 60%, 66%, and 58% of women with factor VII, factor X and combined factor V and VIII deficiency, respectively.[39] Another study assessed the quality of life during menstruation in 99 patients with inherited bleeding disorders, including vWD, carriers of hemophilia A or hemophilia B, and factor XI deficiency, and compared these women with an age-matched control group.[40] This study showed that, although patients with inherited bleeding disorders felt that their health (in general) was very good, they had significantly poorer quality of life (as judged by their professional or social activity) than controls. Quality of life was statistically poorer in patients with vWD, those who had menstrual periods of longer than 8 days, and those who experienced menstrual flooding or passage of clots. Menorrhagia was heavier in vWD patients with a vWF activity below 30 IU/dl than in those with higher levels. Duration of menstruation was significantly longer and episodes of flooding were significantly more common in patients with inherited bleeding disorders than in the control group. Forty-seven percent of patients with inherited bleeding disorders had consultations with their family practitioner or gynecologist for menorrhagia, 36% had medical treatment, and 27% had surgical procedures, including 10 hysterectomies. Postoperative bleeding was also observed in 14%. Another study showed that, among women with menorrhagia and normal pelvic examination and ultrasonography, 17% had an inherited bleeding disorder (13% had vWD and 4% had factor XI deficiency).[41]

Diagnosis of hemophilia A or B carriership and performance or prenatal diagnosis is of paramount importance. The woman must be examined for the clotting factor deficiency (factor VIII or factor IX) after a complete medical history and clinical examination. It must be stressed that a significant increase in clotting factor levels (e.g. factor VIII, vWF) has been reported during pregnancy in normal women as well as in carriers of hemophilia A. In the case of families with hemophilia A, the disease may be due to any of a large number of different mutations of the factor VIII gene. In hemophilia B, wide heterogeneity has been found. Thus the mutation must first be identified in an affected family member; it should then be searched for in the woman who is being investigated for hemophilia carriership. Increasing worldwide use of molecular genetic analysis is enabling accurate carrier detection for hemophiliacs to be made more widely available. DNA polymorphisms in linkage analysis is an accurate method for carrier detection that is applicable to most affected families. For families with severe hemophilia A, the inversion mutation can be sought by most molecular genetics laboratories. For families in whom by these procedures are uninformative, other point mutation screening techniques are available. Dedicated electrophoresis equipment enables these techniques to become more widespread. Genotype assessment based on direct identification of the pathogenic mutation in a chorionic villus sample obtained in the gestational week 11–12 is the most reliable method for prenatal diagnosis and should be used if available.[42,43] Genetic linkage studies of polymorphisms should be the second choice in the assessment of carriers and in prenatal diagnosis.

Carriers of hemophilia should be offered adequate psychosocial support before, during and after the prenatal diagnostic procedures. Carriers who have experienced the complications of hemophilia or its treatment appear to be more in favor of prenatal diagnosis than women whose hemophilic children have received modern treatment without complications.

Carriers of hemophilia A and B require special obstetric care with close liaison with the hemophilia center, and management guidelines should be available and observed. Knowledge of fetal sex is very valuable for management in labor and should be determined antenatally even if the mother declines prenatal diagnosis.

ACQUIRED DISORDERS OF COAGULATION

Acquired disorders of coagulation may be secondary to an underlying systemic disease, or they may originate from iatrogenic interventions or be drug-related. Such disorders usually manifest as mild or severe hemorrhagic syndrome during the course of a known disease, but they may be the first symptom of an underlying disease. The personal and family history are needed for the diagnosis of the origin of the hemorrhagic syndrome, since affected patients have not had previous bleeding episodes. Laboratory tests aim to identify any specific defect of the clotting factors and reveal if the defect is due to reduced production, to increased consumption or clearance, or to inhibition of the activity of a specific clotting factor. Special attention should be given to the development of specific anti-factor VIII antibodies in hemophiliacs, which is an acquired immunological reaction and is discussed later in this chapter.

Specific clotting factor inhibitors

Anti-factor VIII antibodies
Anti-factor VIII antibodies are the most frequently found auto-antibodies in several diseases, including systemic lupus erythematosus, rheumatoid arthritis, and other collagen diseases; syphilis; and drug sensitivity reactions to penicillin. It is also common in the postpartum period and is sometimes seen in elderly patients for no apparent reason. The antibodies are usually Immunoglobulin G. Patients with anti-factor VIII antibodies have mild or severe persistent hemorrhages.

Functionally inhibiting alloantibodies in hemophilia patients treated with factor VIII concentrates may develop. This represents a serious clinical problem since the presence of anti-factor VIII antibodies renders ineffective any substitution therapy with factor VIII concentrates. Inhibitors have been denoted as high response or low response based on the anamnestic response of the antibody to antigenic challenge. Alloantibodies that demonstrate an increase in titer have been termed high-response inhibitors. However, the antibody level that distinguishes high from low response is not defined, with levels of 5 Bethesda units used by some and 10 Bethesda units used by others. In order to establish a more uniform definition, the Factor VIII and Factor IX Subcommittee recommends the use of 5 Bethesda units to differentiate high- and low-response inhibitors. Thus, an antibody that is persistently 5 Bethesda units/ml (BU/ml) despite repeated challenge with substitution factor concentrate should be termed a low-response inhibitor, whereas the term high-response inhibitor should be applied to cases where the inhibitory activities have been >5 BU/ml at any time. Pathological inhibitors of blood coagulation as a cause of postpartum acquired hemostatic failure are rare. Since 1937, 96 cases of postpartum factor VIII inhibitors have been reported. However, it can be associated with very severe bleeding (unexplained excessive or prolonged vaginal bleeding or soft tissue hematomas or bleeding from multiple sites) during the postpartum period and with high morbidity and mortality. Suspicion for the diagnosis of this condition is often low. The risk of developing factor VIII inhibitors is highest after the first delivery, but inhibitors may appear during pregnancy or after several deliveries. Bleeding usually becomes apparent within 3 months of delivery but could be as late as 12 months after delivery. Factor VIII inhibitors may cross the placenta to the fetus and persist for up to 3 months to the infant, usually without bleeding complications.

Anti-factor von Willebrand antibodies (acquired von Willebrand syndrome)
The acquired von Willebrand syndrome (AvWS) is a rare bleeding disorder with laboratory findings similar to those of congenital von Willebrand disease. Moreover, diagnosis of AvWS has been difficult and treatment empiri-

cal. An international registry organized by the International Society on Thrombosis and Hemostasis reported a total of 186 AvWS cases, which were associated with lymphoproliferative disorders (48%), myeloproliferative disorders (15%), neoplasia (5%), immunological disorders (2%), cardiovascular disorders (21%), and miscellaneous disorders (9%).[44,45] Ristocetin cofactor activity (vWF:RCo) or collagen binding activity (vWF:CBA) were usually low in AvWS (median values 20 u/dl), while factor VIII coagulant activity was sometimes normal (median 25 u/dl, range 3–191). Factor VIII and vWF inhibiting activities were present in only a minority of cases (16%). Bleeding episodes in AvWS were mostly of mucocutaneous type (68%).

Most cases of acquired von Willebrand disease are due to a circulating antibody that combines with the high molecular weight multimers of vWF. These vWF multimer-antibody complexes are subsequently cleared from the circulation, either by the reticuloendothelial system or by adsorption onto tumor cells. Clearance results in extremely low functional levels and variable antigenic levels. Mixing studies, which are traditionally used to diagnose factor inhibitors, are useful only if removal of vWF–antibody complexes can be accomplished *in vitro*.[46]

Antibodies against other factors

Acquired inhibitors against other clotting factors are formed in the context of collagen disease, multiple myeloma, amyloidosis, macroglobulinemia, Waldenström's lymphoproliferative diseases, myeloproliferative diseases, solid tumors, and viral or bacterial infections. Patients usually suffer from mild or severe bleeding. Laboratory diagnosis emerges from the prolongation of PT (in the case of anti-factor VII inhibitor, and both PT and aPTT in the case of anti-factor V or anti-factor X inhibitor. Anti-factor XI inhibitors associated with bleeding have also been described.

Anti-factor XII inhibitors and anti-prekallikrein have also been described in autoimmune diseases and in neoplastic diseases, but these autoantibodies do not induce any

significant bleeding. Anti-factor XIII inhibitors are very rare; they occur in cases of congenital deficiency or after treatment with isoniazide. Inhibitors of fibrinogen and fibrinoformation have been described in the context of multiple myeloma and certain myeloproliferative syndromes.

Acquired inhibitors of thrombin are alloantibodies that are formed after use of hemostatic bandages covered with bovine thrombin. The antibodies are of the Immunoglobulin G type. The diagnosis is based on the prolongation of the thrombin time, which is not corrected after the addition of either normal plasma or human thrombin.

Some rare cases with endogenous heparin-like circulating anticoagulants have been reported. The presence of endogenous heparin-like circulating anticoagulants have often been associated with systemic diseases such as multiple myeloma, acquired immunodeficiency syndrome, acute monoblastic leukemia, and systemic mastocytosis. Patients have moderate bleeding tendency and prolonged thrombin clotting time which can be corrected with *in vitro* addition of protamine sulfate or platelet factor 4, whereas the levels of the clotting factors are either normal or somewhat increased. Heparin-like anticoagulant activity of the patients' plasma has been quantified using normal plasma as a substrate and heparin standardization.[47]

Acquired dysfibrinogenemias have been associated with advanced liver disease, including cirrhosis and hepatocellular carcinoma. It is believed that abnormalities of fibrinogen cause impaired fibrin monomer polymerization. Acquired abnormalities that mimic dysfibrinogenemia include multiple myeloma and Waldenström's macroglobulinemia (in which polymerization of the normal fibrin monomers may be impaired by the presence of the paraprotein). Autoimmune diseases may also mimic dysfibrinogenemias because some acquired antibodies inhibit fibrin polymerization or delay fibrinopeptide production. Moreover, hydroxyethyl starch and dextran, may interfere with fibrinogen cleavage and fibrin polymerization and so artificially lower the levels of fibrinogen.[34]

Table 4.10 Causes of acute and chronic DIC	
Acute DIC	**Chronic DIC**
Septicemia and infection	Solid tumors
Fulminant hepatic failure	Liver cirrhosis
Allergic reactions	Allergic reactions
Transplantation	Vasculitis
Heat stroke	Kasabach–Merrit syndrome
Hypothermia	Adult respiratory distress syndrome
Leukemia	Leukemia
Homozygous protein C deficiency	Organ transplantation
Snake bites	Aortic aneurysm/vascular tumors
Polytrauma	Late gestation
Large operations	Hemolysis, elevated liver enzymes and low platelet
Brain injury	count (HELLP) syndrome
Extracorporeal circulation	Retained dead fetus
Fat embolism	Artificial surfaces
Cardiac bypass surgery	
Peritoneovenous shunt	
Amniotic fluid embolism	
Placental abruption	
Septic abortion	
Acute fatty liver	
Uterine rupture	
Toxemia of pregnancy	
Acute hemolytic transfusion reaction	
Massive transfusion	

Disseminated intravascular coagulation

Disseminated intravascular coagulation (DIC) is an acquired syndrome characterized by the uncontrolled widespread activation of coagulation resulting in intravascular fibrin formation and deposition of fibrin in small vessels. The process may be accompanied by secondary fibrinolysis or inhibition of fibrinolysis. Microclot formation and a consequent organ failure or hemorrhagic diathesis may occur. Different diseases as well as clinical conditions associated with DIC are listed in Table 4.10. The diseases in which DIC occurs most frequently are infections (systemic inflammatory response syndrome) and obstetrical complica-

tions.[48] An acute DIC is rare but life-threatening, whereas chronic DIC is relatively frequent and causes attention by bleeding.

DIC is a continuous dynamic process that can be subdivided into three phases:

- compensated activation of the hemostatic system;
- decompensated activation of the hemostatic system; and
- full-blown DIC.

Clinical and laboratory findings in each phase of DIC are summarized in Table 4.11.

Table 4.11   Clinical and laboratory findings of DIC

Phases of DIC	Laboratory data
Phase I: Compensated activation of the hemostatic system **Clinical findings** No symptoms **Laboratory analysis** No measurable consumption of hemostasis components Increased levels of activation markers Increased levels of enzyme–inhibitor complexes	PT, aPTT, thrombin time normal Platelet count normal F1+2, TAT elevated Antithrombin slightly decreased D-dimers increased Soluble fibrin ±
Phase II: Decompensated activation of the hemostatic system **Clinical findings** Bleeding from injuries and venous puncture sites as well as decreased organ function (e.g. kidneys, lungs, liver) **Laboratory analysis** Continuous decrease in platelet count and coagulation factors Continuous increase in activation markers Continuous increase in enzyme–inhibitor complexes	PT, aPTT prolonged or increasing prolongation Thrombin time mostly within normal limits but sometimes slightly prolonged Platelet count, fibrinogen coagulation factors activity, antithrombin decreased or continuously decreasing F1+2, TAT, FDP, D-dimers increased Soluble fibrin increased
Phase III: Full-blown DIC **Clinical findings** Skin bleedings of different sizes, as well as multiple-organ failure **Laboratory analysis** Clearly expressed consumption of hemostatic components	PT, aPTT, thrombin time extremely prolonged or unclottable Platelet count very diminished (<40% of the initial value) Fibrinogen, antithrombin and coagulation factors activities very diminished (<50% of the initial values) F1+2, TAT, FDP, D-dimers very increased Soluble fibrin very increased

F1+2, prothrombin fragments 1, 2; TAT, thrombin-antithrombin complex; FDP, fibrinogen and/or fibrin degradation products. From Muller-Berghaus et al.[48]

Hyperfibrinolysis

Systemic (primary) fibrinolysis is a clinical disorder in which fibrinolytic enzymes circulate in an active form in the blood and attack different clotting factors (mainly factors V or VIII), fibrinogen, and local hemostatic plugs within the vasculature. The large amounts of fibrinogen or fibrin degradation products could inhibit platelet adhesion and aggregation. Fibrinolysis that is limited to the vicinity of a fibrin clot is termed localized or secondary fibrinolysis. Although systemic fibrinolysis is uncommon, bleeding may be very severe, and prompt diagnosis of this syndrome is essential. In general, systemic fibrinolysis occurs when excessive amounts of plasminogen activators accumulate in the blood, fibrinolytic inhibitors are deficient, or the liver is unable to clear plasminogen activators or plasmin. Systemic fibrinolysis may develop during therapeutic thrombolysis with plasminogen activators (e.g. streptokinase, urokinase, tPA). Patients with advanced liver disease and patients in the anhepatic phase of liver transplantation may develop systemic fibrinolysis caused by reduced synthesis of a_2-antiplasmin and deficient clearance of fibrinolytic enzymes. Rarely, chronic systemic fibrinolysis may occur in patients with generalized amyloidosis due to absorption of a_2-antiplasmin to amyloid fibrils along with elevated levels of plasminogen activators. Acute promyelocytic leukemia has been shown to induce systemic fibrinolysis. Cardiovascular surgery with extracorporeal circulation and local fibrinolysis in the prostatic bed may increase fibrinolytic activity and induce systemic fibrinolysis.[49] Finally, rare patients with homozygous a_2-antiplasmin deficiency have a severe bleeding disorder. Heterozygous patients have a less severe phenotype.

Systemic fibrinolysis is explored with the use of euglobulin lysis time (ELT). ELT is a sensitive test, and a positive result (lysis time in <60 minutes) does not necessarily indicate that clinical bleeding is a result of systemic fibrinolysis,

---

Table 4.12 Clinical and laboratory tests for systemic fibrinolysis

Hyperfibrinolytic process	Abnormal tests
Circulating plasminogen activators or plasmin	D-dimers Euglobulin lysis time tPA activity Plasmin antiplasmin complex
Proteolysis of clotting factors by plasmin	D-dimers PT aPTT Fibrinogen
Platelet function impairment	Bleeding time
Lysis of fibrin or fibrinogen	FDP, D-dimers Thrombin clotting time
Consumption of fibrinolytic reactants	Plasminogen a_2-antiplasmin PAI-1, D-dimers

From Hathaway and Goodnight.[49] FDP, fibrinogen and/or fibrin degradation products.

but a negative test makes the diagnosis unlikely. The concentration of fibrinogen is a helpful parameter to estimate the severity of the fibrinolytic process, assuming that other causes of hypofibrinogenemia (as well as DIC) have been excluded. Measurement of fibrinogen degradation products and D-dimers is important. Owing to the proteolysis of factor V and factor VIII by fibrin, prothrombin time and aPTT are prolonged. The most essential laboratory findings in systemic fibrinolysis are summarized in Table 4.12.

CONCLUSION

Accurate diagnosis of congenital bleeding disorders is a multidisciplinary procedure. Owing to the rarity of these disorders, clinical examination and laboratory testing of the patient must be closely connected. The diagnostic precision and the positive predictive value of the tests that investigate blood coagulation abnormalities is strengthened when biological exploration is associated with detailed medical, personal, and family history, as well as with precise clinical information on the hemorrhagic diathesis. Since most of the assays that explore the different

phases of hemostasis and fibrinolysis are sophisticated, elegant, and expensive, the diagnostic procedure must be performed in experienced laboratories that fulfill strict criteria of quality control, pre-analytical standards on blood sampling, plasma preparation and conservation, and rational selection of the reagents and instruments.

Increased awareness among general practitioners, gynecologists, pediatricians, and surgeons about the association between hemorrhagic diathesis and an underlying congenital disorder of blood coagulation and a close cooperation with specialized hematologists is necessary for optimal management of these patients. Unexplained postpartum and postoperative hemorrhage or menorrhagia that does not respond to general measures should alert clinicians to the possibility of bleeding disorders as a causative factor. Moreover, appropriate preoperative assessment and hemostatic control during gynecological procedures, however minor, in collaboration with specialized, experienced laboratories is essential to minimize risks of hemorrhagic complications in women with congenital or acquired disorders of blood coagulation.

REFERENCES

1. Rapaport SI. Preoperative hemostatic evaluation: which tests, if any? *Blood* 1983;**61**:229–31.
2. Makris PE. *Haemostasis*. Thessaloniki, Greece: University Studio Press; 1994.
3. Caen J, Larrieu MJ, Samama M. L'hémostase: méthodes d'exploration et diagnostique pratique. Paris: Expansion Scientifique; 1968.
4. Born JVR, Cross MJ. The aggregation of blood platelets. *J Physiol* 1963;**168**:178–95.
5. Cazenave JP, Hemmendinger S, Beret A *et al.* L'agrégation plaquettaire. Outil d'investigation clinique et d'étude pharmacologique. Méthodologie. *Ann Biol Clin* 1983;**41**:167–79.
6. Lecompte T. Exploration des fonctions plaquettaires en pratique clinique. *Spectra Bio* 1999;**18**: 21–6.
7. Santoro SA, Eby CS. Laboratory evaluation of hemostatic disorders. In: Hoffman R, Benz EJ, Sanford Jr *et al.* (eds), *Hematology. Basic Principles and Practice*, 3rd ed. Churchill Livingstone; 2000:1841–50.
8. Boneau B, Cazenave JP. *Introduction à l'étude de l'hémostase et de la thrombose*, 2nd ed. Reims: Boehringer Ingelheim France, 1997.
9. Samama MM. Exploration d'un syndrome hemorrhagique. Biologie pratique en hemostase et thrombose. Cahier de formation biologie medicale, No 20, September 2000.
10. Cheng HT. APTT revisited: detecting dysfunction in the hemostatic system through waveform analysis. *Thromb Haemost* 1999;**82**:684–7.
11. Rand MD, Lock JB, van't Veer C *et al.* Blood clotting in minimally altered whole blood. *Blood* 1996;**88**:3432–45.
12. Hemker HC, Beguin S. Phenotyping the clotting system. *Thromb Haemost* 2000;**84**:747–51.
13. Salooja N, Perry DJ. Thromboelastography. *Blood Coagul Fibrinolysis* 2001;**12**:327–37.
14. Brandt JT, Triplett DA, Alving B, Scharrer I. Criteria for the diagnosis of lupus anticoagulants: an update. *Thromb Haemost* 1995;**74**:1185–90.

15. Exner T. Diagnostic methodologies for circulating anticoagulants. *Thromb Haemost* 1995;**74**: 338–44.

16. Arnout D, Boutière B, Sampol J. Diagnostic biologique des anticoagulants de type lypique (lupus anticoagulants). *Rev Fr Lab* 1997;**293**:29–35.

17. Bellucci-Sessa S, Caen JP. Inherited platelet disorders. In: Hoffbrand AV, Mewis SM, Tuddenham EGD (eds). *Postgraduate Haematology*, 4th ed. London: Butterworth-Heinemann; 1999;450–70.

18. Nurden A. Inherited abnormalities of platelets. *Thromb Haemost* 1999;**82**:468–80.

19. Cattaneo M, Lecchi A, Randi AM *et al.* Identification of a new congenital defect of platelet function characterized by severe impairment of platelet responses to adenosine diphosphate. *Blood* 1992;**80**:2787–96.

20. Nurden P, Savi P, Heilmann E *et al.* An inherited bleeding disorder linked to a defective interaction between ADP and its receptor on platelets. *J Clin Invest* 1995;**95**:1612–22.

21. Leon C, Vial C, Gachet C *et al.* The P2Y1 receptor is normal in a patient presenting a severe deficiency of ADP-induced platelet aggregation. *Thromb Haemost* 1999;**81**:775–81.

22. Eckly A, Gendrault JL, Hechler B *et al.* Differential involvement of the P2Y 1 and P2Y T receptors in the morphological changes of platelet aggregation. *Thromb Haemost* 2001;**85**:694–701.

23. Hollopeter G, Jantzen HS, Vincent D *et al.* Identification of the platelet ADP receptor targeted by antithrombotic drugs. *Nature* 2001;**409**:202–7.

24. Huizing M, Anikster Y, Gahl WA. Hermansky–Pudlak syndrome and Chediak–Higashi syndrome: disorders of vesicle formation and trafficking. *Thromb Haemost* 2001;**86**:233–45.

25. Favier R, Douay L, Esteneva B *et al.* A novel genetic thrombocytopenia (Paris–Trousseau) associated with platelet inclusions, dysmegacaryopoiesis and chromosome deletion at 11q23. *C R Acad Sci Paris* 1993;**316**:698–701.

26. Antonarakis SE, Rossiter JP, Young M *et al.* Factor VIII gene inversions in severe hemophilia A: results of an international consortium study. *Blood* 1995;**86**:2206–12.

27. Antonarakis SE, Kazazian HH Jr, Tuddenham EGD. Molecular etiology of factor VIII deficiency in hemophilia A. *Hum Mutat* 1995;**5**: 1–22.

28. White GC, Rosendaal F, Aledort LM *et al.* Definitions in Hemophilia. Classification of the severity of hemophilia. On behalf of the Factor VIII and Factor IX Subcommittee of the International Society on Thrombosis and Haemostasis, 2000.

29. Rodeghiem E, Castaman G, Dini E. Epidemiological investigation of the prevalence of von Willebrand's disease. *Blood* 1987;**69**: 454–9.

30. Levy G, Ginsburg D. Getting at the variable expressivity of von Willebrand disease. *Thromb Haemost* 2001;**86**:144–8.

31. Roberts HR, Hoffman M. Other clotting factor deficiencies. InL Hoffman R, benz EJ, Sanford Jr *et al.* (eds). *Hematology. Basic Principles and Practice*, 3rd ed. Churchill Livingstone, 2000:1912–24.

32. Haverkate F, Samama M. Familial dysfibrinogenemia and thrombophilia. Report on a study of the SSC Subcommittee on Fibrinogen. *Thromb Haemost* 1995;**73**:151–61.

33. Matsuda M, Sugo T, Yoshida N *et al.* Structure and function of fibrinogen: insights from dysfibrinogens. *Thromb Haemost* 1999;**82**:283–90.

34. Roberts HR, Stinchcombe TE, Gabriel DA. The dysfibrinogenaemias. *Br J Haematol* 2001;**114**: 249–57.

35. Nichols WC, Seligsohn U, Zivelin A *et al.* Linkage of combined factors V and VIII deficiency to chromosome 18q by homozygosity mapping. *J Clin Invest* 1997;**99**:596–601.

36. Moussalli M, Pipe SW, Hauri HP *et al.* Mannose-dependent endoplasmic reticulum (ER) – Golgi intermediate compartment-53-mediated ER to Golgi trafficking of coagulation factors V and VIII. *J Biol Chem* 1999;**274**:32539–42.

37. Neerman-Arbez M, Johnson KM, Morris MA *et al.* Molecular analysis of the ERGIC-53 gene in 35 families with combined factor V–factor VIII deficiency. *Blood* 1999;**93**:2253–60.

38. Kadir RA, Economides DL, Sabin CA *et al.* Assessment of menstrual blood loss and gynaecological problems in patients with inherited bleeding disorders. *Haemophilia* 1999;**5**:40–84.

39. Economides D, Kadir R, Lee CA. Inherited bleeding disorders in obstetrics and gynaecology. *Br J Obstet Gynaecol* 1999;**106**:5–13.

40. Kadir RA, Sabin CA, Pollard D *et al.* Quality of life during menstruation in patients with inherited bleeding disorders. *Haemophilia* 1998;**4**: 836–41.

41. Kadir RA, Economides DL, Sabin CA *et al.* Frequency of inherited bleeding disorders in women with menorrhagia. *Lancet* 1998;**351**:4 85–99.

42. Goodeve AC. Advances in carrier detection in haemophilia. *Haemophilia* 1998;**4**:358–64.

43. Ljung RC. Prenatal diagnosis of haemophilia. *Haemophilia* 1999;**5**:84–7.

44. Federici AB, Rand JH, Bucciarelli P *et al.* Acquired von Willebrand syndrome: data from an international registry. *Thromb Haemost* 2000;**84**:345–9.

45. Federici AB, Stabile F, Castaman G *et al.* Treatment of acquired von Willebrand syndrome in patients with monoclonal gammopathy of uncertain significance: comparison of three different therapeutic approaches. *Blood* 1998; **92**:2707–11.

46. Rinder MR, Richard RE, Rinder HM. Acquired von Willebrand's disease: a concise review. *Am J Hematol* 1997;**54**:139–45.

47. Tefferi A, Nichols W, Bowie EJW. Circulating heparin-like anticoagulants: report of five consecutive cases and review. *Am J Med* 1990;**88**:184–90.

48. Muller-Berghaus G, ten Cate H, Levi M. Disseminated intravascular coagulation: clinical spectrum and established as well as new diagnostic approaches. *Thromb Haemost* 1999;**82**:706–12.

49. Hathaway WE, Goodnight SH. Systemic fibrinolysis. In: *Disorders of Hemostasis and Thrombosis: A Clinical Guide.* McGraw-Hill; 1993.

5

Inherited thrombophilia

Sam Schulman

Young patients with venous thromboembolism should have an investigation of biochemical and genetic risk factors performed because the chances of identifying an abnormality are higher than in elderly patients with thrombosis and because the diagnosis of inherited thrombophilia may have a significant influence on future management. In addition, for female patients the detection of inherited thrombophilia may have an impact on their choice of birth control and on the management of future pregnancies. Inherited thrombophilia is not only related to deep vein thrombosis and pulmonary embolism but also to certain complications during pregnancy. It is therefore important to have a knowledge of the different variants of inherited thrombophilia and their diagnosis, as well as of the prevention and treatment of thromboembolic complications and how this differs from prevention and treatment in patients without inherited thrombophilia.

CLASSIFICATION

The abnormalities associated with inherited thrombophilia can be classified in different ways. One way is to look at the mechanism through which the condition leads to an increased propensity to form blood clots. It is possible to group the conditions into

- those that cause an insufficient inhibition of blood coagulation (e.g. antithrombin deficiency, protein C or protein S); and

- those that primarily lead to increased procoagulant activity (e.g. increased levels of coagulation factors – factor VIII, factor IX or factor XI – or prothrombin via the G20210A prothrombin polymorphism or factor V Leiden).

Another way of using the mechanism of the conditions as a basis for classification is to divide the abnormalities into

- those that cause an increased thrombin generation; and
- those that cause decreased neutralization of thrombin;[1] this group includes only antithrombin deficiency.

A more practical classification is perhaps according to the diagnostic routine. Thus, although all the causes are inherited, we can say that:

- for some of the abnormalities the genetic defect has not been identified (increased levels of factor VIII and maybe also of factors IX and XI);
- for others a large number of gene defects have been identified, so that genotypic diagnosis is not practical and phenotypic assessment is used instead (antithrombin deficiency, protein C deficiency, protein S deficiency, dysfibrinogenemia); and
- in a few cases a single genetic defect – a

Table 5.1 Conditions associated with inherited thrombophilia

Phenotypic diagnosis – genetic defect not identified

Increased level of factor VIII
Increased level of factor IX*
Increased level of factor XI*

Phenotypic diagnosis – many mutations described

Deficiency of antithrombin
Deficiency of protein C
Deficiency of protein S
Dysfibrinogenemia
Homocysteinuria
Homocysteinemia

Genotypic diagnosis – single nucleotide polymorphism

G1691A factor V (Leiden), causing activated protein C resistance
G20210A prothrombin, causing mild elevation of the prothrombin level

*Described only in an epidemiological study

single nucleotide polymorphism – is present, so that this can be the basis for the diagnostic procedure (G1691A mutation or factor V Leiden, G20210A prothrombin polymorphism).

In addition to the causes mentioned above, homocysteinuria and homocysteinemia have to be taken into account, but their inclusion into any of those classifications is difficult, since these conditions may cause increased coagulation via several mechanisms, which are so far highly speculative.

The conditions that cause inherited thrombophilia are summarized in Table 5.1. A few more causes have been implicated, but only a limited number of cases have been described

and there have been contradictory observations about the association with venous thromboembolism. These conditions are, for example, dysplasminogenemia or hypoplasminogenemia, deficiency of heparin cofactor II, deficiency of histidine-rich glycoprotein, and abnormal thrombomodulin.

The reported prevalence of the different kinds of thrombophilia depends on the selection of the population to be studied. Thus, in studies of truly consecutive patients with venous thromboembolism in which all cases have been investigated, the prevalence is lower than in studies of patients selected for referral to a hemostasis unit. The latter are usually younger and have often a family history of venous thromboembolism. Furthermore, the ethnicity of the population matters for the prevalence of the G1691A mutation and the G20210A prothrombin polymorphism, which are virtually absent in the African and Asian populations. The typical prevalences in a Caucasian population are shown in Table 5.2.

There is a subclassification for thrombophilic defects with several genetic defects associated with a lower plasma level. Generally, a decreased enzymatic activity paralleled by a low antigen level constitutes type I, whereas decreased activity with normal antigen level is considered type II. Type I is the most common variant, but type II may have been missed in some cases if the only screening was by immunological assay.

A large number of genetic defects have been identified for antithrombin, protein C and protein S deficiencies, including many deletions and point mutations. Some of these gene defects cause distinct functional defects if they correspond to a specific binding site in the protein or multiple functional defects (pleiotropic effect). These genetic defects are reported to specific protein databases.[3–5]

ANTITHROMBIN DEFICIENCY

The first description of inherited thrombophilia dates back to 1965 and deals with a patient with antithrombin deficiency. This glycoprotein was previously called antithrombin III, but since the

Table 5.2 Prevalence of inherited thrombophilia in healthy subjects and patients with venous thromboembolism among Caucasians

Inherited thrombophilia	Prevalence in the general population (%)	Prevalence in unselected patients with venous thromboembolism (%)
Antithrombin deficiency	0.02	1–2
Protein C deficiency	0.2–0.4	3–4
Protein S deficiency	Unknown	2
Factor V Leiden (G1691A)	5	20
Prothrombin G20210A	2–3	6
High level of FVIII (>1.5 IU/ml)	11	25
Homocysteinemia (>18.5 μmol/l)	5	10

*Data based on Seligsohn and Lubetsky[1] and Rosendaal[2]

other 'antithrombins' have now been identified as being other proteins with more specific functions, there is only one 'antithrombin'. It belongs to the serine protease family and inactivates thrombin and factors IXa, Xa, XIa and XIIa. This reaction is markedly accelerated by heparin or proteoglycans on the vascular endothelium.

Type I antithrombin deficiency is, in its heterozygous form, associated with a high risk of deep vein thrombosis or pulmonary embolism. Superficial thrombophlebitis or arterial thrombosis are not typical. The homozygous form is probably not compatible with life.[6]

Type II deficiency (reduced activity, normal antigen) may present with fewer symptoms in the heterozygous form, and a few cases of homozygosity for this subtype have been described. Type II functional defects affect the reactive site where thrombin cleaves to form a thrombin–antithrombin complex, or the heparin binding site.

In comparison with other types of thrombophilia, antithrombin deficiency has often been perceived as the most severe disorder. Using markers of activation of the coagulation system, fibrinopeptide A was more elevated in patients with this deficiency than among those with deficiency of protein C or protein S.[7] However,

measurement of prothrombin fragment 1+2 in the same patients showed the opposite pattern.[7] Even so, the clinical impression is that patients with antithrombin deficiency present with symptoms of venous thromboembolism at a younger age than those with other defects[8,9] and that it confers a higher risk of thromboembolism during pregnancy[10] and of fetal loss.[11] Although fatal cases have been described in a few families with antithrombin deficiency, evidence is lacking that this condition should result in a shortening of the life span, as assessed in two large retrospective studies.[12,13]

In the laboratory, screening for antithrombin deficiency is done with a functional assay. In cases of a low level, typing is performed with an immunological assay (by electroimmunoassay or enzyme-linked immunosorbent assay (ELISA)) and crossed immunoelectrophoresis.

The differential diagnosis is acquired antithrombin deficiency which occurs in severe liver disease or during treatment with L-asparaginase (because of decreased synthesis), disseminated intravascular coagulation or massive thrombosis (because of increased consumption), nephrotic syndrome or inflammatory bowel disease (because of loss through leakage), and possibly during treatment with heparin – mainly unfractionated (because of binding to heparin).

PROTEIN C DEFICIENCY

The second thrombophilic entity to be reported was protein C deficiency in 1981.[14] Protein C belongs to the family of vitamin K-dependent glycoproteins and is activated by thrombin to activated protein C (APC). This activated process is enhanced 20,000 times when thrombin is bound to thrombomodulin on endothelial cells in small blood vessels or when protein C is bound to the endothelial protein C receptor which is present mainly in large vessels, especially arteries. APC downregulates thrombin generation by inactivating factor VIIIa and factor Va through selective cleavage. Protein S is a cofactor in this reaction, which takes place on phospholipid surfaces. APC also appears to play a major role in septicemia by modulation of leukocyte functions and reduction of inflammatory response.

In the heterozygous form protein C deficiency is associated with an increased risk of venous thromboembolism as well as superficial thrombophlebitis. Homozygous protein C deficiency manifests itself with purpura fulminans, which is caused by thrombosis in small vessels with accompanying ischemic necrosis of the skin and subcutis.[15] This occurs in the neonatal period or during the first years of life, depending on whether the protein C level is almost undetectable or not. The deficiency does not appear to cause excess mortality.[16]

Type II protein C deficiency may result in a defective activation by thrombin–thrombomodulin, a decreased binding to phospholipids or poor interaction with cofactors or substrates. Among healthy controls, about one in 200 have a low level of protein C, but these people do not suffer from an increased rate of thrombotic manifestations.[17]

The diagnosis of protein C deficiency is based on a functional assay (either amidolytic or clotting) in which protein C is activated to APC by thrombin, thrombin–thrombomodulin complex, or the snake venom Protac. Depending on the assay selected, one of the type II variants may turn out falsely normal. Measurement of protein C antigen is used to verify a type II defect. Other causes of protein C deficiency are medication with vitamin K antagonists, vitamin K deficiency, liver disease or, rarely, a mutation in the γ-glutamylcarboxylase gene.[18]

PROTEIN S DEFICIENCY

In 1984, protein S deficiency was described as another cause of thrombophilia.[19,20] This glycoprotein has several features in common with protein C, since it is also vitamin K-dependent and exerts its inhibiting function together with protein C. Free protein S increases the affinity of APC for negatively charged phospholipid surfaces on the endothelium or platelets, which enhances local complex formation of APC with factor Va and factor VIIIa. Beside its cofactor function, protein S has anticoagulant effects of its own in the free form on the factor IXa–factor VIIIa–phospholipid complex ('tenase') and the factor Va–factor Xa–phospholipid complex ('prothrombinase'). Sixty percent of protein S is bound to the β-chain of C4b-binding protein and so is inactive. Protein S is produced by the liver, endothelial cells, megakaryocytes and the testicular Leydig cells.

The clinical manifestations of protein S deficiency are similar to those of protein C deficiency. The subtypes of protein S deficiency are (depending on the classification system) type I (low total and free antigen, low activity), type II or IIb (normal antigen, low activity) and type III or IIa (low free antigen but normal total antigen, low activity).

Since all subtypes have low free antigen, this is usually the basis for screening, either with an ELISA method or with electroimmunoassay. Functional assays are used, but there is an interference in cases of concomitant APC resistance. Genetic analysis of protein S deficiency has been complicated by the existence of two protein S genes, one an active gene and one a pseudogene, in close proximity to each other on chromosome 3.

The differential diagnosis includes the same entities as mentioned above for protein C deficiency. In addition, the protein S level is reduced during pregnancy and by treatment with estrogens.

APC RESISTANCE

Until 1993, investigations for biochemical defects in patients with venous thromboembolism gave positive results in only about 5% of the cases (i.e. patients who had one of the deficiencies mentioned above). In 1993, patients with resistance to the anticoagulant effect of APC were described;[21] this was shown in 1994 to be the effect of a G1691A point mutation in the factor V gene, resulting in a 506 arginine to glycine replacement.[22] This is called the factor V Leiden mutation and it is by far the most common inherited cause of APC resistance. Factor V is cleaved by APC at arginine 306, arginine 506, and arginine 679; two mutations at the former site – 306 arginine to threonine (factor V Cambridge)[23] and 306 arginine to glycine (factor V Hong Kong)[24] have been reported in a few patients with thrombosis. The factor V Leiden mutation has a single origin about 30,000 years ago and is found only in Caucasians.[25] It is the most common thrombophilic abnormality identified in investigations of patients from this race, and it increases the risk of deep vein thrombosis five fold; superficial thrombophlebitis is also more common. A peculiar feature, repeatedly demonstrated, is that patients with this mutation have a lower risk of developing symptomatic or fatal pulmonary embolism.[26,27] A proposed benefit of this common mutation is reduced intrapartum bleeding in female carriers, which could have provided an improved chance of survival in the premodern era.[28] Homozygous factor V Leiden has a prevalence of 0.06–0.25% and confers a high risk of venous thromboembolism, but otherwise the manifestations are of the same kind as in the heterozygous population.

A mild form of APC resistance has been observed in patients with an A4070G polymorphism in factor V, resulting in a 1299His to Arg replacement, and this feature is associated with nine other polymorphisms constituting the haplotype HR2. Subjects with the R2 allele have an odds ratio of 1.8 for venous thromboembolism.[29]

APC resistance is analyzed with an activated partial thromboplastin time (aPTT) assay with and without addition of APC in order to arrive at a ratio of these two coagulation times. Improved specificity is obtained by using factor V-deficient plasma and normalized ratios. In cases of APC resistance, the factor V Leiden mutation is confirmed with a polymerase chain reaction analysis.

FACTOR II G20210A

Another relatively common point mutation, reported in 1996 and associated with a mildly elevated plasma level of prothrombin and an increased risk of venous thromboembolism, is the G20210A polymorphism in the 3' untranslated region of the prothrombin gene.[30] Heterozygotes have a four-fold increase in the risk of venous thromboembolism. The mechanism whereby this polymorphism affects the prothrombin level has not been elucidated.

The clinical manifestations are similar to those seen with factor V Leiden, but there may be less frequent thrombotic events in the patients who are homozygous for factor II G20210A than in those who are homozygous for factor V Leiden.[31]

INCREASED FACTOR VIII LEVELS

A high plasma concentration of factor VIII but not of von Willebrand factor is an independent risk factor for venous thromboembolism;[32] this finding is independent of the blood group[32] and is not due to an acute phase reaction.[33] Although family studies have revealed concordance between high levels of factor VIII and thrombosis,[34] no genetic defect has so far been identified. Factor VIII levels above 1.5 IU/ml appear to increase the risk of thrombosis almost five-fold.[32]

INCREASED LEVELS OF FACTOR IX OR FACTOR XI

Based on retrospective analyses of samples obtained in the Leiden Thrombophilia Study with more than 400 patients with deep vein thrombosis and as many controls, it was recently reported that an increased antigen level of factor IX[35] or factor XI[36] is an independent risk factor for thrombosis. Whether they are independent from each other was not tested. For patients with a level above the 90th percentile (factor IX, 1.29 IU/ml; factor XI, 1.21 IU/ml) the adjusted odds ratios for thrombosis were 2.5 and 2.2, respectively. As for high factor VIII levels, no genetic explanation has been found, and it cannot yet be concluded with certainty that these thrombophilic defects are inherited. Although a secondary elevation caused by the thrombotic event has not been excluded, samples were obtained 6 months after the event to minimize the influence of acute phase effect.

DYSFIBRINOGENEMIA

Dysfibrinogenemia is a congenital condition associated with abnormal function of fibrinogen and venous thromboembolism. It is rare, since it has been found in only 0.8% of (probably) selected patients with a history of venous thromboembolism.[37] The underlying mechanisms for the thrombotic predisposition are increased levels of thrombin, caused by defective binding of thrombin to the abnormal fibrinogen, and an impaired stimulatory function of abnormal fibrin in fibrinolysis mediated by tissue plasminogen (t-PA).

Several mutations responsible for this dysfunction have been reported. The diagnosis of dysfibrinogenemia is established when a lower chronometrically determined fibrinogen than the immunological value is combined with a prolonged thrombin time. Alternatively, the defect may be identified by demonstration of the mutation.

HOMOCYSTEINURIA AND HOMOCYSTEINEMIA

The severe inherited defects in homocysteine metabolism, cystathionine β-synthase deficiency (with a prevalence of homozygotes of one in 200,000), and the homozygous deficiency of N^5,N^{10}-methylene-tetrahydrofolate reductase (MTHFR) (which occurs in about one in 2,000,000) result in congenital homocysteinuria. Patients develop severe mental retardation, seizures, skeletal deformities, ectopia lentis, premature

vascular disease with severe atherosclerosis, and venous thromboembolism. Heterozygotes with cystathionine β-synthase deficiency have moderately elevated levels of plasma homocysteine, and the prevalence of this form in the general population is 0.3–1.4%. A thermolabile mutant of MTHFR results, in its homozygous form, in a 50% reduction of the enzyme activity, and it is a risk factor for coronary artery disease.[38] The genetic defect is a C to T substitution at nucleotide 677 with an alanine to valine substitution in the protein, which has been found in Caucasians and East Asians but not in Africans.[39] The prevalence of this homozygous form is 5–15%.[40] Although the MTHFR C677T variant causes homocysteinemia only the phenotype, but not the genotype, has been associated with an increased risk of venous thromboembolism.[41,42]

Blood samples for analysis of homocysteine should be obtained from the fasting patient in the morning (because of diurnal variation in levels). The differential diagnosis includes many causes of acquired homocysteinemia (such as low levels of folate, cobalamin or pyridoxine due to dietary deficiency or interaction by methotrexate, anticonvulsants, theophylline, cigarette smoking, pernicious anemia, old age, chronic renal insufficiency, hypothyroidism, and several types of cancer).[40]

HYPOFIBRINOLYSIS

Several defects resulting in a decreased fibrinolytic capacity and therefore, at least theoretically, in an increased risk of thrombosis have been described. However, the cases have been few in number and for some of the defects controversial findings have been reported. Plasminogen is the central zymogen of fibrinolysis, and the defects can be either hypoplasminogenemia (type I) or dysplasminogenemia (type II), both of which have been reported in a few patients with venous thromboembolism. However, in a cohort of 9611 blood donors, all but two of 80 donors or family members with familial deficiency of plasminogen were asymptomatic.[43] Furthermore, in a study of 1192 consecutive patients with thrombosis, 23 had a low level of plasminogen, but 11 of those had other defects or circumstantial risk factors, and investigation of family members did not reveal an increased risk.[44]

The main activator of plasminogen – t-PA – and in turn plasminogen activator inhibitor (PAI)-1 have been extensively studied for their association with venous thromboembolism, and they were not found to be good predictors in healthy people.[45] Recently, the D-allele of an Alu repeat insertion/deletion polymorphism in intron h of the t-PA gene was reported to show an association with venous thromboembolism during pregnancy.[46] PAI-1 has a 4G/5G polymorphism in the promoter region 675 base pairs, upstream from the start of the transcription site. The 4G allele has a significantly higher activity *in vitro*, but the clinical studies have given controversial results. A meta-analysis of nine studies showed that the 4G allele is associated with a slightly increased risk of myocardial infarction,[47] but although this allele was associated with a higher PAI-1 level in patients with venous thromboembolism, the distribution of 4G/5G genotypes was the same as in controls.[48]

Factor XII seems to be of minimal or no importance for the blood coagulation *in vivo*, but it may play a role in the fibrinolytic system by enhancing the release of t-PA. A deficiency of factor XII has been reported as a risk factor for thrombosis[49] and habitual abortions,[50] but confirmation in larger studies is needed.

THROMBOMODULIN DEFECTS

The cell membrane protein thrombomodulin forms complexes with thrombin, which are crucial for a negative feedback on the coagulation by the activation of protein C. Four mutations at different locations in the thrombomodulin gene have been identified in patients with thrombosis.[51] However, family investigations revealed that cosegregation with thromboembolism was incomplete.

TISSUE FACTOR PATHWAY INHIBITOR DEFECTS

The main inhibitor of the factor VII–tissue factor pathway is the tissue factor pathway inhibitor

(TFPI), which first binds and inhibits factor Xa, thereafter forming a larger, quaternary complex with factor VIIa, tissue factor, and calcium. A major part of the TFPI pool is released into the circulation by heparin, and low levels of TFPI after heparin have been reported in a small study of patients with thrombosis; however, a family study did not show cosegregation.[52] In a study of 342 patients with deep vein thrombosis and 5120 blood donors a 536C to T substitution, corresponding to a 151Pro to Leu exchange was associated with thrombosis.

A PROTECTIVE POLYMORPHISM IN FACTOR XIII

In a meta-analysis of five studies on the effect of a G to A transition in exon 2 of the factor XIII gene causing a 34Val to Leu exchange, the odds ratio for venous thromboembolism was 0.58 (95% CI 0.41–0.82).[53] Thus, there seems to be a protective effect of this polymorphism, which previously had been observed in arterial thrombotic disease.

OTHER CANDIDATE DEFECTS

There have been case reports of thrombosis in patients with a deficiency of heparin cofactor II, histidine-rich glycoprotein or factor VII, but confirmation is lacking or even contradictory.

COMMON CLINICAL FEATURES

The typical manifestations of the thrombophilic defects discussed above are deep vein thrombosis and pulmonary embolism, although the latter seems to be less common in patients with factor V Leiden. The risk of these events is summarized in Table 5.3. In pregnant women with or without thrombophilia, the typical location of thrombosis is in the left iliac vein or the left iliofemoral vein. Superficial thrombophlebitis appears to be most prevalent in protein C deficiency and protein S deficiency, followed by factor V Leiden. For most of the defects there have also been case reports on unusual venous thrombotic locations, such as in cerebral, visceral or upper extremity veins. A higher proportion of patients

Table 5.3 The annual incidence of venous thrombosis in various defects

Defect	Annual incidence (% per year)
Antithrombin deficiency (heterozygous)	0.87–1.6
Protein S deficiency	0.5–1.65
Protein C deficiency	0.43–0.72
G20210A prothrombin polymorphism (heterozygous)	0.55
Factor V Leiden (heterozygous)	0.25–0.45

Data from Seligsohn and Lubetsky[1]

with cerebral vein thrombosis seem to have thrombophilic defects compared with those with typical deep vein thrombosis or pulomary embolism.

In all of these defects it is unusual for the first presentation of symptoms to occur in childhood; however, on the other hand, if a neonate suffers from venous thromboembolism or arterial cerebral thrombosis there is a high probability of finding one or more of these defects.

Since several of these causes of venous thromboembolism have a prevalence in the general population of about 5%, there will be a non-negligible number of people with a combination of defects. These patients have a very high risk of thrombosis, as illustrated by some studies.[54,55]

It has now repeatedly been shown that among patients with certain pregnancy complications, there is an over-representation of thrombophilic abnormalities, and again combinations of defects increase the risk further.[56,57] These complications include early fetal loss, stillbirth (fetal loss after 28 weeks gestation), retarded fetal growth, pre-eclampsia, and placental abruption. It can of course be speculated that the pathogenesis of these complications includes thrombosis in the placental blood vessels, at least in some cases.

SCREENING FOR THROMBOPHILIA

Should all patients who have had an episode of venous thromboembolism undergo laboratory investigation? Since the more severe types of inherited thrombophilia, including antithrombin deficiency, protein C deficiency or protein S deficiency are likely to present with clinical manifestations in early adulthood, the chances of finding them in patients over 50 years of age is relatively small. The less severe factor V Leiden and G20210A prothrombin mutation may be discovered in elderly patients, but then again, how much will such a diagnosis affect management? The answer is, probably very little, as demonstrated below. Except for young patients, it is true that those with recurrent thromboembolism, those with a positive clinical family history, and those with atypical thrombotic locations have a high risk of carrying a thrombophilic defect, and these patients are recommended for laboratory investigation.

Should young women be screened before prescription or oral contraceptives or before pregnancy? An illustrative example is screening for the most common defect – factor V Leiden mutation – before prescribing oral contraceptives. The incidence of fatal venous thromboembolism in the UK is 0.1–0.2 per 100,000; with oral contraceptives it is about 0.7 per 100,000. With the eight-fold increased risk of thromboembolism in carriers of the factor V Leiden mutation, the annual incidence of fatal thromboembolism would rise to 5.6 per 100,000. If, in these circumstances, 20,000 women with the factor V Leiden mutation could be identified and refused prescription of oral contraceptives, one life would be saved annually. However, withholding oral contraceptives to all these women would result in a number of disadvantages, including unwanted pregnancies and abortions, as well as associated morbidity and perhaps mortality. Since the prevalence of the mutation is about 5%, 400,000 women would have to be screened to diagnose the number quoted, and with a cost of about $US30 per analysis, the screening to save this life would amount to $US12 million.

A large retrospective study of 72,201 deliveries during 11 years yielded 62 cases with objectively verified venous thromboembolism.[58] Investigation of these women revealed that four were heterozygous for the factor V Leiden mutation. Based on this, it could be estimated that the risk of thrombosis during pregnancy or the puerperium in women with this defect is one in 400–500, which would not favour implementation of screening. That would cost about $US2 million for a cohort of this size, or $US0.5 million per avoided case of thrombosis in factor V Leiden; moreover, this cost takes into account only the screening and not the costs for prophylaxis and monitoring.

Should women who have a family history of uninvestigated thrombosis have laboratory screening? In about half of the patients referred for laboratory investigation, no thrombophilic defect can be demonstrated with available methods. With the recent course of events it may still be expected that many patients in the other half have hitherto unknown genetic abnormalities, which we will not be able to identify. Thus, a negative result may be false and give the woman a misconception that there is no risk in taking oral contraceptives. It is probably better simply to inform her that as long as there is venous thromboembolism in the family there is an increased risk for her as well, and that opting for another mode of anticonception is preferable.

If, on the contrary, somebody is diagnosed with inherited thrombophilia, relatives should be investigated, since there is a 50% chance of finding a defect in each first-degree relative. This is especially important for fertile female relatives, in whom prophylactic strategies will yield the highest benefit.

PROPHYLAXIS AND TREATMENT

The same kind and dose of pharmacological prophylaxis as given to other patients should be given to those with inherited thrombophilia who require surgery, but it is also required in less major procedures. Patients with deficiency of antithrombin constitute a special subset, since the antithrombin level can be reduced by heparin, theoretically leading to an increased risk of thrombosis. Antithrombin concentrate has occasionally been given to these patients for surgery and for the first few days after surgery, but no randomized study has been performed to prove the benefits of this approach. In pregnant women with previous venous thromboembolism, it appears to be safe to abstain from prophylaxis with heparin during pregnancy and to follow closely.[59] However, this is probably not true in patients with a thrombophilic defect. Again, the highest risk seems to be conferred by antithrombin deficiency. Some groups have positive experience from the use of antithrombin concentrate during delivery, when the dose of heparin has to be reduced to avoid bleeding, but others have successfully used only heparin or dextran. It seems from several case series that the dose of heparin regularly used for prophylaxis during pregnancy is not sufficient for women with antithrombin deficiency. Instead, unfractionated heparin at the dose of 15,000 IU twice daily or low molecular weight heparin 5000 IU twice daily is required.

Treatment of established venous thromboembolism in patients with inherited thrombophilia follows the regular guidelines, including most patients with antithrombin deficiency.[60] Only those of the latter group with a lack of prolongation of aPTT in spite of high doses of heparin or with other complicating factors such as septicemia may need antithrombin concentrate.

SECONDARY PROPHYLAXIS

The acute treatment of venous thromboembolism has to be followed up with secondary prophylaxis to avoid rapid recurrences, and this is especially true in the case of patients with inherited thrombophilias. Secondary prophylaxis involves vitamin K antagonists, which impair the function of all vitamin K-dependent coagulation factors (factors II, VII, IX, and X) and inhibitors (protein C and protein S), by the synthesis of hypo-γ-carboxylated variants. In case of a pre-existing deficiency of protein C or protein S, a further rapid drop in the level of these inhibitors can cause an imbalance, with thrombosis in small blood vessels and subcutaneous skin necrosis. Therefore, treatment with vitamin K antagonists should be instituted very gradually in these patients.

Table 5.4 Risk of recurrence of venous thromboembolism in relation to the presence of (presumably) genetic risk factors as found in 14 studies

Number of patients	Index event	Design	Risk factor	Odds ratio (95% CI)
21	Venous thromboembolism	Prospective	Hyperhomocysteinemia	2.5 (1.1–5.7)
22	Venous thromboembolism	Prospective	High factor VIII levels	3.9 (1.4–11)
23	Deep vein thrombosis	Prospective	Factor V Leiden	4.1 (1.0–15)
24	Deep vein thrombosis	Selected pts	Factor V Leiden	1.1 (0.2–6.2)
25	Venous thromboembolism	Prospective	Factor V Leiden	1.3 (0.7–2.4)
26	Deep vein thrombosis	Prospective	Factor V Leiden	2.4 (1.3–4.5)
16	Venous thromboembolism	Prospective	Factor V Leiden	1.3 (0.7–2.5)
10	Deep vein thrombosis	Prospective	Factor V Leiden	0.5 (0.1–1.8)
17	Venous thromboembolism	Retrospective	Factor V Leiden	1.1 (0.7–1.6)
18	Deep vein thrombosis	Retrospective	Factor V Leiden	1.3 (0.7–2.4)
19	Venous thromboembolism	Prospective	Prothrombin G20210A	0.7 (0.2–2.1)
16	Venous thromboembolism	Prospective	Prothrombin G20210A	1.1 (0.3–3.3)
18	Deep vein thrombosis	Retrospective	Prothrombin G20210A	1.7 (0.8–3.5)
17	Deep vein thrombosis	Retrospective	Factor V Leiden and prothrombin G20210A	4.2 (1.5–11.7)

Data from Schulman[61]

The optimal duration of secondary prophylaxis after venous thromboembolism in general is vividly debated, but for the majority 6 months seems to be necessary.[61] For patients with the classical inhibitor deficiencies (antithrombin deficiency, protein C deficiency or protein S deficiency) the risk of recurrence is as high as 10% per year, at least initially,[62] and prolonged prophylaxis is justified; however, it must be reassessed annually with respect to patient compliance, hemorrhagic events, and stability of anticoagulation.[63] For the more common thrombophilic defects, data from several studies are available and have recently been summarized (Table 5.4).[61] For patients with factor V Leiden in the heterozygous form, six out of eight studies did not show a statistically significant increase in the risk of recurrence but two – one of which was a small study – did show an increased risk. This may be true, but the increase is so small that it does not support a change from the routine duration of secondary prophylaxis. For those with the prothrombin G20210A polymorphism, three out of three studies failed to show an increased risk. For those with hyperhomocysteinemia or with high factor VIII levels one study each has demonstrated an increased risk of recurrence, but the optimal kind of secondary prophylaxis requires further investigation. Finally, for the combination of factor V Leiden and the prothrombin polymorphism, the odds ratio for a recurrence is as high as 4.2 (95% CI 1.5–11.7), and these patients need at least as much attention as those with antithrombin deficiency.

CONCLUSION

The number of known inherited thrombophilic defects is steadily increasing, and with this increase our insight into the clinical problems encountered is also increasing. With proper tailoring of the anticoagulant prophylaxis and therapy, these patients can, however, be managed with an acceptably low risk.

REFERENCES

1. Seligsohn U, Lubetsky A. Genetic susceptibility to venous thrombosis. *N Engl J Med* 2001;**344**:1222–31.

2. Rosendaal FR. Venous thrombosis: a multicausal disease. *Lancet* 1999;**353**:1167–73.

3. Lane DA, Bayston T, Olds RJ *et al.* Antithrombin mutation database: 2nd (1997) update. *Thromb Haemost* 1997;**77**:197–211.

4. Reitsma PH, Bernardi F, Doig RG *et al.* Protein C deficiency: a database of mutations. 1995 update. *Thromb Haemost* 1995;**73**:876–89.

5. Gandrille S, Borgel D, Ireland H *et al.* Protein S deficiency: a database of mutations. *Thromb Haemost* 1997;**77**:1201–14.

6. Hakten M, Deniz U, Ozbay G, Ulutin ON. Two cases of homozygous antithrombin III deficiency in a family with congenital deficiency of AT. In: Senzinger H, Vinazzer H, eds. *Thrombosis and Haemorrhagic Disorders*. Wurzburg: Schmitt and Meyer; 1989.

7. Mannucci PM, Tripodi A, Bottasso B *et al.* Markers of procoagulant imbalance in patients with inherited thrombophilic syndromes. *Thromb Haemost* 1992;**67**:200–2.

8. Thaler E, Lechner K. Antithrombin III deficiency and thromboembolism. *Clin Haematol* 1981;**10**:369–90.

9. Hirsh J, Piovella F, Pini M. Congenital antithrombin III deficiency. Incidence and clinical features. *Am J Med* 1989;**87(suppl 3B)**:34S–38S.

10. Conard J, Horellou MH, Van Dreden P *et al.* Thrombosis and pregnancy in congenital deficiencies in AT III, protein C or protein S: study of 78 women. *Thromb Haemost* 1990;**63**:319–20.

11. Preston FE, Rosendaal FR, Walker ID *et al.* Increased fetal loss in women with heritable thrombophilia. *Lancet* 1996;**348**:913–16.

12. Rosendaal FR, Heijboer H, Briët E *et al.* Mortality in inherited antithrombin III deficiency 1830 to 1989. *Lancet* 1991;**337**:260–2.

13. van Boven HH, Vandenbroucke JP, Westendorp RGJ, Rosendaal FR. Mortality and causes of death in inherited antithrombin deficiency. *Thromb Haemost* 1997;**77**:452–5.

14. Griffin J, Evatt B, Zimmerman T *et al. J Clin Invest* 1981;**68**:1370–3.

15. Tripodi A, Franchi F, Krachmalnikoff A, Mannucci PM. Asymptomatic homozygous protein C deficiency. *Acta Haematol* 1990;**83**:152–5.

16. Allaart CF, Rosendaal FR, Noteboom WMP, Brët E. Survival in families with hereditary protein C deficiency, 1820 to 1993. *BMJ* 1995;**311**:910–13.

17. Miletich JP, Sherman I, Broze G. Absence of thrombosis in subjects with heterozygous protein C deficiency. *N Engl J Med* 1987;**57**:44–8.

18. Brenner B, Sanchez-Vega B, Wu SM *et al.* A missense mutation in the γ-glutamyl-carboxylase gene causes combined deficiency of vitamin K dependent blood coagulation factors. *Blood* 1998;**92**:4554–9.

19. Comp P, Esmon C. Recurrent venous thromboembolism in patients with a partial deficiency of protein S. *N Engl J Med* 1984;**311**:1525–8.

20. Schwarz HP, Fischer M, Hopmeier P *et al.* Plasma protein S deficiency in familial thrombotic disease. *Blood* 1984;**64**:1297–300.

21. Dahlbäck B, Carlsson M, Svensson PJ. Familial thrombophilia due to a previously unrecognized mechanism characterized by poor anticoagulant response to activated protein C: prediction of a cofactor to activated protein C. *Proc Natl Acad Sci USA* 1993;**90**:1004–8.

22. Bertina RM, Koeleman BP, Koster T *et al.* Mutation in the blood coagulation factor V associated with the resistance to activated protein C. *Nature* 1994;**369**:64–7.

23. Williamson D, Brown K, Luddington R *et al.* Factor V Cambridge: a new mutation (Arg[306] to Thr) associated with resistance to activated protein C. *Blood* 1998;**91**:1140–4.

24. Chan WP, Lee CK, Kwong YL *et al.* A novel mutation of Arg 306 of factor V gene in Hong Kong Chinese. *Blood* 1998;**91**:1135–9.

25. Zöller B, Hillarp A, Dahlbäck B. Activated protein C resistance caused by a common factor V mutation has a single origin. *Thromb Res* 1997;**85**:237–43.

26. Martinelli I, Cattaneo M, Panzeri D, Mannucci PM. Low prevalence of factor V:Q506 in 41 patients with isolated pulmonary embolism. *Thromb Haemost* 1997;**77**:440–3.

27. Vandenbroucke JP, Bertina RM, Holmes ZR *et al.* Factor V Leiden and fatal pulmonary embolism. *Thromb Haemost* 1998;**79**:511–16.

28. Lindqvist PG, Svensson PJ, Dahlbäck B, Marsál K. Factor V Q[506] mutation (activated protein C

resistance) associated with reduced intrapartum blood loss: a possible evolutionary selection mechanism. *Thromb Haemost* 1998;**79**:69–73.

29. Alhenc-Gelas M, Nicaud V, Gandrille S *et al.* The factor V gene A4070G mutation and the risk of venous thrombosis. *Thromb Haemost* 1999;**81**: 193–7.

30. Poort SR, Rosendaal FR, Reitsma PH, Bertina RM. A common genetic variation in thr 3'-untranslated region of the prothrombin gene is associated with elevated plasma prothrombin levels and an increase in venous thrombosis. *Blood* 1996;**88**:3698–703.

31. Girolami A, Simioni P, Tormene D, Scarano L. Two additional homozygous patients for the 20210 prothrombin polymorphism with no venous thrombosis. *Thromb Res* 1999;**96**:415–17.

32. Koster T, Blann AD, Briët E *et al.* Role of clotting factor VIII in effect of von Willebrand factor on occurrence of deep-vein thrombosis. *Lancet* 1995;**345**:152–5.

33. O'Donnell J, Mumford AD, Manning RA, Laffan M. Elevation of FVIII:C in venous thromboembolism is persistent and independent of the acute phase response. *Thromb Haemost* 2000;**83**:10–13.

34. Kraaijenhagen RA, in 't Anker PS, Koopman MMW *et al.* High plasma concentration of factor VIIIc is a major risk factor for venous thromboembolism. *Thromb Haemost* 2000;**83**:5–9.

35. van Hylckama Vlieg A, van der Linden IK, Bertina RM, Rosendaal FR. High levels of factor IX increase the risk of venous thrombosis. *Blood* 2000;**95**:3678–82.

36. Meijers JCM, Tekelenburg WLH, Bouma BN *et al.* High levels of coagulation factor XI as a risk factor for venous thrombosis. *N Engl J Med* 2000;**342**:696–701.

37. Haverkate F, Samama M. Familial dysfibrinogenemia and thrombophilia. Report on a study of the SSC Subcommittee on Fibrinogen. *Thromb Haemost* 1995;**73**:151–61.

38. Kang SS, Wong PWK, Susmano A *et al.* Thermolabile methylene tetrahydrofolate reductase: an inherited risk factor for coronary artery disease. *Am J Hum Genet* 1991;**48**:536–45.

39. Frosst P, Blom HJ, Milos R *et al.* A candidate genetic risk factor for vascular disease: a common mutation in methylenetetrahydrofolate reductase. *Nature Genet* 1995;**10**:111–13.

40. Welch GN, Loscalzo J. Homocysteine and atherothrombosis. *N Engl J Med* 1998;**338**: 1042–50.

41. den Heijer M, Blom HJ, Gerrits WB *et al.* Is hyper-homocysteinemia a risk factor for recurrent venous thrombosis? *Lancet* 1995;**345**:882–5.

42. Kluitjmans LAJ, den Heijer M, Reitsma PH *et al.* Thermolabile methylenetetrahydrofolate reductase and factor V Leiden in the risk of deep-vein thrombosis. *Thromb Haemost* 1998;**79**:254–8.

43. Tait RC, Walker ID, Conkie JA *et al.* Isolated familial plasminogen deficiency may not be a risk factor for thrombosis. *Thromb Haemost* 1996;**76**:1004–8.

44. Demarmels Biasutti F, Sulzer I, Stucki B *et al.* Is plasminogen deficiency a thrombotic risk factor? A study on 23 thrombophilic patients and their family members. *Thromb Haemost* 1998;**80**:167–70.

45. Ridker PM, Vaughan DE, Stampfer MJ *et al.* Baseline fibrinolytic state and the risk of future venous thrombosis. A prospective study of endogenous tissue-type activator and plasminogen activator inhibitor. *Circulation* 1992;**85**: 1822–7.

46. Hooper WC, El-Jamil M, Dilley A *et al.* The relationship between the tissue plasminogen activator Alu I/D polymorphism and venous thromboembolism during pregnancy. *Thromb Res* 2001;**102**:33–7.

47. Iacoviello L, Burzotta F, Di Castelnuovo A *et al.* The 4G/5G polymorphism of the PAI-1 promoter gene and the risk of myocardial infarction: a meta-analysis. *Thromb Haemost* 1998;**80**:1029–30.

48. Stegnar M, Uhrin P, Peternel P *et al.* The 4G/5G sequence polymorphism in the promoter of plasminogen activator inhibitor-1 (PAI-1) gene: relationship to plasma PAI-1 level in venous thromboembolism. *Thromb Haemost* 1998;**79**: 975–9.

49. Mannhalter C, Fischer M, Hopmeier P, Deutsch E. Factor XII activity and antigen concentrations in patients suffering from recurrent thrombosis. *Fibrinolysis* 1987;**1**:259–63.

50. Braulke I, Pruggmayer M, Melloh P *et al.* Factor XII (Hageman) deficiency in women with habitual abortion: new subpopulation or recurrent aborters? *Fertil Steril* 1993;**59**:98–101.

51. Öhlin AK, Marlar RA. Thrombomodulin gene defects in families with thromboembolic disease: a report on four families. *Thromb Haemost* 1999;**81**:338–44.

52. Kleesiek K, Schmidt M, Götting C *et al.* The 536C to T transition in the human tissue factor pathway inhibitor (TFPI) gene is statistically associated with a higher risk for venous thrombosis. *Thromb Haemost* 1999;**82**:1–5.

53. Alhenc-Gelas M, Reny JL, Aubry ML *et al.* The

FXIII Val 34 Leu mutation and the risk of venous thromboembolism. *Thromb Haemost* 2000;**84**: 1117–18.

54. De Stefano V, Martinelli I, Mannucci PM *et al.* The risk of recurrent deep venous thrombosis among heterozygous carriers of both factor V Leiden and the G20210A prothrombin mutation. *N Engl J Med* 1999;**341**:801–6.

55. Margaglione M, D'Andrea G, Colaizzo D et al. Coexistence of factor V Leiden and factor II A20210 mutations and recurrent venous thromboembolism. *Thromb Haemost* 1999;**82**:1583–7.

56. Preston FE, Rosendaal FR, Walker I *et al.* Increased fetal loss in women with heritable thrombophilia. *Lancet* 1996;**348**:913–16.

57. Kupferminc MJ, Eldor A, Steinman N *et al.* Increased frequency of genetic thrombophilia in women with complications of pregnancy. *N Engl J Med* 1999;**340**:9–13.

58. McColl MD, Ramsay JE, tait RC *et al.* Risk factor for pregnancy associated venous thromboembolism. *Thromb Haemost* 1997;**78**:1183–8.

59. Brill-Edwards P, Ginsberg JS, Gent M *et al.* Safety of withholding heparin in pregnant women with a history of venous thromboembolism. *N Engl J Med* 2000;**343**:1439–44.

60. Schulman S, Tengborn L. Treatment of venous thromboembolism in patients with congenital deficiency of antithrombin III. *Thromb Haemost* 1992;**68**:634–6.

61. Schulman S. Duration of anticoagulants in acute or recurrent venous thromboembolism. *Curr Opin Pulm Med* 2000;**6**:321–5.

62. van den Belt AGM, Sanson BJ, Simioni P *et al.* Recurrence of venous throboembolism in patients with familial thrombophilia. *Arch Intern Med* 1997;**157**:2227–32.

63. Lane DA, Mannucci PM, Bauer KA *et al.* Inherited thrombophilia: part 2. *Thromb Haemost* 1996;**76**:824–34.

6

Acquired thrombophilia: antiphospholipid syndrome and essential thrombocythemia

Guido Finazzi, Monica Galli and Tiziano Barbui

ANTIPHOSPHOLIPID SYNDROME

INTRODUCTION

Antiphospholipid (aPL) antibodies are a wide and heterogeneous group of immunoglobulins that include, among others, lupus anticoagulants (LAs) and anticardiolipin (aCL) antibodies. LAs are acquired inhibitors of coagulation that were first described in patients with systemic lupus erythematosus (SLE). They prolong phospholipid-dependent coagulation reactions,[1] but despite this *in vitro* behavior, LAs are not usually associated with bleeding complications. aCL antibodies react with anionic phospholipid in solid-phase immunoassays and are responsible for the biological false-positive test for syphilis.[2] LAs and aCL antibodies are closely related antibodies, and they are concurrently present in approximately two-thirds of cases.

In the 1990s, work from different laboratories made it clear that LAs and aCL antibodies do not recognize anionic phospholipids, as had long been believed, but plasma proteins bound to suitable anionic surfaces (though not necessarily phospholipid surfaces). Among them, β2-glycoprotein I (β2-GPI) and prothrombin (PT) are the most common and investigated antigenic targets. β2-GPI is required by the great majority of aCL antibodies to react with cardiolipin in immunoassays,[3] whereas LA activity in phospholipid-dependent coagulation tests is caused by both anti-β2-GPI (aβ2-GPI) antibodies[4] and anti-PT (aPT) antibodies.[5] Other proteins recognized by aPL antibodies include activated protein C, protein S, annexin V, low and high molecular weight kininogens, factor XII, and tissue-type plasminogen activator.[6] Since most of these proteins are involved in the regulation of the coagulation processes, it is conceivable that antibodies that reduce their plasma concentration or hamper with their function may produce an imbalance between the procoagulant and anticoagulant systems, thus explaining the increased thrombotic risk of the patients. Despite a wealth of research, however, no definite demonstration of a pathogenetic role for aPL antibodies in the development of thrombosis has yet been given. Indeed, arterial and venous thrombosis and obstetrical complications are the clinical events most commonly associated with aPL antibodies, and it is these that constitute the so-called antiphospholipid syndrome (APS).[7] Two types of APS have been described:

- 'primary' APS, which occurs in the absence of an underlying disease;[8] and
- 'secondary' APS, which is related to SLE, other autoimmune or neoplastic diseases, or other pathological conditions.[9]

Table 6.1 Preliminary criteria for the classification of the antiphospholipid syndrome

Clinical criteria

1. Vascular thrombosis

One or more clinical episodes of arterial, venous, or small vessel thrombosis, in any tissue or organ. Thrombosis must be confirmed by imaging or doppler studies or histopathology, with the exception of superficial venous thrombosis. For histopathological confirmation, thrombosis should be present without significant evidence of inflammation in the vessel wall

2. Pregnancy morbidity

- One or more unexplained deaths of a morphologically normal fetus at or beyond the 10th week of gestation, with normal fetal morphology documented by ultrasound or by direct examination of the fetus; or
- One or more premature births of a morphologically normal neonate at or beyond the 34th week of gestation, because of severe preeclampsia or eclampsia, or severe placental insufficiency; or
- Three or more unexplained consecutive spontaneous abortions before the 10th week of gestation, with maternal anatomic or hormonal abnormalities and paternal and maternal chromosomal causes excluded

Laboratory criteria

1. Anticardiolipin antibody of IgG and/or IgM isotype in blood, present in medium or high titer on two or more consecutive occasions, at least 6 weeks apart, measured by standardized enzyme-linked immunosorbent assay for β2-glycoprotein I-dependent aCL antibodies.

2. Lupus anticoagulants present in plasma on two or more consecutive occasions, at least 6 weeks apart, detected according to the guidelines of the International Society of Thrombosis and Haemostasis (Scientific Subcommittee on Lupus Anticoagulant/Phospholipid-Dependent Antibodies) in the following steps:

- Prolonged phospholipid-dependent coagulation demonstrated on a screening test (e.g. activated partial thromboplastin time, kaolin clotting time, dilute Russell's viper venom time, dilute prothrombin time, testarin time);
- Failure to correct the prolonged coagulation time on the screening test by mixing with normal platelet-poor plasma;
- Shortening or correction of the prolonged coagulation time on the screening test by addition of excess phospholipid; and
- Exclusion of other coagulopathies

Definite Antiphospholipid syndrome is considered to be present if at least one of the clinical criteria and one of the laboratory criteria are met

From Wilson et al.[7]

Arterial and venous thrombosis, including recurrent events, are reported in approximately one-third of patients with aPL antibodies. Arterial thrombosis are mainly cerebrovascular, whereas lower extremity thrombosis and pulmonary embolism are the most common venous events. Clinical obstetric criteria for APS[7] are given in Table 6.1.

Although not included among these criteria – which have been recently set by an international workshop[7] – intrauterine growth retardation, pre-eclampsia, and prematurity are other common obstetric APS-associated events.[10] Overall, the prevalence of obstetric complications in women with aPL antibodies is about 15–20%.[11]

ASSOCIATION BETWEEN OBSTETRIC COMPLICATIONS AND VARIOUS aPL ANTIBODIES

The strength of the association between obstetric complications and aPL antibodies has been estimated by cross-sectional and case-control studies.[12–15] The presence of LAs carries an odds ratio ranging from 3.0 to 4.8, whereas the presence of aCL antibodies carries an odds ratio ranging from 0.86 to 20.0. These figures vary according to the primary or secondary nature of APS, the mother's clinical history, and the titers, isotypes and types of aPL being investigated. The highest risk of pregnancy loss has been reported in SLE patients.[14] A maternal history of pregnancy loss represents a strong risk factor for further adverse obstetric events,[13,15] whereas the presence of LAs or aCL antibodies does not seem to have a negative effect on the outcome of the first pregnancy.[13] Whether or not a relationship between the antibody titer and the risk of obstetric complications exists still has to be clarified.[11,16]

The association of aPL antibodies other than aCL or LAs with fetal loss has been investigated by the Nîmes Obstetricians and Haematologists (NOHA) study.[15] LAs, immunoglobulin (Ig)G (IgG) and IgM aCL, aβ2-GPI, anti-annexin V, and anti-phosphatidylethanolamine (aPE) antibodies were measured in three groups of women (one group with unexplained primary recurrent early fetal loss, one group with explained episodes, and one group with no previous obstetrical accidents). Only LAs, IgG aβ2-GPI, IgG anti-annexin V, and IgM aPE antibodies were found to be independent, retrospective risk factors for unexplained primary early fetal loss. The same markers were prospectively found to be associated with a significant risk of fetal loss during subsequent pregnancies.[15] Such a role, however, has been disputed by other authors.[17,18] At present, the investigation of aPL antibodies other than LAs and aCL is not suggested in the routine work-up of women with obstetric complications.

PATHOGENESIS OF THE OBSTETRIC COMPLICATIONS

Following the first description of intrauterine fetal death associated with placental infarction in a woman with LAs,[19] the hypothesis that thrombotic events that occur in the placental vasculature eventually lead to early abortion or fetal death was raised. Histopathological analysis of aborted placentae has been performed for relatively few women with aPL antibodies. Extensive infarcted areas, a decrease in vasculosyncytial membranes, and an increase in fibrosis and hypovascular villi have been reported.[20,21] These findings are consistent with placental hypoxia. Experimental models of APS induction following mouse immunization with human polyclonal and monoclonal aCL antibodies[21,22] were characterized by low fecundity rate and an increased rate of fetal resorption (equivalent to abortions in humans). These findings support the notion that at least some aPL antibodies may play a role in the pathogenesis of the obstetric complications of APS. The mechanism by which aPL antibodies may cause miscarriages has yet to be defined. Since placental thrombosis is also found in the placentas of women without aPL antibodies, such histopathological abnormalities are thus not specific to APS. Alternative mechanisms that take into account the possibility that aPL antibodies may have a direct adverse effect on the process of embryonic implantation have been proposed. It has recently been shown that IgG from patients with APS bind to trophoblast cells and reduce their *in vitro* invasiveness, differentiation, and gonadotropin secretion.[23–25] Two human monoclonal aPL antibodies (one a β2-GPI-independent IgG and the other a β2-GPI-dependent IgM) reproduced the same effects, which were reversed by interleukin-3 and low-molecular weight heparin, but not by aspirin.[24,25]

TREATMENT OF OBSTETRIC COMPLICATIONS

Thrombosis of the placental vasculature and defective embryonic implantation represent the biological rationale of the efficacy of unfractionated and low molecular weight heparins in the treatment of recurrent early abortions and fetal deaths in women with aPL antibodies. Indeed, heparin, alone or in combination with low-dose aspirin, represents the current standard of treatment for pregnant aPL-positive women to prevent recurrent obstetric complications. The live birth rate for women with APS has been prospectively reported to be as low as 10% (0% in those with LAs and 40% in those with aCL antibodies alone).[26] The combination of heparin plus low-dose aspirin has been demonstrated by randomized, controlled clinical trials to increase the live birth rate significantly, up to 71–80% and to be superior to low-dose aspirin alone (live birth rate about 40%).[27,28] Replacement of unfractionated heparin with low molecular weight heparin produced similar results.[29] Heparin administration is well tolerated and, in general, does not decrease bone density.[30]

Despite the high live birth rate, heparin-treated pregnancies of aPL-positive women are still characterized by an excessive frequency of maternal and fetal complications. Two studies on approximately 200 women reported problems in about 42–50% of the women and in 28–35% of the newborns.[29,31] The most common problems were:

- premature delivery (before the 37th week);
- gestational hypertension;
- antepartum hemorrhage;
- growth retardation; and
- oligohydramnios.

Approximately 50% of the pregnancies underwent Caesarean delivery, which was, in most cases, elective. The outcome for the newborns has been investigated by Ruffatti *et al.*,[32] who evaluated 55 infants born to 53 aPL-positive women. After delivery at 25–40 weeks' gestation, birth weight ranged from 800 to 4000 g and the mean Apgar score was 9.6 at 5 minutes. Twelve newborns needed intensive care treatment because of prematurity, but none had thrombotic complications or malformations, and no aPL-related manifestations developed during a follow-up ranging from 1.3 years to 5.6 years.

Taken together, these findings indicate that heparin plus low-dose aspirin, despite being the treatment of choice of a pregnant aPL-positive woman with a poor obstetric history, still needs to be better calibrated in terms of dosage, duration, and timing of administration (Table 6.2). The randomized clinical trials so far conducted started aspirin as soon as the pregnancy test was positive and introduced heparin when fetal heart activity was noted by ultrasound.[28,29] Therefore, the question remains as to whether this treatment should be commenced even before conception in order to reduce the rate of early abortions. Indeed, little and conflicting experimental data exist as to the effect of heparin and aspirin in facilitating the process of embryonic implantation. The same trials stopped therapy at the 34th week of gestation because of the risk of osteopenia. However, it is now recommended that heparin and low-dose aspirin administration should be continued until delivery in order to reduce the rate of late complications.[33] Again, the best timing and dosage of heparin during labour, in relation to the mother's risk of hemorrhage, has not yet been established. Treatment should be continued during the puerperium only in aPL-positive women with known risk factors for thrombosis.

Pregnant, aPL-positive women should undergo regular platelet counts, at least in the first weeks of heparin administration, owing to the risk of heparin-induced thrombocytopenia. The periodic control of aPL antibody titers during pregnancy does not seem to be helpful, since several factors (including increased plasma levels of some coagulation factors and

Table 6.2 Treatment options of antiphospholipid-positive women during pregnancy

Clinical setting	Treatment of choice	Open questions
First pregnancy	No treatment	Role of low-dose aspirin
To prevent further adverse events in the case of a poor obstetric history (see Wilson et al.[7])	Unfractionated or low molecular weight heparin plus low-dose aspirin	Timing and dosage of heparin Role of high-dose immunoglobulins
To prevent recurrence of thrombosis (independent of the obstetric history)	Unfractionated or low molecular weight heparin at therapeutic dosage	Timing of switch from oral anticoagulation to heparin
Puerperium in the case of previous history of thrombosis	Oral anticoagulation (aiming at a prothrombin time international normalized ratio of 2–3)	

expansion of plasma volume) influence the outcome of such tests. Therefore, the decrease or disappearance of aPL antibodies during pregnancy should not modify the therapeutic policy.

Corticosteroids were the first treatment option for the prevention of recurrent miscarriage in women with aPL antibodies.[34] Their use, however, has come into disfavour inasmuch as clinical studies have demonstrated that corticosteroids are less efficacious than heparin and aspirin and are associated with a high rate of fetal–maternal complications (including prematurity, hypertension, and diabetes mellitus).[35–38]

High-dose immunoglobulin therapy has been reported to be effective in some cases, even though its precise mechanism of action has yet to be elucidated. This treatment has been recently evaluated by a multicenter, placebo-controlled pilot study carried out in 16 aPL-positive women with or without a history of recurrent miscarriages or thromboembolic events.[39] All of the women received heparin and low-dose aspirin and were randomized either to monthly courses of immunoglobulins (1 g/kg body weight for 2 days) or placebo until the 36th week of gestation. The two groups were similar with respect to age, gravidity, number of previous pregnancy losses, and gestational age at the initiation of the treatment. All women delivered live babies after the 32nd week of gestation. No differences were observed in the rates of pre-eclampsia or placental insufficiency. There were fewer cases of fetal growth restriction and admissions to neonatal intensive care units among newborns of the high-dose immunoglobulin treatment group; however, these differences were not statistically significant. A recent meta-analysis failed to demonstrate that intravenous immunoglobulins are of benefit in women with unexplained recurrent miscarriages.[40] Therefore, at the present time intravenous immunoglobulins may be considered only for the treatment of women who cannot receive heparin and low-dose aspirin or for those in whom heparin and low-dose aspirin has proved to be ineffective.

THROMBOSIS DURING PREGNANCY

Although the exact thrombotic risk during pregnancy is not known, particularly in women with no history of thromboembolic events, pregnancy and the puerperium do increase the risk of deep venous thrombosis. It is reasonable that unfractionated or low molecular weight heparin should be given throughout pregnancy to aPL-positive women with a known history of thrombosis in order to reduce the risk of recurrence. Oral anticoagulation may replace heparin after delivery and should be continued during the puerperium. Therapeutic doses must be used in aPL-positive women who were taking oral anticoagulation before pregnancy. The use of heparin or aspirin prophylaxis during pregnancy to prevent a first arterial or venous thrombosis has not been established.

IN VITRO FERTILIZATION AND HORMONE CONTRACEPTION

It is not known whether aPL antibodies are involved in the pathogenesis of infertility. However, since 10–15% of couples of reproductive age suffer from infertility, regardless of their aPL status, it is likely that aPL-positive women will be candidates for ovulation induction, with or without *in vitro* fertilization and embryo transfer. Owing to the high levels of ovarian estrogen (mainly estradiol) caused by gonadotropin stimulation, aPL-positive women undergoing ovulation induction may be subject to an increased thromboembolic risk. Since no case of thrombosis has been reported, such a risk appears to be minor. The proper use of antithrombotic treatment during one or, most commonly, several procedures of ovulation induction and ovum retrieval is not clear; in fact, heparin may increase the risk of ovarian hemorrhage, and it has been suggested that heparin should be discontinued 12–24 hours before the procedure and restarted 6–8 hours after ovum retrieval.[41]

The routine evaluation of aPL antibodies in women undergoing *in vitro* fertilization is not warranted, as pointed out by a recent meta-analysis.[42] Seven studies on more than 2000 women, 703 of whom had at least one abnormal aPL antibody test, failed to report an association between aPL antibodies and reduced success of *in vitro* fertilization.

Hormone contraception increases a woman's thrombotic risk, in particular when other congenital or acquired risk factors for thrombosis are present. Data about the arterial and venous thrombotic risk of aPL-positive women taking oral contraceptives are still limited and conflicting, even though LAs or aCL antibodies do not dramatically increase such a risk.[43]

Experience with hormone replacement therapy is limited, since it has been used only in few women with SLE. Apparently no increase in lupus flares was observed.[44] No data are available about the thrombotic risk, particularly in women with APS.

ESSENTIAL THROMBOCYTHEMIA

INTRODUCTION

Essential thrombocythemia (ET) is a clonal disorder of the multipotential hemopoietic stem cell. It leads to bone marrow hyperplasia, excessive proliferation of megakaryocytes, and a sustained elevation of the platelet count. ET is generally considered a disease of middle age, with median onset between the ages of 50 and 60 years. However, with the advent of automated platelet counting, it is now diagnosed with increasing frequency in younger people, including women of childbearing age. The major cause of mortality and morbidity is thromboembolic complications, which occur more frequently in older subjects and in those with previous thrombosis, but which may be precipitated by concomitant prothrombotic situations such as pregnancy or the puerperium. Chemotherapy is effective in reducing the rate of vascular events but potential leukemogenicity and adverse effects on fertility and fetal growth have been reported.

DIAGNOSTIC CRITERIA

ET should be differentiated from reactive thrombocytoses such as occurs during infectious, inflammatory, or malignant diseases or in association with iron-deficiency anemia or hemolytic anemia or after splenectomy.[45] The

---

Table 6.3 Updated diagnostic criteria for essential thrombocythemia

Platelet count > 600 × 10^9/l

Hematocrit < 40% or normal red blood cell mass (males < 36 ml/kg, females < 32 ml/kg)

Stainable iron in marrow or normal serum ferritin or normal red blood cell mean corpuscular volume (if these measurements suggest iron deficiency, polycythemia vera cannot be excluded unless a trial of iron therapy fails to increase the red blood cell mass into the polycythemic range)

No Philadelphia chromosome or *bcr/abl* gene rearrangement

Collagen fibrosis of marrow either absent or less than one-third of biopsy area without either marked splenomegaly or leukoerythroblastic reaction

No cytogenetic or morphological evidence of a myelodysplastic syndrome

No cause for reactive thrombocytosis

From Murphy et al.[46]

---

distinction between ET and reactive thrombocytosis is clinically relevant since the vascular occlusive risk is much greater in ET than it is in RT. Equally important is the distinction between ET and thrombocytosis associated with other chronic myeloproliferative disorders, such as polycythemia vera, idiopathic myelofibrosis and chronic myeloid leukaemia. At present, there are no tests to establish the diagnosis of ET with certainty, so that the disease remains largely a diagnosis of exclusion, based on a set of diagnostic criteria such as those proposed by the Polycythemia Vera Study Group, which have recently been updated (Table 6.3).[47] Spontaneous megakaryocyte colony formation, abnormal cytogenetics or other markers of clonality, and bone marrow megakaryocytosis have been proposed as positive markers of ET.[47] However, diagnostic systems based on positive criteria are not yet routinely applied, and their predictive value has not been established in appropriate clinical trials.

RISK STRATIFICATION

Even though many patients with ET do not present with symptoms, some 8–84% of patients suffer from either thrombotic or hemorrhagic complications.[48] Thrombosis includes large-vessel obstructions (both arterial and venous) as well as microvascular occlusions. Large-vessel obstruction frequently involves the cerebral arteries, the peripheral and the coronary arteries, and the peripheral veins, the hepatic veins (Budd–Chiari syndrome) and the portomesenteric veins. Microvascular occlusions produce symptoms such as transient cerebral ischemia, migraine, visual dysfunction, digital ischemia and erythromelalgia. Thrombotic events are relatively infrequent below the age of 40 years and have the highest incidence in patients over the age of 60 years.[49] A prior history of thrombosis has also been found to be a significant risk factor for subsequent vascular complications.[49] Despite the identification of a broad array of specific structural, biochemical and metabolic platelet defects, no parameter of hemostasis has been shown to reliably herald a thrombotic tendency in patients with ET.[50]

Hemorrhagic events are less frequent than thrombosis and may occur either spontaneously or following trauma. Skin bruising and recurrent bleeding from mucous membranes or the digestive tract are more common in patients with platelet counts in excess of 1500 × 10^9/l and this may be related to an acquired deficiency of von Willebrand's factor (vWF).[51] The number of circulating platelets decreases the concentration of plasma large vWF multimers, which may compromise hemostasis at high platelet counts. Serious bleeding may be triggered by aspirin treatment. ET can be classified into two categories according to the risk of bleeding and thrombosis (Table 6.4). This risk stratification should be carefully considered before the patient's treatment is decided.[48,52]

Table 6.4 Risk stratification in essential thrombocythemia

Low risk

Age < 60 years, *and*

No history of thrombosis, *and*

Platelet count < 1500 × 10⁹/l

High risk

Age ≥ 60 years, *or*

A previous history of thrombosis, *or*

Platelet count ≥ 1500 × 10⁹/l

Correction of cardiovascular risk factors (smoking, obesity) is recommended in all patients

GENERAL RECOMMENDATIONS FOR MANAGEMENT

Young asymptomatic subjects with platelet counts in the range of 600–1500 × 10⁹/l are at lower risk and can be followed without cytoreductive treatment. In one prospective study, the incidence of major thrombotic events in this category of untreated ET patients was not statistically different from that of a group of normal subjects matched for age and sex.[53] Nevertheless, major thrombotic events can occur in a small percentage of 'lower-risk' cases. The risk–benefit of low-dose aspirin in the primary prevention of thrombosis is uncertain and is yet to be tested in appropriate clinical trials. For 'high-risk' patients, hydroxyurea (plus aspirin in the case of ischemia or thrombosis) is the treatment of choice because its efficacy in preventing thrombotic complications has been proven in a randomized clinical trial.[54] However, the possible long-term leukemogenicity of this drug, as well as that of other effective cytoreductive agents such as busulphan and pipobroman, remains a major concern.[55,56] Anagrelide and interferon-α could overcome this worry, but their efficacy has been demonstrated only in lowering the platelet count; clinical studies aimed at documenting additional clinical benefit in ET are needed.[57,58]

ET IN PREGNANCY

Epidemiology and clinical course

ET may jeopardize the outcome of pregnancy. In a review of the literature dealing with 57 women and 106 pregnancies (mostly untreated with cytoreductive drugs), the success rate was 57% (60 live births) and the rate of miscarriage 43% (46 miscarriages).[59] The most frequent complication was spontaneous abortion during the first trimester of pregnancy in 36% (38 abortions out of 106 pregnancies). Other complications, such as intrauterine death and stillbirth, which occurred in 6% (7 out of 106), premature delivery in 8% (8 out of 106), pre-eclampsia in 4% (4 out of 106), and fetal growth retardation in 4% (4 out of 106), were less common. These figures should be compared with the complication rate expected in normal pregnancies.[60] Spontaneous abortion occurs in 5% of all pregnancies in the first 12 weeks and in another 10–12% up to 24th week. Intrauterine death after 24 weeks and stillbirth are observed in about 2% of all pregnancies with considerable variations according to area, sex and race. The rate of premature delivery (birth between the 24th and 37th week or birth weight < 2.5 kg) is about 6%. Thus, the risks to the fetus in ET pregnancies appear to be at least twice that expected in normal pregnancies. The outcome of pregnancies in studies including at least five cases is summarized in Table 6.5.

When evaluating the literature it is important to bear in mind that most reports deal with single cases or small numbers and that there may be a tendency to report patients with complications rather than those with an uncomplicated course. Studies of consecutive series of patients observed in single institutions may overcome this bias.[61–63] In a retrospective analysis of 34 pregnancies seen in 18 ET patients at the Mayo Clinic, Rochester, Minnesota, USA, 17 (50%) resulted in live birth and 17 in unsuccessful pregnancies (see Table 6.5).[61] Abortion could not be predicted from history of disease complication, preconception platelet counts or the presence or absence of specific therapy during pregnancy. In other studies, however, the proportion of live birth was higher in patients who received an active treatment. In a retrospective study of nine

Table 6.5 Essential thrombocythemia and pregnancy: literature review of original report on five or more pregnancies

Reference	Number of patients	Number of pregnancies	Number (%) of live births	Number of unsuccessful pregnancies		
				Elective abortions	Spontaneous abortions	Miscarriage-associated complications
Beressi et al.[61]	18	34	17 (50)	2	12	1 ectopic pregnancy 1 abruptio placentae 1 stillbirth
Bangerter et al.[63]	9	17	11 (65)	0	6	0
Pagliaro et al.[62]	9	15	9 (60)	1	2	3 intrauterine deaths
Falconer et al.[70]	2	12	2 (17)	0	10	0
Bellucci et al.[71]	3	11	4 (36)	0	6	1 abruptio placentae
Kaaja and Leinonen et al.[72]	2	10	3 (30)	0	6	1 intrauterine death
Beard et al.[73]	6	9	8 (89)	0	1	0
Randi et al.[74]	5	6	6 (100)	0	0	0
Millard et al.[75]	3	5	2 (40)	0	2	1 stillbirth

women with 15 pregnancies, live births were observed in 60% of cases, but the success rate increased to 100% in the seven cases treated with aspirin and subcutaneous heparin during pregnancy.[62] More recently, Bangerter et al.[63] retrospectively evaluated treatment and outcome of 17 pregnancies in nine consecutive ET patients observed between 1988 and 1998. Eleven (65%) pregnancies resulted in live birth and six (35%) ended in spontaneous abortion. Six women received low-dose aspirin during pregnancy; in five of these cases, this was followed by low molecular-weight heparin until the end of the sixth week postpartum. This treatment was correlated with a more favorable outcome (100% live births) compared with no treatment (45%, p = 0.04).

Maternal thrombotic or hemorrhagic complications are uncommon. Willoughby et al.[64] evaluated the outcome of 121 pregnancies; they reported that one patient had experienced a major postpartum haemorrhage, 5% had a minor hemorrhagic event, two had minor thrombotic events and three had major thrombotic events. However, a rate of major thrombotic events of 1–2% per year has been reported in nonpregnant patients with ET in this age group,[54] as has occasional severe hemorrhage (particularly when the platelet count is above $1000 \times 10^9/l$).

The platelet count generally shows a progressive decline during pregnancy in ET patients. This decrease seems to be greater than the reduction seen in normal pregnancies, which is due to an increase in blood volume. The mechanism is not known, but it could be related to placental or fetal production of a factor that downregulates platelet production.[65] In the postpartum period, the platelet count returns to the previous increased level and a rebound thrombocytosis may be observed in some patients. This increases the probability of vascular complications.[64]

Management

Antithrombotic drugs have been widely used in the management of pregnancy in ET. The rationale for their use comes from the evidence that placental infarction caused by thrombosis seems to be the most consistent pathological event. In general, there is an increased incidence of recurrent fetal loss in almost all congenital and acquired thrombophilic disorders.[66] Conceivably, the presence of a disease with a thrombotic diathesis may exacerbate the physiological prothrombotic and hypofibrinolytic state of normal pregnancy.

Aspirin

Among antithrombotic agents, aspirin seems the most advantageous, although the evidence for its efficacy is both retrospective and based on small numbers of patients.[59,63] Aspirin (75–100 mg once daily) should be started before pregnancy to facilitate placentation and fetal development. Bleeding complications are rare events. Particular attention should be paid to patients with platelet counts above $1000 \times 10^9/l$ since (as mentioned above) the risk of bleeding is higher and may be enhanced by aspirin. The drug should not be stopped before delivery because severe thrombotic events may occur in the postpartum period despite anticoagulation with heparin or warfarin after discontinuation of aspirin.[64]

Low molecular weight heparin

The successful use of low molecular weight heparins in other pregnancies in which there is a high risk of thrombosis[67] has drawn attention to the possibility of it being used in selected ET patients, such as those with previous thrombotic events or other associated thrombophilic conditions. Compared with unfractionated heparin, low molecular weight preparations have the advantages of a single daily administration and, possibly, a lower risk of heparin-induced thrombocytopenia and osteoporosis. A limited experience with the use of low molecular weight heparin (2500 anti-Xa units subcutaneously once daily) in five women with ET was encouraging.[63] The drug was started 1 week before labor and given for 6 weeks postpartum, with the dose immediately before delivery omitted. No thrombotic or drug-related complications were observed.

Myelosuppressive drugs

Myelosuppressive drugs to reduce the platelet count should preferably be avoided in pregnancy, particularly in the first trimester because:

- their safety is uncertain and none of the drugs has a product licence for use in pregnancy;
- the expected natural fall of the platelet count during pregnancy may reduce the need for cytoreduction;
- there is no demonstrated association between platelet count and the risk of complications of pregnancy.

However, the need for cytoreduction should be considered in selected high-risk situations such as previous or current thrombosis, major bleeding or a pregnancy complication that might have been caused by ET, and progressive rising of platelet count above $1500 \times 10^9/l$ while not on cytoreductive therapy.

If cytoreduction is given, interferon-α is probably the safest option.[68,69] There are no reports of teratogenic effects in animals or adverse effects in humans, but some evidence suggests that IFN-α may decrease fertility. The usual starting dose is 3 million IU daily, but the amount of drug required usually falls during pregnancy as the platelet count declines. Fever and flu-like symptoms are experienced by most patients and usually require contemporaneous administration of paracetamol. IFN-α was found to be associated with weakness, myalgia, weight loss, hair loss, severe depression and gastrointestinal and cardiovascular symptoms when given to non-pregnant patients in a recent review of 273 cases, and it was terminated in 25% of cases, owing to side effects.[58]

Hydroxyurea is best avoided at the time of conception and in pregnancy. While the outcome of a small number of pregnancies has been published – and these are mainly without fetal complications – one stillbirth and one malformed infant have been reported after exposure to hydroxyurea.[60] Teratogenicity in animals has also been reported.

Anagrelide is not recommended in women who are or may become pregnant.[57] This drug may cause fetal harm, including severe thrombocytopenia. Five women became pregnant while on anagrelide treatment at doses of 1–4 mg/day.[60] Treatment was stopped as soon as it was realized that they were pregnant and all delivered normal babies.

In conclusion, evidence-based recommendations for the most appropriate treatment of pregnancy in women with ET are limited, since only anedoctal data or retrospective studies are available, and clinical judgment for individual patient care must be based on scanty information in the literature.

REFERENCES

1. Mackie IJ, Donohoe S, Machin SJ. Lupus anticoagulant measurement. In: Khamashta MA, ed. *Hughes' Syndrome*. London: Springer; 2000:214–24.
2. Loizou S, McCrea JD, Rudge AC, *et al*. Measurement of anticardiolipin antibodies by an enzyme-linked immunosorbent assay: standardization and quantitation of results. *Clin Exp Immunol* 1985;**62**:739–44.
3. Galli M, Comfurius P, Maassen C, *et al*. Anticardiolipin antibodies (ACA) directed not to cardiolipin but to a plasma protein cofactor. *Lancet* 1990;**335**:1544–7.
4. Galli M, Comfurius P, Barbui T, *et al*. Anticoagulant activity of β2–glycoprotein I is potentiated by a distinct subgroup of anticardiolipin antibodies. *Thromb Haemost* 1992;**68**:297–300.
5. Galli M, Beretta G, Daldossi M, *et al*. Different anticoagulant and immunological properties of anti-prothrombin antibodies in patients with antiphospholipid antibodies. *Thromb Haemost* 1997;**77**:486–91.
6. Galli M, Non β2–glycoprotein I cofactors for antiphospholipid antibodies. *Lupus* 1996;**5**:388–92.
7. Wilson A, Gharavi AE, Koike T, *et al*. International consensus statement on preliminary classification criteria for definite antiphospholipid syndrome: report of an international workshop. *Arthritis Rheum* 1999;**42**:1309–11.

8. Asherson RA, Khamashta MA, Ordi-Ros J, *et al.* The 'primary' antiphospholipid syndrome: major clinical and serological features. *Medicine* 1989;**68**:366–74.

9. Alarcon-Segovia D, Deleze M, Oria CV, *et al.* Antiphospholipid antibodies and the antiphospholipid syndrome in systemic lupus erythematosus: a review of 500 consecutive cases. *Medicine* 1989;**68**:353–65.

10. Lockshin MD. Pregnancy loss and antiphospholipid antibodies. *Lupus* 1998;**7**:S86–S89.

11. Lynch A, Marlar R, Murphy J, *et al.* Antiphospholipid antibodies in predicting adverse pregnancy outcome. A prospective study. *Ann Intern Med* 1994;**120**:470–5.

12. Barbui T, Cortelazzo S, Galli M, *et al.* Antiphospholipid antibodies in early repeated abortions: a case-controlled study. *Fertil Steril* 1988;**50**:589–92.

13. Infante-Rivard C, David M, Gauthier R, Rivard GE. Lupus anticoagulant, anticardiolipin antibodies, and fetal loss. *N Engl J Med* 1991;**325**:1063–6.

14. Ginsberg JS, Brill-Edwards P, Johnston M, *et al.* Relationship of antiphospholipid antibodies to pregnancy loss in patients with systemic lupus erythematosus: a cross-sectional study. *Blood* 1992;**80**:975–80.

15. Gris JC, Quéré I, Sanmarco M, *et al.* Antiphospholipid and antiprotein syndromes in non-thrombotic, non-autoimmune women with unexplained recurrent primary early foetal loss. The Nimes Obstetricians and Haematologists Study – NOHA. *Thromb Haemost* 2000;**84**:228–36.

16. Balash J, Reverter JC, Creus M, *et al.* Human reproductive failure is not a clinical feature associated with β2-glycoprotein I antibodies in anticardiolipin and lupus anticoagulant seronegative patients (the antiphospholipid/cofactor syndrome). *Hum Reprod* 1999;**14**:1956–9.

17. Franklin RD, Hollier N, Kutteh WH, *et al.* β2-glycoprotein I as a marker of antiphospholipid syndrome in women with recurrent pregnancy loss. *Fertil Steril* 2000;**73**:531–5.

18. Nilsson IM, Astedt B, Hedner U, Berezin D. Intrauterine death and circulating anticoagulant ('antithromboplastin'). *Acta Med Scand* 1975;**197**:153–9.

19. De Wolf F, Carreras LO, Moerman P, *et al.* Decidual vasculopathy and extensive placental infarction in a patient with repeated thromboembolic accidents, recurrent fetal loss, and a lupus anticoagulant. *Am J Obstet Gynecol* 1982;**142**:829–34.

20. Out HJ, Kooijman CD, Bruinse HW, Derksen RH. Histopathological findings in placentae from patients with intra-uterine fetal death and antiphospholipid antibodies. *Eur J Obstet Gynecol Reprod Biol* 1991;**41**:179–86.

21. Blank M, Cohen J, Toder V, Shoenfeld Y. Induction of anti-phospholipid syndrome in naive mice with mouse lupus monoclonal and human polyclonal anti-cardiolipin antibodies. *Proc Natl Acad Sci USA* 1991;**88**:3069–73.

22. Bakimer R, Fishman P, Blank M, *et al.* Induction of primary antiphospholipid syndrome in mice by immunization with a human monoclonal anticardiolipin antibody (H-3). *J Clin Invest* 1992;**89**:1558–63.

23. Di Simone N, Meroni PL, Del Papa N, *et al.* Antiphospholipid antibodies affect trophoblast gonadotropin secretion and invasiveness by binding directly and through adhered β2-glycoprotein I. *Arthritis Rheum* 2000;**43**:140–50.

24. Di Simone N, Caliandro D, Castellani R, *et al.* Low-molecular weight heparin restores in-vitro trophoblast invasiveness and differentiation in presence of immunoglobulin G fractions obtained from patients with antiphospholipid syndrome. *Hum Reprod* 1999;**14**:489–95.

25. Di Simone N, Caliandro D, Castellani R, *et al.* Interleukin-3 and human trophoblast: in vitro explanations for the effect of interleukin in patients with antiphospholipid syndrome. *Fertil Steril* 2000;**73**:1194–2000.

26. Rai RS, Clifford K, Cohen H, Regan L. High prospective fetal loss rate in untreated pregnancies of women with recurrent miscarriage and antiphospholipid antibodies. *Hum Reprod* 1995;**10**:3301–4

27. Kutteh WH. Antiphospholipid antibody-associated recurrent pregnancy loss: treatment with heparin and low-dose aspirin is superior to low-dose aspirin alone. *Am J Obstet Gynecol* 1996;**174**:1584–9.

28. Rai R, Cohen H, Dave M, Regan L. Randomized controlled trial of aspirin and aspirin plus heparin in pregnant women with recurrent miscarriages associated with phospholipid antibodies (or antiphospholipid antibodies). *BMJ* 1997;**314**:253–7.

29. Backos M, Rai R, Baxter N, *et al.* Pregnancy complications in women with recurrent miscarriage associated with antiphospholipid antibodies treated with low dose heparin and aspirin. *Br J Obstet Gynaecol* 1999;**106**:102–7.

30. Backos M, Rai R, Thomas E, *et al*. Bone density changes in pregnant women treated with heparin: a prospective, longitudinal study. *Hum Reprod* 1999;**14**:2876–80.

31. Ruffatti A, Orsini A, Di Leonardo L, *et al*. A prospective study of fifty-three consecutive calcium heparin treated pregnancies in patients with antiphospholipid antibody-related fetal loss. *Clin Exp Rheum* 1997;**15**:499–504.

32. Ruffatti A, Dalla Barba B, Del Ross T, *et al*. Outcome of fifty-five newborns of antiphospholipid-positive mothers treated with calcium heparin during pregnancy. *Clin Exp Rheum* 1998;**16**:605–10.

33. Rai R. Obstetric management of antiphospholipid syndrome. *J Autoimmun* 2000;**15**:203–7.

34. Lubbe WF, Butler WS, Palmer SJ, Liggins GC. Fetal survival after prednisone suppression of maternal lupus-anticoagulant. *Lancet* 1983;**i**:1361–3.

35. Cowchock FS, Reece EA, Balaban D, *et al*. Repeated fetal losses associated with antiphospholipid antibodies: a collaborative randomized trial comparing prednisone with low-dose heparin treatment. *Am J Obstet Gynecol* 1992;**166**:1318–23.

36. Silver RK, McGregor SN, Sholl JS, *et al*. Comparative trial of prednisone plus aspirin versus aspirin alone in the treatment of anticardiolipin-positive obstetric patients. *Am J Obstet Gynecol* 1993;**169**:1411–17.

37. Lockshin MD, Druzin Ml, Qamar T. Prednisone does not prevent recurrent fetal death in women with antiphospholipid antibody. *Am J Obstet Gynecol* 1989;**160**:439–43.

38. Laskin CA, Bombardier C, Hannah ME, *et al*. Prednisone and aspirin in women with autoantibodies and unexplained recurrent fetal loss. *N Engl J Med* 1997;**337**:148–53.

39. Branch DW, Peaceman AM, Druzin M, *et al*. A multicenter, placebo-controlled pilot study of intravenous immune globulin treatment of antiphospholipid syndrome during pregnancy. *Am J Obstet Gynecol* 2000;**182**:122–7.

40. Daya S, Gunby J, Porter F, *et al*. Critical analysis of intravenous immunoglobulin therapy for recurrent miscarriage. *Hum Reprod Update* 1999;**5**:475–82.

41. Udoff LC, Branch DW. Management of patients with antiphospholipid antibodies undergoing *in vitro* fertilization. *J Autoimmun* 2000;**15**:209–11.

42. Homstein MD, Davis OK, Massey JB, *et al*. Antiphospholipid antibodies and in vitro fertilization success: a meta-analysis. *Fertil Steril* 2000;**73**:330–3.

43. Petri M, Robinson C. Oral contraceptives and systemic lupus erythematosus. *Arthritis Rheum* 1997;**40**:797–803.

44. Arden NK, Lloyd ME, Spector TD, Hughes GRV. Safety of hormone replacment therapy (HRT) in systemic lupus erythematosus. *Lupus* 1994;**3**:11–13.

45. Barbui T, Finazzi G. Thrombocytosis. In: Loscalzo J, Schafer AL, eds.*Thrombosis and Hemorrhage*, 2nd ed. Baltimore:Williams and Wilkins; 1998:665–79.

46. Murphy S, Peterson P, Iland H, *et al*. Experience of the Polycythemia Vera Study Group with essential thrombocythemia: a final report on diagnostic criteria, survival, and leukemic transition by treatment. *Semin Hematol* 1997;**34**:29–39.

47. Pearson TC. Diagnosis and classification of erythrocytosis and thrombocytosis. In: Green AR, Pearson TC, eds. *Myeloproliferative Disorders. Baillieres Clin Haematol* 1998;**11**:695–720.

48. Barbui T, Finazzi G. Management of essential thrombocythemia. *Crit Rev Oncol Hematol* 1999;**29**:257–66.

49. Cortelazzo S, Viero P, Finazzi G, *et al*. Incidence and risk factors for thrombotic complications in a historical cohort of 100 patients with essential thrombocythemia. *J Clin Oncol* 1990;**8**:556–62.

50. Finazzi G, Budde U, Michiels JJ. Bleeding time and platelet function in essential thrombocythemia and other myeloproliferative syndromes. *Leuk Lymphoma* 1996;**22 (suppl 1)**:71–78.

51. Van Genderen PJJ, Michiels JJ, van der Poel-van de Luytgaarde SCPAM, *et al*. Acquired von Willebrand disease as a cause of recurrent mucocutaneous bleeding in primary thrombocythemia: relationship with platelet count. *Ann Hematol* 1994;**69**:81–4.

52. Tefferi A. Risk-based management in essential thrombocytemia. In: *Hematology*. ASH Education Program Book; 1999:172–7.

53. Ruggeri M, Finazzi G, Tosetto A, *et al*. No treatment for low-risk essential thrombocythemia: results from a prospective study. *Br J Haematol* 1998;**103**:772–7.

54. Cortelazzo S, Finazzi G, Ruggeri M, *et al*. Hydroxyurea for patients with essential thrombocythemia and a high risk of thrombosis. *N Engl J Med* 1995;**332**:1132–6.

55. Finazzi G, Barbui T. Treatment of essential thrombocythemia with special emphasis on leukemogenic risk. *Ann Hematol* 1999;**78**:389–92.

56. Finazzi G, Ruggeri M, Rodeghiero F, *et al*. Second malignancies in patients with essential thrombocythemia treated with busulfan and hydroxyurea: long-term follow-up of a randomized clinical trial. *Br J Haematol* 2000;**110**:577–83.

57. Tefferi A, Silverstein MN, Petitt RM, *et al*. Anagrelide as a new platelet-lowering agent in essential thrombocythemia: mechanism of action, efficacy, toxicity, current indication. *Semin Thromb Haemost* 1997;**23**:379–84.

58. Lengfelder E, Griesshammer M, Hehlmann R. Interferon-alpha in the treatment of essential thrombocythemia. *Leuk Lymphoma* 1996;**22 (suppl 1)**:135–42.

59. Griesshammer M, Heimpel H, Pearson TC. Essential thrombocythaemia and pregnancy. *Leuk Lymphoma* 1996;**22 (suppl 1)**:57–63.

60. Griesshammer M, Bergmann L, Pearson T. Fertility, pregnancy and the management of myeloproliferative disorders. In: Green AR, Pearson TC, eds. *Myeloproliferative Disorders. Baillieres Clin Haematol* 1998;**11**:859–74.

61. Beressi AH, Tefferi A, Silverstein MN, *et al*. Outcome analysis of 34 pregnancies in women with essential thrombocythemia. *Arch Intern Med* 1995;**155**:1217–22.

62. Pagliaro P, Arrigoni L, Muggiasca ML, *et al*. Primary thrombocythemia and pregnancy. Treatment and outcome in fifteen cases. *Am J Hematol* 1996;**53**:6–10.

63. Bangerter M, Guthner C, Beneke H, *et al*. Pregnancy in essential thrombocythemia: treatment and outcome of 17 pregancies. *Eur J Hematol* 2000;**65**:165–9.

64. Willoughby SJB, Fairhead S, Woodcock BE, *et al*. Postpartum thrombosis in primary thrombocythemia. *Eur J Haematol* 1997;**59**:121–3.

65. Jones E, Mosesson M, Thomason J, *et al*. Essential thrombocythaemia in pregnancy. *Obstet Gynecol* 1988;**71**:501–3.

66. Brenner B. Inherited thrombophilia and pregnancy loss. *Thromb Haemost* 1999;**82**:634–40.

67. Brenner B, Hoffman R, Blumenfeld Z, *et al*. Gestational outcome in thrombophilic women with recurrent pregnancy loss by enoxaparin. *Thromb Haemost* 2000;**83**:693–7.

68. Spilberg O, Shimon I, Sofer O, *et al*. Transient normal platelet count and decreased requirement for interferon during pregnancy in essential thrombocythemia. *Br J Haematol* 1996;**92**:491–3.

69. Delage R, Demers C, Cantin G, *et al*. Treatment of essential thrombocythemia during pregnancy with Interferon-α. *Obstet Gynecol* 1996;**87**:814–17.

70. Falconer J, Pineo G, Blahey W, *et al*. Essential thrombocythemia associated with recurrent abortions and fetal growth retardation. *Am J Hematol* 1987;**25**:347.

71. Bellucci S, Janvier M, Tobelem G, *et al*. Essential thrombocythemia. Clinical evolutionary and biological data. *Cancer* 1986;**58**:2440–7.

72. Kaaja RJ, Leinonen PJ. Successful pregnancies after recurrent abortions in mild essential thrombocythemia. *Acta Obstet Gynecol Scand* 1998;**77**:1022–3.

73. Beard J, Hillmen P, Anderson CC, *et al*. Primary thrombocythemia in pregnancy. *Br J Haematol* 1991;**77**:371–4.

74. Randi ML, Barbone E, Rossi C, *et al*. Essential thrombocythemia and pregnancy: a report of six normal pregnancies in five untreated patients. *Obstet Gynecol* 1994;**83**:915–17.

75. Millard FE, Hunter CS, Anderson M, *et al*. Clinical manifestations of essential thrombocythemia in young adults. *Am J Hematol* 1990;**33**:27–31

7

Gene targeting of coagulation factors and embryogenesis

Hartmut Weiler and Berend Isermann

INTRODUCTION

The advent of gene targeting technology has made it feasible to alter, in a precisely controlled fashion, the function of specific genes in complex model organisms such as laboratory mice. Gene targeting allows the achievement of a complete loss (or 'knockout') of gene function, and the study of the physiological consequences of the mutation in an intact animal. Over the past decade, the gene knock-out approach has been used in mice to ablate the genes for almost all currently known coagulation factors, fibrinolytic enzymes, and regulators of coagulation and fibrinolysis, resulting in a generation of knockout mice with precisely defined defects in the hemostatic mechanism. Such a complete absence of function and antigen expression is extremely rare in humans – or, as is the case for most factors, has not been observed at all. Many genetically altered mice constitute animal models for hemostatic disorders associated with bleeding or thrombosis.

The analysis of knockout mice has led to the recognition that some, but not all, coagulation factors control critical processes during embryonic development. This observation is the focus of this chapter, which reviews the phenotypic consequences of disruption of individual hemostatic components and also discusses those knockout models that exhibit defects in embryonic hemostasis, blood vessel development, and placental function.

Figure 7.1 gives an overview of the consequences of factor deficiency on the *in utero* survival of completely factor-deficient knockout mice. In each case, the mother is a heterozygous carrier of the knockout mutation, and factor levels in the maternal blood are correspondingly reduced compared with those of a normal mouse. The completely factor-deficient embryos originate from mating heterozygous parents. Heterozygous deficiency of any of the factors does not compromise fertility or reproductive performance.

This survey reveals several interesting facts.

First, the earliest defects observed in any of the knockout models do not occur before approximately day 8 after fertilization. This developmental stage in mice is approximately equivalent to the second to third week of pregnancy in humans. Thus, it appears that complete factor deficiency of the embryo (or a heterozygous defect in the parents) does not interfere with the initial successful establishment of pregnancy and implantation.

Secondly, disruption of the hemostatic mechanism by complete elimination of embryonic platelets[1] or fibrinogen[2] is entirely compatible with development of the fetus to term and birth. Therefore, a defect in the formation of a fibrin–platelet aggregate as the putative physiological endpoint of hemostasis does not interfere with embryogenesis. However, fibrinogen deficiency is incompatible with female reproduction, and mice

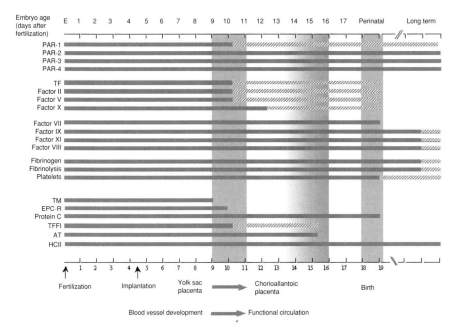

Figure 7.1 Survival of knock-out mice with coagulation factor deficiency. The intrauterine survival of knockout mice that lack the components indicated on the left is plotted over time. The embryonic age in days (E1–E18) denotes the elapsed time after fertilization. Critical developmental hallmarks are given at the bottom of the figure: implantation of the blastocyst in the uterus takes place around 4.5 days after fertilization. Birth occurs between 17.5 and 19.5 days after fertilization. Time windows underlaid in grey highlight stages in development during which the absence of coagulation factors or regulators causes embryonic death. Solid bars indicate normal survival, hatched bars denote partial survival.

that lack platelets or fibrinogen suffer from serious bleeding complications.

Thirdly, neither plasminogen nor the plasmin-generating fibrinolytic enzymes tissue-type plasminogen activator (tPA) and urokinase-type plasmingen activator (uPA) perform an essential function during mouse embryogenesis.[3,4] Mice with a disabled fibrinolytic system experience thrombosis in later life.

Fourthly, the abrogation of factors that regulate the initiation and maintenance of coagulation has rather divergent effects. Inactivation of the gene encoding tissue factor (TF) causes fatal developmental defects. In contrast, the only known genuine ligand for TF, factor VII, appears dispensable for proper intrauterine growth and development. About half of the knockout embryos that lack factors X or V or prothrombin (factor II) die in early mid-gestation. The remaining factor-deficient embryos survive to birth

without obvious developmental defects, yet succumb to fatal bleeding in early life. On the other hand, complete deficiency of factors VII,[5] VIII[6] (hemophilia A), IX[7] (hemophilia B), or XI,[8] does not affect embryogenesis but does cause bleeding of variable severity after birth. Thus, the inability to assemble the thrombin-generating prothrombinase complex of factor Va and Xa, as well as the elimination of prothrombin, its substrate, has much more severe consequences than the functional inactivation of the other factors of the common coagulation pathway.

Fifthly, disruption of natural anticoagulant mechanisms has severe consequences on intrauterine survival. Elimination of the genes that encode tissue factor pathway inhibitor (TFPI) or antithrombin, or disruption of the protein C-dependent anticoagulant pathway results in intrauterine death or a fatal thrombotic diathesis at birth. However, the phenotypic manifestation of mutations in anticoagulant pathways – the time of death – and the cause of developmental failure vary substantially in each of these knockout models.

DEFICIENCIES THAT CAUSE FAILURE OF INTRAUTERINE DEVELOPMENT

Defects in mouse embryos that lack a functional TF gene[9–11] become evident 9–10 days after fertilization and may cause embryonic death before 11.5 days. Embryos that completely lack TF (TF–/– or TF-null embryos) appear bloodless, small, and necrotic. Large, extravascular pools of blood accumulate in the yolk sac cavity, suggesting that the primary cause of death is a massive hemorrhagic event in the vasculature of the yolk sac that drains the embryonic circulatory system of blood. Occasionally, similar hemorraghic blood pools are seen in the pericardium. Yolk sac hemorrhage is associated with abnormalities in the vascular architecture of the yolk sac, such as the absence of large vitelline vessels, a comparably irregular plexus of enlarged capillaries, and a paucity of perivascular mesenchymal cells in the vascular wall. The severity of the defects seen in TF–/– embryos is strongly influenced by additional genes that vary between different strains of laboratory mice. Indeed, if the C57Bl/6 mouse strain is used for the analysis of TF knockout mice, a small fraction of TF–/– embryos survive to birth without signs of intrauterine hemorrhage or vascular abnormalities, although these TF–/– mice do experience severe hemorrhage in early life.

Curiously, disruption of the TFPI-gene has consequences that are almost identical to those of the elimination of the TF gene.[12] The majority of TFPI knockout embryos die between 9.5 and 10.5 days after fertilization. Just like TF-deficient mice, the embryos that lack TFPI exhibit pools of free blood in the yolk sac cavity and the pericardial sac and have histological abnormalities in the architecture of the blood vessels of the yolk sac. As with TF knockout mice, some of the TFPI–/– mice manage to escape early embryonic death. However, most TFPI–/– mice that survive beyond 10.5 days after fertilization exhibit severe bleeding later on (because of a consumptive coagulopathy) and do not survive to birth.

Bearing in mind that initiation of coagulation requires formation of a complex between TF and factor VIIa, it is surprising that mice devoid of factor VII develop normally.[5] In striking contrast to the severe developmental defects seen in TF–/– mice, there is no intrauterine loss of factor VII-deficient animals, the vasculature is well developed and functional, and 100% of knockout animals survive to birth. Seventy percent of factor VII-null newborn mice succumb to fatal intra-abdominal bleeding within 24 hours after birth, and the remaining animals die before reaching an age of 4 weeks.

The absence of coagulation factor V leads to a partial block of intrauterine development that occurs in early mid-gestation (days 9–10 after fertilization).[13] Approximately half of the mutant embryos somehow bypass this developmental bottleneck but then die from massive neonatal hemorrhage within hours after birth. Those mutant mice that fail to progress through normal development are already lagging behind in their developmental progress by 9.5 days after fertilization and exhibit abnormalities in the architecture of the yolk sac vasculature that resemble, to some extent, the defects seen in TF-deficient mice. However, whereas TF-deficient mice suffer from massive yolk sac hemorrhage, no bleeding or loss of vascular integrity in the yolk sac was seen in factor V-null mice.

The phenotype of mice that lack prothrombin closely resembles the pathology seen in TF and TFPI knockout mice.[14,15] At 9–10 days after fertilization, a significant portion of prothrombin-null mice are delayed or arrested in development and appear pale. Both bleeding into the yolk sac cavity and abnormal vascular architecture of the yolk sac have been described in prothrombin –/– mice, but these defects do not necessarily seem to occur together or at the same time: one research group observed the same vascular abnormalities as described in TF–/– mice but no bleeding.[14] In an independent study, hemorrhage into the yolk sac cavity was seen, yet vascular morphology was described as unremarkable.[15] As with other embryonic lethal factor deficiencies, a fraction of prothrombin–/– mice manage to escape early death. Depending on the specific mouse strain used for these experiments, these 'survivors' either die later in gestation or are born – yet again, live-born prothrombin-deficient mice develop fatal hemorrhagic events and die within a few days of birth.

Total deficiency of the blood coagulation factor X causes mid-gestation embryonic death (between 11.5 and 12.5 days after fertilization) in about one-third of mutant embryos.[16] The remaining embryos survive to birth without any evident complications. The majority of live-born factor X–/– mice develop fatal intra-abdominal, subcutaneous, and intracranial hemorrhage within the first 3 weeks after birth. Both the time of death and the phenotypically observable anomalies in factor X–/– mice differ from those seen in animals that lack TF, TFPI, factor V, factor II, or the thrombin receptor protease-activated receptor 1 (PAR-1). First, in mice lacking these factors, grossly observable defects are clearly already present at 9.5 days after fertilization, while factor X-deficient mice appear normal at that time. Secondly, the integrity of the yolk sac vasculature seems largely preserved in factor X–/– mice, although there is evidence for severe hemorrhage into brain ventricles. However, it has not yet been determined if the rapid death and resorption of mutant embryos is caused by fulminant failure of the placental circulation.

In mice, the thrombin receptor PAR-1 is not essential for thrombin-mediated platelet activation, but it conveys thrombin-dependent signaling events in a variety of cell types, including endothelial cells and fibroblasts. Disruption of the PAR-1 gene[17] causes a developmental defect that kills roughly half of the mutant embryos, whereas the other half survives to term. Early in embryogenesis (at 9 days after fertilization) virtually all PAR-1 knockout mice show a delay in overall growth and developmental progress; these delays affect both the embryo proper and the extraembryonic tissues that form the early placenta. The condition of half of the mutant embryos deteriorates rapidly after this, leading to a total arrest of growth, a cessation of the heart beat, and abortion. However, the remaining PAR-1–/– mice seem to recover completely from this early challenge, resume normal

growth by 11.5 days after fertilization, and develop into grossly normal adult mice. Neither hemorrhage nor vascular abnormalities has been described for PAR-1 knockout mice.

Abrogation of antithrombin function causes embryonic lethality in late mid-gestation, between 15 and 16 days after fertilization.[18] In contrast to mice with the coagulation factor deficiencies discussed above, the penetrance of the lethal phenotype is complete, and no antithrombin–/– mice survive to term. The defects in these animals include widespread tissue necrosis associated with fibrin deposition in the heart and liver, as well as severe subcutaneous and intracranial hemorrhage. These anomalies were attributed to a severe consumptive coagulopathy resulting from uncontrolled activity of the coagulation system.[18]

Gene targeting has been used to disrupt two different components of the protein C anticoagulant pathway – protein C itself and thrombomodulin (TM), the essential cofactor for the activation of protein C. Mice that lack protein C survive to term and are born alive, but they exhibit a severe and fatal consumptive coagulopathy at birth.[19] Although protein C deficiency does not cause embryonic death, early signs of thrombosis, such as focal tissue necrosis and hemorrhage, are already evident *in utero* around 12.5 days after fertilization and then increase in severity until birth. Ablation of the TM gene has much more severe consequences on fetal development than protein C deficiency. TM–/– mice uniformly succumb to a complete early mid-gestation growth arrest (at 8.5 days after fertilization), followed by the rapid resorption of all mutant embryos within 24 hours.[20] This early time of developmental failure precedes the occurrence of defects in all other knockout models in which the hemostatic system function is affected, and indeed it occurs before the establishment of a functional vascular system within the embryo. The growth arrest and abortion of TM–/– mice is caused by a failure of placental trophoblast function, since the development of TM–/– mice proceeds normally as long as TM expression is selectively maintained only in this particular cell type.[21] However, these mice with partially restored TM function succumb to a lethal consumptive coagulopathy. Assuming that the developmental function of TM does indeed involve the activation of protein C, the discrepancy between the phenotype of mice that lack either protein C or TM might reflect the fact that protein C produced by the (heterozygous, protein C-deficient) mother is readily available for interaction with TM expressed on placental surfaces that are exposed to maternal blood. On the other hand, TM, a transmembrane molecule, cannot be supplied via the mother's blood. Later on, within the embryonic vasculature, the absence of either embryonic protein C or TM has almost identical consequences. The secondary coagulopathy in TM- or protein C-deficient mice is easily explained by the loss of anticoagulant function of the protein C pathway, and indeed it occurs roughly at the same time (12.5 days after fertilization) in both knockout models. However, the absence of TM from the placental trophoblast does not seem to cause placental thrombosis, and the mechanism that underlies the arrest in embryonic growth remains to be clarified (see below).

DEVELOPMENTAL FAILURE DUE TO LOSS OF INTEGRITY OF THE YOLK SAC VASCULATURE

The developmental abnormalities in embryos that lack TF, TFPI, prothrombin, and factor V all occur roughly at the same time (9–10 days after fertilization) and seem to affect primarily the functional integrity of the yolk sac vasculature. The consequences of prothrombin and TF deficiency are virtually identical, suggesting that TF-mediated generation of proteolytically active thrombin is required for proper function of the yolk sac circulation. Deficiency of at least one other critical factor required for thrombin generation, factor V, produces a similar, albeit not identical, phenotype. While there is pronounced yolk sac hemorrhage in mice that lack TF or TFPI, bleeding is not necessarily associated with prothrombin deficiency and is absent in factor V–/– mice. The similar phenotype of mice carrying these mutations suggests that they affect a common pathway of thrombin generation, that is congruent with their well-established function in the context of the coagulation reaction (see Figure 7.2).

Thus, although thrombin formation seems necessary for establishment or maintenance of vascular integrity (or both), its function may not be limited to preventing fatal blood loss. Indeed, the embryonic defects in mice that lack the thrombin receptor PAR-1 are not accompanied by bleeding; nevertheless they result in developmental arrest. Assuming that thrombin is indeed the physiologically relevant activator of PAR-1, one may conclude that the generation of thrombin and its subsequent action on PAR-1 regulate a critical process in development. The divergent consequences of disrupting either thrombin-generation or its interaction with PAR-1 suggest that the thrombin-generating pathway affects developmental processes through multiple mechanisms, including hemostasis and initiation of cellular signaling events by activated coagulation proteases. The actual chain of events that leads to the death of affected embryos remains somewhat unclear. For example, lethal hemorrhage could be caused by a failure to establish vascular integrity secondary to abnormalities in blood vessel development, but the loss of vascular integrity could also be triggered by hemostatic failure.

The elucidation of the specific mechanisms and their interactions with developmental processes are an area of ongoing research. A number of questions are being addressed:

- What is the precise mechanism by which coagulation activation preserves vascular function?
- Why does elimination of the blood clotting inhibitor TFPI produce the same consequences as elimination of its target, TF (the initiator of blood clotting)?
- Why are mice that lack factor X or factor VII spared from the developmental disasters that occur at mid-gestation in the other mouse models?
- What allows at least some of the mice that lack prothrombin, TF, factor V, or PAR-1 to complete embryogenesis successfully?

One possible explanation for the lack of developmental defects in factor X knockout mice or factor VII knockout mice might be derived from

Contact activation pathway   **Extrinsic pathway**

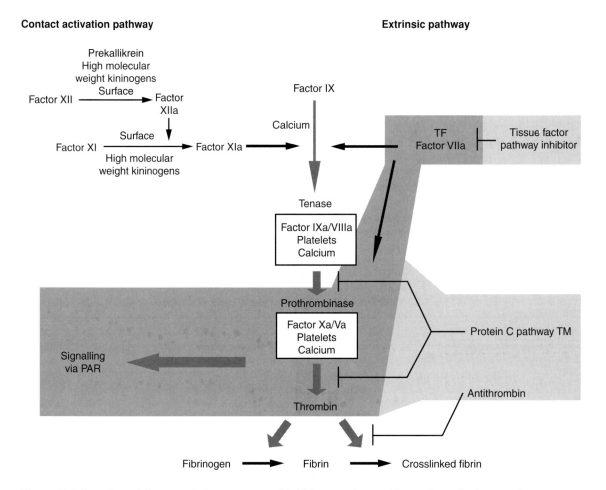

Figure 7.2 Overview of the coagulation system and inhibitory pathways. Tissue factor is the membrane-associated initiator of blood clotting. In normal circumstances, TF is not present on cells in contact with blood, such as blood vessel endothelium. Coagulation is triggered by loss of the endothelial barrier between bloodborne factor VII and cells that express tissue factor. The ensuing formation of proteolytically active TF-factor VIIa complexes results in activation of coagulation factors IX and X, thereby initiating localized thrombin generation. TFPI regulates the proteolytic activity of the TF-factor VIIa complex via formation of a ternary complex between TF, factor VIIa, factor Xa, and TFPI. The inhibitory action of TFPI depends on the presence of activated factor X. This mechanism allows only for a short-lived triggering of the coagulation cascade that effects an initial burst of thrombin generation. The subsequent amplification and maintenance of thrombin production occurs in a TF-independent manner via the Tenase-complex (composed of calcium ions, phospholipid, factor IXa, and factor VIIIa) and prothrombinase complex (composed of calcium ions, phospholipid, factor Va, and factor Xa). The activity of the coagulation system is balanced by various natural anticoagulant mechanisms, including antithrombin and the protein C pathway. Antithrombin is a circulating proteinase inhibitor that forms complexes in a heparin-dependent manner with several activated coagulation factors, most importantly factor Xa and thrombin; these coagulation factors are inactivated upon formation of the complexes with antithrombin. The protein C pathway is initiated by the formation of a complex between thrombin and endothelial membrane-bound TM. TM-associated thrombin converts circulating protein C into enzymatically active protein C, which then, together with the non-enzymatic cofactor protein S proteolytically, degrades activated coagulation factors Va and VIIIa. Destruction of these key components of the thrombin generating tenase and prothrombinase complexes causes a downregulation of thrombin production. Pathways that are presumed to be critical for embryonic development are highlighted in grey.

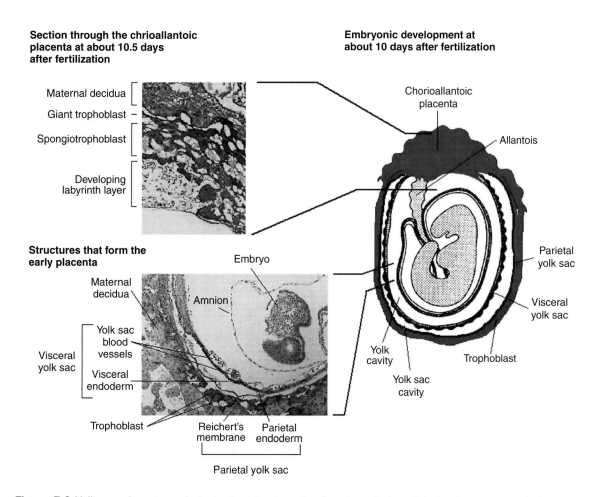

Figure 7.3 Yolk sac placenta and chorioallantoic placenta. Overview of placental structures present between 8.5 and 10 days after fertilization. The term 'yolk sac placenta' denotes the early placental structures that mediate exchange of nutrients and metabolites between mother and fetus until the chorioallantoic placenta is completely established. The early yolk sac placenta consists of an outer trophoblast layer apposed to a thick extracellular membrane (Reichert's membrane) that is produced by underlying parietal endoderm cells. These layers constitute the maternal aspect of the yolk sac cavity, which is bordered on the fetal aspect by the yolk sac membranes. These consist of visceral endoderm, a secretory–resorptive epithelium with liver-like function, and, attached to the fetal aspect of the visceral endoderm, the mesenchyme containing the yolk sac vasculature. The yolk sac is separated from the amnion that surrounds the embryo by the yolk cavity. The chorioallantoic or (definite) placenta is formed where the embryonic allantois contacts the chorionic plate (at about 8.75 days after fertilization). It is established by proliferation and differentiation of specialized embryonic trophoblast populations, by invasion of these trophoblast layers by fetal blood vessels originating from the allantois, and by remodeling of maternal blood vessel in contact with the trophoblast. During this process, maternal blood vessels become discontinuous, and the mother's blood is in direct contact with trophoblast cells, in close proximity to the outer aspect of fetal blood vessels. The formation of the chorioallantoic placenta as a major route of exchange between maternal blood and embryonic blood vessels occurs between 8.5 and 11.5 days after fertilization.

the fact that the levels of most coagulation factors produced by the embryo are substantially lower than those in adult mice,[22] yet they are sufficient to maintain embryonic hemostasis. Conceivably, even trace amounts of some factors that might be transferred from the mother[5] to the embryo might suffice to compensate for the lack of factor production in the embryo. The low abundance of clotting factors in the embryo might also explain why a lack of TFPI produces the same effect than the lack of TF: in the absence of TFPI, unfettered TF-initiated thrombin formation might rapidly deplete the limiting amount of prothrombin, thus reproducing the effect of prothrombin deficiency. Indeed, combined deficiency of factor VII and TFPI cures the developmental defect seen in TFPI−/− mice.[22] However, the same study raises concerns about the validity of the 'maternal transfer concept' to explain the lack of developmental defects in factor VII knockout mice.

It is a common theme in all of these knockout models that developmental defects occur only in a subpopulation of factor-deficient mice. Partial lethality might arise from a stochastic (or 'chance') compensatory process that could, for example, reflect the efficiency of maternal factor transfer. Alternatively, functional defects in the yolk sac circulation might be compensated to some extent by perfusion via the chorioallantoic placenta, which provides an alternative route for nutrient supply to the embryo. Establishment of the chorioallantoic placenta occurs between 9.5 and 10.5 days after fertilization, and slight variations in the timing of this process could lead to the rescue of some of the factor-deficient embryos. The variable survival of factor-deficient mice clearly has a genetic component, since the fraction of surviving animals varies depending on the genetic composition of the mouse strain. Characterization of these genetic traits will probably identify additional genes that interact with the physiological pathway that maintains vascular function in the yolk sac.

Regardless of the precise mechanism and the details of coagulation factor function in early mouse embryogenesis, the results from the knockout studies suggest that deficiency of TF, TFPI and factors II, V, and X is incompatible with

proper development of the fetus. Despite certain differences in embryology between mice and humans, a functional yolk sac vascular plexus is also formed during human embryogenesis. Since a complete lack of the above critical factors has never been observed in humans, their critical developmental function may have been conserved in evolution. The above studies highlight the notion that activation of the coagulation system not only results in the formation of a blood clot but also elicits cellular responses via engagement of receptors that sense the presence of activated coagulation factors. It seems safe to predict that the insights gained from the study of the developmental function of coagulation factors will also shed light on their role in vascular function during physiological and pathophysiological hemostasis and thrombosis.

DEFICIENCIES THAT AFFECT PLACENTAL FUNCTION

A body of evidence suggests that activation of the blood coagulation system is precisely controlled during pregnancy in order to maintain placental function as a prerequisite for fetal health and to minimize the risk of pregnancy-associated thrombotic complications for the mother. Both humans and mice exhibit a similar type of placentation (hemochorial placentation), which results in the direct contact of maternal blood with the surface of embryonic trophoblast cells.[23] (For a summary of placental development, see Figure 7.3.) Maintenance of the hemostatic balance in the microenvironment of the fetal–maternal interface requires the interaction of regulatory molecules that are expressed on the embryonic trophoblast surface with coagulation factors that are supplied via the mother's blood. The analysis of mice that lack the coagulation components TF, fibrinogen, and TM has revealed that this interplay between fetal and maternal hemostasis is critical for a successful outcome to a pregnancy. This section briefly describes the anomalies that occur in the placenta of mice with altered function of TF, fibrinogen, or TM.

Afibrinogenemia – the complete lack of fibrinogen – does not impair mouse embryogenesis, but it does cause bleeding complications of varying severity in later life, sometimes with fatal consequences.[2] Fibrinogen-deficient mice are fertile, but pregnancy has fatal consequences for the female mice – about 10 days after fertilization, such mice exhibit severe and ultimately fatal placental hemorrhage. The onset of these complications coincides with critical physiological alterations of the placental vasculature that result in a loss of blood vessel integrity. Under the influence of growth factors such as vascular endothelial growth factor, maternal blood vessels in the decidua are expanded and remodeled, resulting in the formation of large blood sinuses in close proximity to the embryonic trophoblast. Eventually, the embryonic trophoblast invades the maternal blood vessel, breaching the integrity of the maternal endothelial lining and establishing direct contact with maternal blood.[23,24] While a normal mouse manages to avoid severe blood loss at this stage of pregnancy, afibrinogenemic mice with a disabled hemostatic mechanism are unable to contain the ensuing bleeding. It is of note that placental defects associated with hemorrhage also occur in mice that lack the β3-integrin constituting part of the platelet fibrinogen receptor. These mice also show anomalies in the architecture of the labyrinth layer of the placenta, including necrosis and narrowing of vascular spaces; these anomalies lead to the death of the fetus.[25]

As described above, the complete absence of TF disrupts the establishment or maintenance of vascular integrity in the mouse yolk sac circulation. This defect can be corrected by expression of a transgenic tissue factor 'minigene' that encodes human TF. The procoagulant potency of the TF transgene is only about 1% of that conveyed by the normal mouse TF gene product, but this low activity suffices to compensate for the absence of the endogenous mouse TF.[26] Despite the rescue from early death, 'low TF' mice exhibit two distinct types of placental defects at later developmental stages. First, about half of the 'low TF' females succumb to a fatal mid-gestation hemorrhage, but only if the mother was carrying offspring that are similarly deficient in TF expression. Analysis of placentae formed by a 'low TF' embryo in a 'low

TF' mother shows structural abnormalities in the labyrinth trophoblast layer, enlarged maternal blood lacunae, free blood pools, and placental hemorrhage. These results suggest that placental hemostasis is co-ordinately and co-operatively regulated by both maternal and embryonic TF. The second defect manifests itself as fatal postpartum uterine bleeding in 'low TF' females. In contrast to mid-gestation hemorrhage, postpartum death occurs regardless of whether the embryo expresses normal levels of TF. This finding demonstrates that normal levels of TF expression in the maternal decidua and uterine epithelium are required (and sufficient) to prevent the massive hemorrhage associated with parturition. The cause–effect relationship between structural abnormalities in the placenta, and the mechanism of TF function in this context are still under investigation. It is not clear whether the role of TF in the above processes is limited to the initiation of coagulation or whether it involves some additional pathway such as the regulation of cell–cell interaction, cellular adhesion, or factor VII-dependent cell signaling.

Experiments testing the interaction of fibrinogen, TF, and TM suggest that the placental and developmental defects seen in mice that lack these factors are difficult to explain solely in the context of hemostasis (authors' observations).

In order to determine if the death and resorption of TM-deficient mice can be prevented by inhibition of thrombosis, pregnant females carrying TM–/– embryos were anticoagulated with heparin. Surprisingly, heparin anticoagulation completely blocked the rapid resorption of TM knockout embryos, but it did not prevent the growth arrest of mutant mice. Exactly the same effect was observed if the TM-deficient mice were carried by a mother that lacked fibrinogen or by a 'low TF' female (the embryo itself expressing fibrinogen and TF). In each case, resorption was blocked, but the arrest of growth persisted. This observation indicates that the formation of fibrin at the fetal–maternal interface, via TF-initiated thrombin generation, mediates the resorptive process that accompanies early mid-gestation abortion, but not the growth arrest of TM knockout mice. Carrying these experiments one step further, embryos that are 'low TF' and simultaneously TM-deficient were generated by crossbreeding. The reduced TF expression by the embryonic trophoblast was sufficient to prevent both the resorption and the growth arrest of TM−/− mice. On the other hand, the absence of TM did not prevent the mid-gestation defects caused by reduced expression of TF. This non-reciprocal complementation of defects in mice that lack both TM (which inhibits blood coagulation) and TF (which initiates blood clotting) provides a convincing argument in favor of a non-hemostatic role for TF.

Future results from investigations into the precise mechanism of action of these hemostatic regulators are very likely to highlight a link between altered hemostasis or thrombophilia and adverse pregnancy outcome. The current concept focuses on placental blood vessel thrombosis, which is thought to cause perfusion insufficiency, intrauterine growth retardation, placental rupture, and, in extreme cases, fetal wastage. The analysis of mouse knockout models strongly suggests that dysregulation of the blood coagulation mechanism at the fetal–maternal interface compromises placental development and induces the resorption of embryos through mechanisms that are distinct from vascular thrombosis. It will be interesting to explore if placental growth and function are indeed modulated by the engagement of protease-activated receptor systems that sense the excessive generation of activated coagulation factors.

REFERENCES

1. Shivdasani RA, Rosenblatt MF, Zucker-Franklin D, et al. Transcription factor NF-E2 is required for platelet formation independent of the actions of thrombopoietin/MGDF in megakaryocyte development. Cell 1995;**81**:695–704.
2. Suh TT, Holmback K, Jensen NJ, et al. Resolution of spontaneous bleeding events but failure of pregnancy in fibrinogen-deficient mice. Genes Dev 1995;**9**:2020–33.
3. Bugge TH, Flick MJ, Daugherty CC, Degen JL. Plasminogen deficiency causes severe thrombosis but is compatible with development and reproduction. Genes Dev 1995;**9**:794–807.
4. Carmeliet P, Schoonjans L, Kieckens L, et al. Physiological consequences of loss of plasminogen activator gene function in mice. Nature 1994;**368**:419–24.
5. Rosen ED, Chan JC, Idusogie E, et al. Mice lacking factor VII develop normally but suffer fatal perinatal bleeding. Nature 1997;**390**:290–4.
6. Bi L, Lawler AM, Antonarakis SE, et al. Targeted disruption of the mouse factor VIII gene produces a model of haemophilia A. Nat Genet 1995;**10**:119–21.
7. Lin HF, Maeda N, Smithies O, et al. A coagulation factor IX-deficient mouse model for human hemophilia B. Blood 1997;**90**:3962–6.
8. Gailani D, Lasky NM, Broze GJ. A murine model of factor XI deficiency. Blood Coagul Fibrinolysis 1997;**8**:134–44.
9. Bugge TH, Xiao Q, Kombrinck KW, et al. Fatal embryonic bleeding events in mice lacking tissue factor, the cell-associated initiator of blood coagulation. Proc Natl Acad Sci USA 1996;**93**: 6258–63.
10. Carmeliet P, Mackman N, Moons L, et al. Role of tissue factor in embryonic blood vessel development. Nature 1996;**383**:73–5.
11. Toomey JR, Kratzer KE, Lasky NM, et al. Targeted disruption of the murine tissue factor gene results in embryonic lethality. Blood 1996;**88**:1583–7.
12. Huang ZF, Higuchi D, Lasky N, Broze GJ. Tissue factor pathway inhibitor gene disruption produces intrauterine lethality in mice. Blood 1997;**90**:944–51.
13. Cui J, O'Shea KS, Purkayastha A, et al. Fatal haemorrhage and incomplete block to embryogenesis in mice lacking coagulation factor V. Nature 1996;**384**:66–8.
14. Xue J, Wu Q, Westfield LA, et al. Incomplete embryonic lethality and fatal neonatal hemorrhage caused by prothrombin deficiency in mice. Proc Natl Acad Sci USA 1998;**95**:7603–7.
15. Sun WY, Witte DP, Degen JL, et al. Prothrombin deficiency results in embryonic and neonatal lethality in mice. Proc Natl Acad Sci USA 1998;**95**:7597–602.
16. Dewerchin M, Liang Z, Moons L, et al. Blood coagulation factor X deficiency causes partial

embryonic lethality and fatal neonatal bleeding in mice. Thromb Haemost 2000;**83**:185–90.

17. Connolly AJ, Ishihara H, Kahn ML, *et al*. Role of the thrombin receptor in development and evidence for a second receptor. *Nature* 1996;**381**:516–19.

18. Ishiguro K, Kojima T, Kadomatsu K, *et al*. Complete antithrombin deficiency in mice results in embryonic lethality. *J Clin Invest* 2000;**106**:873–8.

19. Jalbert LR, Rosen ED, Moons L, *et al*. Inactivation of the gene for anticoagulant protein C causes lethal perinatal consumptive coagulopathy in mice. *J Clin Invest* 1998;**102**:1481–8.

20. Healy AM, Rayburn HB, Rosenberg RD, Weiler H. Absence of the blood-clotting regulator thrombomodulin causes embryonic lethality in mice before development of a functional cardiovascular system. *Proc Natl Acad Sci USA* 1995;**92**:850–4.

21. Isermann B, Hendrickson SB, Hutley K, *et al*. Tissue-restricted expression of thrombomodulin in the placenta rescues thrombomodulin-deficient mice from early lethality and reveals a secondary developmental block. *Development* 2001;**128**:827–38.

22. Chan JC, Carmeliet P, Moons L, *et al*. Factor VII deficiency rescues the intrauterine lethality in mice associated with a tissue factor pathway inhibitor deficit. *J Clin Invest* 1999;**103**:475–82.

23. Pijnenborg R, Robertson WB, Brosens I, Dixon G. Review article: trophoblast invasion and the establishment of haemochorial placentation in man and laboratory animals. *Placenta* 1981;**2**:71–91.

24. Cross JC, Werb Z, Fisher SJ. Implantation and the placenta: key pieces of the development puzzle. *Science* 1994;**266**:1508–18.

25. Hodivala-Dilke KM, McHugh KP, Tsakiris DA, *et al*. Beta3-integrin-deficient mice are a model for Glanzmann thrombasthenia showing placental defects and reduced survival. *J Clin Invest* 1999;**103**:229–38.

26. Erlich J, Parry GC, Fearns C, *et al*. Tissue factor is required for uterine hemostasis and maintenance of the placental labyrinth during gestation. *Proc Natl Acad Sci USA* 1999;**96**:8138–43.

8

Oral contraceptives and cardiovascular disease

Ivan Bank, Saskia Middeldorp and Martin H Prins

INTRODUCTION

The introduction of oral contraceptives in the late 1950s has altered society and has even led to radical demographic alterations. Currently, combined oral contraceptives are the most effective and most easily reversible method of contraception. They have the best 'pearl index' (i.e. the number of pregnancies occurring despite the use of contraception in 100 women during 1 year).[1,2] Oral contraceptives are also used for other indications, such as treatment of menstrual disorders. The widespread use of oral contraceptives has given rise to concerns about possible side effects, especially cardiovascular disease. Initial case reports on fatal thromboembolic disease in young women who used oral contraceptives have led to a multitude of studies that have assessed the risk of venous and arterial disease in relation to the use of these drugs,[3–5] as well as assessing the potential underlying hemostatic and metabolic mechanisms. This chapter reviews the epidemiology of cardiovascular disease in relation to the use of oral contraceptives, as well as the presently known underlying mechanisms of cardiovascular disease in oral contraceptive users.

Types of oral contraceptives

Hormonal contraceptives are female sex steroids. They can take the form of a synthetic estrogen combined with a synthetic progesterone (progestagen) or of a progestagen only. They are mostly administered orally, but they are sometimes given intramuscularly. The combinations of estrogens and progestagens have their contraceptive effect by selective inhibition of pituitary function that results in inhibition of ovulation. The combined agents also produce a change in cervical mucus and in the motility and secretion in the tubes, decreasing the likelihood of conception and implantation. Use of progestagens alone does not always inhibit ovulation but does produce the latter effects.

Combined oral contraceptives are often classified according to the type of progestagens. The so-called first-generation pills contain norethisterone (acetate), lynesterol, ethynodiolacetate or norethynodrel; they are not used any more. The presently available oral contraceptives are second-generation pills, which contain norgestrel, levonorgestrel or norgestrinone, and third-generation combined oral contraceptives, which contain desogestrel, norgestimate or gestodene. The second- and third-generation progestagens are combined with 20–50 µg ethinyl estradiol ('sub-50 pills').

EPIDEMIOLOGY OF ORAL CONTRACEPTIVES AND CARDIOVASCULAR DISEASE

Oral contraceptives and venous disease

Risk of deep venous thrombosis and pulmonary embolism
Venous thromboembolism is a common disorder, with an overall annual incidence in Western

populations of 2–3 per 1000. The incidence increases with age.[6] In young women, venous thromboembolism is the most common cardiovascular event. Its reported incidence varies between 0.4 and 1.5 per 10,000 women–years in women aged 25–29 years, and between 0.6 and 3.0 per 10,000 women–years in the group aged 40–44 years.[7,8] Lower limb deep venous thrombosis and pulmonary embolism are the most common presenting features, but a partial or complete occlusion of a vein by a thrombus may also occur at other sites.

Since the first report that suggested a relationship between oral contraceptives and the occurrence of venous thromboembolism in a 40-year-old woman, many studies on this potential association have been performed.[4] Table 8.1 summarizes recent epidemiological studies of the risk of venous thromboembolism in women who use the contraceptive pill compared with non-users. For users of first-generation pills, the risk of

venous thromboembolism is between three and six times higher than it is for non-users. It has been consistently reported that the use of second-generation pills is associated with a two- to fourfold increase; this risk is increased three- to twelvefold when third-generation pills are used. The risk of venous thromboembolism seems more enhanced by the use of third-generation contraceptives, than by second-generation oral contraceptives, with reported odds ratios varying from 1.3 to 4.4. The absolute risk for venous thromboembolism in women using second-generation or third-generation oral contraceptives is estimated to be, respectively, between 1.6 and 3.1 per 10,000 women/year and between 2.9 and 5.0 per 10,000 women/year.[9,10] The increase in risk is most pronounced in 'first-time' users, and it decreases over time, because susceptible women possibly develop venous thromboembolism shortly after they have started using oral contraceptives.[11,12] There are no data avail-

Table 8.1 Risk of venous thromboembolism for women using different generations of oral contraceptives versus non-users

First-generation	Second-generation	Third-generation	Third-generation versus second	Study number
Odds ratio (95% CI)	Odds ratio (95% CI)	Odds ratio (95% CI)	Odds ratio	
—	3.5 (2.6–4.7)	9.1 (5.6–14.7)	2.6	104
3.4 (1.4–7.9)	3.6 (2.5–5.1)	7.4 (4.2–12.9)	2.1	105
—	2.8 (2.1–3.8)	12.2 (4.8–31.4)	4.4	105
—	—	—	1.9	9
6.2 (3.8–10.2)	3.6 (2.6–4.8)	5.3 (3.8–7.3)	1.5	106
5.7 (3.4–9.4)	3.2 (2.3–4.3)	4.8 (3.4–6.7)	1.5	107
—	—	—	1.3	10
—	1.8 (1.1–2.9)	3.2 (2.3–4.4)	1.8	11
—	3.3 (1.9–5.7)	8.7 (3.9–19.0)	2.6	108
—	1.7 (0.3–10.5)	4.4 (1.0–18.7)	2.6	109
—	—	—	3.5	12
—	—	—	1.9	110
—	—	—	2.3	110
—	3.6 (0.9–15.0)	7.6 (2.8–20.9)	2.1	111

able on the risk of recurrence of venous thromboembolism in relation to continued use of oral contraceptives after a first episode.

The risk of oral contraceptive-related venous thromboembolism in high-risk women

Since the baseline risk for venous thromboembolism in women with inherited thrombophilia is increased, it is important to estimate the additional increase in risk caused by the use of oral contraceptives in this population. The risk of venous thromboembolism in women with inheritable thrombophilic defects is found to be strongly enhanced by the use of oral contraceptives. Heterozygous factor V Leiden carriers who use oral contraceptives have an approximately 30-fold increased risk compared with women who do not carry the mutation and do not use the pill.[13–15] The same kind of interaction has been reported for women with deficiency of protein C, protein S or antithrombin and for heterozygous carriers of the prothrombin 20210A mutation, with odds ratios varying 6.4 and 16.3.[16,17] For women with increased levels of factor VIII (a known risk factor for venous thromboembolism), the increase in risk during the use of oral contraceptives has been found to be merely additive (as opposed to multiplicative), with an odds ratio of 10.3 compared with women with normal factor VIII levels who did not use the pill.[18]

In terms of absolute risk, the incidence has been found to be between 0.5% (95% CI 0.1–1.4) and 2.0% (95% CI 0.3–7.2) per year of pill use in women with the factor V Leiden mutation, and 4.3% (95% CI 1.4–9.7) per year in women with deficiency of protein C, protein S or antithrombin.[17,19] At present, such absolute risk estimates are not available in women with the prothrombin mutation. In women with factor VIII levels above 150% of normal levels who use the pill, the absolute risk has been calculated to be approximately 6 in 10,000, based on a baseline estimate of 0.7 per 10,000 women.[18]

Risk of cerebral venous sinus thrombosis

Cerebral venous sinus thrombosis is a very rare but serious and potentially lethal disease with an estimated absolute risk in premenopausal women of four per 1,000,000.[20] The best-known

risk factors are trauma; autoimmune disease; pregnancy; the puerperium; inherited thrombophilic risk factors; and the use of oral contraceptives.[20–23]

Oral contraceptives increase the risk of cerebral vein thrombosis in women approximately 20-fold.[20,24] As for deep vein thrombosis or pulmonary embolism, there appears to be a multiplicative interaction between use of oral contraceptives and hereditary thrombophilia. One study found an odds ratio of 34 for cerebral vein thrombosis in women with either factor V Leiden or protein C deficiency who also used the pill, whereas in another study an odds ratio as high as 149.3 (31.0–711.0) in women with the prothrombin mutation who used oral contraceptives has been reported (both studies provided a comparison with women without a defect who did not use the pill).[20,24] Furthermore, women who use third-generation combined oral contraceptives have been found to be at an even higher (twofold increased) risk of venous sinus thrombosis compared with women who use second-generation preparations.[25]

Oral contraceptives and arterial disease

Risk of myocardial infarction

Myocardial infarction is caused by irreversible necrosis of the heart muscle that results from prolonged ischemia. Nearly all cases of myocardial infarction are due to the formation of an acute thrombus that obstructs an atherosclerotic lesion. Men are affected more often than women (the overall ratio is 4:1). However, before the age of 40 years the ratio is about 8:1, whereas beyond the age of 50 years it decreases to 1:1.[26,27] Next to the increase in age, cigarette smoking is an important risk factor for myocardial infarction in women.[28] Although past use of oral contraceptives does not seem to increase the risk of this disease, many studies found a clear association between the current use of the pill and myocardial infarction.[5,29–34] In women who use any type of low-dose oral contraceptive, the relative risk of myocardial infarction is 2.6 (1.7–3.8).[35] Although some data indicate that the relative risk of myocardial infarction in third-generation oral contraception users is not increased in relation to non-users, this finding could not be established in two large case-control studies.[34,36,37]

There is an important interaction with other risk factors for arterial cardiovascular disease, such as smoking and hypertension, and the use of oral contraceptives in relation to the risk of myocardial infarction. In a large multicenter case-control study in women aged 35–44 years, the risk of death due to myocardial infarction was 69 per 100,000 in heavy smokers who used combined oral contraceptives versus 0.1 per 100,000 in non-smoking women who did not use oral contraceptives.[33] However, the risk of myocardial infarction attributable to combined oral contraceptives alone is much lower than the risk attributable to smoking alone or to the combination of the two.[8] Alternatively, oral contraceptives could make atherosclerotic coronary arteries more prone to arterial spasm.[38,39]

The use of progestagens alone is not associated with an increased risk of myocardial infarction.[40]

Risk of ischemic stroke
The incidence of ischemic stroke in females aged 18–44 years is about 4.3–5.4 per 100,000 women–years.[41–43] A fatal ischemic stroke occurs in less than 0.5 per 100,000 women under 45 years of age. Since the first case-report that raised this issue, many researchers have studied the association between ischemic stroke and use of oral contraceptives.[5,42,44–47]

One of the first case-control studies exploring the relationship between use of the pill and ischemic stroke found a relative risk of ischemic stroke of 3.1 (95% CI 1.1–8.6) in a population using high-dose estrogen pills.[48] A worldwide study by the World Health Organization revealed a relative risk of ischemic stroke in females who use oral contraceptives of approximately 3.0 (1.7–5.6) compared with non-users, both in developed and developing countries.[49] A recent meta-analysis of 16 adequate studies investigating the risk of ischemic stroke in low-dose oral contraception users calculated a relative risk of 1.9 (1.3–2.7) in studies that were

controlled for smoking and hypertension.[50] No significant difference in the risk of ischemic stroke between women using second- or third-generation preparations could be detected.

The use of progestagen-only contraceptives does not increase the risk of ischemic stroke.[40,51]

Risk of hemorrhagic stroke
Approximately 10% of strokes are due to hemorrhages into the brain parenchyma, the subarachnoid space, or both, and another 10% are due to subarachnoid hemorrhage.[52]

The incidence of hemorrhagic stroke is higher in women than in men and is estimated to be 5.6 per 100,000 women–years in women aged 15–44 years.[53–55] High-dose oral contraceptives have been reported to be associated with an increased risk of intracerebral hemorrhage,[56–58] although this risk seems to be lower or not increased at all in women using low-dose estrogen oral contraceptives (reported relative risks range from 1.14 to 2.5).[49,54] The risk of hemorrhagic stroke may be higher among users of the pill who are already at higher risk of hemorrhagic stroke because of unruptured aneurysms, hypertension or smoking.[35,44,49,54,59,60] Data on potential differences between the effects of second- and third-generation pills on the risk of hemorrhagic stroke are not available.

POTENTIAL MECHANISMS OF THE EFFECT OF ORAL CONTRACEPTIVES ON CARDIOVASCULAR RISK

Effects of oral contraceptives on hemostasis

Hemostasis is mediated by the coagulation system, which leads to the production of fibrin, and the fibrinolytic system, which is responsible for its degradation. Within both systems, several regulating mechanisms are known to maintain an optimal balance between coagulation and fibrinolysis in different situations. Oral contraceptives influence the concentrations and activities of many factors of both coagulation and fibrinolysis.[61–63]

Coagulation is initiated by the tissue factor–factor VIIa complex (the extrinsic pathway), which leads (by the activation of factor X) to the formation of the key enzyme thrombin; thrombin converts fibrinogen to fibrin. The extrinsic pathway is inhibited by tissue factor pathway inhibitor (TFPI). Furthermore, thrombin is generated via the intrinsic route (i.e. factors IXa and VIIIa – also called the tenase complex) and factors Xa and Va (also called the prothrombinase complex). Thrombin activity (and thus fibrin formation) is regulated by natural anticoagulants (i.e. antithrombin) and the protein C pathway, consisting of protein C and protein S. Antithrombin is the primary inhibitor of thrombin and factor Xa, but it also forms an irreversible complex with other activated coagulation factors. In the presence of thrombomodulin, thrombin activates protein C; activated protein C, together with its cofactor protein S, inactivates factors Va and VIIIa. This results in a downregulation of thrombin generation.

In the presence of fibrin, the fibrinolytic system is initiated when tissue plasminogen activator (t-PA) binds to plasminogen, which is then converted to its active form, plasmin. Plasmin degrades fibrin, resulting in the dissolution of the clot. The activity of plasminogen activators is inhibited by the plasminogen activator inhibitors, PAI-1 and PAI-2.

Furthermore, the coagulation and fibrinolytic systems are linked by thrombin-activatable fibrinolysis inhibitor (TAFI). Thrombin activates TAFI, which then downregulates fibrinolysis by inhibiting the binding between fibrin and plasminogen.

Effects on coagulation and the anticoagulant system

During the use of oral contraceptives, the concentrations of many clotting factors are increased, including factors VII, VIII, factor X and fibrinogen.[61,64,65] Moreover prothrombin fragment 1+2 (a marker of thrombin formation) is known to increase during oral contraceptive use.[65,66] In the natural anticoagulant pathway, the concentrations of protein S, and to a lesser extent antithrombin, are reduced in plasma of women using the pill.[64,67] Furthermore, the ability of activated protein C to downregulate

coagulation by inactivating factors V and VIII diminishes during the use of oral contraceptives, as can be assessed by assays that measure activated protein C resistance.[68–70]

Although initially it was assumed that most of these effects are dose-dependent results of the estrogenic component of oral contraceptives, it is now clear that the progestagenic component importantly modulates this effect.[71–73] In a crossover study, it was demonstrated that third-generation oral contraceptives (containing desogestrel) induce greater increases in factor VII and prothrombin than second-generation oral contraceptives (containing levonorgestrel) and a more significant decrease in factor V.[66] However, no difference in markers of thrombin generation was found between the two generations of agent. Interestingly, there were clear differences between both pills with respect to their effects on the anticoagulant pathways – with use of the third-generation oral contraceptives, total and free protein S were both markedly more decreased and activated protein C resistance was more pronounced.[74,75]

EFFECTS ON THE FIBRINOLYTIC SYSTEM

Increased fibrinolytic activity is observed during the use of combined oral contraceptives, as measured by increased concentrations of plasminogen, tissue plasminogen activator, plasmin–antiplasmin complexes and fibrin degradation products.[61] Progestagens seem to modulate the fibrinolysis-enhancing effect of estrogens.[76,77] However, in overall functional tests of the fibrinolytic system, no enhanced fibrinolysis is observed. This is probably attributable to a downregulation of fibrinolytic activity by extra thrombin generation by the coagulation system via increased concentrations of TAFI. This inhibition of fibrinolysis is induced more by third-generation than second-generation oral contraceptives.[78]

EFFECTS OF ORAL CONTRACEPTIVES ON RISK FACTORS FOR ARTERIAL DISEASE

Well-known risk factors for atherosclerosis include:

- dyslipidemias;
- hypertension;
- cigarette smoking;
- diabetes mellitus;
- obesity;
- lack of physical activity.

The use of combined oral contraceptives influences most of these factors.

Effects on lipid metabolism

In the exogenous pathway of lipid metabolism, absorbed cholesterol and triglycerides are incorporated into chylomicrons and transported into the venous circulation, where they become hydrolyzed by lipoprotein lipase and release fatty acids into muscle cells and adipose tissue. Metabolic remnants are absorbed by the liver, which can release them as free cholesterol or bile acids back into the intestine.

In the endogenous pathway, very low density protein (VLDL) particles are released by the liver into the circulation. Assimilation of VLDL residues result in cholesterol-rich low density lipoproteins (LDL), that can be taken up by extrahepatic cells or by the liver. Cholesterol released into the circulation is transported by high density lipoprotein (HDL) particles, which return cholesterol to the liver for excretion into the bile tract.

Elevated levels of triglycerides (carried mostly as VLDL) and elevated LDL levels promote atherosclerosis, while HDL is thought to protect against atherosclerosis.[79–81]

Estrogens and androgens have different effects on lipid metabolism. While estrogens lower LDL and elevate HDL and triglycerides, androgens and androgenic progestins do the opposite by reducing HDL and elevating LDL, mostly by interfering with hepatic lipase.[82–85] In addition, low HDL levels seem to increase the atherosclerotic risk in women more than in men.[86] Oral contraceptives containing third-generation progestagens (i.e. those with the lowest androgenic activity) are associated with a net beneficial lipid profile (i.e. lower LDL and higher HDL concentrations than in non users).[87] In contrast, in women using second-generation combined oral contraceptives, the LDL concentration remains similar but the HDL concentration is substantially reduced.[87] The beneficial effect of third-generation oral contraceptives on the lipid profile was an important reason for developing and marketing these newer combined oral contraceptives.

Effects on carbohydrate metabolism

Diabetes mellitus is an important risk factor for atherosclerosis, although the effects of diabetes alone are difficult to assess. Many patients with diabetes also have secondary dyslipidemia and are often obese or hypertensive. Combined oral contraceptives increase levels of fasting insulin and C-peptide, as well as the amount of insulin needed to cope with a standardized sugar load, indicating increased resistance to insulin.[87,88] Insulin resistance has also been associated with an increased risk of coronary heart disease.[89,90] The use of oral contraceptives does not lead to an increased risk of diabetes mellitus later in life.[91,92]

Effects on blood pressure

Hypertension is associated with the development of atherosclerosis, but also with premature death, non-lethal strokes, myocardial infarction, retinal damage and kidney damage.[93] Arterial pressure and blood flow to the tissues are controlled by cardiac output and vascular resistance, both of which are influenced by the sympathic nervous system and the renin–angiotensin–aldosterone system.[94] Hypertension may occur whenever there is an imbalance among the cardiac output, the volume of the vascular system and the vascular resistance. Oral contraceptives cause small increases in cardiac output, leading to higher systolic and diastolic blood pressure and increased heart rate. Hypertension is relatively unusual among users of oral contraceptives, although nearly 5% of women using higher-dose oral contraceptives develop hypertension.[95–97] The effects are possibly dose-related and mainly induced by the estrogenic component, which can affect levels of renin substrate, although the data are conflicting.[98–100] Blood pressure usually normalizes after discontinuation of oral contraceptives.

Interaction between other risk factors and oral contraceptives

Although smoking is not a risk factor for venous thromboembolism, it is an important risk factor for arterial disease, especially in pill users who are over 35 years of age. These women have an increased risk of death from arterial cardiovascular events of up to 20 times compared with women who do not use the pill and do not smoke.[33,101] The attributable risk of oral contraceptives in non-smoking women is estimated to be 1.4 per 100,000, whereas it is 8.7 per 100,000 in women who smoke.[8]

Obesity is a risk factor for coronary artery disease. A modest weight gain is an adverse effect of oral contraceptives in clinical practice, in particular associated with the use of combined agents that contain androgen-like progestagens (second-generation oral contraceptives).[102] Nevertheless, significant weight gain in combination with the use of oral contraceptives leading to an increase in arterial (and venous) disease has not been shown in studies. Weight gain can be controlled by changing to preparations that contain lower amounts of progestagens.[103]

CLINICAL IMPLICATIONS

Clinical decisions on the use of oral contraceptives in women who are at a high risk of vascular disease should consider the benefits of these hormonal preparations (including better contraceptive qualities than other methods of contraception and beneficial effects on menstrual disorders) in relation to the documented risks and the preferences of the woman seeking advice.

For women with a past history of venous thromboembolism, most clinicians will try to avoid the use of hormonal contraception and seek alternative contraceptive methods, such as the newest generation of intrauterine devices.

For women without inherited thrombophilic conditions who had a first thrombotic event after a strong temporary risk factor (e.g. trauma, surgery, immobilization), cautious use of oral contraceptives could be considered.

Whether female carriers of inherited thrombophilic factors who do not have a history of venous thromboembolism are wise to use oral contraceptives remains a matter of individual counseling based on the known risk estimates. The use of second-generation combined oral contraceptives is definitely preferred to the use of third-generation preparations because of the higher risk of venous thromboembolism during use of the third-generation preparations. Since arterial cardiovascular diseases are relatively uncommon in premenopausal women, guidelines for prescription of combined oral contraceptives in women with arterial disease will be controversial. However, almost all women who develop arterial disease are older or have other risk factors such as smoking and hypertension. Thus, alternative contraceptive methods could be considered in these women. Since there is hardly any evidence that third-generation combined oral contraceptives induce a lower increase in the risk of arterial cardiovascular disease, there does not, at present, seem to be a strong indication to prefer these preparations in high-risk women.

In general, counseling women at increased risk of venous or arterial vascular diseases with regard to the use of oral contraceptives should be done individually and seems more important than an absolute 'yes' or 'no'.

In summary third-generation oral contraceptives cause an increased risk of venous thromboembolism compared with second-generation preparations, which is probably due to a stronger negative effect on the natural anticoagulant and antifibrinolytic system. This effect is even more pronounced in women with hereditary risk factors for venous thromboembolism.

The use of combined oral contraceptives is also associated with an increased risk of arterial cardiovascular disease, in particular myocardial infarction and stroke. However, this risk seems to be limited to older women who also have other risk factors such as smoking and hypertension.

Furthermore, the attributable risk of oral contraception on this risk is much lower than, for instance, smoking itself. Although third-generation oral contraceptives have a beneficial effect on lipid profiles, this is not translated into a lower increase in risk in most studies.

In general, the increases in the risk of cardiovascular diseases associated with the use of oral contraceptives has to be balanced against the advantages of these drugs, especially in view of the absolute baseline estimates of cardiovascular diseases, which are generally low in women of child-bearing age.

REFERENCES

1. Mladenovic D, Grcic R, Pestelek B, Kapor M. Critical dosages for oral contraceptives. *J Int Med Res* 1977;**5**:276–80.
2. Trussell J, Hatcher RA, Cates WJ, *et al.* Contraceptive failure in the United States: an update. *Stud Fam Plann* 1990;**21**:51–4.
3. Inman WH, Vessey MP, Westerholm B, Engelund A. Thromboembolic disease and the steroidal content of oral contraceptives. A report to the Committee on Safety of Drugs. *BMJ* 1970;**2**:203–9.
4. Jordan WM. Pulmonary embolism. *Lancet* 1961;**2**:1146–7.
5. Boyce J, Fawcett JW, Noall EWP. Coronary thrombosis and Conovid. *Lancet* 1963;**1**:111–12.
6. Nordstrom M, Lindblad B, Bergqvist D, Kjellstrom T. A prospective study of the incidence of deep-vein thrombosis within a defined urban population. *J Intern Med* 1992;**232**:155–60.
7. Lidegaard O, Milsom I. Oral contraceptives and thrombotic diseases: impact of new epidemiological studies. *Contraception* 1996;**53**:135–9.
8. Farley TM, Meirik O, Chang CL, Poulter NR. Combined oral contraceptives, smoking, and cardiovascular risk. *J Epidemiol Community Health* 1998;**52**:775–85.
9. Jick H, Jick SS, Gurewich V, *et al.* Risk of idiopathic cardiovascular death and nonfatal venous thromboembolism in women using oral contraceptives with differing progestagen components. *Lancet* 1995;**346**:1589–93.
10. Farmer RD, Lawrenson RA, Thompson CR, *et al.* Population-based study of risk of venous thromboembolism associated with various oral contraceptives. *Lancet* 1997;**349**:83–8.
11. Lidegaard O, Edstrom B, Kreiner S. Oral contraceptives and venous thromboembolism. A case-control study. *Contraception* 1998;**57**:291–301.
12. Herings RM, Urquhart J, Leufkens HG. Venous thromboembolism among new users of different oral contraceptives. *Lancet* 1999;**354**:127–8.
13. Vandenbroucke JP, Koster T, Briet E, *et al.* Increased risk of venous thrombosis in oral-contraceptive users who are carriers of factor V Leiden mutation. *Lancet* 1994;**344**:1453–7.
14. Hellgren M, Svensson PJ, Dahlback B. Resistance to activated protein C as a basis for venous thromboembolism associated with pregnancy and oral contraceptives. *Am J Obstet Gynecol* 1995;**173**:210–13.
15. Andersen BS, Olsen J, Nielsen GL, *et al.* Third generation oral contraceptives and heritable thrombophilia as risk factors of non-fatal venous thromboembolism. *Thromb Haemost* 1998;**79**: 28–31.
16. Martinelli I, Taioli E, Bucciarelli P, *et al.* Interaction between the G20210A mutation of the prothrombin gene and oral contraceptive use in deep vein thrombosis. *Arterioscler Thromb Vasc Biol* 1999;**19**:700–3.
17. Simioni P, Sanson BJ, Prandoni P, *et al.* Incidence of venous thromboembolism in families with inherited thrombophilia. *Thromb Haemost* 1999;**81**:198–202.
18. Bloemenkamp KW, Helmerhorst FM, Rosendaal FR, Vandenbroucke JP. Venous thrombosis, oral contraceptives and high factor VIII levels. *Thromb Haemost* 1999;**82**:1024–7.
19. Middeldorp S, Henkens CM, Koopman MM, *et al.* The incidence of venous thromboembolism in family members of patients with factor V Leiden mutation and venous thrombosis. *Ann Intern Med* 1998;**128**:15–20.
20. de Bruijn SF, Stam J, Koopman MM, Vandenbroucke JP. Case-control study of risk of cerebral sinus thrombosis in oral contraceptive users and in [correction of who are] carriers of hereditary prothrombotic conditions. The Cerebral Venous Sinus Thrombosis Study Group. *BMJ* 1998;**316**:589–92.
21. Bousser MG, Chiras J, Bories J, Castaigne P. Cerebral venous thrombosis—a review of 38 cases. *Stroke* 1985;**16**:199–213.
22. Ameri A, Bousser MG. Cerebral venous thrombosis. *Neurol Clin* 1992;**10**:87–111.

23. Deschiens MA, Conard J, Horellou MH, Ameri A, *et al.* Coagulation studies, factor V Leiden, and anticardiolipin antibodies in 40 cases of cerebral venous thrombosis. *Stroke* 1996;**27**:1724–30.

24. Martinelli I, Sacchi E, Landi G, *et al.* High risk of cerebral-vein thrombosis in carriers of a prothrombin-gene mutation and in users of oral contraceptives. *N Engl J Med* 1998;**338**:1793–7.

25. de Bruijn SF, Stam J, Vandenbroucke JP. Increased risk of cerebral venous sinus thrombosis with third-generation oral contraceptives. Cerebral Venous Sinus Thrombosis Study Group. *Lancet* 1998;**351**:1404.

26. Gillum RF. Trends in acute myocardial infarction and coronary heart disease death in the United States. *J Am Coll Cardiol* 1994;**23**:1273–7.

27. Goddale F, Thomas WA, O'Neal RM. Myocardial infarction in women. *Arch Patholol* 1960;**69**: 599–609.

28. Mant D, Villard-Mackintosh L, Vessey MP, Yeates D. Myocardial infarction and angina pectoris in young women. *J Epidemiol Community Health* 1987;**41**:215–19.

29. Mann JI, Vessey MP, Thorogood M, Doll SR. Myocardial infarction in young women with special reference to oral contraceptive practice. *BMJ* 1975;**2**:241–5.

30. Engel HJ, Engel E, Lichtlen PR. Coronary atherosclerosis and myocardial infarction in young women: role of oral contraceptives. *Eur Heart J* 1983;**4**:1–6.

31. Stampfer MJ, Willett WC, Colditz GA, *et al.* A prospective study of past use of oral contraceptive agents and risk of cardiovascular diseases. *N Engl J Med* 1988;**319**:1313–17.

32. Croft P, Hannaford P. Risk factors for acute myocardial infarction in women. Evidence from the Royal College of General Practitioners' oral contraception study. *BMJ* 1989;**298**:165–8.

33. Anonymous. Acute myocardial infarction and combined oral contraceptives: results of an international multicentre case-control study. WHO Collaborative Study of Cardiovascular Disease and Steroid Hormone Contraception. *Lancet* 1997;**349**:1202–9.

34. Lewis MA, Heinemann LA, Spitzer WO, *et al.* The use of oral contraceptives and the occurrence of acute myocardial infarction in young women. Results from the Transnational Study on Oral Contraceptives and the Health of Young Women. *Contraception* 1997;**56**:129–40.

35. Farley TM, Collins J, Schlesselman JJ. Hormonal contraception and risk of cardiovascular disease. An international perspective. *Contraception* 1998;**57**:211–30.

36. Heinemann LA, Lewis MA, Thorogood M, *et al.* Case-control study of oral contraceptives and risk of thromboembolic stroke: results from International Study on Oral Contraceptives and Health of Young Women. *BMJ* 1997;**315**:1502–4.

37. Dunn N, Thorogood M, Faragher B, *et al.* Oral contraceptives and myocardial infarction: results of the MICA case-control study. *BMJ* 1999;**318**: 1579–83.

38. Collins P, Rosano GM, Sarrel PM, *et al.* 17 beta-Estradiol attenuates acetylcholine-induced coronary arterial constriction in women but not men with coronary heart disease. *Circulation* 1995;**92**:24–30.

39. Gilligan DM, Quyyumi AA, Cannon RO. Effects of physiological levels of estrogen on coronary vasomotor function in postmenopausal women. *Circulation* 1994;**89**:2545–51.

40. Anonymous. Cardiovascular disease and use of oral and injectable progestogen-only contraceptives and combined injectable contraceptives. Results of an international, multicenter, case-control study. World Health Organization Collaborative Study of Cardiovascular Disease and Steroid Hormone Contraception. *Contraception* 1998;**57**:315–24.

41. Schwartz SM, Siscovick DS, Longstreth WTJ, *et al.* Use of low-dose oral contraceptives and stroke in young women. *Ann Intern Med* 1997;**127**:596–603.

42. Petitti DB, Sidney S, Quesenberry CPJ, Bernstein A. Incidence of stroke and myocardial infarction in women of reproductive age. *Stroke* 1997;**28**:280–3.

43. Lis Y, Spitzer WO, Mann RD. A concurrent cohort study of oral contraceptive users from the VAMP research bank. *Pharmacoepidemiol Drug Saf* 1993;**2**:51–63.

44. Anonymous. Oral contraceptives and stroke in young women. Associated risk factors. *JAMA* 1975;**231**:718–22.

45. Longstreth WTJ, Swanson PD. Oral contraceptives and stroke. *Stroke* 1984;**15**:747–50.

46. Thorogood M, Mann J, Murphy M, Vessey M. Fatal stroke and use of oral contraceptives: findings from a case-control study. *Am J Epidemiol* 1992;**136**:35–45.

47. Poulter NR, Chang CL, Farley TM, *et al.* Effect on stroke of different progestagens in low oestrogen dose oral contraceptives. WHO Collaborative Study of Cardiovascular Disease and Steroid Hormone Contraception. *Lancet* 1999;**354**:301–2.

48. Vessey MP, Doll R. Investigation of relation between use of oral contraceptives and throm-

boembolic disease. A further report. *BMJ* 1969;**2**:651–7.

49. Anonymous. Haemorrhagic stroke, overall stroke risk, and combined oral contraceptives: results of an international, multicentre, case-control study. WHO Collaborative Study of Cardiovascular Disease and Steroid Hormone Contraception. *Lancet* 1996;**348**:505–10.

50. Gillum LA, Mamidipudi SK, Johnston SC. Ischemic stroke risk with oral contraceptives: a meta-analysis. *JAMA* 2000;**284**:72–8.

51. Lidegaard O. Oral contraception and risk of a cerebral thromboembolic attack: results of a case-control study. *BMJ* 1993;**306**:956–63.

52. Kunitz SC, Gross CR, Heyman A, *et al*. The pilot Stroke Data Bank: definition, design, and data. *Stroke* 1984;**15**:740–6.

53. Longstreth WTJ, Nelson LM, Koepsell TD, van Belle G. Clinical course of spontaneous subarachnoid hemorrhage: a population-based study in King County, Washington. *Neurology* 1993;**43**:712–18.

54. Petitti DB, Sidney S, Bernstein A, *et al*. Stroke in users of low-dose oral contraceptives. *N Engl J Med* 1996;**335**:8–15.

55. Johnston SC, Selvin S, Gress DR. The burden, trends, and demographics of mortality from subarachnoid hemorrhage. *Neurology* 1998;**50**: 1413–18.

56. Petitti DB, Wingerd J. Use of oral contraceptives, cigarette smoking, and risk of subarachnoid haemorrhage. *Lancet* 1978;**2**:234–5.

57. Beral V. Mortality among oral-contraceptive users. Royal College of General Practitioners' Oral Contraception Study. *Lancet* 1977;**2**:727–31.

58. Vessey MP, Lawless M, Yeates D. Oral contraceptives and vascular disease. *Epidemiol Rev* 1989;**11**:241–3.

59. Sacco RL, Wolf PA, Bharucha NE, *et al*. Subarachnoid and intracerebral hemorrhage: natural history, prognosis, and precursive factors in the Framingham Study. *Neurology* 1984;**34**: 847–54.

60. Johnston SC, Colford JMJ, Gress DR. Oral contraceptives and the risk of subarachnoid hemorrhage: a meta-analysis. *Neurology* 1998;**51**:411–18.

61. Kluft C, Lansink M. Effect of oral contraceptives on haemostasis variables. *Thromb Haemost* 1997; **78**:315–26.

62. Beller FK, Ebert C. Effects of oral contraceptives on blood coagulation. A review. *Obstet Gynecol Surv* 1985;**40**:425–36.

63. Fotherby K, Caldwell AD. New progestogens in oral contraception. *Contraception* 1994;**49**:1–32.

64. Bonnar J. Coagulation effects of oral contraception. *Am J Obstet Gynecol* 1987;**157**:1042–8.

65. Quehenberger P, Loner U, Kapiotis S, *et al*. Increased levels of activated factor VII and decreased plasma protein S activity and circulating thrombomodulin during use of oral contraceptives. *Thromb Haemost* 1996;**76**:729–34.

66. Middeldorp S, Meijers JM, Van den Ende AE, *et al*. Effects on coagulation of levonorgestrel- and desogestrel-containing low dose oral contraceptives: a cross-over study. *Thromb Haemost* 2000;**84**:4–8.

67. Schafer AI. Hypercoagulable states: molecular genetics to clinical practice. *Lancet* 1994;**344**:1739–42.

68. Meinardi JR, Henkens CM, Heringa MP, van der Meer J. Acquired APC resistance related to oral contraceptives and pregnancy and its possible implications for clinical practice. *Blood Coagul Fibrinolysis* 1997;**8**:152–4.

69. Rosing J, Tans G, Nicolaes GA, *et al*. Oral contraceptives and venous thrombosis: different sensitivities to activated protein C in women using second- and third-generation oral contraceptives. *Br J Haematol* 1997;**97**:233–8.

70. Curvers J, Thomassen MC, Nicolaes GA, *et al*. Acquired APC resistance and oral contraceptives: differences between two functional tests. *Br J Haematol* 1999;**105**:88–94.

71. Bottiger LE, Boman G, Eklund G, Westerholm B. Oral contraceptives and thromboembolic disease: effects of lowering oestrogen content. *Lancet* 1980;**1**:1097–101.

72. Kuhl H. Effects of progestogens on haemostasis. *Maturitas* 1996;**24**:1–19.

73. Winkler UH. Effects on hemostatic variables of desogestrel- and gestodene-containing oral contraceptives in comparison with levonorgestrel-containing oral contraceptives: a review. *Am J Obstet Gynecol* 1998;**179**:S51–S61.

74. Rosing J, Middeldorp S, Curvers J, *et al*. Low-dose oral contraceptives and acquired resistance to activated protein C: a randomised cross-over study. *Lancet* 1999;**354**:2036–40.

75. Tans G, Curvers J, Middeldorp S, *et al*. A randomized cross-over study on the effects of levonorgestrel- and desogestrel-containing oral contraceptives on the anticoagulant pathways. *Thromb Haemost* 2000;**84**:15–21.

76. Sabra A, Bonnar J. Hemostatic system changes induced by 50 micrograms and 30 micrograms estrogen/progestogen oral contraceptives. Modification of estrogen effects by levonorgestrel. *J Reprod Med* 1983;**28**:85–91.

77. Levi M, Middeldorp S, Buller HR. Oral contraceptives and hormonal replacement therapy cause an imbalance in coagulation and fibrinolysis which may explain the increased risk of venous thromboembolism. *Cardiovasc Res* 1999;**41**:21–4.

78. Meijers JM, Middeldorp S, Tekelenburg W, *et al.* Increased fibrinolytic activity during use of oral contraceptives is counteracted by an enhanced factor XI-independent down regulation of fibrinolysis. A randomized cross-over study of two low-dose oral contraceptives. *Thromb Haemost* 2000;**84**:9–14.

79. Carlson LA, Bottiger LE. Ischaemic heart-disease in relation to fasting values of plasma triglycerides and cholesterol. Stockholm prospective study. *Lancet* 1972;**1**:865–8.

80. Castelli WP, Doyle JT, Gordon T, *et al.* HDL cholesterol and other lipids in coronary heart disease. The cooperative lipoprotein phenotyping study. *Circulation* 1977;**55**:767–72.

81. Stein O, Stein Y. Atheroprotective mechanisms of HDL. *Atherosclerosis* 1999;**144**:285–301.

82. Burkman RT, Zacur HA, Kimball AW, *et al.* Oral contraceptives and lipids and lipoproteins: Part II–Relationship to plasma steroid levels and outlier status. *Contraception* 1989;**40**:675–89.

83. Krauss RM, Roy S, Mishell DRJ, *et al.* Effects of two low-dose oral contraceptives on serum lipids and lipoproteins: differential changes in high-density lipoprotein subclasses. *Am J Obstet Gynecol* 1983;**145**:446–52.

84. Wahl P, Walden C, Knopp R, *et al.* Effect of estrogen/progestin potency on lipid/lipoprotein cholesterol. *N Engl J Med* 1983;**308**:862–7.

85. Nikkilä EA, Tikkanen MJ, Kuusi T. Effects of progestins on plasma lipoproteins and hepatic-releasable lipases. In: Bardin CW, Milgran E, Mauvais-Jarvis P, eds. *Progesterone and Progestins.* New York: Raven Press; 1983:411–20.

86. Jacobs DRJ, Mebane IL, Bangdiwala SI, *et al.* High density lipoprotein cholesterol as a predictor of cardiovascular disease mortality in men and women: the follow-up study of the Lipid Research Clinics Prevalence Study. *Am J Epidemiol* 1990;**131**:32–47.

87. Godsland IF, Crook D, Simpson R, *et al.* The effects of different formulations of oral contraceptive agents on lipid and carbohydrate metabolism. *N Engl J Med* 1990;**323**:1375–81.

88. Godsland IF, Walton C, Felton C, *et al.* Insulin resistance, secretion, and metabolism in users of oral contraceptives. *J Clin Endocrinol Metab* 1992;**74**:64–70.

89. Pyorala K, Savolainen E, Kaukola S, Haapakoski J. Plasma insulin as coronary heart disease risk factor: relationship to other risk factors and predictive value during 9½–year follow-up of the Helsinki Policemen Study population. *Acta Med Scand Suppl* 1985;**701**:38–52.

90. Godsland IF, Stevenson JC. Insulin resistance: syndrome or tendency? *Lancet* 1995;**346**:100–3.

91. Duffy TJ, Ray R. Oral contraceptive use: prospective follow-up of women with suspected glucose intolerance. *Contraception* 1984;**30**:197–208.

92. Hannaford PC, Kay CR. Oral contraceptives and diabetes mellitus. *BMJ* 1989;**299**:1315–16.

93. Prentice RL. On the ability of blood pressure effects to explain the relation between oral contraceptives and cardiovascular disease. *Am J Epidemiol* 1988;**127**:213–19.

94. Hypertension. In: Kaplan NM, Braunwold E, eds. *Heart Disease: A Textbook of Cardiovascular Medicine,* 4th ed. Philadelphia: WB Saunders; 1992:62–79.

95. Kovacs L, Bartfai G, Apro G, *et al.* The effect of the contraceptive pill on blood pressure: a randomized controlled trial of three progestogen–oestrogen combinations in Szeged, Hungary. *Contraception* 1986;**33**:69–77.

96. Nichols M, Robinson G, Bounds W, *et al.* Effect of four combined oral contraceptives on blood pressure in the pill-free interval. *Contraception* 1993;**47**:367–76.

97. Dong W, Colhoun HM, Poulter NR. Blood pressure in women using oral contraceptives: results from the Health Survey for England 1994. *J Hypertens* 1997;**15**:1063–8.

98. Weir RJ. Effect on blood pressure or changing from high to low dose steroid preparations in women with oral contraceptive induced hypertension. *Scott Med J* 1982;**27**:212–15.

99. Wilson ES, Cruickshank J, McMaster M, Weir RJ. A prospective controlled study of the effect on blood pressure of contraceptive preparations containing different types and dosages of progestogen. *Br J Obstet Gynaecol* 1984;**91**:1254–60.

100. Anonymous. The WHO multicentre trial of the vasopressor effects of combined oral contraceptives: 2. Lack of effect of estrogen. Task Force on Oral Contraceptives. WHO Special Programme of Research, Development and Research Training in Human Reproduction. *Contraception* 1989;**40**:147–56.

101. Anonymous. Further analyses of mortality in oral contraceptive users. Royal College of General

Practitioners' Oral Contraception Study. *Lancet* 1981;**1**:541–6.

102. Darney PD. OC practice guidelines: minimizing side effects. *Int J Fertil Menopausal Stud* 1997;**42**(suppl 1):158–69.

103. London RS. The new era in oral contraception: pills containing gestodene, norgestimate, and desogestrel. *Obstet Gynecol Surv* 1992;**47**:777–82.

104. Anonymous. Effect of different progestagens in low oestrogen oral contraceptives on venous thromboembolic disease. World Health Organization Collaborative Study of Cardiovascular Disease and Steroid Hormone Contraception. *Lancet* 1995;**346**:1582–8.

105. Anonymous. Venous thromboembolic disease and combined oral contraceptives: results of international multicentre case-control study. World Health Organization Collaborative Study of Cardiovascular Disease and Steroid Hormone Contraception. *Lancet* 1995;**346**:1575–82.

106. Lewis MA, Heinemann LA, MacRae KD, *et al.* The increased risk of venous thromboembolism and the use of third generation progestagens: role of bias in observational research. The Transnational Research Group on Oral Contraceptives and the Health of Young Women. *Contraception* 1996;**54**:5–13.

107. Spitzer WO, Lewis MA, Heinemann LA, *et al.* Third generation oral contraceptives and risk of venous thromboembolic disorders: an international case-control study. Transnational Research Group on Oral Contraceptives and the Health of Young Women. *BMJ* 1996;**312**:83–8.

108. Bloemenkamp KW, Rosendaal FR, Buller HR, *et al.* Risk of venous thrombosis with use of current low-dose oral contraceptives is not explained by diagnostic suspicion and referral bias. *Arch Intern Med* 1999;**159**:65–70.

109. Vasilakis C, Jick SS, Jick H. The risk of venous thromboembolism in users of postcoital contraceptive pills. *Contraception* 1999;**59**:79–83.

110. Jick H, Kaye JA, Vasilakis-Scaramozza C, Jick SS. Risk of venous thromboembolism among users of third generation oral contraceptives compared with users of oral contraceptives with levonorgestrel before and after 1995: Cohort and case-control analysis. *BMJ* 2000;**321**:1190–5.

111. Parkin L, Skegg DC, Wilson M, *et al.* Oral contraceptives and fatal pulmonary embolism. *Lancet* 2000;**355**:2133–4.

9

Hormone replacement therapy and venous thrombosis

Geneviève Plu-Bureau and Jacqueline Conard

INTRODUCTION

Hormone replacement therapy (HRT) was initially administered because women had clinical manifestations of estrogenic deprivation due to cessation of ovarian activity. At first, HRT was given to prevent osteoporosis, improve quality of life, and sometimes to prevent myocardial infarction.[1] However, HRT may be associated with deleterious side effects on the breast and veins.

This chapter reviews the effects of menopause on the risk of thrombosis and on hemostasis parameters, the various HRT regimens, and epidemiological studies on the venous risk and the changes in hemostasis variables that can affect such a risk.

MENOPAUSE, RISK OF THROMBOSIS, AND MODIFICATIONS OF HEMOSTASIS

Menopause leads to a loss of the cardiovascular protection that is present in fertile women, but not to an increased risk of venous thrombosis. It should be noted that age alone also influences the risk of venous thrombosis.[2]

The Northwick Park Heart Study is the first and only longitudinal relationship between hemostasis parameters and the menopause.[3,4] After adjustment for age, significant increases in factor VII (14.9%, $p < 0.0001$), antithrombin (5.1%, $p < 0.005$), and fibrinogen (0.41 g/l,

$p < 0.0001$) were associated with natural menopause in 362 women. The same trends were observed in the case of artificial menopause but the results were not statistically significant because of the small number of subjects ($n = 28$).

Several cross-sectional studies have been published: Prospective Cardiovascular Munster study (PROCAM),[5] the Paris study,[6,7] Atherosclerosis Risk In Communities (ARIC),[8,9] Healthy Women,[10] Scottish Heart Health,[11] Whitehall II,[12] Framingham,[13] Finrisk Haemostasis,[14] and Thrombocheck.[15] In most studies, menopause was associated with an increase in factor VII, fibrinogen, and plasminogen activator inhibitor (PAI)-1, changes considered to be deleterious for cardiovascular risk but not venous risk. Antithrombin levels were in fact higher[4,10] or unchanged.[3,9] Physical exercise induced an increase in fibrinolysis, a finding confirmed in physically active menopausal women.[16] In addition, a factor VII polymorphism (Arg353Gln), which is present in a small proportion of women, was not associated with the expected increase in factor VII during menopause.[17]

In summary, menopause is not associated with an increased risk of venous thromboembolic events (VTE). Significant increases in fibrinogen and PAI-1 may be associated with an increased cardiovascular risk. Physical exercise and genetic status may also be important.

HRT AND THE RISK OF VENOUS THROMBOEMBOLISM

HRT regimens

HRT is the administration of an estrogen, and sometimes a progestogen. The estrogen may be conjugated equine estrogens (CEE) derived from the urine of pregnant mares. These estrogens are called 'natural' but they are not of human origin and are a mixture of about 10 different estrogen derivatives. They are used mostly in the USA. In Europe, the synthetic natural estradiol is more often used. It can be administered either orally or by transdermal, subcutaneous, vaginal, or (more recently) intranasal route. A progestogen is added to the estrogen to avoid endometrial cancer, usually as a natural progesterone or medroxy-progesterone acetate (MPA), norethisterone acetate (NETA), chlormadinone acetate, promegestone, nomegestrol acetate, or didrogesterone.

The estrogen and the progestogen may be administered together or not, continuously or not. In France, the estrogen is usually administered for 25 days and the progestogen for 10 or 25 days every month, resulting in monthly withdrawal bleedings. Daily continuous administration of the estrogen and the progestogen is frequently associated with amenorrhea.

Epidemiological studies

The risk of VTE during HRT was considered because of the risk reported with hormonal oral contraception. Since HRT was administered to compensate for decreased estrogen levels and to mimic the premenopausal hormonal status, it was not expected to increase the risk of thrombosis. Results of the different epidemiological studies have been evaluated and reviewed.[18,19] Before 1996, no increased risk of VTE had been observed (Table 9.1).[20-23] After 1996, results showed an increased risk,[24-28] a relative risk close to 2 and a combined risk of 2.1 (95% CI 1.2–3.8).[19] The increased risk is higher in the first year of

Table 9.1 HRT and risk of VTE. Results of studies published before and after 1996

Study	Year of recruitment	Study design	Relative risk
Before 1996			
Collaborative Drug Surveillance Program[20]	1972	Case–control	2.3 (95% CI 0.6–8.0)
Petitti et al.[21]	1969–1971	Case–control	0.7 (95% CI 0.2–2.5)
Devor et al.[22]	1980–1987	Case–control	0.6 (95% CI 0.2–1.8)
Nachtigall et al.[23]	1965–1975	Randomized trial	0.8 (95% CI 0.4–1.6)
After 1996			
Daly et al.[24]	1990–1993	Case–control	3.6 (95% CI 1.8–7.0)
Jick et al.[25]	1980–1994	Case–control	3.3 (95% CI 1.4–7.8)
Grodstein et al.[26]	1976–1992	Cohort	2.1 (95% CI 1.2–3.8)
Perez-Gutthann et al.[27]	1991–1994	Nested case–control	2.1 (95% CI 1.3–3.6)
Varas-Lorenzo et al.[28]	1985–1991	Nested case–control	2.3 (95% CI 1.0–5.3)
Hulley et al.[29]	1993–1998	Randomized trial	2.8 (95% CI 1.5–5.5)
Høibraaten et al.[32]	1990–1996	Case–control	1.2 (95% CI 0.76–1.94)
Høibraaten et al.[42]	1996–1998	Randomized trial*	4.7 (p = 0.04)

*Risk of recurrent venous thromboembolism

Table 9.2 HRT and risk of VTE according to the duration of treatment

Study	Duration of HRT (months)	Number of cases	Relative risk (95% CI)
Daly et al.[24]	1–12	14	6.7 (2.1–21.3)
	13–36	16	4.4 (1.6–11.9)
	37–60	4	1.9 (0.5–7.8)
	> 60	10	2.1 (0.8–6.1)
Jick et al.[25]	< 12	4	6.7 (1.5–30.8)
	12–60	3	2.8 (0.6–11.7)
	> 60	11	4.4 (1.6–12.2)
Grodstein et al.[26]	< 60	12	2.6 (1.2–5.2)
	> 60	10	1.9 (0.9–4.0)
Perez-Gutthann et al.[27]	1–6	14	4.6 (2.5–8.4)
	6–12	8	3.0 (1.4–6.5)
	> 12	13	1.1 (0.6–2.1)
Hulley et al.[29]	1–12	13	3.29 (1.1–10.1)
	13–24	8	4.1 (0.9–19.3)
	25–36	7	2.4 (0.6–9.3)
	37–60	6	2.1 (0.2–8.2)
Høibraaten et al.[32]	< 12	19	3.5 (1.5–8.2)
	> 12	26	0.7 (0.4–1.1)

HRT and decreases after that (Table 9.2).[24–27] No difference was observed between treatments with estrogens administered with progestogens or unopposed estrogens. After discontinuation of HRT, the risk returns to that of non-users.

A randomized, double-blind, placebo-controlled trial (Heart and Estrogen–progestin Replacement Study (HERS)) has studied the effect of conjugated equine estrogens (0.625 mg) and medroxyprogesterone acetate (2.5 mg) or placebo in 2763 women who had established coronary disease but no previous VTE.[29] No significant difference was observed for the primary outcome of the study, namely non-fatal myocardial infarction or death due to coronary heart disease. In contrast, a significant increased risk of VTE was observed, especially during the first years of treatment. The risk was increased in women who had lower extremity fractures (relative hazard 18.1, 95% CI 5.4–60.4), women who had cancer (3.9, 95% CI 1.6–9.4), 90 days after inpatient surgery (4.9, 95% CI 2.4–9.8), and women undergoing non-surgical hospitalization (5.7, 95% CI 3.0–10.8).[30] Interestingly, the risk was decreased with aspirin (0.5, 95% CI 0.2–0.8) and statins (0.5, 95% CI 0.2–0.9).[30]

In the Estrogen Replacement and Athero-sclerosis (ERA) study (a double-blind, randomized, placebo-controlled clinical trial), the effects of HRT on the progression of coronary athero-sclerosis in women were examined.[31] A similar trend of VTE risk was found in the treated groups (0.625 mg conjugated estrogen alone or plus 2.5 mg medroxyprogesterone acetate) and the placebo group, but it was not significant because of the small sample size.

In these studies the estrogens used were mainly conjugated equine estrogens associated with

Table 9.3 HRT and risk of VTE according to the route of administration

Study	Route of administration	Number of cases	Relative risk (95% CI)
Daly et al.[24]	Oral	37	4.6 (2.1–10.1)
	Transdermal	5	2.0 (0.5–7.6)
Perez-Gutthann et al.[27]	Oral	20	2.1 (1.3–3.6)
	Transdermal	7	2.1 (0.9–4.6)

medroxyprogesterone acetate. In a more recent study, estradiol (mainly oral) was also associated with an increased risk of VTE, which was significant only during the first year of treatment.[32]

Information about the non-oral mode of administration is scanty. No significant difference was found, but the number of women receiving this therapy was too small to draw any firm conclusions (Table 9.3).[24,27]

In summary, HRT with conjugated equine estrogens and oral estrogens are associated with an increased risk of VTE in women who have no prior history (and who were excluded from the epidemiological studies). However, the absolute risk is low but is higher during the first year of treatment. Progestogen does not seem to have a role in this risk. More information about the risk of estradiol administered by the transdermal route is needed.

HRT and hemostasis

The influence of HRT on hemostasis has been mostly studied in observational studies[9–11,13,14,33–36]

Table 9.4 HRT and hemostasis: main results in cross-sectional studies

Authors	Study design	Sample size	Age (years)	Fibrinogen	Factor VII	PAI-I	Other factors
Meilhan et al.[10]	Cross-sectional	207	49–56	↓	→		↓ antithrombin, → plasminogen
Lee et al.[11]	Cross-sectional	4837	25–64	↓			
Scarabin et al.[33]	Cross-sectional	259	45–54	→	↓	↓	
Nabulsi et al.[34]	Cross-sectional	4958	45–64	↓	↑	→	↓ antithrombin, → D-dimers
Shahar et al.[9]	Nested case–control	288					↓ tissue plasminogen activator antigen
Manolio et al.[35]	Cross-sectional	2955	≥ 65	↓	↑		
Gebara et al.[13]	Cross-sectional	749				↓	↓ tissue plasminogen activator antigen
Salomaa et al.[14]	Cross-sectional	1202	45–64	↓	→		
Meilhan et al.[36]	Cross-sectional	273	65–82	↓		↓	

↓: decrease; ↑: increase; →: no change

Study	Sample size	Age (years)	Treatment	Results
Caine et al.[37]	29	43–69	1. CEE 0.625 mg 2. CEE 1.25 mg 3. Placebo	F1+2 ↑ dose dependent AT; PS ↓ dose dependent FPA ↑ in group 1 & 2
PEPI[38]	875	45–64	1. Placebo 2. CEE 0.625 mg 3. CEE 0.625 mg + MPA10 mg 4. CEE 0.625 mg + MPA2.5 mg 5. CEE 0.625 mg + progesterone	Fibrinogen ↑ in placebo Not increased in other groups
Conard et al.[39]	47	Mean 52	1. Placebo 2. Estradiol 1 mg + NA 2.5 mg 3. Estradiol 5.5 mg + NA 3.75 mg	Plasminogen ↑ in treated groups No change in fibrinogen, antithrombin, protein S, F1+2, PC
Italian study[40]	255	Mean 52	1. TTS Estradiol 50 mg + MPA (cyclic) 2. TTS Estradiol 50 mg + MPA (continuous) 3. Placebo	Fibrinogen, antithrombin, protein S, factor VIII: ↓ in group 2
Scarabin et al.[41]	45	45–64	1. Estradiol 2 mg + progesterone 2. Estradiol gel + progesterone 3. No HRT	Antithrombin, PAI, tissue plasminogen activator antigen: ↓ in group 1 F1 + 2: ↑ in group 1 Fibrinogen, factor VII, D-dimer: →
Høibraaten et al.[42]	140	< 70	1. Estradiol 2 mg + NETA 1 mg 2. Placebo	F1 + 2, TAT, D-dimer: ↑ in group 1 Fibrinogen, factor VIII: no change Antithrombin, PC, TFPI: ↓ in group 1

Table 9.5 HRT and hemostasis: results of randomized controlled trials

↓: decrease; ↑: increase; →: no change

and in a small number of controlled randomized trials (Tables 9.4 and 9.5).[37–42] Several modifications of coagulation and fibrinolysis parameters have been observed during HRT,[43] including profibrinolytic and procoagulant effects. HRT induces a profibrinolytic effect by decreasing PAI-1 levels and decreasing fibrinogen levels or preventing the menopause-associated increase in fibrinogen levels.[38] Thus, HRT may counteract the effect of menopause and can be considered beneficial for cardiovascular risk.

Other changes observed during HRT (decreases in antithrombin, protein S and tissue factor pathway inhibitor (TFPI) levels) have a procoagulant effect and can be considered deleterious for VTE risk.[10,34,37,40–42,44] In addition, coagulation activation markers (fibrinopeptide A, prothrombin fragment 1.2, and D-dimers) are also increased during HRT,[37,41,42] suggesting an imbalance between the regulatory mechanisms.

Modifications of factor VII are not homogeneous during HRT – increased levels as well as decreased or stable levels have been reported. A possible explanation for this is the presence in some women of a polymorphism that is associated with an absence of HRT-induced and postmenopausal increases in factor VII levels, in contrast with the increased levels observed in women who are not carriers of this polymorphism.[17] This explanation could suggest that HRT has no specific effect on factor VII levels.

Conjugated equine estrogens have been studied more extensively than estradiol. Oral and transdermal routes of administration of the estradiol have been compared in a small open study[45] and in a randomized controlled study of a relatively small number of women.[41] Changes in antithrombin, protein S and prothrombin fragment 1.2 levels observed with the oral route were similar to those observed with conjugated equine estrogens. In contrast, there were no significant changes with the transdermal route, possibly because the first liver passage is avoided. Transdermal estradiol also improves the anticoagulant response to activated protein C.[46] These results may mean that the transdermal route has no deleterious effect on the VTE risk but it may lack the cardiovascular protection if fibrinogen and fibrinolysis parameters are surrogate end-points.

The influence of the progestogens associated with a same dose and type of estrogen has rarely been studied. In one study,[47] different doses of NETA and megestrol acetate were combined with the same dose of estradiol. The highest dose of NETA was associated with a decrease in antithrombin and factor VII levels. Some progestogens may reverse the effect of the estrogen (e.g. nomegestrol acetate may increase

antithrombin levels and counteract the decrease in antithrombin levels caused by the estrogen).[45,47]

In summary, menopause is not associated with modifications of hemostasis compatible with an increased risk of VTE. In contrast, conjugated equine estrogens and oral estradiol, but not transdermal estradiol, induce hypercoagulability, a potential risk factor for VTE.

HRT in women at risk of venous thrombo-embolism

It may be expected that the risk of VTE during HRT is higher in women who have had previous thrombosis or a congenital thrombophilia. This could explain, at least partly, the increased risk during the first year of treatment. Coagulation tests were performed in women who developed thrombosis during one of the epidemiological studies.[48] The relative risk of thrombosis was higher in women with antithrombin less than 90% (OR 3.33, 95% CI 1.15–9.65), protein C less than 80% (OR 2.93, 95% CI 1.06–8.14), acquired activated protein C resistance (OR 4.06, 95% CI 1.62–10.21), factor IX above 150% (2.34, 95% CI 1.26–4.35), and D-dimers above 250 µg/ml (3.84, 95% CI 1.99–7.42). The risk from HRT in women with known congenital thrombophilia is presently unknown but, by analogy, it is probably higher than in the general population of women.

A randomized, double-blind study was recently done in women with a history of deep vein thrombosis; 71 women were treated with 2 mg oral estradiol associated with 1 mg norethisterone acetate, while 69 women received a placebo.[49] The primary outcome was recurrent VTE. The study was prematurely terminated, owing to an increased occurrence of VTE in the treated group compared with placebo (10.7% versus 2.3%). Simultaneously, studies demonstrating an increased risk in women without previous thrombosis were published.

In summary, women with previous VTE or coronary heart disease have a higher risk of VTE during HRT that contains conjugated equine estrogens or oral estradiol. Women with congenital thrombophilia may also be at higher risk.

Information about transdermal estradiol in these women is needed.

OTHER HORMONAL TREATMENTS FOR THE MENOPAUSE

Since estrogen-containing treatments should be avoided in some women, other treatments have been proposed. Among them are drugs with tissue-specific effects, known as selective estrogen receptor modulators. Tamoxifen, used initially to prevent the recurrence of breast cancer, was also found to protect against osteoporosis. Raloxifene produces estrogen agonistic effects in some tissues and estrogen antagonistic effects in others.

In two of three randomized trials for the primary prevention of breast cancer by tamoxifen, an increased risk of VTE was observed in treated women compared with women receiving placebo.[50–52] Raloxifene at two doses (60 mg and 120 mg) was compared with placebo in a multicenter trial for the prevention of osteoporotic fractures in 7705 osteoporotic women below 81 years of age.[53] An increased risk of VTE was observed in women receiving raloxifene (RR 3.1, 95% CI 1.5–6.2). Tibolone is a steroid hormone with tissue-specific activity combining estrogenic, progestogenic, and androgenic activities. Information about the risk of thrombosis during tibolone is limited,[24] but coagulation risk factors for VTE (antithrombin and protein S levels) are not modified and a marked profibrinolysis has been noted.[54]

The effect of phytoestrogens on the risk of thrombosis or hemostasis variables is presently unknown.[55]

CONCLUSION

HRT with conjugated equine estrogens or oral estradiol is associated with an increased risk of VTE. The risk is higher in women who are at risk before starting HRT (e.g. women with previous VTE, women with congenital thrombophilia), and this type of HRT should be avoided in such at-risk women. More information is needed about the risk of the transdermal route of estradiol administration. Randomized trials are under way; the Women's Health Initiative is scheduled to yield results by 2005 and the first results of the Women's International Study of Long Duration Oestrogen after Menopause in 14 countries are expected in 2012. At present, the authors are aware of a French multicenter case–control study (Estrogen and Thromboembolism Risk (ESTHER) study under the auspices of Institut National de la Santé et de la Recherche Médicale (INSERM)) looking at HRT and the risk of VTE and focusing on the impact of the mode of administration of the estrogen.

The question of screening for thrombophilia before HRT may be raised. In women with no personal or family history of VTE, screening does not seem to be required. In women with no personal history but a positive family history, no screening is required if there have been previous uneventful pregnancies or use of oral contraception. In contrast, screening for thrombophilia may be justified in women who have had no pregnancy and who have not taken any oral contraception but who have a positive family history of VTE at a young age.

REFERENCES

1. Manson JE, Martin KA. Postmenopausal hormone-replacement therapy. *N Engl J Med* 2001;**345**:34–40.
2. Anderson FA Jr, Wheeler HB, Goldberg RJ, *et al.* A population-based perspective of the hospital incidence and case-fatality rates of deep vein thrombosis and pulmonary embolism. The Worcester DVT Study. *Arch Intern Med* 1991;**151**:933–8.
3. Meade TW, Haines AP, Imeson JD, *et al.* Menopausal status and haemostatic variables. *Lancet* 1983;**1**:22–4.
4. Meade TW, Dyer S, Howarth DJ, *et al.* Antithrombin III and procoagulant activity: sex differences and effect of menopause. *Br J Haematol* 1990;**74**:77–81.
5. Balleisen L, Bailey J, Epping PH, *et al.* Epidemiological study on factor VII, factor VIII and fibrinogen in an industrial population: I. Baseline data on the relation to age, gender,

body-weight, smoking, alcohol, pill-using, and menopause. *Thromb Haemost* 1985;**54**:475–9.

6. Scarabin PY, Bonithon-Kopp C, Bara L, *et al*. Relationship between plasminogen activator inhibitor activity and menopausal status. *Fibrinolysis* 1990;**4**:233–6.

7. Scarabin PY, Bonithon-Kopp C, Bara L, *et al*. Factor VII activation and menopausal status. *Thromb Res* 1990;**57**:227–34.

8. Folsom AR, Wu KK, Davis CE, *et al*. Population correlates of plasma fibrinogen and factor VII, putative cardiovascular risk factors. *Atherosclerosis* 1991;**91**:191–205.

9. Shahar E, Folsom AR, Salomaa VV, *et al*. Relation of hormone-replacement therapy to measures of plasma fibrinolytic activity. *Circulation* 1996;**93**:1970–5.

10. Meilhan EN, Kuller LH, Mattews KA, *et al*. Hemostatic factors according to menopausal status and use of hormone replacement therapy. *Ann Epidemiol* 1992;**2**:445–55.

11. Lee AJ, Lowe GDO, Smith WCS, *et al*. Plasma fibrinogen in women: relationships with oral contraception, the menopause and hormone replacement therapy. *Br J Haematol* 1993;**83**:616–21.

12. Brunner EJ, Marmot MG, White IR, *et al*. Gender and employment grade differences in blood cholesterol, apolipoproteins and haemostatic factors in the Whitehall II study. *Atherosclerosis* 1993;**102**:195–207.

13. Gebara OCE, Mittleman MA, Sutherland P, *et al*. Association between increased estrogen status and increased fibrinolytic potential in the Framingham Offspring Study. *Circulation* 1995;**91**:1952–8.

14. Salomaa V, Rasi V, Pekkanen J, *et al*. Association of hormone therapy with hemostatic and other cardiovascular risk factors. The FINRISK hemostasis study. *Arterioscler Thromb Vasc Biol* 1995;**15**:1549–55.

15. Scarabin PY, Vissac AM, Kirzin JM, *et al*. Population correlates of factor VII. Importance of age, sex, and menopausal status as determinants of activated factor VII. *Arterioscler Thromb Biol* 1996;**16**:1170–6.

16. DeSouza CA, Parker Jones P, Seals DR. Physical activity status and adverse age-related differences in coagulation and fibrinolytic factors in women. *Arterioscler Thromb Vasc Biol* 1998;**18**:362–8.

17. Meilhan E, Ferrell R, Kiss, *et al*. Genetic determination of coagulation factor VIIc levels among

healthy middle-aged women. *Thromb Haemost* 1995;**73**:623–5.

18. Douketic JD, Ginsberg JS, Holbrook A, *et al*. A re-evaluation of the risk for venous thromboembolism with the use of oral contraceptives and hormone replacement therapy. *Arch Intern Med* 1997;**157**:1522–30.

19. Oger E, Scarabin PY. Assessment of the risk of venous thromboembolism among users of hormone replacement therapy. *Drugs Aging* 1999;**14**:55–61.

20. Boston Collaborative Drug Surveillance Program. Surgically confirmed gallbladder, venous thromboembolism, and breast tumors in relation to postmenopausal estrogen therapy. *N Engl J Med* 1974;**290**:15–19.

21. Petitti DB, Wingerd J, Pellegrin F, Ramcharan S. Risk of vascular disease in women. Smoking, oral contraceptives, non-contraceptive estrogens and other factors. *JAMA* 1979;**242**:1150–4.

22. Devor M, Barrett-Connor E, Renvall M, *et al*. Estrogen replacement therapy and the risk of venous thrombosis. *Am J Med* 1992;**92**:275–84.

23. Nachtigall LE, Natchigall RH, Natchigall RD, Beckman EM. Estrogen replacement therapy. A prospective study in the relationship to carcinoma and cardiovascular and metabolic problems. *Obstet Gynecol* 1979;**54**:74–9.

24. Daly E, Vessey MP, Hawkins MM, *et al*. Risk of venous thromboembolism in users of hormone replacement therapy. *Lancet* 1996;**348**:977–80.

25. Jick H, Derby LE, Myers MW, *et al*. Risk of hospital admission for idiopathic venous thromboembolism among users of postmenopausal estrogens. *Lancet* 1996;**348**:981–3.

26. Grodstein F, Stampfer MJ, Goldhaber SZ, *et al*. Prospective study of exogenous hormones and risk of pulmonary embolism in women. *Lancet* 1996;**348**:983–7.

27. Perez-Gutthann S, Garcia Rodriguez LA, Castellsague JC, Duque Oliart A. Hormone replacement therapy and risk of venous thromboembolism: population based case-control study. *BMJ* 1997;**314**:796–800.

28. Varas-Lorenzo C, Garcia Rodriguez LA, Cattaruzzi C, *et al*. Hormone replacement therapy and the risk of hospitalization for venous thromboembolism: a population-based study in southern Europe. *Am J Epidemiol* 1998;**147**:387–90.

29. Hulley S, Grady D, Busch T, *et al*. for the Heart and Estrogen/progestin Replacement Study (HERS) Research Group. Randomized trial of estrogen plus progestin for secondary prevention

of coronary heart disease in postmenopausal women. *JAMA* 1998;**280**:605–13.

30. Grady D, Wenger NK, Herrington D, *et al.* Postmenopausal hormone therapy increases risk for venous thromboembolic disease. The Heart and Estrogen/progestin Replacement Study. *Ann Intern Med* 2000;**132**:689–96.

31. Herrington DM, Reboussin DM, Brosnihan B, *et al.* Effects of estrogen replacement on the progression of coronary-artery atherosclerosis. *N Engl J Med* 2000;**343**:522–9.

32. Høibraaten E, Abdelnoor M, Sandset PM. Hormone replacement therapy with estradiol and risk of venous thromboembolism. A population based case control study. *Thromb Haemost* 1999;**82**:1218–21.

33. Scarabin PY, Plu-Bureau G, Bara L, *et al.* Haemostatic variables and menopausal status: influence of hormone replacement therapy. *Thromb Haemost* 1993;**70**:584–7.

34. Nabulsi AA, Folsom AR, White A, *et al.* Association of hormone replacement therapy with various cardiovascular risk factors in postmenopausal women. The Atherosclerosis Risk in Communities Study Investigators. *N Engl J Med* 1993;**328**:1069–75.

35. Manolio TA, Furberg CD, Shemanski L, *et al.* Associations of postmenopausal estrogen use with cardiovascular disease and its risk factors in older women. *Circulation* 1993;**88**:2163–71.

36. Meilhan EN, Cauley JA, Tracey RP, *et al.* Association of sex hormones and adiposity with plasma levels of fibrinogen and PAI in postmenopausal women. *Am J Epidemiol* 1996;**143**:159–66.

37. Caine YG, Bauer KA, Barzegar S, *et al.* Coagulation activation following estrogen administration to postmenopausal women. *Thromb Haemost* 1992;**68**:392–5.

38. PEPI. Effects of estrogen and estrogen/progestin regimens on heart risk factors in postmenopausal women. The Postmenopausal Estrogen/ Progestin Interventions (PEPI) Trial. The writing group for the PEPI Trial. *JAMA* 1995;**273**:199–208.

39. Conard J, Denis C, Basdevant A, *et al.* Cardiovascular risk factors and combined estrogen-progestin replacement therapy: a placebo-controlled study with nomegestrol acetate and estradiol. *Fertil Steril* 1995;**64**:957–62.

40. Writing Group for the Estradiol Clotting Factors Study. Effects on haemostasis of hormone replacement therapy with transdermal estradiol and oral sequential medroxyprogesterone acetate: a 1-year, double-blind, placebo-controlled study. *Thromb Haemost* 1996;**75**:476–80.

41. Scarabin PY, Alhenc-Gelas M, Plu-Bureau G, *et al.* Effects of oral and transdermal estrogen/progesterone regimens on blood coagulation and fibrinolysis in postmenopausal women. A randomized controlled trial. *Arterioscler Thromb Vasc Biol* 1997;**17**:3071–8.

42. Høibraaten E, Ovigstad E, Andersen TO, *et al.* The effects of hormone replacement therapy (HRT) on hemostatic variables in women with previous venous thromboembolism: results from a randomized, double-blind, clinical trial. *Thromb Haemost* 2001;**85**:775–81.

43. Meade TW. Hormone replacement therapy and haemostatic function. *Thromb Haemost* 1997;**78**:765–9.

44. Douketis JD, Gordon M, Johnston M, *et al.* The effects of hormone replacement therapy on thrombin generation, fibrinolysis inhibition, and resistance to activated protein C: prospective cohort study and review of literature. *Thromb Res* 2000;**99**:25–34.

45. Conard J, Samama M, Basdevant A, *et al.* Differential AT III-response to oral and parenteral administration of 17β-estradiol. *Thromb Haemost* 1983;**49**:245.

46. De Mitrio V, Marino R, Cicinelli E, *et al.* Beneficial effects of postmenopausal hormone replacement therapy with transdermal estradiol on sensitivity to activated protein C. *Blood Coagul Fibrinolysis* 2000;**11**:175–82.

47. Sporrong T, Mattsson LA, Samsioe G, *et al.* Haemostatic changes during continuous oestradiol–progestogen treatment of postmenopausal women. *Br J Obstet Gynaecol* 1990;**97**:939–44.

48. Lowe G, Woodward M, Vessey M, Rumely A, Gough P, Daly E. Thrombotic variables and risk of idiopathic venous thromboembolism in women aged 45–64 years. Relationship to hormone replacement therapy. *Thromb Haemost* 2000;**83**:530–5.

49. Hoibraaten E, Ovigstad E, Arnesen H, *et al.* Increased risk of recurrent venous thromboembolism during hormone replacement therapy: results of the randomized, double-blind, placebo-controlled estrogen in venous thromboembolism trial (EVTET). *Thromb Haemost* 2000;**84**:961–7.

50. Powles T, Eeles R, Ashley S, *et al.* Interim analysis of the incidence of breast cancer in the Royal Marsden Hospital Tamoxifen Randomised Chemoprevention Trial. *Lancet* 1998;**352**:98–101.

51. Veronesi U, Maisonneuve P, Costa A, *et al.* Prevention of breast cancer with tamoxifen: preliminary findings from the Italian Randomised Trial Among Hysterectomised Women. *Lancet* 1998;**352**:93–7.

52. Fisher B, Costantino JP, Wickerham DL, *et al.* Tamoxifen for prevention of breast cancer: report of the National Surgical Adjuvant Breast and Bowel Project P-1 Study. *J Natl Cancer Inst* 1998;**90**:1371–88.

53. Cummings SR, Eckert S, Krueger KA, *et al.* The effect of raloxifene on risk of breast cancer in postmenopausal women: results from the MORE randomized trial. *JAMA* 1999;**281**:2189–97.

54. Winkler UH, Altkemper R, Kwee B, Helmond FA, Coelingh Bennink HJT. Effects of tibolone and continuous combined hormone replacement therapy on parameters in the clotting cascade: a mulicenter, double-blind, randomized study. *Fertil Steril* 2000;**74**:10–19.

55. Glazier G, Bowman MA. A review of the evidence for the use of phytoestrogens as a replacement for traditional estrogen replacement therapy. *Arch Intern Med* 2001;**161**:1161–72.

10

Ovarian hyperstimulation and thrombosis

Anne Gompel, Delphine P Levy and Jacqueline Conard

Ovarian hyperstimulation syndrome (OHSS) is usually a complication of ovulation induction or ovarian stimulation during *in vitro* fertilization (IVF) treatment. Thrombosis is a rare occurrence during OHSS, however, it may be very severe and it can cause death. When it does occur, it is often when OHSS is already improving, and it may occur in the absence of severe OHSS.

OVULATION INDUCTION

Conventional ovulation induction is usually indicated in anovulatory conditions or 'unexplained' infertility in the presence of normal sexual intercourse or insemination. Various regimens can be administered, including antiestrogens such as clomiphene citrate, gonadotropins such as human menopausal gonadotropin (hMG) or follicular stimulating hormone (FSH) to control follicular growth, or human chorionic gonadotropin (hCG) to trigger ovulation and for luteal support. Pulsatile gonadotropin releasing hormone (GnRH) can also be administered to patients with hypothalamic amenorrhea. The aim is to obtain recruitment and maturation of one or, at most, two follicles. Antiestrogens very rarely result in OHSS, which is mainly observed in women with the polycystic ovary syndrome. Pulsatile GnRH is never complicated by OHSS and should be used as often as possible. However, its indica-

tions are restricted to clomiphene-unresponsive hypothalamic amenorrhea. Treatments with hMG–FSH and hCG are usually incriminated when OHSS and multiple pregnancy occur.

The predominant indication for ovulation induction is now assisted reproductive technologies (ART) for IVF. Long or short protocols can be used, with combinations of GnRH analogs and exogenous gonadotropins (FSH or hMG) before oocyte recovery. FSH or hMG stimulate follicular selection and growth. GnRH analogs preclude the possibility of a precocious surge in luteinizing hormone (LH). Induction of ovulation is ensured by hCG, and oocyte recovery is performed 36 hours after hCG administration. Luteal support by administration of progesterone is safer than hCG injections, which can increase the risk of OHSS. The aim of this procedure, also called 'controlled ovarian hyperstimulation', is the recruitment and maturation of up to 15–20 follicles. After *in vitro* fecundation, two or three embryos are replaced while the others are frozen for subsequent transfer cycles. Moderate to severe OHSS may ensue from this procedure, especially when pregnancy is established.

The protocols for ovulation induction, especially those that include gonadotropin administration, increase serum estrogen levels, but the increases are much faster and greater after regular IVF procedures.[1]

THE OVARIAN HYPERSTIMULATION SYNDROME

Before the introduction of ART, the incidence of OHSS with conventional ovulation induction was 8–23% for mild OHSS (grade 1), 1–8% for moderate OHSS (grade 2) and < 1% for severe OHSS (grade 3).[2–4] During ART, moderate OHSS was reported to occur in 3–4% of cases, with the severe form occurring in 0.5–5% of cycles.[5,6] OHSS can have different clinical presentations, staged in three main grades according to severity (Table 10.1).

The underlying mechanism for the clinical manifestations of OHSS is an increase in vascular permeability at the ovarian level. An important extravascular exudative fluid shift occurs, leading to hypovolemia, oliguria or anuria, electrolyte imbalance, and hemoconcentration. A resulting stimulation of the renal renin–angiotensin system worsens the hemodynamic modifications. Adult respiratory distress syndrome, renal failure, and death have been reported secondary to hemodynamic alterations.[7] Thromboembolic complications may also be associated with the hemodynamic features of the syndrome, and are provoked by hemoconcentration. Deaths from cerebrovascular thrombosis have been reported (see below).

OHSS occurrence is mainly dependent on hCG administration, either exogenously, for the induction of ovulation, or endogenously, when pregnancy is established. This explains the fact that OHSS is far more common during pregnancy cycles, especially in the cases of multiple pregnancies. In consequence, during conventional ovulation induction treatments, hCG injection is withheld when serum estradiol levels reach > 4,300 pmol/l (1200 pg/ml) or more than two dominant follicles are seen at ultrasonography. This implies strict monitoring in order to decrease the risk of OHSS. During IVF, conditions indicating the possibility of OHSS include preovulation estradiol serum levels > 12,675 pmol/l (3500 pg/ml) as well as the development of more than 25 small or intermediate-sized follicles. Avoiding or postponing (coasting) hCG administration when the ovaries have been hyperstimulated can often prevent OHSS. Risk factors for OHSS include the existence of polycystic ovaries at ultrasound (seen in 40% of patients undergoing IVF procedures), young age (often male factor couple

Table 10.1 Grades of OHSS			
	Pathophysiology	**Clinical signs**	**Ultrasound findings**
Grade 1 (mild)	Fluid accumulation	Weight gain, abdominal distension and discomfort	Enlarged ovaries (>5 cm in diameter)
Grade 2 (moderate)	Further fluid accumulation	Nausea and vomiting dyspnea	Further ovarian enlargment (8–12 cm in diameter), ascites
Grade 3 (severe)	Intravascular volume contraction, decreased cardiac output, decreased central venous pressure	Tense ascites, severe dyspnea, compromised circulation	Pleural and pericardial effusions, hepatorenal failure

OHSS, ovarian hyperstimulation syndrome

infertilities), and a brisk ovarian responsiveness to stimulation. OHSS is also more common when ovarian stimulation protocols include gonadotropins and long-acting GnRH-agonist pituitary suppression (resulting from higher doses of gonadotropins and usually involving young patients). Whether the inclusion of LH in the ovarian stimulation protocol increases the occurrence of OHSS is still a matter of debate.[8]

The mechanism of OHSS involves rapid angiogenesis at the ovarian level and an increase in capillary permeability, together with rapid ovary enlargement.[7] The observed increase in ovarian size is due to follicular growth and secondary luteal cysts, which contribute, together with ascites, to the increase in intra-abdominal pressure. In some cases, removing ascites fluid may improve the clinical features of the syndrome.[9] Many possible candidates have been suggested as playing a role in the development of OHSS. The causative role of estradiol was initially discussed, since the severity of the syndrome is correlated with plasma estradiol levels. However, OHSS could not be reproduced when rabbits were treated with estradiol. Indeed, the increase in estradiol is linked to the number of follicles and reflects only the intensity of the stimulation. Furthermore, ovarian hyperstimulation without OHSS has been described in the absence of pregnancy in patients with pituitary gonadotropic adenoma.[10] Histamine, serotonin, and prostaglandins have also been implicated, though without any convincing demonstration of a predominant role. At this time, several other factors also seem fundamental, including the ovarian renin–angiotensin system, various cytokines, and vascular endothelial growth factor (VEGF).

Strong evidence suggests that the ovarian renin–angiotensin system plays a major role in the pathophysiology of OHSS. Prorenin, which can be locally activated, and angiotensin II are both present and active in the ovary. Prorenin production is under the control of LH and hCG, and several reports have correlated level of prorenin, number of follicles, and dose of hCG injected during IVF treatment cycles with severity of OHSS and plasma levels of renin and aldosterone.[6,7] In addition to the renin–angio-

tensin system, alternative mediators may also play a role in the genesis of OHSS, involving immune activation and release of vasoactive substances such as prostaglandins (PGs), the secretion of which is increased by estradiol and angiotensin II. Recent work has demonstrated the expression of various cytokines (interleukin (IL)-1, IL-6, tumor necrosis factor-α, IL-2, and IL-8) in the oocyte and early embryo, in addition to their production from local macrophages and monocytes and their correlation with the clinical manifestations of OHSS.[6,7] VEGF, a potent vasoactive and angiogenetic protein, has also been reported to be considerably increased in the serum of patients with severe OHSS, and, moreover, to depend on hCG administration.[11,12] All these factors probably contribute to the vascular alterations seen in OHSS.

THROMBOEMBOLIC MANIFESTATIONS OF OHSS

Venous and arterial thromboembolic manifestations have been reported during conventional ovulation induction in OHSS, initially by Crooke et al.[13] and also by Mozes et al.[14] Since then, most of the reported cases have been observed after ART.[15,16] Prevalence of thromboembolism has been estimated to one in 128 cases of severe OHSS; since OHSS is estimated to occur in 0.5–5% of cycles, the risk of a thrombotic event in ART could be one in 2650–6400 cycles.[16]

Seventy cases of arterial or venous thromboembolic events complicating OHSS have been reported so far in the literature.[16–26] Thromboses are essentially venous and, for unknown reasons, unusual sites such as jugular or upper limb veins are frequently involved. Indeed, 34 cases (49%) concerned these locations or the cerebral veins. Pulmonary embolism was infrequent. Eighteen of the cases were arterial (26%). Thrombosis does not occur at the same time as OHSS, but 6–70 days after hCG injection.[16–26] The mean observed delay is longer for venous thrombosis (38 days) than for arterial thrombosis (14 days). OHSS was associated with 75% of the cases of thrombosis and pregnancy with 80.4%.

Few fatal or severe thrombotic events associated with ovarian stimulation have been reported: a fatal thrombosis of the carotid artery,[14] a massive pulmonary embolism,[15] amputation of the lower limb after thrombosis of the femoral artery,[14] amputation of the forearm after thrombosis of the axillary artery recurring after thromboarterectomy,[25] coma, tetraplegia, and aphasia.[27]

ESTRADIOL, HEMOSTATIC CHANGES AND THROMBOSIS

The role of estradiol in coagulation is emphasized by the higher risk of thromboembolic disease in pregnancy.[28] Pregnancy is associated with an increase in several coagulation factors (fibrinogen, factor VII, factor VIII, and von Willebrand factor), decrease in antithrombin (AT) and protein S, and modifications of fibrinolysis (increased plasminogen and plasminogen activator inhibitors PAI-1 and PAI-2) levels.[29] These changes may result in a hypercoagulable state, reaching its maximum during the last trimester of pregnancy.

Most studies involving women undergoing ovulation induction reported an increase in platelet count and coagulation factor levels. An increase in fibrinogen and factor V was first reported in two women.[30] An increase in von Willebrand factor, a decrease in antithrombin and reduced fibrinolytic activity were also reported.[31–33] Lox et al. compared coagulation and fibrinolysis during hMG stimulation, with or without GnRH analog suppression, followed by hCG injection.[34] After hCG injection, levels of all coagulation factors (factors V, VII, VIII, IX, XI, and XII) increased and prothrombin time (PT) and activated partial thromboplastin time (aPTT) were shortened but remained in the normal range. Biron et al. reported an increase in coagulation activation and inflammation markers only after hCG administration.[35] The following changes were observed: increase in fibrinogen, prothrombin fragment 1+2, thrombin–antithrombin complexes, and D-dimers; decrease in coagulation inhibitors AT, protein C, and protein S. No change in reactivity of activated protein C was observed.[35,36]

In severe ovarian hyperstimulation syndrome (OHSS), Kodama et al. suggested that the plasma kinin system could contribute to the hypercoagulation state by increasing hemoconcentration and causing activation of coagulation and fibrinolysis.[37] A procoagulant activity of blood monocytes, mediated by tissue factor expression, has also been reported.[38] In a study of 40 women, 13 developed a severe form of OHSS followed by seven pregnancies (58%).[39] They were compared with a group of 10 women with a low estradiol (three pregnancies, 27%) and 17 women with a high estradiol level (five pregnancies, 29%). Tests of the coagulation and fibrinolytic systems were performed on days 0, 2, 4, 6, 8, and 10 after hCG administration. In addition, blood samples were collected beyond day 10, at 1-week intervals for 4 weeks in women with OHSS, and results were compared with the occurrence of pregnancy. Alterations in fibrinogen, AT, and markers of coagulation activation were more marked in OHSS than in women with high or low estrogen levels. Interestingly, elevation of coagulation activation markers persisted for 3 weeks or more after the onset of OHSS, but only in women who became pregnant.

MECHANISMS OF THROMBOSIS

The pathogenesis of these thrombotic events can be explained in part by the hypercoagulable state caused by OHSS, but it remains more obscure in the absence of OHSS. Most of the observed cases of thromboembolism were associated with OHSS and hemoconcentration as demonstrated by an increase in hematocrit. However, some cases were associated with a state of hemodilution. Increase in blood viscosity and coagulation factors are probably the main predisposing factors for thrombosis. In addition, immobilization of the patients during OHSS could be an additional risk factor. Hyperestrogenism certainly plays a role, contributing to the hypercoagulable state even in the absence of OHSS. Some modifications of coagulation may be associated with hyperestrogenism, such as an increase in fibrinogen and other coagulation factors and a decrease in coagulation inhibitors. However, fibrinogen levels were either correlated[35] or not[39] with estrogen levels. The increase in fibrinogen could also be related to the increase in C-reactive protein resulting from inflammation.[35] The change in estradiol between baseline and hyperstimulation correlated with the change in activated protein C (APC) resistance.[40]

As stated above, thrombosis usually occurs after a lag time following OHSS. It is not clear which factors act to promote the delayed thrombotic events. Pregnancy is well known for increasing the incidence of thrombosis and it may explain the occurrence of thrombosis in women with OHSS when they become pregnant. However, coagulation modifications are progressive and most of the thrombotic events occur during the last trimester of pregnancy or postpartum. Relative stasis of the legs and increase in intra-abdominal pressure may decrease the venous return. These events can explain venous thrombosis of the lower extremities. However, thromboses related to OHSS are mostly observed in the upper limb vessels or the head and neck vessels. Internal jugular vein thrombosis, which is often reported in OHSS, is very rare in the general population, even in women with familial thrombophilia in the absence of anatomical abnormalities, severe infections, or trauma.

Vascular and inflammatory changes described in OHSS may contribute to the hypercoagulable state, and the risk may be further increased in women with congenital thrombophilia or antiphospholipid syndrome. Thrombophilia has been detected in seven cases – antithrombin deficiency in one case with deep vein thrombosis,[41] protein S deficiency in one case with deep vein thrombosis[42] and one case with internal jugular vein thrombosis,[26] factor V Leiden mutation in three cases,[26,43] and factor II 20210A mutation in one case with internal jugular vein thrombosis.[26] Thrombophilia is probably more common than reported in women who experience thrombosis related to OHSS, since a complete coagulation screening is not performed in all women and the most common thrombophilias, namely factor V Leiden and factor II 20210A mutations, have

been known only since 1994 and 1996 respectively.

Elevated anticardiolipin antibodies have been reported in only two cases.[44,45] No prospective study has been performed on ovulation induction in women with system lupus erythematosus (SLE). Bruce and Laskin recently reported that they did not observe any case of SLE in 535 women who underwent several cycles of controlled ovarian hyperstimulation.[46] However, complicated consequences of 12 ovulation induction procedures, especially with gonadotropins, performed in eight women with SLE have been published to date by various teams.[47–49] It should be emphasized that antiphospholipid (aPL) antibodies were present in six of the seven patients tested, but they were not associated with the classical manifestations of the antiphospholipid syndrome. After the first treatment, recovery was achieved in all women but one who had an SLE flare associated with stenosis of the inferior vena cava and left renal vein, leading to pulmonary hypertension in the presence of anticardiolipin antibodies. Rechallenge was performed in four cases, leading in three to a severe SLE flare and one death from probable pulmonary embolism in the presence of anticardiolipin antibodies.[49]

THERAPEUTIC AND PREVENTION ISSUES

Prevention of OHSS depends on strict ovulation monitoring in standard ovulation induction. In IVF cycles where hyperstimulation is an aim, the issue is more complicated. Some authors propose the use of albumin; however, thrombosis can still occur despite its use.[27] Glucocorticoids are potent inhibitors of cytokine synthesis, but in a randomized controlled trial, Tan et al.[50] found no protective effect for corticosteroids started just after oocyte retrieval (at an initial dosage of 30 mg daily for 5 days, then quickly stopped within 5 days). To be effective this therapy may need to be started earlier or maintained for longer. In the future, specific anticytokine regimens may become available. Recently a rapid decrease in both serum estradiol concentration and ovarian size has been achieved with a high-dose GnRH antagonist.[51]

Prophylactic administration of heparin is advised in cases of severe OHSS, especially if there is an increased hematocrit or an increased risk of thrombosis, but there is no prospective study evaluating its efficacy. However, recommendations have been proposed.[3,15,16,26,52] It must be remembered that hyperstimulated ovaries are at high risk of hemorrhagic complications; therefore, indications for ovulation induction should be carefully tested in these women.[53] When prophylactic anticoagulation is administered in a woman with severe OHSS, it may be recommended to prolong the treatment during the first month of pregnancy since pregnancy and OHSS are associated with a hypercoagulable state. If a woman has a known thrombophilia or a history of venous thrombosis, the feasibility of IVF might be questioned, especially in thrombophilias at very high risk of thrombosis such as antithrombin deficiency or when the previous thrombosis was accompanied by a massive pulmonary embolism. In these women, when ovulation induction is considered feasible, heparin prophylaxis may be administered from the beginning of the procedure with a transitory interruption for oocyte retrieval, or started after retrieval and prolonged during pregnancy. The advocated doses correspond to 'high risk' prophylaxis.[26] Controlled studies are needed to determine the more appropriate protocol and doses.

Screening for thrombophilia could be planned before ovulation induction in patients with a personal or family history of venous thromboembolism. The screening includes PT and aPTT for the detection of circulating anticoagulant, AT, protein C, and protein S assays, resistance to activated protein C, and factor II 20210A mutation.

In cases of anovulation, antiestrogens constitute the first line of treatment. Standard doses should be used (100 mg of clomiphene) and care should be given in the presence of features of polycystic ovary syndrome, with a stringent follow-up by ultrasonography, estradiol monitoring, and clinical evaluation of weight and blood pressure. When this treatment fails, in cases of amenorrhea pulsatile GnRH should be preferred to gonadotropins, since it does not involve any risk of OHSS. Gonadotropins should be used sparingly and with continuous and careful clinical and biological control. In such cases, especially in SLE and antiphospholipid syndrome independently or during IVF, the authors currently maintain hydroxychloroquine, give a preventative dose of prednisone (0.5 mg/kg per day) and start subcutaneous unfractionated heparin or low molecular weight heparin at nearly therapeutic doses (such as enoxaparin 40 mg every 12 hours) on day 1 of controlled ovarian stimulation for at least several weeks.[53] Heparin is temporarily withheld after the morning administration on the day before oocyte retrieval, and it is started again, in association with aspirin (100 mg per day), immediately after this retrieval. In patients with prior antiphospholipid-related thrombotic events, the authors maintain heparin throughout any resultant pregnancy and for 1 month postpartum. The use of elastic stockings is strongly encouraged. In women with prior asymptomatic antiphospholipids and in those who are antiphospholipid-free, the administration of prophylactic doses (enoxaparin 40 mg once daily) for 2–3 months after the IVF procedure is probably sufficient.

Low molecular weight heparin is particularly suitable in this setting because it does not cross the placenta and, compared with unfractionated heparin, it appears to cause less osteoporosis with long-term use and less heparin-induced thrombocytopenia, a condition sharing similarities with antiphospholipid-related thrombocytopenia. The ideal dosage is unknown.

CONCLUSION

Thrombosis is a rare but sometimes severe or fatal event during ovulation induction. Its clinical presentation and pathophysiology remains mostly obscure. The prevention of severe OHSS may partly prevent thrombosis but attention should now be concentrated on the risk factors of venous thrombosis. The appropriate prophylaxis regimen is also yet to be defined.

REFERENCES

1. Meirow D, Laufer N, Schenker JG. Ovulation induction and *in vitro* fertilization. *Gynecol Endocrinol* 1993;**6**:211–24.

2. Schenker JG, Weinstein D. Ovarian hyperstimulation syndrome: a current survey. *Fertil Steril* 1978;**30**:255–68.

3. Jacobs HS, Agrawal R. Complications of ovarian stimulation. *Baillieres Clin Obstet* 1998;**12**:565–79.

4. Whelan JG, Vlahos NF. The ovarian hyperstimulation syndrome. *Fertil Steril* 2000;**73**:883–96.

5. MacDougall MJ, Tan SL, Balen A, Jacobs HS. A controlled study comparing patients with and without polycystic undergoing in-vitro fertilization. *Hum Reprod* 1993;**8**:233–7.

6. Simon A, Revel A, Hurwitz A, Laufer N. The pathogenesis of ovarian hyperstimulation syndrome: a continuing enigma. *J Assist Reprod Genet* 1998;**15**:202–9.

7. Elchalal U, Schenker JG. The pathophysiology of ovarian hyperstimulation syndrome: view and ideas. *Hum Reprod* 1997;**12**:1129–37.

8. Levy DP, Navarro JM, Schattman GL, Davis OK, Rosenwaks Z. The role of LH in ovarian stimulation: exogenous LH: let's design the future. *Hum Reprod* 2000;**15**:2258–65.

9. Borenstein R, Elchalal U, Lunenfeld B, Shoham Schwartz Z. Severe ovarian hyperstimulation syndrome: a reevaluated therapeutic approach. *Fertil Steril* 1989;**51**:791–5.

10. Christin-Maitre S, Rongieres-Bertrand C, Kottler ML, *et al.* A spontaneous and severe hyperstimulation of the ovaries revealing a gonadotroph adenoma. *J Clin Endocrinol Metab* 1998;**83**:3450–3.

11. Krasnow JS, Berga SL, Gusik DS, Zeleznik AJ, Yeo KT. Vascular permeability factor and vascular endothelial growth factor in ovarian hyperstimulation syndrome: a preliminary report. *Fertil Steril* 1996;**65**:552–5.

12. Abramov Y, Barak V, Nisman B, Schenker JG. Vascular endothelial growth factor plasma levels correlate with the clinical picture in severe ovarian hyperstimulation syndrome. *Fertil Steril* 1997;**67**:261–5.

13. Crooke AC, Butt WR, Carrington SP. Pregnancy in women with secondary amenorrhoea with human gonadotrophins. *Lancet* 1964;**1**:184–8.

14. Mozes M, Bogokowsky H, Antebi E, Lunenfeld B, Rabau E, Serr DM. Thromboembolic phenomena after ovarian stimulation with human gonadotrophins. *Lancet* 1965;**2**:1213–15.

15. Bénifla JL, Conard J, Naouri M, *et al.* Syndrome d'hyperstimulation ovarienne et thrombose. *J Gynecol Obstet Biol Reprod* 1994;**23**:778–83.

16. Stewart JA, Hamilton PJ, Murdoch AP. Thromboembolic disease associated with ovarian stimulation and assisted conception techniques. *Hum Reprod* 1997;**12**:2167–73.

17. Stewart JA, Hamilton PJ, Murdoch AP. Upper limb thrombosis associated with assisted conception treatment. *Hum Reprod* 1997;**12**:2174–5.

18. Moutos DM, Miller MM, Mahadevan MM. Bilateral internal jugular venous thrombosis complicating severe ovarian hyperstimulation syndrome after prophylactic albumin administration. *Fertil Steril* 1997;**68**:174–6.

19. Aboulghar MA, Mansour RT, Serour GI, Amin YM. Moderate ovarian hyperstimulation syndrome complicated by deep cerebrovascular thrombosis. *Hum Reprod* 1998;**13**:2088–91.

20. Todros T, Carmazzi CM, Bontempo S, Gaglioti P, Donvito V, Massobrio M. Spontaneous ovarian hyperstimulation syndrome and deep vein thrombosis in pregnancy. *Hum Reprod* 1999;**14**:2245–8.

21. Loret de Mola JR, Kiwi R, Austin C, Goldfarb JM. Subclavian deep vein thrombosis associated with the use of recombinant follicle-stimulation hormone (Gonal-F) complicating mild ovarian hyperstimulation syndrome. *Fertil Steril* 2000;**73**:1253–5.

22. Tang OS, Ng EH, Cheng PW, Ho PC. Cortical vein thrombosis misinterpreted as intracranial haemorrhage in severe ovarian hyperstimulation syndrome. *Hum Reprod* 2000;**15**:1913–16.

23. Ludwig M, Felberbaum RE, Diedrich K. Deep vein thrombosis during administration of HMG for ovarian stimulation. *Arch Gynecol Obstet* 2000;**263**:139–41.

24. Belaen B, Geerinckx K, Vergauwe P, Thys J. Internal jugular vein thrombosis after ovarian stimulation. *Hum Reprod* 2001;**16**:510–12.

25. Mancini A, Milardi D, Di Pietro ML, *et al.* A case of forearm amputation after ovarian stimulation for *in vitro* fertilization–embryo transfer. *Fertil Steril* 2001;**76**:198–200.

26. Arya R, Shehata HA, Patel RK, *et al.* Internal jugular vein thrombosis after assisted conception therapy. *Br J Haematol* 2001;**115**:153–155.

27. Humbert G, Delaunay P, Leroy J. Accident vasculaire cérébral au cours d'un traitement par les gonadotrophines. *Nouv Presse Med* 1973;**2**:28–30.

28. Greer IA. Thrombosis in pregnancy. *Lancet* 1999;**353**:1258–65.

29. Eldor A. Thrombophilia, thrombosis and pregnancy. *Thromb Haemost* 2001;**86**:104–11.

30. Phillips LL, Gladstone W, Vande Wiele R. Studies of the coagulation and fibrinolytic systems in hyperstimulation syndrome after administration of human gonadotropins. *J Reprod Med* 1975;**14**:138–43.

31. Kim HC, Kemmann E, Shelden RM, Saidi P. Response of blood coagulation parameters to elevated endogenous 17β-estradiol levels induced by human menopausal gonadotropins. *Am J Obstet Gynecol* 1981;**140**:807–10.

32. Aune B, Hoie KE, Oian P, Holst N, Osterud B. Does ovarian stimulation for in-vitro fertilization induce a hypercoagulable state? *Hum Reprod* 1991;**7**:925–7.

33. Todorow S, Schricker ST, Siebzehnruebl ER, *et al.* von Willebrand factor: an endothelial marker to monitor in-vitro fetilization patients with ovarian hyperstimulation syndrome. *Hum Reprod* 1993;**8**:2039–46.

34. Lox C, Cañez M, DeLeon F, Dorsett J, Prien S. Hyperestrogenism induced by menotropins alone or in conjunction with luprolide acetate in *in vitro* fertilization cycles: the impact of hemostasis. *Fertil Steril* 1995;**63**:566–70.

35. Biron C, Galtier-Dereure F, Rabesandratana H, *et al.* Hemostasis parameters during ovarian stimulation for *in vitro* fertilization: results of a prospective study. *Fertil Steril* 1997;**67**:104–9.

36. Wramsby ML, Bokarewa MI, Blomback M, Bremme AK. Response to activated protein C during normal menstrual cycle and ovarian stimulation. *Hum Reprod* 2000;**15**:795–7.

37. Kodama H, Takada S, Fukuda J, *et al.* Activation of plasma kinin system correlates with severe coagulation disorders in patients with ovarian hyperstimulation syndrome. *Hum Reprod* 1997;**12**:891–95.

38. Balasch J, Reverter JC, Fabregues F, Tassies D, Ordinas A, Vanrell JA. Increased unduced monocyte tissue factor expression by plasma from patients with severe ovarian hyperstimulation syndrome. *Fertil Steril* 1996;**66**:608–13.

39. Kodama H, Fukuda J, Karube H, Matsui T, Shimizu Y, Tanaka T. Status of the coagulation and fibrinolytic systems in ovarian hyperstimulation syndrome. *Fertil Steril* 1996;**66**:417–23.

40. Curvers J, Nienhuis SJ, Nap AW, Hamulyak K, Evers JLH, Rosing J. Activated protein C resistance during *in vitro* fertilization treatment. *Eur J Obstet Gynecol Reprod Biol* 2001;**95**:222–4.

41. Kligman I, Noyes N, Benadiva CA *et al.* Massive deep vein thrombosis in a patient with antithrombin III deficiency undergoing ovarian stimulation for *in vitro* fertilization. *Fertil Steril* 1995;**63**:673–6.

42. Boulieu D, Ninet J, Pinede L, *et al.* Thrombose veineuse précoce de siège inhabituel, en début de grossesse après stimulation ovariennne. *Contracept Fertil Sex* 1989;**17**:725–7.

43. Horstkamp B, Lubke M, Kentenich H, *et al.* Internal jugular vein thrombosis caused by resistance to activated protein C as a complication of ovarian hyperstimulation after in-vitro fertilization. *Hum Reprod* 1996;**11**:280–2.

44. Ellis MH, Ben Nun I, Rathaus V, Wermer M, Shenkman L. Internal jugular vein thrombosis in patients with ovarian hyperstimulation syndrome. *Fertil Steril* 1998;**69**:140–2.

45. Birdsall MA, Lockwood GM, Ledger WL, Johnson PM, Chamley LW. Antiphospholipid antibodies in women having in-vitro fertilization. *Hum Reprod* 1996;**11**:1185–9.

46. Bruce IN, Laskin CA. Sex hormones in systemic lupus erythematosus: a controversy for modern times. *J Rheumatol* 1997;**24**:1461–3.

47. Le Thi Huong D, Wechsler B, Piette JC, *et al.* Risks of ovulation-induction therapy in systemic lupus erythematosus. *Br J Rheumatol* 1996;**35**:1184–6.

48. Ben-Chetrit A, Ben-Chetrit E. Systemic lupus erythematosus induced by ovulation induction treatment. *Arthritis Rheum* 1994;**37**:1614–17.

49. Casoli P, Tumiati B, La Sala G. Fatal exacerbation of systemic lupus erythematosus after induction of ovulation. *J Rheumatol* 1997;**24**:1639–40.

50. Tan SL, Balen A, Hussein E, Campbell S, Jacobs HS. The use of glucocorticoids for the prevention of ovarian hyperstimulation syndrome: a prospective randomized study. *Fertil Steril* 1992;**58**:378–83.

51. De Jogn D, Macklon NS, Mannaerts BM, Coelingh Bennink HJ, Fauser BC. High dose gonadotrophin-releasing hormone antagonist (Garinelix) may prevent ovarian hyperstimulation syndrome caused by ovarian stimulation for in-vitro fertilization. *Hum Reprod* 1998;**13**:573–5.

52. Verdy E. Evaluation du risque thromboembolique avant stimulation ovarienne: quel bilan? Quell prévention. *Gynecol Obstet Fertil* 2000;**12**:875–9.

53. Weschler B, Huong DT, Vautier-Brouzes D, Lefevre G, Gompel A, Piette JC. Can we advise ovulation induction in patients with SLE? *Scand J Rheumatol* 1998;**107** Suppl:53–9.

11

Haemostasis in normal pregnancy

Katarina Bremme

INTRODUCTION

Changes in blood coagulation and fibrinolysis during pregnancy create a state of hypercoagulability.[1,2] This phenomenon, probably caused by hormonal changes, protects the woman from fatal haemorrhage during delivery but predisposes her to thromboembolism. There are significant data suggesting that oestradiol-induced triglyceride alteration is responsible for these changes in coagulation and fibrinolysis.[3]

Hypercoagulation may be due to increased platelet aggregation, increased concentration of coagulation factors, decreased levels of coagulation inhibitors or decreased fibrinolytic capacity. Antithrombin, protein C and protein S are important coagulation inhibitors. Antithrombin inactivates thrombin, factors Xa, IXa and XIIa, kallikrein and plasmin; protein C, when activated, degrades factors Va and VIIIa and has profibrinolytic properties. Protein C is activated by thrombin on the endothelial cell in the presence of thrombomodulin, and its anticoagulant activity requires the non-enzymatic cofactor, protein S, which exists in plasma as a free protein and as a complex with the complement component C4b-binding protein. Only free protein S functions as a cofactor.[4]

Two specific fibrinolytic inhibitors of plasminogen activators (i.e. plasminogen activator inhibitor (PAI)-1 and (PAI)-2) are increased in plasma during pregnancy.[5] The former is also present in platelets, endothelial cells and the placenta; PAI-2 is the main inhibitor from the placenta.[6] Although there is a positive correlation between thrombin-activatable fibrinolysis inhibitor (TAFI) antigen levels and age in the female population, the mean value of TAFI was not influenced by pregnancy.[7]

The presence of D-dimers, which are specific plasmin degradation products of cross-linked fibrin, suggests ongoing fibrin deposition in the uteroplacental vasculature, followed by fibrin degradation.[6] The existence of low levels of soluble fibrin (fibrin monomers) also supports the hypothesis that fibrin has been formed.[8,9] Another indicator of hypercoagulation in normal pregnancy is the presence of thrombin–antithrombin complexes, formed as soon as thrombin appears in the circulation[10] and increased levels of prothrombin fragment 1 + 2.[11]

COAGULATION AND FIBRINOLYSIS DURING NORMAL PREGNANCY

Platelets

Maintenance of normal function of the blood vessels and a non-thrombotic state requires endothelial integrity. Platelets circulate as non-adhesive discs filled with potentially vasoactive material and they do not interact with the normal blood vessel wall. The endothelial cell is a source of von Willebrand factor (vWF), which binds to the platelet surface, resulting in platelet adhesion. Prostacyclin (prostaglandin $(PG)I_2$) is the principal prostanoid synthesized by blood vessels; it is a powerful vasodilator and a potent inhibitor of platelet aggregation, and it is in balance with the production by platelets of thromboxane, a vasoconstrictor and powerful aggregating agent.

There have been conflicting reports concerning the platelet count during normal pregnancy.[2] The advent of automated platelet counts has led to the recognition that, during late pregnancy, many healthy women become thrombocytopenic by conventional criteria (platelet count $< 150 \times 10^9/l$).[12] In a 1-year population-based surveillance study involving 4382 full-term women, maternal platelet counts were performed. At delivery, 7.3% had platelet counts $< 150 \times 10^9/l$,[13] a finding confirmed in another study (11.6%).[14] Women with gestational thrombocytopenia do not require alteration of their treatment, and healthy pregnant women with a platelet count $> 115 \times 10^9/l$ in late pregnancy do not require further investigation during pregnancy.[14] According to Bremme *et al.*,[15] platelet counts were significantly lower at 24 weeks' pregnancy than in week 12. The increase in mean platelet volume[16,17] also suggests that a compensated state of progressive platelet destruction occurs during the third trimester.

Low-grade chronic intravascular coagulation within the uteroplacental circulation is part of the physiological response to pregnancy. Thus, normal pregnancy is associated with a degree of enhanced platelet destruction, which is compensated for by increased production. When subjects with a normal pregnancy were compared to non-pregnant controls, O'Brien *et al.*[18] demonstrated a significantly lower platelet count and an increase in circulating platelet aggregates and *in vitro* hypoaggregability. This suggests the occurrence of platelet activation, which causes *in vivo* platelet aggregation followed by exhaustion of platelets. Additional evidence of *in vivo* activation in late pregnancy is supported by increased concentration of β-thromboglobulin (β-TG) in the second and third trimester of pregnancy compared with first trimester and non-pregnant age-matched controls.[19]

Thromboxane A_2 is the major product of arachidonic acid metabolism in platelets and a potent vasoconstrictor and platelet aggregating agent. Since it has a short half-life, it is normally measured as its stable hydration product, thromboxane B_2. Thromboxane biosynthesis was determined in normal pregnant subjects by measurement of its major urinary and plasma metabolites, 2,3-dinorthromboxane B_2 and 11-dehydrothromboxane B_2. Urinary 2,3-dinor-thromboxane B_2 increased early in pregnant subjects compared with non-pregnant and postpartum subjects period and remained elevated throughout pregnancy. Similarly, plasma and urinary 11-dehydrothromboxane B_2 increased in pregnancy.[20]

Enhancement of the generalized hypercoagulable state is detected in advance of raised plasma levels of β-TG and increased urinary excretion of thromboxane in apparently healthy women using whole blood cytometry to confirm the sensitivity of the assay. Measuring the endogenous production of PGI_2, assessed by 2,3-dinor-6-keto-$PGF_{1\alpha}$, seems to be more accurate as a marker for early dysfunction.[21] Flow cytometric analysis of platelets from normal pregnant women shows an enhanced degranulation response to adenosine disphosphate *in vitro* compared with age matched non-pregnant women.[22,23] Compensated, accelerated intravascular coagulation may be necessary for the maintenance of the uterine placenta interface and for preparation for the haemostatic challenge of delivery.[24]

Coagulation system

During pregnancy there are significant increases in the concentration of coagulation factors V, VII, VIII, IX, X, XII and vWF and a particularly pronounced increase in plasma fibrinogen.[1,2,25,26] The plasma fibrinogen concentration increases from non-pregnant levels of about 2.5–4.0 g/l in the first trimester to as high as 6.0 g/l in late pregnancy and labour as a result of increased synthesis. Factor VII may be increased as much as 10-fold.[2,27] vWF and factor VIII are increased in late pregnancy, the coagulation activity being about twice that in the nonpregnant state. The rise in factor IX concentration during pregnancy is small,[27] as is the decrease in factor XI (with concentrations down to 60–70% of the non-pregnant value), reaching a nadir at term.[28] There is a gradual fall in fibrin-stabilizing factor XIII, reaching 50% of the normal non-pregnant value at term after an initial increase at the beginning of pregnancy.[29] Factors II and V do not change in pregnancy.[2] The prothrombin complex (factors II, VII and X) is highest (prothrombin time shortest) in mid-pregnancy and it remains high in the third trimester. This increase probably reflects an increase in factors VII and X.[1,2]

Antithrombin
Antithrombin (AT) levels are significantly higher in women than men; they increase with age in women and are negatively associated with the use of female hormones. Although some earlier studies[30] have indicated a modest decrease in antithrombin towards the end of pregnancy, other studies with more specific functional assays have shown normal levels throughout pregnancy, with some decrease during delivery.[1,2,15,31,32]

Protein C, thrombomodulin and protein S
The protein C level remains normal during normal pregnancy.[33–36] By following the same women through pregnancy and using a functional method, a slight increase in the second trimester and at 5 weeks postpartum was found, but the levels were within non-pregnant normal range.[37,38]

Thrombomodulin (TM) represents a major determinant of the antithrombogenicity of the vessel wall. It shifts thrombin activity from procoagulant to anticoagulant by triggering the pwerful anticoagulant protein C system and by directly inhibiting fibrin formation, platelet aggregation and factor V activation.[39] TM also has a role in fibrinolysis, acting as the cofactor of plasma cocarboxypeptidase B. A soluble form of TM exists in plasma and urine, and this form can be used as a marker of endothelial damage, though it also originates from other platelets.

Neutrophil activation triggers endothelial TM proteolysis and increases TM levels in the last weeks of gestation.[40] TM levels increase continuously during pregnancy, in early pregnancy being barely different from non-pregnant values and with a rapid decrease postpartum.[41]

Protein S normally exists in plasma in two forms – the functionally active, free form and the form complexed with C4B-binding protein (which is functionally inactive). Although a fall in free protein S levels in pregnancy is physiological it is questionable whether this contributes to the hypercoagulable state of pregnancy and the increased incidence of thromboembolism. However, a further fall in free protein S levels during pregnancy in women with heterozygous congenital protein S deficiency may exacerbate the thrombotic tendency. Gilabert *et al.*[34] found a significant decrease in the levels of free and total protein S in the second trimester, and the levels remained low throughout pregnancy. Malm *et al.*[42] found a decreased level in the first trimester, with still lower levels in the second trimester, but there are no further significant changes during the third trimester.[36] Bremme *et al.*[15] also found a decreased level of free protein S in weeks 12–15 (0.26 µg/ml) with a significant decrease in week 24 (0.17 µg/ml) and a significantly lower level week 35 although numerically only down to 0.14 µ/ml. The values for both total protein S and free protein S in pregnancy are below normal ranges for non-oral contraceptive-using women as early as 6–11 weeks of gestation.[31]

Activated protein C resistance and factor V Leiden
The term activated protein C (APC) resistance has been used to describe the phenomenon by which plasma fails to be anticoagulated by the addition of APC *in vitro*, even in the presence of normal protein S function.[43] APC sensitivity is reduced during pregnancy[44] and, at term, 45% of pregnant women have an APC sensitivity ratio below the 95th percentile for the normal range for non-pregnant women of similar age.[45] Lower ratios in the classic APC resistance test have been reported during pregnancy, and this phenomenon has been called 'acquired' APC resistance.[46–48]

When 28 parous women without previous miscarriage, pregnancy complications or thrombotic events and non-carriers of the Arg 506 Gln mutation in FV, where investigated throughout a normal pregnancy a suppression of APC response was observed which reached lowest values by week 28.[49] The reduction in the APC ratio was directly related to its value in the non-pregnant state, being most pronounced in the women with the highest APC ratio before pregnancy. A low APC ratio early in pregnancy was observed in subjects who subsequently developed pre-eclampsia.[50] In another study, 38% of subjects who had no evidence of factor V Leiden or cardiolipin antibodies, showed a low APC ratio in the third trimester of pregnancy and had significant lower birth weights than subjects with a normal APC ratio.[31]

The vast majority of patients with familial APC resistance have the same mutation in their factor V gene (1691 G→A).[51] This so-called FV Leiden mutation is extremely prevalent (2–7%) in populations of European extraction but much less common or even absent in other populations. In a prospective study to investigate the prevalence of APC resistance among pregnant women, the overall prevalence was 11% (270 out of 2480), with seven women (0.3%) carrying the factor V:Q506 allele in its homozygous form and 263 women being heterozygous.[52] The prevalence of the factor Leiden mutation in APC resistance is around 85% in non-pregnant patients.

Women with pre-existing resistance to APC may develop a more pronounced defect during pregnancy. Retrospective studies show factor V Leiden-associated APC resistance and fetal death in all trimesters, fetal growth restriction, early-onset pre-eclampsia and HELLP (hemolysis, elevated liver enzymes, and low platelet count) syndrome.[53,54] Limited information exists to determine whether the APC resistance acquired during pregnancy confers the same risk as factor V Leiden-related APC resistance.[55] In the Leiden thrombophilia study a dose–response relationship was observed between the sensitivity to APC and the risk of thrombosis in non-factor V Leiden-mutated subjects.[55] This study also indicated that in carriers of the factor V Leiden mutation, the risk of thrombosis was about three times higher than in subjects with normal factor V gene and low APC sensitivities. In pregnancy about 50% of women acquire activated protein C resistance,[56] as detected by the standard

activated partial prothrombin time (aPTT)-based assay but none of these women had thromboembolic complications.

Little is known about the cause of the lowered APC ratio. The overall prevalence of APC resistance was 11% in a prospective study in Malmö, Sweden, and it was characterized by an eight-fold higher risk of venous thromboembolism but a lower rate of profuse intrapartum hemorrhage ($p = 0.02$).[52] One group found a negative covariance between the classic APC ratio and factor VIII at delivery.[45] The low APC ratio preceded an increase in factor VIII, which suggested that high levels of factor VIII during pregnancy could have been a result of its protection from inactivation and its accumulation in the circulation. The correlation became weaker in the course of pregnancy, losing significance by week 32.[49] Changes in free protein S concentration are unlikely to contribute significantly to the development of APC resistance during pregnancy. In a longitudinal and prospective study on healthy pregnant women, Kjellberg et al.[37] were unable to find any correlation between the total change in the classic APC ratio and the total changes in factor VIII, fibrinogen or protein S.

Protein C inhibitor (PCI) decreases during pregnancy.[57] He et al.[58] confirmed that PCI levels gradually decreased during pregnancy to reach a minimum in week 32, remaining on the same low level in week 37. Moreover, the PCI decrease corresponded to increases in APC resistance (Figure 11.1). This phenomenon implies that consumption of active PCI is directly involved in the mechanism of acquired APC resistance.

A modified APC resistance test, which includes sample dilution in factor V-deficient plasma before the aPTT-based assay, has been developed and shown to be useful in screening for factor V Leiden in patients on oral anticoagulants or with phospholipid. The modified APC test is more useful in detecting factor V Leiden mutation during pregnancy, since the classic APC test may give a false-positive result, especially in late pregnancy. Prior dilution of the patient's plasma with factor V-deficient plasma increases the specificity of the APC resistance test for factor V Leiden by minimizing the contribution of other factors.

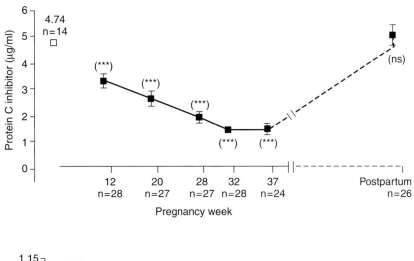

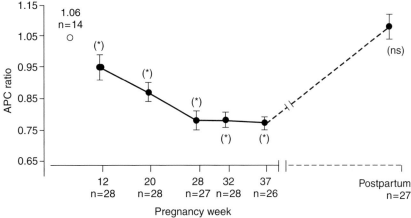

Figure 11.1 Levels (mean ± standard error) of protein C inhibitor and APC ratio during normal pregnancy and postpartum compared with those of healthy non-pregnant women. The Student's t-test (unpaired) was used for comparisons with the reference levels in the healthy young non-pregnant women: protein C inhibitor, 4.74 ± 0.48 µg/ml; APC ratio, 1.06 ± 0.19 µg/ml (mean ± standard error). ***$p < 0.001$; *$p < 0.05$; ns, $p > 0.05$. The changes between week 37 and postpartum could not be described. From He et al.[70]

Anti-phospholipid antibodies

Phospholipid antibodies (PLa) could exert a procoagulant effect by inhibiting the phospholipid-dependent activation of the protein-C–protein-S degradation of activated factor V. A reduced response to APC ratio was found in PLa-positive more often than in PLa-negative samples ($p < 0.005$) and was more common in the samples with lupus anticoagulants (LA) than in samples with cardiolipin antibodies (Cla).[59] A lack of correlation between the PLa level and the APC ratio was found in women who were negative for PLa and in those who were positive for PLa,[60] which implies that autoimmune reaction against phospholipid and APC response have different regulation mechanisms in healthy women.[49]

Cla occur only rarely (2.2%) in normal subjects, including pregnant women,[61] although reports put the figure between 0.5 and 6.2% of Cla and between 0 and 1.2% of LA.[62,63] Adverse pregnancy outcomes are not an invariable consequence of a positive test, and therapy is not always required to achieve normal outcomes. In a study of 700 low-risk pregnant women, 18 had phospholipid antibodies but, unlike the evidence from patients with antiphospholipid syndrome, there was not an association between antibody titre and adverse outcome.[61] Testing of pregnant women is therefore not recommended if not clinically indicated.[63] Screening of PLa in thrombosis-prone women during pregnancy is, however, indicated since the dosage of anticoagulant might need to be increased in PLa-positive women.[64]

Fibrinolysis

Plasma fibrinolytic activity is reduced during pregnancy, remains low during labour and delivery and returns to normal within 1 hour of placental delivery.[2] The rapid return of systemic fibrinolytic activity to normal following delivery of the placenta and the fact that the placenta contains inhibitors that block fibrinolysis suggest that inhibitors of fibrinolysis during pregnancy are mediated through the placenta.[65]

Tissue plasminogen activator (t-PA) activity decreased during pregnancy,[66] owing not only to the gradual and threefold increase in PAI-1 but also to the increasing levels of PAI-2.[6,67]

PAI-2 was originally discovered in the human placenta. Its plasma level generally becomes detectable only during pregnancy. Since villous cells are the source of PAI-2,[68,69] changes in the amount of placental tissue may influence its level in plasma.[70,72] In other words, a positive correlation between PAI-2 concentrations and placental weights is found. The concentration of PAI-2 varies with birth weights,[70–72] indicating the dependency not only on quantity and quality of the placental tissues but also on fetal growth.

At about week 8 of normal pregnancy, plasma PAI-2 may reach a level of 10 µg/l and then gradually increase until term.[68] In two patients with the diagnosis of hydatidiform mole, no PAI-2 was detected in the plasma (Figure 11.2).[70] Others have reported similar findings, as well as weak immunohistochemical staining of PAI-2 in the trophoblastic epithelium. Thus, the presence of the fetal tissues and their healthy state are of importance for the regulation of plasma PAI-2 levels. Despite the high levels of PAI-1 and PAI-2, an increased

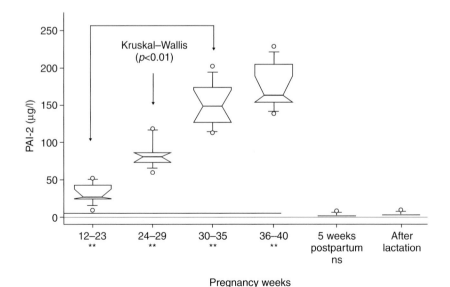

Figure 11.2 The levels of plasma PAI-2 during varying gestational periods, 5 weeks postpartum and after lactation in normal pregnant women. ** = $p<0.01$; ns, $p>0.05$; statistical method, Kruskal–Waxis. From He et al.[70]

level of the fibrinolytic degradation product D-dimer was found in third-trimester samples, suggesting that fibrinolysis still protects the women.[73]

Thrombin-activatable fibrinolysis inhibitor (TAFI) is a recently described fibrinolysis inhibitor; when activated, it removes the carboxyterminal lysine residues from fibrin and thus slows clot lysis by decreasing activation of plasminogen by t-PA on the fibrin network. The mean value of TAFI is not influenced by pregnancy.[7] Thus excessive activation of TAFI may constitute an additional contributing factor to thromboembolic complications and, since the level is not influenced by gestation, it could even be used in pregnant women.[74]

CHANGES IN COAGULATION AND FIBRINOLYSIS FOLLOWING DELIVERY

The increase in clotting activity at the time of parturition is probably related to expulsion of the placenta and release of thromboplastic substances at the site of separation,[75] and it may predispose to the development of deep vein thrombosis. The changes in the hemostatic mechanism during the puerperium are the same as those observed after extensive surgery,[76] determined on the basis of an increase in fibrinopeptide A ($p < 0.001$), β-thromboglobulin ($p < 0.001$) and platelet factor 4 ($p < 0.001$).[24] The mean platelet counts decreased slightly ($p < 0.05$) at the time of placental delivery but when measured shortly postpartum after uncomplicated vaginal delivery the platelet count remain unchanged, although it would be expected to decrease after a Caesarean section delivery.[77] The platelet count increased on days 2–5 ($p < 0.01$) postpartum, but the time to peak values is between 6–14 days.[78]

Plasma antithrombin levels decrease significantly after Caesarean delivery but not after vaginal delivery. The significant rise starts almost at once after normal delivery and lasts at least 2 weeks. A rise in protein C levels is shown immediately after delivery and still 3 days postpartum.[31,79] According to Gilabert et al.,[75] the level of protein S (total and free) increased significantly after delivery from the first day of the puerperium; in the study Malm et al.,[42] total protein S had normalized in the first week postpartum. Free protein S is not normalized 5 weeks postpartum,[38] and 8 weeks postpartum 15% of the women still have levels below the reference range for non-pregnant women.[37] Thus, the free fraction of protein S does not seem to reach the non-pregnant value within 8 weeks postpartum, which might be taken into consideration when evaluating thrombophilia.

Increasing thrombin-antithrombin complex (TAT) levels during labour and delivery indicated generation of thrombin, which was mainly inactivated by antithrombin. During normal delivery, the median TAT level increased from 4.1 to 7.8 times that of the median normal reference level,[80] while 1–2 days after delivery, the median TAT level was 2.5 times the median normal reference. Three weeks after delivery blood coagulation and fibrinolysis were generally normalized. Coagulation, measured as increased factor VIII activity, and levels of vWF antigen, fibrinogen and fibrinopeptide A is normalized 3–4 weeks after delivery. Until then, the increased level of coagulation variables were counteracted by an increase in antithrombin. The fibrinolytic system is triggered immediately after placental separation. The increase in PAI-2 during pregnancy is almost linear; at term, levels of 100–300 µg/l have been reported, followed by a decrease to undetectable levels within about 1 week after delivery.[5,6] Analyses from samples taken before the women left hospital (mean 2.4 days postpartum) showed that PAI-1 had already decreased to the non-pregnant level and that PAI-2 was reduced to 28% of the level in the third trimester.[37] In another study, the levels seemed to start to decrease between week 35 and parturition. High levels occurred in one woman 5 weeks postpartum after lactation.[15] An increased level, not yet well understood, has been found in some normal women and men.

The number of cases of venous thromboembolism around delivery accounts for a large proportion of all cases related to pregnancy.[81] The observed risk around delivery corresponds to the prothrombotic state of the coagulation system accompanying pregnancy apparent in the third trimester and highest around delivery and declining, but still substantially elevated, during the puerperium. After the puerperium, during the first year post partem, the decreased risk of venous thrombosis may be associated with lower levels of estrogen among lactating women.

The peak in clotting and platelet activity seems to occur immediately after placental delivery, whereas the peak in fibrinolytic activity is seen during the first 3 hours postpartum.[24] This is reflected by an increase in fibrin–fibrinogen degradation products and D-dimer levels. The difference in clotting and fibrinolytic activity at the time of parturition may be used to ensure maximum coagulation at the time of delivery (Figure 11.3).

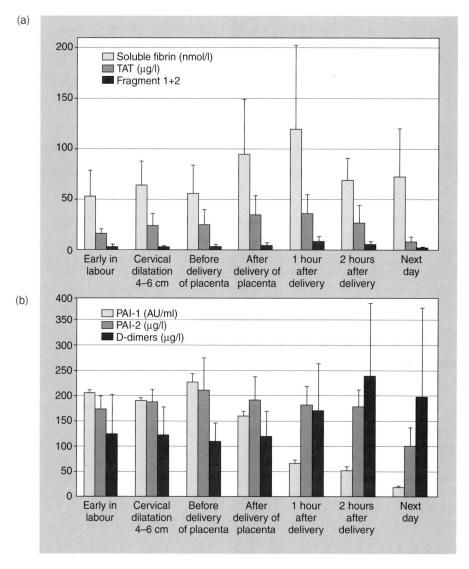

Figure 11.3 Haemostatic indices (mean ± SD) in normal pregnant women during delivery (n = 16). (a) Coagulation activity measured with soluble fibrin, thrombin–antithrombin complex and fragment 1+2 shows maximum values 1 hour after delivery. (b) Fibrinolytic activity measured with PAI-1, PAI-2 and D-dimers shows maximum values 2 hours after delivery.

QUANTITATION OF THE HAEMOSTATIC PROBLEMS ASSOCIATED WITH PREGNANCY

The exact mechanism whereby prothrombotic and lipid abnormalities lead to pregnancy failure is unknown. This may result from thrombosis of the placental vessels and stimulation of an inflammatory response from the endothelium. Stimulation of an inflammatory response results in secretion of proadhesive molecules and cytokines from the endothelium and alteration of the anticoagulant protein C system on the endothelial surface. Hypercoagulability can be biochemically defined as a condition of procoagulant imbalance caused by heightened activity of coagulation enzymes in the absence of laboratory and clinical signs of fibrin formation. This situation may be detected by measuring plasma markers of coagulation activation. An increase in the markers of activation of the endothelium is a feature of normal pregnancy, but heightened activation is associated with disorders of pregnancy such as pre-eclampsia. To identify this imbalance in the haemostatic system and to locate the underlying causes, there are many laboratory tests.

Normal pregnancy is associated with major changes in the coagulation and fibrinolytic system that takes care of the haemostatic challenge of delivery and also maintains placental function during pregnancy. The effect is an increased thrombotic potential, which is most marked around term and in the immediate postpartum period. The changes in the coagulation system in normal pregnancy are consistent with a continuing low-grade process of coagulant activity.[24] The finding that fibronectin values did not increase with advancing gestational age in normal pregnancy[82–84] but were significantly increased in samples from women with severe pre-eclampsia suggest that maternal vascular endothelial cell injury is an early and specific sign of the pathogenesis of pre-eclampsia.[81] It is interesting that fibronectin levels were not increased, indicating that despite the low-grade disseminated intravascular coagulation in normal pregnancy there was no evidence of endothelial damage (in contrast to disorders such as preeclampsia where low grade disseminated

intravascular coagulation is associated with endothelial injury).[84] Under electron microscopy, fibrin is deposited in the intervillous space of the placenta and in the walls of spiral arteries that supply the placenta. The increased levels of fibrinogen and coagulation factors during pregnancy are probably a compensatory response to local utilization. The resulting hypercoagulability is advantageous in meeting the sudden demand for haemostatic components at placental separation. The concentration of the coagulation inhibitors antithrombin and protein C remained within normal levels, whereas the mean level of free protein S showed a significant decrease from 0.26 U/ml in early pregnancy to 0.14 U/ml in week 35. At the same time, soluble fibrin levels increased from 9.2 to 13.4 nmol/l and thrombin–antithrombin complexes increased from 3.1 to 7.1 µg/l; both are indicators of thrombin activity. A concurrent increase in the levels of the fibrinolytic inhibitors PAI-1 and PAI-2 (from 7.4 to 37.8 AU/ml and 31 to 160 µg/l, respectively suggests a decrease in fibrinolytic activity. However, the levels of fibrin D-dimer (i.e. fibrin split products) also increased in parallel, from 91 to 198 µg/l, suggesting that fibrinolysis is present. Thus, a balance normally exists, which is probably why thrombotic events are rare during pregnancy (Figures 11.4 and 11.5).[15]

Thrombin generation

Thrombin, the key enzyme that converts fibrinogen to fibrin, is in a 1:1 complex inactivated by the inhibitor antithrombin. Therefore, the generation of thrombin–antithrombin complexes is a marker of thrombin formation. A significant and gradual increase, which reached doubled values in the third trimester, was described.[71] TAT complex levels higher than reference values have been reported to be present in 50% of women during the first trimester, and all subjects show elevated levels in the second and third trimesters. The levels were within reference values at 5 weeks postpartum.[15] A significant positive correlation between gestational age and elevated factor fragment 1+2 has also been shown. The observed rise in prothrombin fragment 1+2 between the first and second

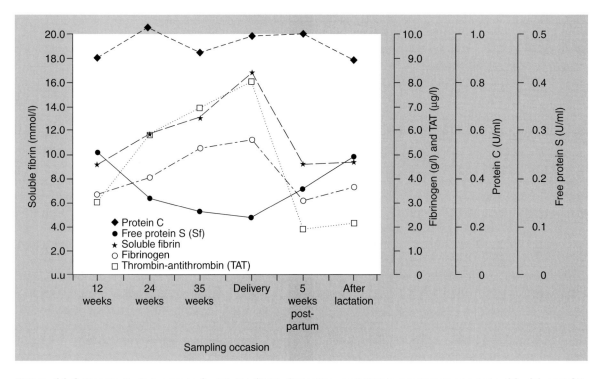

Figure 11.4 Protein C, free protein S, soluble fibrin, fibrinogen and TAT in pregnancy at weeks 12, 24 and 35, delivery, 5 weeks postpartum and after lactation. From Bremme et al.[15]

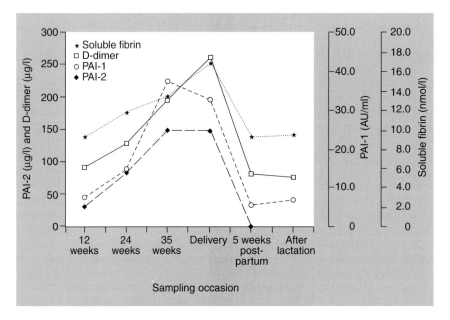

Figure 11.5 Soluble fibrin, D-dimer, PAI-1 and PAI-2 in pregnancy at weeks 12, 24 and 35, delivery, 5 weeks postpartum and after lactation. From Bremme et al.[15]

trimesters indicates that a degree of activation of coagulation occurs relatively early in normal pregnancy.[31,85] Prothrombin fragment 1+2 was increased three times (to 3.14 nmol/l) in pregnancy week 38 and was still elevated 1 week postpartum compared with weeks 10–15 of pregnancy (0.97 nmol/l), but it normalized in week 8 postpartum.[37] Delorme et al.[86] have shown that 'pregnant plasma' in in vitro experiments is capable of more rapid and elevated generation of thrombin than non-pregnant plasma. This result, in combination with evidence of an increase in prothrombin activation and TAT complex formation, suggests that heightened thrombin generation is a feature of normal pregnancy.

Fibrin formation is known to be essential for normal placental implantation. Since thrombin has both procoagulant and anticoagulant, it is not clear whether enhanced thrombin generation of pregnancy contributes to a prothrombotic state. Using a more specific method than Wallmo et al.,[8] Bremme et al.,[15] found sporadically elevated levels of soluble fibrin with increasing frequency throughout pregnancy. This may be due to the increased availability of several coagulation proteins, such as fibrinogen and prothrombin complex factors. Although a higher concentration of plasma soluble fibrin was observed in many of the women with pregnancy complications, no clear correlation to the outcome of pregnancy was obtained. Whether or not plasma-soluble fibrin is of any value, either diagnostically or in the treatment of patients with pregnancy complications, remains to be shown.[38,87]

He et al.[88] were thus interested in establishing a method for screening the overall haemostatic potential in plasma (OHPP). A fibrin time curve was made via spectrophotometric registration of fibrin generation and lysis in plasma, to which exogenous thrombin and tissue-type plasminogen activator had been added. The area under the curve, calculated by the sum of absorbance, varied in correlation to the concentrations of platelets or purified pro- or anticoagulants – tissue factor, vWF, fibrinogen, antithrombin and PAI-1.

The sum of absorbance offers information about the combined effects of coagulation and fibrinolysis in the blood sample. This, determi-

nation of the sum of absorbance has opened up the possibility for monitoring the overall hemostatic potential in plasma. Preliminary results were satisfactory; the levels of OHPP, expressed as the sums of absorbance, were higher in normal pregnant women than in the controls and were even higher in pre-eclamptic patients than in uncomplicated pregnant women, which corresponds to the different grades of hypercoagulability in the three groups. The normal pregnant women had a lower median sum of absorbance than the pre-eclampsia patients, although it was higher than that of the normal controls ($p < 0.001$).[88] Preliminary results show increasing values of OHPP during pregnancy, confirming the usefulness of the method (Figure 11.6).

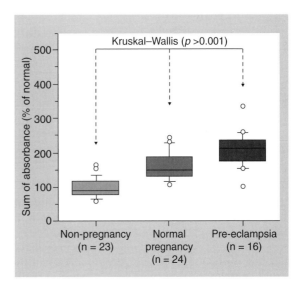

Figure 11.6 Box-plots of the sums of absorbance in groups of young, healthy non-pregnant women and pregnant women with or without pre-eclampsia. The pregnant women with or without pre-eclampsia were sampled in gestational weeks 35–38. The box-plots indicate the 10th, 25th, 50th, 75th and 90th percentiles. The 50th percentile of the individual values are contained within the box. Values either above the 90th or below the 10th percentiles are represented by small open circles; statistical method, Kruskal–Wallis. From He et al.[88]

REFERENCES

1. Bonnar J. Haemostasis and coagulation disorders in pregnancy. In: Bloom AL, Thomas DP, eds. *Haemostasis and Thrombosis*. Edinburgh: Churchill Livingstone; 1987:570–84.
2. Stirling Y, Woolf L, North WRS, *et al.* Haemostasis in normal pregnancy. *Thromb Haemost* 1984;**52**:176–82.
3. Sattar N, Greer IA, Rumley A, *et al.* A longitudinal study of the relationships between haemostatic, lipid and oestradiol changes during normal human pregnancy. *Thromb Haemost* 1999;**81**:71–5.
4. Dahlbäck B. Protein S and C4b-binding protein: components involved in the regulation of the protein C anticoagulant system. *Thromb Haemost* 1991;**66**:49–61.
5. Kruithof E, Tran-Thang C, Gudinchet A, *et al.* Fibrinolysis in pregnancy: a study of plasminogen activator and inhibitors. *Blood* 1987;**69**:460–6.
6. Wright JG, Cooper P, Åstedt B, *et al.* Fibrinolysis during normal human pregnancy: complex inter-relationships between plasma levels of tissue plasminogen activator and inhibitors and the euglobulin clot lysis time. *Br J Haematol* 1988;**69**:253–8.
7. Chetaille P, Alessi MC, Kouassi D, *et al.* Plasma TAFI antigen variations in healthy subjects. *Thromb Haemost* 2000;**83**:902–5.
8. Wallmo L, Karlsson K, Teger-Nilsson AC. Fibrinopeptide A and intravascular coagulation in normotensive and hypertensive pregnancy and parturition. *Acta Obstet Gynaecol Scand* 1984;**63**:637–40.
9. van Wersch JWJ, Ubachs JMH. Blood coagulation and fibrinolysis during normal pregnancy. *Eur J Clin Chem Clin Biochem* 1991;**29**:45–50.
10. Collen D, De Cock F, Verstraete M. Quantitation of thrombin-antithrombin III complexes in human blood. *Eur J Clin Invest* 1977;**7**:407–11.
11. Cerneca F, Ricci G, Simeone R, *et al.* Coagulation and fibrinolysis changes in normal pregnancy. Increased levels of procoagulants and reduced levels of inhibitors during pregnancy induce a hypercoagulable state, combined with a reactive fibrinolysis. *Eur J Obstet Gynecol Reprod Biol* 1997;**73**:31–6.
12. Burrows RF, Kelton JG. Thrombocytopenia at delivery: a prospective survey of 6715 deliveries. *Am J Obstet Gynecol* 1990;**162**:731–4.
13. Sainio S, Kekomäki R, Riikonen S, Teramo K. Maternal thrombocytopenia at term: a population-based study. *Acta Obstet Gynecol Scand* 2000;**79**:744–9.
14. Shehata N, Burrows R, Kelton J. Gestational thrombocytopenia. *Clin Obstet Gynecol* 1999;**42**:327–34.
15. Bremme K, Östlund E, Almqvist I, *et al.* Enhanced thrombin generation and fibrinolytic activity in the normal pregnancy and the puerperium. *Obstet Gynecol* 1992;**80**:132–7.
16. Wallenburg HCS, van Kessel PH. Platelet lifespan in normal pregnancy as determined by a non-radio-isotopic technique. *Br J Obstet Gynaecol* 1978;**85**:33–6.
17. Fay RA, Hughes AO, Farron NT. Platelets in pregnancy. Hyperdestruction in pregnancy. *Obstet Gynecol* 1983;**61**:238–40.
18. O'Brien WF, Saba HI, Knuppel RA, Scerbo JC, Cohen GR. Alterations in platelet concentration and aggregation in normal pregnancy and preeclampsia. *Am J Obstet Gynecol* 1986;**155**:486–90.
19. Douglas JT, Shah M, Lowe GDO. Plasma fibrinopeptide A and beta-thromboglobulin in pre-eclampsia and pregnancy hypertension. *Thromb Haemost* 1982;**47**:54–5.
20. Fitzgerald DJ, Mayo G, Catella F, *et al.* Increased thromboxane biosynthesis in normal pregnancy in mainly derived from platelets. *Am J Obstet Gynecol* 1987;**157**:325–30.
21. Mills JL, Der Simonian R, Raymond E, *et al.* Prosacyclin and thromboxane changes predating clinical onset of preeclampsia. *JAMA* 1999;**282**:356–62.
22. Janes SL, Goodall AH. Flow cytometric detection of circulating activated platelets and platelet hyper-responsiveness in pre-eclampsia and pregnancy. *Clin Sci* 1994;**86**:731–9.
23. Gatti I, Tenconi PM, Guarneri D, *et al.* Hemostasis parameters and platelet activation by flow-cytometry in normal pregnancies: a longitudinal study. *Int J Clin Lab Res* 1994;**24**:217–19.
24. Gerbasi FR, Bottoms S, Farag A, Mammen E. Increased intravascular coagulation associated with pregnancy. *Obstet Gynecol* 1990;**75**:385–9.
25. Letsky EA. *Coagulation Problems During Pregnancy*. Edinburgh: Churchill Livingstone; 1985.
26. Greer IA. Haemostasis and thrombosis in pregnancy. In: Bloom AL, Forbes CD, Thomas DP, Tuddenham EGD, eds. *Haemostasis and Thrombosis* 3rd ed. Edinburgh: Churchill Livingstone; 1994:987–1015.
27. Beller FK, Ebert C. The coagulation and fibrinolytic enzyme systems in normal pregnancy

and the puerperium. *Eur J Obstet Gynecol Reprod Biol* 1982;**13**:177–97.

28. Hellgren M, Blombäck M. Studies on blood coagulation and fibrinolysis in pregnancy, during delivery and in the puerperium. *Gynaecol Obstet Invest* 1981;**12**:141–54.

29. Persson BL, Stenberg P, Holmberg L, Astedt B. Transamidating enzymes in maternal plasma and placenta in human pregnancies complicated by intrauterine growth retardation. *J Dev Physiol* 1980;**2**:37–46.

30. Weiner CP, Brandt J. Plasma antithrombin III activity in normal pregnancy. *Obstet Gynecol* 1980;**56**:601–3.

31. Clark P, Brennand J, Conkie JA, *et al.* Activated protein C sensitivity. Protein C, protein S and coagulation in normal pregnancy. *Thromb Haemost* 1998;**79**:1166–70.

32. Weenink GH, Treffers PE, Kahle LH, ten Cate JW. Antithrombin III in normal pregnancy. *Thromb Res* 1982;**26**:281–7.

33. Gonzales R, Alberca J, Vicente V. Protein C levels in late pregnancy, postpartum and in women on oral contraceptives. *Thromb Res* 1985;**39**:637–40.

34. Gilabert J, Fernandez JA, Espana F, *et al.* Physiological coagulation inhibitors (protein S, protein C and antithrombin III) in severe preeclamptic states and in users of oral contraceptives. *Thromb Res* 1988;**49**:319–29.

35. Aznar J, Gilabert J, Estellé A, Espana F. Fibrinolytic activity and protein C in preeclampsia. *Thromb Haemost* 1986;**55**:314–7.

36. Faught W, Garner P, Jones G, Ivey B. Changes in protein C and protein S levels in normal pregnancy. *Am J Obstet Gynecol* 1995;**172**:147–50.

37. Kjellberg U, Andersson N-E, Rosén S, *et al.* APC resistance and other haemostatic variables during pregnancy and puerperium. *Thromb Haemost* 1999;**81**:527–31.

38. Bremme K, Blombäck M. Monitoring of a woman with protein C deficiency during pregnancy and the effects of heparin. *Thromb Haemorrh Disord* 1992;**5**:11–15.

39. Esmon CT. The roles of protein C and thrombomodulin in the regulation of blood coagulation. *J Biol Chem* 1989;**264**:4743–6.

40. Boffa MC, Valsecchi L, Fausto A, *et al.* Predictive value of plasma thrombomodulin in preeclampsia and gestational hypertension. *Thromb Haemost* 1998;**79**:1092–5.

41. de Moerloose P, Mermillod N, Amiral J, Reber G. Thrombomodulin levels during normal pregnancy at delivery and in the postpartum. Comparison with tissue type plasminogen activator and plasminogen activator inhibitor-1. *Thromb Haemost* 1998;**79**:554–6.

42. Malm J, Laurell M, Dahlbäck B. Changes in the plasma levels of vitamin K-dependent protein C and S and of C4b-binding protein during pregnancy and oral contraception. *Br J Haematol* 1988;**68**:437–43.

43. Dahlbäck B, Carlsson M, Svensson PJ. Familial thrombophilia due to a previously unrecognized mechanism characterized by a poor anticoagulant response to activated protein C. *Proc Natl Acad Sci USA* 1993;**94**:1004–8.

44. Cumming PC, Tait RC, Fildes S, *et al.* Development of resistance to activated protein C during pregnancy. *Br J Haematol* 1995;**90**:725–7.

45. Mathonnet F, de Mazancourt P, Bastenaire B, *et al.* Activated protein C sensitivity ratio in pregnant women at delivery. *Br J Haematol* 1996;**92**:244–6.

46. Vasse M, Leduc O, Borg FY, *et al.* Resistance to activated protein C: evaluation of three functional assays. *Thromb Res* 1994;**76**:47–59.

47. Bokarewa MI, Bremme K, Blombäck M. Arg 506 Gln mutation in factor V and risk of thombosis during pregnancy. *Br J Haematol* 1996;**92**:473–8.

48. Walker MC, Garner PR, Keely EJ, *et al.* Changes in activated protein C resistance during normal pregnancy. *Am J Obstet Gynecol* 1997;**177**:162–9.

49. Bokarewa MI, Wrambsy M, Bremme K, Blombäck M. Variability of the response to activated protein C during normal pregnancy. *Blood Coagul Fibrinolysis* 1997;**8**:239–44.

50. Clark P, Sattar M, Walker ID, Greer IA. The Glasgow Outcome, APCR and Lipid (GOAL) pregnancy study: significance of pregnancy associated activated protein. *Thromb Haemost* 2001;**85**:30–5.

51. Bertina RM, Koeleman BPC, Koster T, *et al.* Mutation in blood coagulation factor V associated with resistance to activated protein C. *Nature* 1994;**369**:64–7.

52. Lindqvist PG, Svensson PJ, Marsal K, *et al.* Activated protein C resistance (FV:Q506) and pregnancy. *Thromb Haemost* 1999;**81**:532–7.

53. Kupfermine MJ, Eldor A, Steinman N, *et al.* Increased frequency of genetic thrombophilia in women with complications of pregnancy. *N Engl J Med* 1999;**340**:9–13.

54. Brenner B, Mandel H, Lanir N, Younis J, Rothbart H, Ohel G. Activated protein C resistance can be associated with recurrent fetal loss. *Br J Haematol* 1997;**97**:551–4.

55. de Visser MCH, Rosendaal FR, Bertina RM. A

reduced sensitivity for protein C in the absence of factor V Leiden increases the risk of venous thrombosis. *Blood* 1999;**93**:1271–6.

56. Fassett MJ, Bohn YC, Kuo J, Wing DA. Longitudinal evaluation of activated protein C resistance among normal pregnancies of Hispanic women. *Am J Obstet Gynecol* 2000;**182**:1433–6.

57. Espana F, Gilabert J, Aznar J, *et al.* Complexes of activated protein C with alpha 1-antitrypsin in normal pregnancy and in severe preeclampsia. *Am J Obstet Gynecol* 1991;**164**:1310–16.

58. He S, Wramsby M, Bokarewa *et al.* Decrease in protein C inhibitor activity and acquired APC resistance during normal pregnancy. *J Thromb Thrombolysis* 2000;**9**:277–81.

59. Bokarewa MI, Bremme K, Falck G, *et al.* Studies on phospholipid antibodies, APC-resistance and associated mutation in the coagulation factor V gene. *Thromb Res* 1995;**78**:193–200.

60. Bokarewa MI, Wramsby M, Bremme K. Reactivity against phospholipids during pregnancy. *Hum Reprod* 1998;**13**:2633–5.

61. Lockwood CJ, Romero R, Feinberg RF, *et al.* The prevalence and biologic significance of lupus anticoagulant and anticardiolipin antibodies in a general obstetric population. *AM J Obstet Gynecol* 1989;**161**:369–73.

62. Perez MC, Wilson WA, Brown HL, Scopelitse E. Anticardiolipin antibodies in unselected pregnant women in relationship to pregnancy outcome. *Perinatology* 1991;**11**:33–6.

63. Harris EN, Spinnato JA. Should anticardiolipin tests be performed in otherwise healthy pregnant women? *Am J Obstet Gynecol* 1991;**165**:1272–7.

64. Bremme K, Lind H, Blombäck M. The effect of prophylactic heparin treatment on enhanced thrombin generation in pregnancy. *Obstet Gynecol* 1993;**81**:78–83.

65. Wiman B, Csemiczky G, Marsk L, Robbe H. The fast inhibitor of tissue plasminogen activator in plasma during pregnancy. *Thromb Haemost* 1984;**52**:124–6.

66. Ishii A, Yamada R, Hamada H. t-PA activity in peripheral blood obtained from pregnant women. *J Perinat Med* 1994;**22**:113–17.

67. Lecander I, Åstedt B. Isolation of a new specific plasminogen activator inhibitor from pregnancy plasma. *Br J Haematol* 1986;**62**:221–8.

68. Booth NA. The natural inhibitors of fibrinolysis. In: Bloom AL, Forbes CS, Thomas DP, Tuddenham EGD, eds. *Haemostasis and Thrombosis*. Edinburgh: Churchill Livingstone; 1994:699–717.

69. Åstedt B, Hågerstrand I, Lecander I. Cellular localisation in placenta of placental type plasminogen activator inhibitor. *Thromb Haemost* 1986;**56**:63–5.

70. He S, Bremme K, Almqvist I, Blombäck M. Decrease in plasminogen activator inhibitor type 2 related more to placental function and intrauterine fetal growth than to severity of preeclampsia. *Hyperten Pregnancy* 1996;**15**:171–82.

71. de Boer K, ten Cate JW, Sturk A, *et al.* Enhanced thrombin generation in normal and hypertensive pregnancy. *Am J Obstet Gynecol* 1989;**160**:95–100.

72. Estellé A, Gilabert J, Espana F, *et al.* Fibrinolytic parameters in normotensive pregnancy with intrauterine fetal growth retardation and in severe preeclampsia. *Am J Obstet Gynecol* 1991;**165**:138–42.

73. Francaalanci I, Comeglio P, Liotta AA, *et al.* D-dimer concentrations during normal pregnancy, as measured by Elisa. *Thromb Res* 1995;**78**:399–405.

74. van Tilburg NH, Rosendaal FR, Bertina RM. Thrombin activatable fibrinolysis inhibitor and the risk for deep vein thrombosis. *Blood* 2000;**95**:2855–9.

75. Gilabert J, Aznar J, Parilla JJ, *et al.* Alterations in the coagulation and fibrinolysis system in pregnancy, labour and puerperium, with special reference to a possible transitory state of intravascular coagulation during labour. *Thromb Haemost* 1978;**40**:387–96.

76. Ygge J. Changes in blood coagulation and fibrinolysis during the puerperium. *Am J Obstet* 1969;**104**:2–12.

77. Dahlstrøm BL, Nesheim BI. Postpartum platelet count in maternal blood. *Acta Obstet Gynecol Scand* 1994;**73**:695–7.

78. Aune B, Jesdal K, Oian P. Late onset postpartum thrombocytosis in preeclampsia. *Acta Obstet Gynecol Scand* 1999;**78**:866–70.

79. Mannucci PM, Vigano S, Botasso B. Protein C antigen during pregnancy, delivery and the puerperium. *Thromb Haemost* 1984;**52**:217.

80. Andersson T, Lorentzen B, Høgdahl H, *et al.* Thrombin–Inhibitor complexes in the blood during and after delivery. *Thromb Res* 1996;**82**:109–17.

81. Salonen Ros H. *Pre-eclampsia and other circulatory diseases during pregnancy: etiological aspects and impact on demale offspring.* Thesis, Stockholm, Sweden, 2001.

82. Ballegeer V, Sptiz B, Kieckens L, *et al.* Predictive value of increased plasma levels of fibronectin in

gestational hypertension. *Am J Obstet Gynecol* 1989;**161**:432–6.

83. Brubaker DB, Ross MG, Marinoff D. The function of elevated plasma fibronectin in preeclampsia. *Am J Obstet Gynecol* 1992;**166**:526–31.

84. Deng L, Bremme K, Hansson LO, Blombäck M. Plasma levels of von Willebrand factor and fibronectin as markers of persisting endothelial damage in preeclampsia. *Obstet Gynecol* 1994;**84**:941–5.

85. Comeglio P, Fedi S, Liotta AA. Blood clotting activation during normal pregnancy. *Thromb Res* 1996;**84**:199–202.

86. Delorme MA, Burrows RF, Ofosu FA, Andrew M. Thrombin regulation in mother and fetus during pregnancy. *Semin Thromb Hemost* 1992;**18**:81–90.

87. Östlund E, Bremme K, Wiman B. Soluble fibrin in plasma as a sign of activated coagulation in patients with pregnancy complications. *Acta Obstet Gynaecol Scand* 1998;**77**:165–98.

88. He S, Bremme K, Blombäck M. A laboratory method for determination of overall haemostatic potential in plasma: Method Design and preliminary results. *Thromb Res* 1999;**96**:145–56.

12

Inherited thrombophilia and gestational venous thromboembolism

Jacqueline Conard and Marie-Hélène Horellou

INTRODUCTION

Thrombophilia is associated with an increased risk of venous thromboembolism (VTE).[1-4] Thrombosis may be idiopathic but it is more often associated with an environmental risk factor. Women have more risk factors than men: pregnancy, severe ovarian hyperstimulation, oral contraception, hormone replacement therapy for symptoms of the menopause. These factors are frequently present when the first episode of VTE occurs.

Although the risk of VTE is increased in pregnant women compared with non-pregnant women, the risk is still low.[5] Some conditions increase the risk of thrombosis, such as higher age of the mother, Caesarean delivery, bed rest during pregnancy, obesity, previous VTE, an acquired abnormality (e.g. lupus anticoagulant), or an hereditary coagulation abnormalities (e.g. thrombophilia). Consequently, an anticoagulant treatment may be considered during pregnancy. The selection of treatment depends on compatibility with pregnancy, the type of thrombophilia, and any previous history of thrombosis in the patient. Recommendations of the Fifth American College of Chest Physicians (ACCP) about the prevention and treatment of venous thrombosis in pregnant women were published during 2001.[6] However, recommendations may change when new information becomes available.

RISK OF THROMBOSIS IN THROMBOPHILIC WOMEN

The main congenital causes of VTE (thrombophilia) are: deficiency in antithrombin (AT, previously named AT III), deficiency of protein C (PC), protein S (PS), activated protein C resistance (APC resistance) associated with factor V Leiden mutation, and prothrombin 20210A variant.[1-4] Other modifications have also been considered as risk factors for venous thrombosis: increased levels of factors VIII,[7,8] IX,[9] or XI,[10] and hypofibrinolysis related to increased levels of the thrombin activatable fibrinolysis inhibitor.[11] Hyperhomocysteinemia and homozygosity for the methylenetetrahydrofolate reductase (MTHFR) C677T mutation are also important. At present, an alteration in hemostasis is found in about 40% of patients with a family history of VTE. Consequently, an unknown cause of thrombophilia may be suspected in another 60% of patients.

Thrombophilias are associated with an increased risk of VTE. The risk is about 50-fold for AT deficiency, 15-fold for PC deficiency, two-fold for PS deficiency, three- to eight-fold for factor V Leiden, and two-fold or less for prothrombin 20210A and hyperhomocysteinemia.[3] Thrombosis may be spontaneous, but it is often associated with surgery, immobilization, oral contraception, hormone replacement therapy, or pregnancy.[3] Age and blood group are also risk factors of thrombosis.

Although the different thrombophilia have similar clinical manifestations, they differ by their frequency, and there is a heterogeneity of clinical expression. Indeed, factor V Leiden is the most common abnormality in Caucasian subjects, being present in 20% of unselected patients with venous thrombosis and in about 5% in the general population in Europe. AT deficiency is less common (about 1% of patients and 0.02% of healthy subjects). Deficiencies in PC or PS and factor II 20210A have an intermediate frequency. Combined deficiencies (especially heterozygous factor V Leiden and FII 20210A) are relatively common.

The magnitude of the risk of thrombosis in the different thrombophilias is difficult to assess. The probands (index patients) usually have a history of thrombotic episodes, so their inclusion in studies causes an overestimation of the risk. The evaluation of the risk of thrombosis may be more appropriate in the relatives. However, it should be realized that bias may also exist. Indeed, the relatives who are the most concerned to be tested are those who have already experienced thrombosis and also include more women than men, for various reasons (e.g. women may be more anxious to know whether they will transmit the abnormality to their children or less reluctant to have blood sampled than men). In addition, when considering the results of the different studies, it must be remembered that factor V Leiden was first detected in 1994 and prothrombin 20210A in December 1996, and these factors may not have been taken into account in some studies.

A retrospective cohort family study has focused on 513 relatives from 233 thrombophilic families in which the proband had at least one VTE episode.[12] The aim of the study was to assess the risk of VTE in individuals with AT, PC or PS deficiency, or APC resistance. The overall incidence of VTE in the group of relatives was 0.52 but it was higher in AT deficiency (1.07) than in PC deficiency (0.54) or PS deficiency (0.50), and APC resistance had the lowest incidence (0.30). Women had the peak incidence in a younger age than men (21–40 years versus 41–60 years). The first episode was frequently associated with oral contraceptives (11%) or puerperium (21%). The

lower risk attributed to factor V Leiden carriers than to PC-deficient carriers was not found in another study.[13] The risk of the prothrombin 20210A variant seems close to the risk of factor V Leiden or slightly lower.[4,14,15]

Some patients have more than one thrombophilia, in which case one of the abnormalities is usually factor V Leiden, since it is the most common. It is suggested that individuals with combined defects are at a higher risk.[1,4,12,15,16]

Homozygous defects may also been observed. Homozygous AT deficiency has only been found for type II heparin binding site deficiency. It seems that homozygous type I AT deficiency or type 2 RS or PE are not compatible with life. Homozygous PC deficiency and homozygous PS deficiency are rare. They have been detected in neonates with purpura fulminans or massive thromboses[4] and in young adults with skin necrosis at the introduction of oral anticoagulants.[17] Homozygous factor V Leiden or prothrombin 20210A mutations are more common and homozygous patients have a higher risk than heterozygous patients, although the difference is not well documented.[15,18]

In summary, thrombophilia is a risk factor for thrombosis, but the risk is not the same in the various thrombophilias. The risk of thrombosis is relatively low in heterozygous factor V Leiden carriers who do not have any other thrombophilia or acquired risk factor. In carriers of the factor II 20210A mutation, the risk seems about the same as in factor V Leiden carriers. In contrast, the risk of thrombosis is the highest in AT deficiency (except in type II heparin binding site deficiency), in combined thrombophilias, and in homozygous patients. Risk situations such as surgery, immobilization, or pregnancy and treatments such as oral contraception are frequently associated with episodes of thrombosis.

RISK OF PREGNANCY-ASSOCIATED VTE IN WOMEN WITH THROMBOPHILIA

The incidence of pregnancy-associated VTE in the general population is estimated at less than one thrombosis per 1000 pregnancies.[5] This is the incidence that is most frequently reported, although the incidence may vary significantly.

There is a good evidence that VTE is more common in the last trimester of pregnancy than in the first or second trimesters and that it is more common postpartum than during pregnancy. These findings have been discussed in the literature, but in some studies women who had VTE during the first trimester (and who consequently received therapeutic doses of anticoagulant for the rest of the pregnancy and postpartum) may not have been excluded for calculations of the risk during the second or third trimester, leading to an underestimation of the risk in the last trimester. The same factor may be responsible for the lower postpartum risk in some studies in that women who had VTE during pregnancy may not have been excluded for postpartum analysis of the results. In addition, VTE may occur after discharge from hospital following delivery.

Various factors have been demonstrated to increase the risk of pregnancy-related VTE:[5]

- age over 35 years;
- immobilization during pregnancy;
- Caesarean section, especially when performed in emergency;
- a personal history of VTE; and
- thrombophilia.

Findings from studies

A number of studies have looked at the risks of VTE in pregnancy and in relatives of women with a history of pregnancy-related VTE.

Studies including propositi and relatives with thrombophilia (Table 12.1)

The risk of pregnancy-related thrombosis has been studied retrospectively in the absence of anticoagulant prophylaxis in AT-, PC-, and PS-deficient women (Table 12.1).[19,20] In these two earliest studies, the risk of deep vein thrombosis or pulmonary embolism (i.e. superficial vein thrombosis was excluded) during pregnancy and postpartum in women with AT, PC, or PS deficiency ranged from 24% to 28%. AT-deficient women had a high risk during pregnancy (14%[19] and 40%[20]) and in the postpartum period (22%[19] and 6%[20]), while PS-deficient

women had a low risk during pregnancy (0%[19] and 5%[20]) and a higher risk in the postpartum period (16%[19] and 22%[20]) (Table 12.2). In these retrospective studies, the women were either the probands or the relatives and they were included irrespective of whether they had had a previous thrombosis before pregnancy. Not all thrombotic episodes were documented by an objective diagnostic test.

Studies restricted to relatives (Tables 12.1 and 12.2)

In a study excluding the probands and including only family members who had no history of VTE, the incidence of thrombotic events confirmed by objective diagnostic testing was low (2%) but still higher than in the normal population (an eight-fold increased risk) (see Tables 12.1 and 12.2).[21] However, the absolute risk in carriers of AT, PC, or PS deficiency was relatively low: seven thrombotic events out of 169 pregnancies (4.1%); two of these events occurred third trimester and the others occurred postpartum. The reported risk was lower in women with factor V Leiden than in AT-, PC-, or PS-deficient carriers (RR 4.2, 95% CI 0.5–148 versus RR 8.2, 95% CI 1.2–184).[22] The incidence of VTE was similar in two studies that included families of factor V Leiden carriers.[22,23] The confidence intervals are wide, possibly owing to a different risk in one of the three deficiencies, namely AT deficiency.[22] In factor V Leiden carriers, the number of events are small and they are mainly postpartum. The large confidence interval for this mutation may also be related to the absence of knowledge about the prothrombin 20210A mutation.[22,23]

Studies in patients receiving prophylaxis

It might be pointed out that the risk of thrombosis during pregnancy has also been estimated in prospective cohort studies in patients receiving some prophylaxis.[24,25] In a prospective study of asymptomatic carriers of PC or PS congenital deficiency, eight pregnancies were followed.[24] Prophylaxis was administered during pregnancy in PC-deficient women but not in PS-deficient women: a superficial vein thrombosis was observed in one carrier of PC deficiency,

Table 12.1 Risk of pregnancy-associated deep vein thrombosis or pulmonary embolism during pregnancy and postpartum in thrombophilic women

	Study	Selection of subjects	Females n	Pregnancies n	Deep vein thrombosis or pulmonary embolism n (%)
AT, PC or PS deficiency	Conard et al., 1990[19]	Propositi and relatives History of VTE or not No prophylaxis	77	155	37 (24%)
	Pabinger and Schneider, 1996[20]	Propositi and relatives History of VTE or not No prophylaxis	71	176	49 (28%)
	Friederich et al., 1996[21]	Relatives No previous VTE No combined deficiency	169	7 (4%)	
Factor V Leiden	Simioni et al., 1999[22]	Relatives No combined defect		157	3 (2%)
	Middledorp et al., 1998[23]	Relatives		235	5 (2%)

Table 12.2 Risk of pregnancy-associated deep vein thrombosis or pulmonary embolism in the various thrombophilias

Study	Subjects	AT	PC	PS	Factor V Leiden	Factor V Leiden plus factor II 20210A
Conard et al., 1990[19]	Pregnancies (n)	50	74	31		
	VTE	18 (36%)	14 (20%)	5 (16%)		
	During pregnancy	7 (14%)	3 (4%)	0 (0%)		
	Postpartum	11 (22%)	12 (16%)	5 (16%)		
Pabinger and Schneider, 1996[20]	Pregnancies, (n)	45	60	71		
	VTE	21 (46%)	9 (15%)	19 (27%)		
	During pregnancy	18 (40%)	6 (10%)	4 (5%)		
	Postpartum	3 (6%)	3 (5%)	15 (22%)		
Friederich et al., 1996[21]	Pregnancies (n)	33	60	76		
	VTE	1 (3%)	1 (1.7%)	5 (7%)		
	During pregnancy	1	1	0		
	Postpartum	0	0	5		
Middledorp et al., 1998[23]	Pregnancies (n)				235 (heterozygous)	
	VTE				5 (2%)	
	During pregnancy				1	
	Postpartum				4	
Samama et al., 1997[27]	Pregnancies (n)				20 (homozygous)	
	VTE				5 (25%)	
	During pregnancy				3	
	Postpartum				2	
Middledorp et al., 2001[28]	Pregnancies (n)				24 (homozygous)	
	VTE				4 (17%)	
	During pregnancy				2	
	Postpartum				2	
Martinelli et al., 2001[26]	Pregnancies (n)				19 (homozygous)	50
	VTE				3 (16%)	2 (4%)
	During pregnancy				1 (3rd trim)	0
	Postpartum				2	2

and no episodes were observed in carriers of PS deficiency. Prophylactic treatment was suggested for 6 weeks after delivery in all the PC- and PS-deficient women: one pulmonary embolism occurred in one of PC deficiency carrier 1 week after a postpartum 4-week prevention. Consequently, in patients with no previous thrombosis, it has been shown that the use of a continuous anticoagulant prophylaxis does not seem warranted, but adequate prophylaxis should be administered during risk situations.[24] Similar conclusions were drawn from the other prospective study.[25]

Studies in women with thrombophilia
Studies that have looked at small groups of patients with combined factor V Leiden and prothrombin 20210A heterozygous mutations or homozygous factor V Leiden mutation have found that the pregnancy-related risk of thrombosis is higher than in normal subjects or heterozygous patients. In 21 women with both mutations, two thromboses were observed in 50 pregnancies (4%), with a relative risk of 9.2 (95% CI 0.8–103.2).[26] In homozygous factor V Leiden carriers, the incidence of thrombosis is very similar in three studies: 20% (5 of 20),[26] 16% (3 of 19),[27] and 17% (4 of 24);[28] the relative risk was 41.3 (95% CI 4.1–419.7).[26] In a multicenter study, the first episode of thrombosis in 34 homozygous carriers of factor V Leiden mutation was associated with pregnancy in 13 women but the total number of pregnancies in these women is not mentioned.[18]

Summary of study findings
Pregnancy is a frequent risk factor associated with VTE in women with thrombophilia. The risk is significantly increased in the postpartum period in all thrombophilias but differs during pregnancy. Women with AT deficiency or homozygous or combined thrombophilias are considered at higher risk. Asymptomatic heterozygous carriers of the factor V Leiden or prothrombin 20210A mutations have the lowest risk. The real magnitude of the risk is difficult to assess. Indeed, in the first reported studies, the risk was probably overestimated, owing to the selection of patients (propositus or relatives,

with or without thrombosis before pregnancy) and to the criteria of diagnosis of thrombosis, which were probably made on purely clinical grounds in some patients. In subsequent studies, family members only were included. Finally, there are a few recent prospective studies in asymptomatic patients, but they are small-sized and patients received an anticoagulant prophylaxis during pregnancy or the postpartum period only. Thus, the risk exists but the magnitude of the risk is still not well defined.

Consequently, prophylaxis of VTE during pregnancy should be adapted according to the type of thrombophilia, the recognized risk factors of VTE (such as age, obesity, number of previous pregnancies, and the presence or absence of previous thrombosis).

FREQUENCY OF THROMBOPHILIA IN WOMEN WITH PREGNANCY-ASSOCIATED VTE

Screening for thrombophilia has been performed in women who experienced VTE associated with pregnancy (Tables 12.3 and 12.4). A retrospective study was conducted in 62 women who had an objectively confirmed venous thrombosis related to pregnancy, and a thrombophilia screening was done in 50 of the women.[29] In an extension of this study, a prothrombin 20210A mutation was found in five subjects out of 55.[30] AT deficiency was identified in 12%, protein C deficiency in 2% and a factor V Leiden mutation in 8%, leading to an approximate risk for women with the defects of 1 in 2.8 in type I AT deficiency, 1 in 42 in type II AT deficiency, 1 in 113 in protein C deficiency, and 1 in 437 in factor V Leiden mutation. According to the authors of these studies, the results do not lend support to the random screening for the mutation in early pregnancy.

In a case-control study, the association between pregnancy-related thrombosis and the factor V Leiden or factor II 20210A mutations and MTHFR C677T polymorphism has been evaluated.[31] Ten out of 42 cases (23.8%) and 4 of 213 controls (without a history of thrombosis) (1.9%; OR 16.3, 95% CI 4.8–54.9) had factor V Leiden mutation; 13 cases (31%) and nine

Table 12.3 Genetic risk factors in pregnancy-related VTE

Study	Type of study	VTE n	Type of thrombophilia		Risk	
McColl et al., 1997[29]	Retrospective	50	AT deficiency	6 (12%)	1 in 2.8	type I
					1 in 42	type II
			PC deficiency	1 (2%)	1 in 113	
			Factor V Leiden	4 (8%)	1 in 437	
Grandone et al., 1998[31]	Case-control	42	Factor V Leiden	10 (24%)	16.3	(CI 4.8–54.9)
			Factor II 20210A	13 (31%)	10.2	(CI 4–25.9)
			MTHFR*	12 (29%)	2.1	(CI 1–4.5)
Gerhardt et al., 2000[32]	Case-control	119	Factor V Leiden	52 (44%)	9.3	(CI 5.1–16.9)
			Factor II 20210A	20 (17%)	15.2	(CI 4.2–52.6)
			Both	11 (9.3%)	107	
			MTHFR*	11 (9.6%)	—	
McColl et al., 2000[30]	Retrospective	75	AT deficiency type I	4/75	282	(CI 31–2532)
			AT deficiency type II	3/75	28	(CI 5.5–142)
			Factor V Leiden	7/75	4.5	(CI 2.1–14.5)
			Factor II 20210A	5/55	4.4	(CI 1.2–16)
			MTHFR*	3/52	0.45	(CI 0.13–1.58)

*Homozygous

controls (4.2%; OR 10.2, 95% CI 4.0–25.9) had the prothrombin mutation; 12 cases (28.6%) and 34 controls (16%; OR 2.1, OR 1.0–4.5) were homozygous for MTHFR. It is suggested that these mutations should be screened for in women with a personal history of venous thrombosis related to pregnancy or the postpartum period.

In another study, the role of genetic factors was evaluated in 119 consecutive women with a history of objectively diagnosed VTE during pregnancy and the puerperium and 233 normal women.[32] Women were screened for inherited and acquired modifications of blood coagulation. In the patients, they found a prevalence of factor V Leiden of 43.7% compared with 7.7% in the normal women (RR 9.3, 95% CI 5.1–16.9), a prevalence of factor II 20210A mutation of 16.9% compared with 1.3% (RR 15.2, 95% CI 4.2–52.6), a prevalence of both factor V Leiden and FII 20210A mutation of 9.3% compared with 0%. The risk of thrombosis in carriers of the mutations was calculated in a multivariate analysis, assuming an overall risk of 1 in 1500 pregnancies. The authors of this paper suggest that the risk of thrombosis is 0.2% in factor V Leiden carriers, 0.5% in FII 20210A mutation carriers, and 4.6% in carriers of both mutations.[32]

In this study, deficiencies in AT, protein C, and protein S were also detected but their inherited origin is uncertain. An AT deficiency was found in 2 out of 131 normal women, which is much higher than the expected prevalence of 0.02% in the normal population. The relative risk reported for antithrombin deficiency was 10.4 (95% CI 2.3–62.5), which is close to the risk of FII 20210A mutation. This result is unexpected because in clinical practice, AT deficiencies are at a much higher risk.

In a study of 112 consecutive women who had a first episode of deep vein thrombosis at a reproductive age, 74 had thrombosis associated with oral contraceptive use and 19 with pregnancy or the postpartum period.[33] In this last group, none was a carrier of prothrombin 20210A (out of the 14 detected), eight were carriers of factor V Leiden (out of 24 detected), and one had both mutations (out of four detected).

In a prospective study of 125 pregnant women with a history of a single episode of venous thrombosis, the safety of withholding heparin prophylaxis was studied.[34] It was found that among the 51 women in whom thrombophilia was detected or who had a previous idiopathic thrombosis, three (5.9%) had an antepartum recurrence (95% CI 1.2–16.2). In contrast, among the 44 women who had no thrombophilia and a previous thrombosis associated with a temporary risk factor, no antepartum thrombosis occurred.

In summary, in women who experience thrombosis during pregnancy or postpartum, thrombophilia is frequently detected, and screening for thrombophilia is justified in these women. If the screening is performed at the time of pregnancy-related thrombosis, it should be remembered that pregnancy induces changes in hemostatic parameters, especially a decrease in PS levels. The PS level may remain low for 6 weeks after delivery. Thus, the diagnosis of congenital deficiency of PS must be confirmed well after delivery and preferably in association with a family study.

PREVENTION OF VTE IN PREGNANT WOMEN WITH THROMBOPHILIA

Oral anticoagulants cross the placenta and may be responsible for embryopathy and fetal hemorrhage.[6] Unfractionated heparin has for a long time been considered as the anticoagulant of choice during pregnancy because it does not cross the placenta but it may induce allergy, heparin-induced thrombocytopenia, and also a decrease in AT levels and osteoporosis when administered for long periods. Low molecular weight heparin is now the most commonly used anticoagulant during pregnancy because it does not cross the placenta and has fewer side-effects than unfractionated heparin. In addition, it has the advantage of easier administration – one injection per day for prevention or two injections per day for treatment, meaning less discomfort for the patient and often the possibility of self-administration. The tolerance of low molecular weight heparin is considered satisfactory.[35,36] In some women with a history of heparin-induced thrombocytopenia or allergy, danaparoid has been administered during pregnancy.[37,38]

Table 12.4 Pregnancy or postpartum related thrombosis and thrombophilia

Study	Type of thrombophilia	Cases n	During pregnancy n	Postpartum
McColl et al., 1997[29]	AT deficiency	6	1st trimester: 3 2nd trimester: 1 3rd trimester: 1	2 (both type II)
McColl et al., 1997[29]	PC deficiency	1		1
McColl et al., 1997[29]	Factor V Leiden	4	1st trimester: 1 (previous DVT) 3rd trimester: 2	
Grandone et al., 1998[31]		3	1	2
McColl et al., 2000[30]		6	1st trimester: 3 (1 with previous VTE, 1 homozygous plus immobility) 3rd trimester: 2	1
Grandone et al., 1998[31]	Factor II 20210A	5	0	5
McColl et al., 2000[30]		4	1st trimester: 1 3rd trimester: 1	2 (both Caesarean deliveries)
Grandone et al., 1998[31]	Factor V Leiden plus factor II 20210A	6	1	5
McColl et al., 2000[30]		1	3rd trimester: 1 (previous VTE)	

Recommendations were published in the *British Journal of Obstetrics and Gynaecology* in 1999;[39] they follow the suggestions presented by the Working Group of the International Society of Thrombosis and Haemostasis. Other recommendations have been published in *Chest* in 2001[6] by the American College of Chest Physicians; all those concerning prophylaxis in women with previous VTE or thrombophilia (or both) are grade 1C, which means they are 'weak', being the result of observational studies, and they may change when new information becomes available. Unlike the previous ACCP recommendations published in 1998, repeated screening with noninvasive tests for deep venous thrombosis, such as compression ultrasound, is no longer justified. In addition, the higher risk of AT-deficient women is now recognized. Finally, low molecular weight heparin has become the anticoagulant of choice during pregnancy and is tending to replace unfractionated heparin. It is surprising that there is no mention in these recommendations of the benefit of elastic stockings in pregnant women at risk of thrombosis.

Authors' comments on current recommendations

The authors make some comments here about the American College of Chest Physicians recommendations, taking into account information from the publications and from their personal experience. The only present consensus is to recommend heparin or warfarin for 6 weeks postpartum in all pregnant women at risk of thrombosis (i.e. because they have had a previous VTE or are carriers of a thrombophilia). The recommendations for management during pregnancy are less stringent.

Thrombophilic women without a personal history of VTE
- American College of Chest Physicians recommendations are clinical surveillance or low-dose heparin (5000 U every 12 hours) or prophylactic low molecular weight heparin throughout pregnancy. The indication for active prophylaxis is stronger in AT-deficient women than in other thrombophilias.

- Comments: clinical surveillance is probably sufficient in women with PS deficiency and in heterozygous carriers of factor V Leiden or prothrombin 20210A variant, but it does not seem appropriate for women with AT deficiency. In the latter, low molecular weight heparin (40 mg or a higher dose once a day) are probably required throughout pregnancy.

Thrombophilic women with a history of VTE before pregnancy
For women who are pregnant after a single episode of VTE:

- American College of Chest Physicians recommendations are clinical surveillance or low-dose unfractionated heparin (5000 U every 12 hours) or moderate-dose unfractionated heparin (adjusted to target a peak anti-factor Xa level of 0.1–0.3 U/ml) or prophylactic low molecular weight heparin (40 mg or 5000 U or adjusted dose to target a peak anti-factor Xa level of 0.2–0.6 U/ml). The indication for active prophylaxis is stronger in AT-deficient women.
- Comments: clinical surveillance alone seems insufficient in AT-deficient women. Low molecular weight heparin is now replacing unfractionated heparin in most countries. It is not clearly mentioned in the recommendations whether the prophylaxis should be administered throughout the pregnancy or only for part of the pregnancy. In AT-deficient women, prophylaxis throughout pregnancy is probably justified, but in other thrombophilias prophylaxis during the third trimester only might be sufficient. Clearly, there is an urgent need of studies in these patients.

For women who are pregnant after multiple episodes of VTE and in women on long-term oral anticoagulants:

- American College of Chest Physicians recommendations are that, since there is a risk of embryopathy between 6 and 12 weeks' gestation, and assuming there is no risk before week 6, women are counseled to perform a pregnancy test as soon as possible. If the test is positive, oral anticoagulants are replaced by heparin. Adjusted dose of unfractionated heparin (target: activated partial thromboplastin time in the therapeutic range) or low molecular weight heparin (target peak anti-factor Xa 0.2–0.6 U/ml) are recommended.

- Comments: Replacement of oral anticoagulants by heparin before conception had been proposed but the duration of exposure to heparin was prolonged and the risk of osteoporosis was consequently increased: this option has now been abandoned. In these patients, long-term oral anticoagulation is recommenced in the postpartum period.

Pregnancy in women with personal history of VTE but no known thrombophilia
- American College of Chest Physicians recommendations: in women who have a single previous VTE in association with a transient risk factor but who have no known thrombophilia, clinical surveillance may be sufficient. Indeed, no recurrent thrombosis was observed during pregnancy in 44 women in the only available prospective study of women in this category who received no antepartum prophylaxis.[34]
- Comments: the risk may depend on the location of thrombosis (e.g. calf vein or proximal vein), as may the sequelae.

Scandinavian studies have previously showed that prophylaxis may be indicated during the last trimester of pregnancy.[40]

Summary of prophylaxis recommendations

Anticoagulant prophylaxis may be required during pregnancy and postpartum in women with thrombophilia. It is advisable to administer prophylaxis throughout pregnancy in AT-deficient women and for 6 weeks postpartum in women with a congenital deficiency in AT, PC or PS, a factor V Leiden or prothrombin 20210A mutation, and previous VTE. Information is lacking about prophylaxis during pregnancy in thrombophilias other than AT deficiency, with or without previous thrombosis, the dose of anticoagulant to be administered, and its duration (i.e. throughout pregnancy or only during part of the pregnancy).

CONCLUSION

Pregnancy is frequently associated with the first episode of VTE in women with thrombophilia. However, systematic screening for thrombophilia is not warranted in every woman before pregnancy, although it may be in women who have a family history of VTE at a young age. When a pregnant woman has a known thrombophilia, the appropriate anticoagulant prophylaxis is still uncertain in most cases, and there is a need for further studies.

REFERENCES

1. Lane DA, Mannucci PM, Bauer KA, *et al*. Inherited thrombophilia: part 1. *Thromb Haemost* 1996;**76**:651–62.
2. Lane DA, Mannucci PM, Bauer KA, *et al*. Inherited thrombophilia: part 2. *Thromb Haemost* 1996;**76**:824–34.
3. Rosendaal FR. Risk factors for venous thrombotic disease. *Thromb Haemost* 1999;**82**:610–19.
4. Seligsohn U, Lubetsky A. Genetic susceptibility to venous thrombosis. *N Engl J Med* 2001;**344**:1222–31.
5. Greer IA. Thrombosis in pregnancy: maternal and fetal issues. *Lancet* 1999;**353**:1258–65.
6. Ginsberg JS, Greer I, Hirsh J. Use of antithrombotic agents during pregnancy. *Chest* 2001;**119**:122S–131S.
7. Koster T, Blann AD, Briet E, Vandenbroucke JP, Rosendaal FR. Role of clotting factor VIII in effect of von Willebrand factor on occurrence of deep vein thrombosis. *Lancet* 1995;**345**:152–5.
8. Kraaijenhagen RA, Anker PS, Koopman MMW, *et al*. High plasma concentration of factor VIIIc is a major risk factor for venous thromboembolism. *Thromb Haemost* 2000;**83**:5–9.
9. Van Hylckama Vlieg A, Van Der Linden IK, Bertina RM, Rosendaal FR. High levels of factor

IX increase the risk of venous thrombosis. *Blood* 2000;**95**:3678–82.

10. Meijers JCM, Tekelenburg WLH, Bouma BN, Bertina RM, Rosendaal DF. High levels of coagulation factor XI as a risk factor for venous thrombosis. *N Engl J Med* 2000;**342**:696–701.

11. Tilburg NHV, Rosendaal FR, Bertina RM. Thrombin activatable fibrinolysis inhibitor and the risk for deep vein thrombosis. *Blood* 2000;**95**:2855–9.

12. Bucciarelli P, Rosendaal FR, Tripodi A, *et al*. Risk of venous thromboembolism and clinical manifestations in carriers of antithrombin, protein C, protein S deficiency, or activated protein C resistance. *Arterioscler Thromb Vasc Biol* 1999;**19**:1026–33.

13. Lensen RPM, Rosendaal FR, Koster T, *et al*. Apparent different thrombotic tendency in patients with factor V Leiden and protein C deficiency due to selection of patients. *Blood* 1996;**88**:4205–8.

14. Martinelli I, Bucciarelli P, Margaglione M, De Stefano V, Castaman G, Mannucci PM. The risk of venous thromboembolism in family members with mutations of the genes of factor V or prothrombin or both. *Br J Haematol* 2000;**111**: 1223–9.

15. Emmerich J, Rosendaal FR, Cattaneo M, *et al*. Combined effect of factor V Leiden and prothrombin 20210A on the risk of venous thromboembolism. *Thromb Haemost* 2001;**86**: 809–16.

16. De Stefano V, Martinelli I, Mannucci PM, *et al*. The risk of recurrent deep venous thrombosis among heterozygous carriers of both factor V Leiden and G20210A prothrombin mutation. *N Engl J Med* 1999;**341**:214–15.

17. Conard J, Horellou MH, Van Dreden P, *et al*. Homozygous protein C deficiency with late onset and recurrent coumarin induced skin necrosis. *Lancet* 1992;**339**: 743–4.

18. The Procare Group. Comparison of thrombotic risk between 85 homozygotes and 481 heterozygotes carriers of the factor V Leiden mutation: retrospective analysis from the Procare Study. *Blood* 2000;**11**:511–18.

19. Conard J, Horellou MH, Van Dreden P, Lecompte T, Samama M. Thrombosis and pregnancy in congenital deficiencies in AT III, protein C or protein S: study of 78 women. *Thromb Haemost* 1990;**63**:319–20.

20. Pabinger I, Schneider B. Thrombotic risk in hereditary antithrombin III, protein C and protein S deficiency. *Arterioscler Thromb Vasc Biol* 1996;**16**:742–8.

21. Friederich PW, Sanson BJ, Simioni P, *et al*. Frequency of pregnancy-related venous thromboembolism in anticoagulant factor-deficient women: implications for prophylaxis. *Ann Intern Med* 1996;**125**:955–60.

22. Simioni P, Sanson BJ, Prandoni P, *et al*. Incidence of venous thromboembolism in families with inherited thrombophilia. *Thromb Haemost* 1998; **81**:198–202.

23. Middeldorp S, Henkens CMA, Koopman MMW, *et al*. The incidence of venous thromboembolism in family members of patients with factor V Leiden mutation and venous thrombosis. *Ann Intern Med* 1998;**128**:15–20.

24. Pabinger I, Kyrle PA, Heistinger M, Eichinger S, Wittmann E, Lechner K. The risk of thromboembolism in asymptomatic patients with protein C and protein S deficiency: a prospective cohort study. *Thromb Haemost* 1994;**71**:441–5.

25. Sanson BJ, Simioni P, Tormene D, *et al*. The incidence of venous thromboembolism in asymptomatic carriers of a deficiency of antithrombin, protein C or protein S: a prospective cohort study. *Blood* 1999;**94**:3702–6.

26. Martinelli I, Legnani C, Bucciarelli P, Grandone E, De Stefano V, Mannucci PM. Risk of pregnancy-related venous thrombosis in carriers of severe inherited thrombophilia. *Thromb Haemost* 2001;**86**:300–3.

27. Samama M, Conard J, Nassiri, S, Horellou MH, Arkam R, Elalamy I. Comparaison de deux groupes de 22 femmes homozygotes ou hétérozygotes pour la mutation du facteur V Leiden. *Bull Acad Natl Med* 1997;**181**:919–37.

28. Middledorp S, Libourel EJ, Hamulyak K, van der Meer J, Buller HR. The risk of pregnancy-related venous thromboembolism in women who are homozygous for factor V Leiden. *Br J Haematol* 2001;**113**:553–55.

29. McColl MD, Ramsay JE, Tait RC, *et al*. Risk factors for pregnancy associated venous thromboembolism. *Thromb Haemost* 1997;**78**:1183–8.

30. McColl MD, Ellison J, Reid F, Tait RC, Walker ID, Greer IA. Prothrombin 20210 G→A, MTHFR C677T mutations in women with venous thromboembolism associated with pregnancy. *Br J Obstet Gynaecol* 2000;**107**:565–9.

31. Grandone E, Margaglione M, Colaizzo D, *et al*. Genetic susceptibility to pregnancy-related venous thromboembolism: roles of factor V Leiden, prothrombin G20210A, and methylene-

tetrahyfolate reductase C677T mutations. *Am J Obstet Gynecol* 1998;**179**:1324–8.

32. Gerhardt A, Scharf RE, Beckmann MW, *et al.* Prothrombin and factor V mutations in women with a history of thrombosis during pregnancy and the puerperium *N Engl J Med* 2000;**342**:374–80.

33. Martinelli I, Taioli E, Bucciarelli P, Akhavan S, Mannucci PM. Interaction between the G20210A mutation of the prothrombin gene and oral contraceptive use in deep vein thrombosis. *Arterioscler Thromb Vasc Biol* 1999;**19**:700–3.

34. Brill-Edwards P, Ginsberg J, Gent Michael, *et al.* Safety of withholding herapin in pregnant women with a history of venous thromboembolism. *N Engl J Med* 2000;**343**:1439–44.

35. Sanson BJ, Lensing AWA, Prins MH, *et al.* Safety of low-molecular-weight heparin in pregnancy: a systematic review. *Thromb Haemost* 1999;**81**:668–72.

36. Lepercq J, Conard J, Borel-Derlon A, *et al.* Venous thromboembolism during pregnancy: a retrospective study of enoxaparin safety in 624 pregnancies. *Br J Obstet Gynaecol* 2001;**108**:1134–40.

37. Macchi L, Sarfati R, Guicheteau M, *et al.* Thromboembolic prophylaxis with danaparoid (Orgaran®) in a high-thrombosis-risk pregnant woman with a history of heparin-induced thrombocytopenia (HIT) and Widal's disease. *Clin Appl Thromb Hemost* 2000;**6**:187–9.

38. Harrison SJ, Rafferty I, McColl MD. Management of heparin allergy during pregnancy with danaparoid. *Blood Coag Fibrinol* 2001;**12**:157–9.

39. McColl MD, Walker ID, Greer IA. The role of inherited thrombophilia in venous thromboembolism associated with pregnancy. *Br J Obstet Gynaecol* 1999;**106**:756–66.

40. Hellgren M, Hahn L. Thromboprophylaxis during pregnancy. *Am J Obstet Gynecol* 1989;**160**:90–4.

13

Diagnosis prevention and treatment of gestational venous thromboembolism

Ian A Greer

INTRODUCTION

Pulmonary thromboembolism (PTE) remains a major cause of maternal mortality and is the most common direct cause of maternal death in the United Kingdom.[1] Deep venous thrombosis (DVT) underlies PTE. Many DVTs are not recognized clinically and are identified only at autopsy after a maternal death. DVT is also associated with a significant risk of further thrombosis and deep venous insufficiency. The need for adequate diagnosis and treatment of thromboembolic disease in pregnancy has been highlighted by the UK Confidential Enquiries into Maternal Deaths.[1] The recent developments in diagnosis, prevention and treatment of venous thromboembolism (VTE) in pregnancy are examined in this chapter.

THE PROBLEM OF GESTATIONAL VENOUS THROMBOEMBOLISM

In order to prevent and treat VTE, it is critical to understand the extent of the problem, the risk factors and the mechanism of thrombosis. The incidence of antenatal DVT has been estimated at 0.615 per 1000 maternities in women under 35 years of age and at 1.216 per 1000 maternities in women over 35 years of age.[2] For postpartum DVT, the incidence has been estimated at 0.304 per 1000 maternities in women under 35 years of age and 0.72 per 1000 maternities in women over 35 years of age. Although antenatal DVT is more common than postpartum DVT,[2,3] the event rate is higher in the puerperium making it the time of greatest risk. Almost 40% of postpartum DVTs present after the woman's discharge from hospital, but complete data on postpartum DVT are difficult to obtain since many cases present to non-obstetric services. The UK Confidential Enquiries, however, provide accurate data for fatal PTE. Maternal mortality from PTE has fallen dramatically over the past 50 years and the greatest reduction in mortality has been in those events that occur after vaginal delivery. Recently, an increase in fatalities after vaginal delivery[1] has highlighted the need for thromboprophylaxis after vaginal delivery in women at increased risk. Mortality from PTE after Caesarean delivery, and during the antenatal and intrapartum period have changed little from the early 1950s despite major advances in identification of risk, thromboprophylaxis and diagnostic and therapeutic intervention over this same period. Thus, prevention and optimal management of VTE remains important to contemporary obstetric practice.

RISK FACTORS FOR VTE IN PREGNANCY

The common risk factors for VTE in pregnancy (Table 13.1) are:[4]

- age over 35 years;
- obesity;
- operative delivery (especially emergency Caesarean delivery in labour);

Table 13.1 Common risk factors for VTE in pregnancy
Age over 35 years
Caesarean delivery, particularly as an emergency in labour
Obesity
Thrombophilia
Past history of VTE
Gross varicose veins
Current infection or inflammatory process (e.g. active inflammatory bowel disease, urinary tract infection)
Pre-eclampsia
Immobility (e.g. bed rest, lower limb fracture)
Long distance travel
Hyperemesis gravidarum and dehydration
Significant current medical problem (e.g. nephrotic syndrome)
Paraplegia

- thrombophilia; and
- a family or personal history of thrombosis suggestive of an underlying thrombophilia. Additional risk factors include gross varicose veins, immobility, paraplegia, dehydration, infective and inflammatory conditions such as inflammatory bowel disease and urinary tract infection, pre-eclampsia, major obstetric haemorrhage such as placental abruption, and concomitant medical conditions such as nephritic syndrome. It should be noted that problems such as hyperemesis in which the woman may be dehydrated and immobile represent a significant risk. Increasingly, long-distance travel is seen as an important risk factor.

LONG-TERM MORBIDITY FROM VTE

A previous VTE is associated with an increased risk of future VTE. There is also a high risk of deep venous insufficiency developing: 80% of women with VTE develop post-thrombotic syndrome and over 60% have objectively confirmed deep venous insufficiency following a treated DVT.[5] Gestational DVT appears to carry the same risk of deep venous insufficiency as non-gestational DVT.[5] The risk of developing venous insufficiency after DVT is greater than with PTE (odds ratio 10.9 (95% CI 4.2–28.0) for DVT compared with 3.8 (95% CI 1.2–12.3 after PTE).[5] This may be due to the clot clearing from the leg veins in those with PTE leading to less extensive damage to the deep venous system.

PATHOLOGICAL MECHANISMS FOR GESTATIONAL VTE

Virchow's triad of hypercoagulability, venous stasis and vascular damage all occur in the course of normal pregnancy. There are increased levels of coagulation factors such as von Willebrand's factor, factor VIII and fibrinogen. Almost 40% of pregnant women acquire resistance to activated protein C, an endogenous anticoagulant, and a reduction in protein S (the co-factor for protein C) is seen in normal pregnancy.[6] Fibrinolysis is physiologically impaired in pregnancy by increased levels of plasminogen activator inhibitors 1 and 2, the latter being produced by the placenta.[7] In the non-pregnant situation, high levels of factor VIII and resistance to activated protein C have been associated with an increased risk of VTE. These physiological changes in the haemostatic and fibrinolytic systems in pregnancy may explain, at least in part, the increased risk of thrombosis. Relative venous stasis is a normal feature of pregnancy, and a substantial reduction in flow occurs by the end of the first trimester, progressing to around a 50% reduction by 25–29 weeks' gestation; flow reaches a nadir at 36 weeks[8] and takes around 6 weeks to return to normal, non-pregnant flow rates. Some degree of endothelial damage to pelvic vessels can occur during the course of vaginal or abdominal delivery.

Almost 90% of gestational-associated DVT occurs on the left side in contrast to the non-pregnant situation, where only 55% of DVT occur on the left.[4,9] The underlying explanation for this is not established, but it may reflect some compression of the left iliac vein by the right iliac artery and the ovarian artery, which cross the vein on the left side only. More than 70% of gestational DVTs are located in the ileofemoral region, compared with only around 9% in the non-pregnant patient, in whom calf vein DVTs are common. Ileofemoral DVTs are more likely to embolize and lead to PTE than calf vein thromboses. Lower abdominal pain can be a presenting feature of DVT in pregnancy. This pain may be due to the opening up of a peri-ovarian collateral circulation or thrombosis extending into the pelvic veins, and it is usually associated with a mild fever and leukocytosis. This presentation may cause diagnostic confusion, and DVT may be mistaken for other intra-abdominal problems such as appendicitis.

THROMBOPHILIA AND GESTATIONAL VENOUS THROMBOSIS

A congenital or acquired thrombophilia is found in around 50% of patients with gestational VTE. The congenital thrombophilias currently recognized include deficiencies of the endogenous anticoagulant proteins, antithrombin, protein C and protein S and abnormalities of procoagulants, particularly factor V Leiden and the prothrombin gene variant. Hyperhomocysteinaemia has been linked to VTE in the non-pregnant situation.[10] Hyperhomocysteinaemia can be associated with homozygosity for a variant of the methylene-tetrahydrofolate reductase gene (MTHFR C677T), sometimes called the thermolabile variant, although the genotype itself is not directly linked to venous thrombosis. Around 10% of people in European populations are homozygous for this common genetic variant. However, such homozygotes do not appear to be at increased risk of gestational VTE.[11–13] Clinical events in homozygotes are likely to reflect not just the genotype, but also a relative deficiency of B vitamins such as folic acid. The absence of an association of this genotype with gestational VTE may reflect the gestationally related physiological reduction in homocysteine levels or the effects of folic acid supplements that are now widely taken by women during pregnancy.

Deficiencies of antithrombin, protein C and protein S, in which the major components of the body's endogenous anticoagulant system are defective or deficient as a result of quantitative or qualitative defects, are uncommon (Table 13.2). They have a combined prevalence of less than 1%,[14] although the prevalence of protein S deficiency is not well established. Investigation of gestational VTE reveals one of these defects in less than 10% of cases. Factor V Leiden is functionally manifest as resistance to activated protein C, the endogenous anticoagulant that inactivates factor Va and factor VIIIa by proteolytic cleavage. Resistance is due to a single point mutation in the factor V gene. This alteration in factor V at the cleavage site results in a potentially hypercoagulable effect because the activated factor V cannot be broken down by activated protein C. Factor V Leiden occurs in 2–7% of western European populations (see Table 13.2),[14] and is usually identified in 20–40% of women with a gestational (or non-gestational) VTE.[15] Activated protein C resistance is acquired in around 40% of pregnancies,[6] possibly as a result of increases in factor V and factor VIII. It can also be seen with other thrombophilic problems such as antiphospholipid antibody syndrome and genetic abnormalities other than factor V, although the latter is uncommon. Prothrombin 20210A, the prothrombin gene variant, occurs in about 2% of the population. This genotype is expressed as elevated plasma

Table 13.2 Prevalence rates for congenital thrombophilia in European populations

Thrombophilic defect	Prevalence (%)
Antithrombin deficiency	0.25–0.55
Protein C deficiency	0.20–0.33
Factor V Leiden heterozygosis	2–7
Prothrombin 20210A heterozygosis	2
MTHFR C677T homozygosis	10

prothrombin levels. It appears to increase the risk of venous thrombosis by a factor of three.[16] Prothrombin 20210G can be found in around 6% of patients with VTE and has been reported in almost 20% of those with a strong family history of VTE.[16] Gestational VTE has been linked to this genotype.[13,17]

Potentially thrombophilic abnormalities are common, affecting at least 15% of Western populations,[18,19] and underlying around 50% of gestational VTE. Yet only around one in 1000 of pregnancies are complicated by a VTE. Thus, thrombophilia alone, even in conjunction with the gestational changes in haemostasis and thrombosis, does not invariably lead to thrombosis. This is because clinical thrombosis in women with thrombophilia is a multicausal event resulting from the interaction between congenital and acquired risk factors.[19] The likelihood of thrombosis depends on the thrombophilia, whether more than one thrombophilia is present, whether previous VTEs have occurred, and whether additional risk factors such as obesity are present.

It is important to consider the level of risk of gestational thrombosis in women with thrombophilia to guide the need for thromboprophylaxis. Much of our existing knowledge comes from observational studies of symptomatic thrombophilic kindreds. This will overestimate the risk for previously asymptomatic women with thrombophilia and also for asymptomatic families in whom a thrombophilia has been identified coincidentally. For example, initial estimates for the risk of gestational VTE without anticoagulant therapy have been found to range from 32% to 60% in antithrombin-deficient women.[14,20-22] Estimates for the risk of gestational thrombosis vary between 3% and 10% for protein C deficiency and between 0% and 6% for protein S deficiency during pregnancy, rising to 7–19% and 7–22%, respectively, postpartum.[14] Factor V Leiden has been reported in up to 46% of women investigated for gestational VTE.[23]

These data reflect the prevalence in symptomatic women and do not provide information on the risk of thrombosis in previously asymptomatic women with thrombophilia. Several recent studies have provided estimates for the risk of gestational thrombosis in the more common thrombophilias.

Gerhardt et al.[12] assessed 119 women with thromboembolism in pregnancy and 233 controls for the presence of thrombophilia. The relative risk for thrombosis in pregnancy after adjusting for other key variables was 6.9 (95% CI 3.3–15.2) with factor V Leiden, 9.5 (95% CI 2.1–66.7) with prothrombin G20210A and 10.4 (95% CI 2.2–62.5) for antithrombin deficiency. Combined defects substantially increase risk, with an odds ratio estimated at 107 for the combination of factor V Leiden and prothrombin G20210A. Additional risk factors such as obesity were present in 25% of the cases compared with 11% of controls. Women with recurrent events were more likely to have an underlying combined thrombophilia. This study also provided a positive predictive value for each thrombophilia assuming an underlying rate of VTE of 0.66 per 1000 pregnancies, consistent with estimates from Western populations.[18] The likelihood of a VTE occurring in pregnancy was estimated at 1:500 for factor V Leiden, 1:200 for prothrombin 20210A and 4.6:100 for these defects combined. A retrospective study of 72,000 pregnancies, in which women with venous thrombosis were assessed for thrombophilia[4] and in which the underlying prevalence of these defects in the population was known, found that the risk of thrombosis was 1:437 for factor V Leiden, 1:113 for protein C deficiency, 1:2.8 for type 1 (quantitative) antithrombin deficiency and 1:42 for type 2 (qualitative) antithrombin deficiency. This study was extended[13] and reported an odds ratio of 4.4 (95% CI 1.2–16) for prothrombin G20210A, 4.5 (95% CI 2.1–14.5) for factor V Leiden, 282 (95% CI 31–2532) for type 1 antithrombin deficiency (quantitative deficiency) and 28 (95% 5.5–142) for type 2 antithrombin deficiency (qualitative deficiency) (Table 13.3). These data are valuable in determining whether to use thromboprophylaxis in pregnancy.

SCREENING FOR CONGENITAL THROMBOPHILIA IN PREGNANCY

There is currently no justification for universal screening of all pregnant women for congenital thrombophilia. The natural history of many

Table 13.3 Risk of VTE in pregnancy with thrombophilia

Thrombophilic defect	Odds ratio (95% CI) for VTE in pregnancy*	Relative risk (95% CI) for VTE in pregnancy†
Type 1 antithrombin deficiency (quantitative deficiency)	282 (31–2532)	N/A
Type 2 antithrombin deficiency (qualitative deficiency)	28 (5.5–142)	N/A
Antithrombin deficiency (activity < 80%)	N/A	10.4 (2.2–62.5)
Factor V Leiden heterozygosis	4.5 (2.1–14.5)	6.9 (3.3–15.2)
Prothrombin 20210A heterozygosis	4.4 (1.2–16)	9.5 (2.1–66.7)
MTHFR C677T homozygosis	0.45 (0.13–1.58)	No increase in risk (relative risk not reported)

*Based on a retrospective study of 93,000 pregnancies in which odds ratios were calculated by screening women with VTE in pregnancy for thrombophilia and relating this to the known prevalence of these defects in the population[12]

†Based on a study of 119 women with thromboembolism in pregnancy and 233 controls for the presence of congenital thrombophilia;[12] relative risk was calculated after logistic regression to adjust for age, body mass index, oral contraceptive use, protein C activity, protein S activity, Factor V Leiden, prothrombin G20210A, MTHFR 677TT and antithrombin activity

thrombophilias in pregnancy, particularly in asymptomatic women, has not been established, and the need for (and nature of) any intervention is not known. It is also uncertain whether this approach to screening would be cost-effective. However, there is a case for offering screening to women who have gestational VTE or a personal or family history of VTE, since around half of these women will have a thrombophilic defect.[18] Although the requirement for antenatal thromboprophylaxis may be uncertain in some forms of thrombophilia, such as asymptomatic factor V Leiden, there is a consensus view that women with a personal history of VTE and an underlying thrombophilic trait should receive thromboprophylaxis during pregnancy and, in particular, the puerperium.[24]

THROMBOPROPHYLAXIS FOR GESTATIONAL VTE: PRACTICAL ISSUES

The management of the woman with a single previous event is controversial. This is because of the wide variation in risk that has been reported, with risks of 1–13% in various studies.[25–28] The higher estimate has led many clinicians to use pharmacological prophylaxis with heparin or low molecular weight heparin during pregnancy and the puerperium. However, these estimates of risk have significant limitations. For example, objective testing was not used in all cases, some of the studies were retrospective and the prospective studies had relatively small sample sizes. Brill-Edwards *et al.* have recently conducted a prospective study of 125 pregnant women with a single previous objectively diagnosed VTE.[29] No heparin was given antenatally but anticoagulants, usually warfarin following an initial short course of heparin or low molecular weight heparin, was given for 4–6 weeks postpartum. The overall rate for recurrent antenatal VTE was 2.4% (95% CI 0.2–6.9). Interestingly, none of the 44 women (95% CI 0.0–8.0) who did not have an underlying thrombophilia and whose previous VTE had been associated with a temporary risk

Table 13.4 Management of gestational VTE

Clinical situation	Suggested management
Single previous VTE associated with a transient risk factor and no additional current risk factors, such as obesity	**Antenatal** Surveillance or prophylactic doses of low molecular weight heparin (e.g. enoxaparin 40 mg daily or dalteparin 5000 units daily), with or without graduated elastic compression stockings 　　Discuss decision about antenatal low molecular weight heparin with the woman **Postpartum** Anticoagulant therapy for at least 6 weeks (e.g. enoxaparin 40 mg daily or dalteparin 5000 units daily or warfarin (target INR 2–3) with low molecular weight heparin overlap until the INR is ≥ 2.0) with or without graduated elastic compression stockings
Single previous idiopathic VTE or single event associated with pregnancy or the combined oral contraceptive pill or single previous VTE with underlying thrombophilia and not on long-term anticoagulant therapy, or single previous VTE and additional current risk factor(s) (e.g. morbid obesity, nephrotic syndrome)	**Antenatal** Prophylactic doses of low molecular weight heparin (e.g. enoxaparin 40 mg daily or dalteparin 5000 units daily) with or without graduated elastic compression stockings; note that there is a strong case for more intense low molecular weight heparin therapy in antithrombin deficiency (specialist advice recommended). **Postpartum** Anticoagulant therapy for at least 6 weeks (e.g. enoxaparin 40 mg daily or dalteparin 5000 units daily or warfarin (target INR 2–3) with low molecular weight heparin overlap until the INR is ≥ 2.0) with or without graduated elastic compression stockings
More than one previous episode of VTE, with no thrombophilia and not on long-term anticoagulant therapy	**Antenatal** Prophylactic doses of low molecular weight heparin (e.g. enoxaparin 40 mg daily or dalteparin 5000 units daily) plus graduated elastic compression stockings **Postpartum** Anticoagulant therapy for at least 6 weeks (e.g. enoxaparin 40 mg daily or dalteparin 5000 units daily or warfarin (target INR 2–3) with low molecular weight heparin overlap until the INR is ≥ 2.0) plus graduated elastic compression stockings

Table 13.4 continued	
Clinical situation	**Suggested management**
Previous episode(s) of VTE in women receiving long-term anticoagulants (e.g. for underlying thrombophilia)	**Antenatal** Switch from oral anticoagulants to low molecular weight heparin (the dose will be greater than that used for routine prophylaxis and will depend on the thrombophilia or type of previous events. Specialist advice is required) by 6 weeks gestation, plus graduated elastic compression stockings **Postpartum** Resume long-term anticoagulants with low molecular weight heparin overlap until INR in prepregnancy therapeutic range, plus graduated elastic compression stockings
Thrombophilia (confirmed laboratory abnormality) but no prior VTE	**Antenatal** Surveillance or prophylactic low molecular weight heparin with or without graduated elastic compression stockings. The indication for pharmacological prophylaxis in the antenatal period is stronger in antithrombin-deficient women than in the other thrombophilias and it is also stronger in symptomatic kindred than asymptomatic kindred **Postpartum** Anticoagulant therapy for at least 6 weeks (e.g. enoxaparin 40 mg daily or dalteparin 5000 units daily or warfarin (target INR 2–3) with low molecular weight heparin overlap until the INR is ≥ 2.0) with or without graduated elastic compression stockings

factor developed a VTE, whereas 5.9% (95% CI 1.2–16%) of the women who were found to have an underlying thrombophilia or whose previous VTE had been idiopathic had a recurrent event.

These data suggest that women with a single previous event associated with a temporary risk factor and without a thrombophilia should not routinely receive antenatal pharmacological thromboprophylaxis. Graduated elastic compression stockings can be used as an alternative treatment in women for whom a clearcut indication for anticoagulation is not present. Postpartum, such women should receive anticoagulant therapy for at least 6 weeks (e.g. enoxaparin 40 mg daily, dalteparin 5000 IU daily, or warfarin (target international normalized ratio (INR) 2–3) with low molecular weight heparin overlap until the INR is ≥ 2.0) with or without graduated elastic compression stockings (Table 13.4).

In women with a single previous VTE and an underlying thrombophilia, women in whom the VTE was idiopathic or women with additional risk factors such as obesity or nephrotic syndrome, there is clearly a much stronger case for pharmacological prophylaxis, although this will depend, in part, on the severity of the event and the type of underlying thrombophilia. Antenatally these women should be considered for prophylactic doses of low molecular weight heparin (e.g. enoxaparin 40 mg daily or dalteparin 5000 IU daily) with or without graduated elastic compression stockings. There is a strong case for more intense low molecular weight heparin therapy in the presence of antithrombin deficiency, although many women with previous VTE and antithrombin deficiency will already be on long-term anticoagulant therapy. Postpartum anticoagulant therapy for at least 6 weeks as desribed above is recommended (see Table 13.4).

For the woman who has had more than one previous VTE, who has no identifiable thrombophilia and who is not on long-term anticoagulant therapy, there is a considerable consensus of opinion that she should receive antenatal pharmacological thromboprophylaxis, usually with low molecular weight heparin or unfractionated heparin. This is usually started from the midpoint of the pregnancy, or earlier if one or more of the past events was gestational or if there are additional risk factors present in the first trimester (such as obesity or hyperemesis gravidarum). It may also be prudent to provide graduated elastic compression stockings from the time of diagnosis of pregnancy and to consider the use of low-dose aspirin, even though its efficacy is not entirely clear, until low molecular weight heparin is started. Postpartum, she should receive at least 6 weeks' pharmacological prophylaxis with low molecular weight heparin, the target INR is 2–3 and low molecular weight heparin should be continued until the INR is ≥ 2. A longer duration of postpartum prophylaxis may be required for women with additional risk factors.

The woman with one or more previous episodes of VTE receiving long-term anticoagulants (e.g. because of underlying thrombophilia) should switch from oral anticoagulants to treatment doses of low molecular weight heparin (e.g. dalteparin 200 IU/kg every 24 hours or enoxaparin 1 mg/kg every 12 hours) by 6 weeks' gestation, and she should be fitted with graduated elastic compression stockings. Postpartum she should resume long-term anticoagulants with low molecular weight heparin overlap until the INR is therapeutic (>2). She should continue to use graduated elastic compression stockings.

Where a woman has thrombophilia confirmed on laboratory testing but no prior VTE, surveillance or prophylactic low molecular weight heparin, with or without graduated elastic compression stockings, can be used antenatally. The indication for pharmacological prophylaxis in the antenatal period is stronger in antithrombin-deficiency than in the other thrombophilias, and it is also stronger in symptomatic kindred than in asymptomatic kindred. Postpartum these women should receive anticoagulant therapy for at least 6 weeks as described above, with or without graduated elastic compression stockings.

DIAGNOSIS OF GESTATIONAL VTE

Objective diagnosis of VTE in pregnancy is essential in all women with symptoms or signs that could be compatible with VTE. Failure to identify VTE places the mother's life at risk, while unnecessary treatment will expose her not only to anticoagulants but also will label her as having had a VTE. This can have an impact on her future healthcare, such as contraception and thromboprophylaxis in future pregnancies. Maternity hospitals should have a protocol for the objective diagnosis of suspected VTE during pregnancy.

The clinical features of DVT include:

- leg pain or discomfort (especially on the left);
- swelling;
- tenderness;
- increased temperature and oedema;
- lower abdominal pain; and
- elevated white cell count.

Features suggestive of PTE include:

- dyspnoea;
- collapse;
- chest pain;
- haemoptysis;
- faintness;
- raised jugular venous pressure;
- focal signs in the chest.

These features of PTE are sometimes combined with the symptoms and signs of DVT.

The clinical diagnosis of VTE during pregnancy is unreliable, particularly since problems such as leg swelling and discomfort are common features of normal pregnancy. In a study of consecutive pregnant women presenting with a clinical suspicion of DVT, the diagnosis was confirmed in less than 10%. This compares with around 25% of diagnoses being confirmed in the non-pregnant situation.[30–32] Around 30% of patients presenting with possible PTE outside pregnancy have the diagnosis confirmed,[33,34] but the number of positive results following investigation appears to be substantially lower in pregnancy,[28] perhaps because of a lower threshold for investigation.

Real-time or duplex ultrasound is the main diagnostic tool[35] for DVT. If the diagnosis is confirmed, anticoagulant treatment should be commenced or continued. In non-pregnant subjects, the pre-test clinical probability of DVT modifies both the positive predictive value and the negative predictive value of objective diagnostic tests.[36,37] A negative ultrasound result with a low level of clinical suspicion suggests that anticoagulant treatment can be discontinued or withheld. With a negative ultrasound report and a high level of clinical suspicion, the pregnant woman should be anticoagulated and the ultrasound repeated in 1 week, or X-ray venography should be considered. If repeat testing is negative, anticoagulant treatment should be discontinued.[38] If PTE is suspected, both a ventilation–perfusion (V–Q) lung scan and a bilateral duplex ultrasound leg examination should be performed. If the V–Q scan reports a 'medium' or 'high' probability of

PTE, anticoagulant treatment should be continued. With a 'low' probability of PTE on V–Q scan but a positive ultrasound for DVT, anticoagulant treatment should be continued. If a V–Q scan reports a low risk of PTE and there are negative leg ultrasound examinations, yet there is a high level of clinical suspicion, anticoagulant treatment should be continued with repeat testing in 1 week (V–Q scan and leg ultrasound examination). If the clinical probability of PTE is high, then even if the V–Q scan shows 'low' probability and the leg ultrasound examination is negative, alternative imaging techniques should be considered (e.g. pulmonary angiography or magnetic resonance imaging; helical computerized tomography).[38] Similarly, if the chest X-ray has abnormalities that lead to difficulties in the diagnosis of PTE using V–Q scanning, then alternative imaging techniques are warranted (Table 13.5). The radiation dose from investigations such as V–Q scanning, chest X-ray and limited venography is modest[39] and considered to pose a negligible risk to the fetus, particularly when set in the context of the risk from PTE. Thus objective diagnostic testing should not be withheld because of concern about fetal radiation exposure.

D-dimer measurements in plasma are now used as a screening test for VTE in the non-pregnant woman, in whom it has a high negative predictive value.[35] Outside pregnancy, a low level of D-dimer suggests the absence of VTE, and further objective tests are not required. An increased level of D-dimer suggests that VTE may be present, and an objective diagnostic test should be performed. In pregnancy D-dimer levels can be increased owing to the physiological changes in the coagulation system, and also if there is a concomitant problem such as pre-eclampsia. Thus elevated D-dimer levels in pregnancy are not necessarily consistent with VTE, and objective diagnostic testing is required. However, a low level of D-dimer in pregnancy is likely to suggest the absence of VTE. Since there is limited information on the efficacy and safety of D-dimer screening for VTE in pregnancy, firm guidance cannot yet be given.

Table 13.5 Treatment after results of investigations for gestational VTE	
Suspected DVT A negative ultrasound venography result with a low level of clinical suspicion	Anticoagulant treatment can be discontinued or withheld
Suspected DVT A negative ultrasound venography report and a high level of clinical suspicion	The woman should be anticoagulated and the ultrasound repeated in 1 week, or X-ray venography should be considered. If repeat testing is negative, anticoagulant treatment should be discontinued
Suspected PTE The V–Q scan reports a 'medium' or 'high' probability of PTE	Anticoagulant treatment should be continued
Suspected PTE A 'low' probability of PTE on V–Q scan but positive ultrasound venography for DVT	Anticoagulant treatment should be continued
Suspected PTE A V–Q scan reports a low risk of PTE and there are negative leg ultrasound venography examinations, yet there is a high level of clinical suspicion	Anticoagulant treatment should continue with repeat testing in 1 week (V–Q scan and leg ultrasound venography examination)
Suspected PTE If the clinical probability of PTE is high, yet the V–Q scan shows 'low' probability and leg ultrasound venography examination is negative	Consider alternative imaging techniques such as pulmonary angiography or magnetic resonance imaging or helical computerized tomography

SCREENING FOR THROMBOPHILIA IN WOMEN WITH AN ACUTE GESTATIONAL VTE

It is important to be aware of the effects of pregnancy and thrombosis on the results of a thrombophilia screen. For example, protein S levels fall in normal pregnancy, making it virtually impossible to make a diagnosis of protein S deficiency during pregnancy. Activated protein C resistance occurs in around 40% of pregnancies, and anticardiolipin antibodies can also influence the result of this test. Antithrombin may be reduced when a thrombus is present and in nephrotic syndrome, and protein C and protein S are reduced in patients with liver disease. Genotyping for factor V Leiden and prothrombin G20210A are not influenced by pregnancy or current thrombosis. Factor V Leiden is associated with an increase in risk of VTE, and this increase is largely due to DVT. Outside pregnancy, the prevalence of underlying factor V Leiden in PTE is around half of that of DVT.[40] This differs from other thrombophilias such as prothrombin G20210A, in which there is no difference in the underlying prevalence of DVT and that of PTE. It has been proposed that factor V Leiden is associated with a more adherent and stable thrombus possibly owing to increased local thrombin generation, and that this stability reduces the likelihood of embolization. Whether this applies to pregnant women with factor V Leiden is not clear.

ANTICOAGULANTS IN PREGNANCY

Treatment and prophylaxis of gestational VTE centres on the use of unfractionated heparin or low molecular weight heparin, because of the fetal hazards of warfarin.[41] Although warfarin is not secreted in breast milk in clinically significant amounts and is safe to use during lactation, it crosses the placenta and is a known teratogen. Warfarin embryopathy (mid-face hypoplasia, stippled chondral calcification, scoliosis, short proximal limbs and short phalanges) may occur with exposure to the drug between 6 and 9 weeks' gestation and the incidence has been estimated at around 5%.[41] The risk of embryopathy may be dose-dependent, with an increased risk when the dose of warfarin is greater than 5 mg/day.[42]

In addition to warfarin embryopathy, there is the possibility of problems arising as a result of fetal bleeding. Since the fetal liver is immature and levels of vitamin K-dependent coagulation factors are low, maternal warfarin therapy maintained in the therapeutic range will be associated with excessive fetal anticoagulation and therefore potential haemorrhagic complications in the fetus. Warfarin should be avoided beyond 36 weeks' gestation[41,43] because of the excessive haemorrhagic risk to both mother and fetus.

Neither unfractionated heparin[44] nor low molecular weight heparin[45,46] crosses the placenta and there is thus no risk of teratogenesis or fetal haemorrhage. Systematic reviews suggest that these agents are safe for the fetus.[47] Heparins are not secreted in breast milk and can be used during lactation. However, prolonged use of unfractionated heparin can be associated with symptomatic osteoporosis, allergy and heparin-induced thrombocytopenia.[48] In contrast, low molecular weight heparins[48] appear to carry less risk of osteoporosis.

Heparin-induced thrombocytopenia is a serious side effect that is associated with extensive venous thrombosis; it usually occurs between 5 and 15 days after the institution of heparin.[49] The risk has been estimated at between 1% and 3% with unfractionated heparin and is substantially lower with low molecular weight heparin.[50]

Allergic reactions usually take the form of itchy, erythematous lesions at the injection sites. Switching between heparin preparations may be helpful; however, cross-reactivity can occur. Allergic reactions should be distinguished from faulty injection technique with associated bruising.

Low molecular weight heparin is now widely used in the pregnant situation for thromboprophylaxis because of its better side effect profile than unfractionated heparin and its once-daily dosing.[47,51–56]

Dextran has been used for peripartum thromboprophylaxis, particularly during Caesarean delivery, but there is a risk of maternal anaphylactoid reactions, which have been associated with uterine hypertonus, profound fetal distress, and a high incidence of fetal death or profound neurological damage.[57] Thus, dextran should be avoided in pregnancy.

Graduated elastic compression stockings are effective in outside pregnancy and in view of the pregnancy-related changes in the venous system, they could be of value in pregnancy. They may act by preventing overdistension of veins, thereby preventing endothelial damage and exposure of subendothelial collagen.[58] Other mechanical techniques, such as intermittent pneumatic compression, are of value for prophylaxis during Caesarean delivery and immediately postpartum.

Hirudin, a direct thrombin inhibitor, is used in outside pregnancy for treatment of heparin-induced thrombocytopenia; it has also been used for postoperative prophylaxis. Since it crosses the placenta, it should not be used in pregnancy. Its use has been reported in a lactating mother because of heparin-induced thrombocytopenia, and hirudin was not detectable in breast milk.[59]

Aspirin has been found in a meta-analysis to have a beneficial effect in the prevention of DVT.

Unlike heparin, its effectiveness in pregnancy remains to be established, but it is likely to offer some benefit. Its effectiveness is likely to be less than that of unfractionated heparin and low molecular weight heparin.[60] In women who are unable to take heparin or in whom the balance of risk is not considered sufficient to merit heparin, it may be useful. Low-dose (60–75 mg daily) aspirin is not associated with adverse pregnancy outcome in the second and third trimesters.[61,62]

MANAGEMENT OF ACUTE GESTATIONAL VTE

When a VTE is suspected, treatment with unfractionated heparin or low molecular weight heparin should be given until the diagnosis is excluded by objective testing, unless anticoagulation is contraindicated. Graduated elastic compression stockings should also be used (along with leg elevation for DVT). Traditionally, unfractionated heparin has been used in the initial management of VTE.[63] In non-pregnant patients with clinically suspected PTE, treatment with anticoagulants (intravenous heparin and warfarin) reduces the risk of further thromboembolism compared with no treatment.[64] Descriptive reports show a high risk of recurrent VTE and death when heparin is withheld from patients with suspected or proven VTE, compared with the low risks with heparin treatment.[65,66] Trials of unfractionated heparin in acute DVT have shown that failure to achieve the lower limit of the target therapeutic range of the aPTT ratio (1.5) is associated with up to a 15-fold increase in the risk of recurrent VTE.[67] The use of the activated partial thromboplastin time (aPTT) to monitor unfractionated heparin can be technically problematic, particularly in late pregnancy when an apparent heparin resistance occurs, owing to increased fibrinogen and factor VIII. In this situation, the anti-factor Xa level may be useful as a measure of heparin dose (target range 0.35–0.7 μ/ml).[63]

The properties of low molecular weight heparin allow the use of fixed-dose, subcutaneous treatment in the acute treatment of VTE, so minimizing or avoiding the need for monitoring. Meta-analyses of randomized controlled trials in non-pregnant subjects have compared low molecular weight heparin with unfractionated heparin in the initial treatment of DVT.[68,69] Low molecular weight heparin was found to be more effective than unfractionated heparin (with a lower mortality) and it was also associated with a lower risk of haemorrhagic complications. For PTE, low molecular weight heparin is as effective as unfractionated heparin in non-pregnant subjects.[70] Low molecular weight heparin has been used for the initial management of VTE in pregnancy[53,71] and has been recommended for this purpose in published clinical guidelines.[24]

Occasionally for life-threatening PTE or when a massive DVT threatens limb viability, thrombolytic therapy may be required. Experience is limited and there is a risk of major haemorrhage if systemic thrombolysis is used around the time of delivery or postpartum.[72]

With intravenous unfractionated heparin, a bolus of 5000 IU given over about 5 minutes is used; this is followed by continuous intravenous infusion of 1000–2000 IU/hour. The dose is adjusted by monitoring the aPTT, with a therapeutic target ratio of 1.5–2.5 times the mean laboratory control value.[72] Protocols for heparin dose adjustment according to aPTT results are useful since they improve the achievement of therapeutic target ranges.[63,73] If anti-factor Xa measurements are to be used to monitor heparin, the target range for the anti-factor Xa level is 0.35–0.70 IU/ml. In a meta-analysis of randomized controlled trials, 12–hourly subcutaneous unfractionated heparin was found to be as effective, and at least as safe, as intravenous unfractionated heparin in the prevention of recurrent thromboembolism in non-pregnant patients with acute DVT.[74] When administered subcutaneously, unfractionated heparin is given in subcutaneous injections of 15,000–20,000 IU every 12 hours, after an initial intravenous bolus of 5000 IU. The dose should be adjusted to maintain the mid-interval aPTT at 1.5–2.5 times the control.[72]

In non-pregnant patients, once-daily administration is recommended for acute treatment of VTE with low molecular weight heparin (e.g. enoxaparin 1.5 mg/kg once daily, dalteparin

10,000–18,000 units once daily, depending on body weight, or tinzaparin 175 units/kg once daily). However, in view of the alterations in the pharmacokinetics of dalteparin and enoxaparin during pregnancy,[75,76] a twice-daily dosage regimen for these low molecular weight heparins in the treatment of VTE in pregnancy is used (enoxaparin 1 mg/kg twice daily or dalteparin 100 units/kg twice daily up to a maximum of 18,000 units in 24 hours has been recommended).[71] These doses have also been used to treat VTE outside pregnancy.

With both unfractionated heparin and low molecular weight heparin, the platelet count should be monitored 4–8 days after treatment commences, then about once a month to detect heparin-induced thrombocytopenia, which is associated with further thrombotic complications. Pregnant women who develop heparin-induced thrombocytopenia and who require continuing anticoagulant therapy should be managed with a heparinoid,[77] danaparoid sodium, or if post-partum with warfarin, with danaparoid continued until the INR is in the therapeutic range.

As warfarin is contraindicated in pregnancy, subcutaneous unfractionated heparin or low molecular weight heparin is used for maintenance treatment of VTE in pregnancy.[24,71] Low molecular weight heparin appears to be superior to aPTT-monitored unfractionated heparin in the maintenance treatment of VTE in pregnancy because of the simpler therapeutic regimen. Women can be taught to self-inject and can be managed as outpatients once the acute event is controlled. Arrangements should be made to allow safe disposal of needles and syringes. Outpatient follow-up for assessment of platelets (and peak anti-factor Xa levels if required) during treatment should be arranged. Therapeutic doses of heparin should be employed (i.e. an adjusted-dose regimen of subcutaneous unfractionated heparin to achieve a target aPTT ratio of 1.5–2.5 times the control value) or low molecular weight heparin administered subcutaneously every 12 hours to achieve a peak anti-factor Xa activity 3–4 hours after an injection of 0.4–1.0 units/ml. In a prospective randomized controlled trial in non-

pregnant patients, a 47% recurrence rate of VTE was reported when thromboprophylactic doses of unfractionated heparin (5000 IU every 12 hours) were used after initial management with intravenous unfractionated heparin.[78]

The duration of therapeutic anticoagulant treatment in the non-pregnant situation is usually 6 months. Since pregnancy is associated with prothrombotic changes in the coagulation system and venous flow, it would appear prudent to apply this same duration of treatment to gestational VTE. If the VTE occurs early in the pregnancy, then provided that there are no additional risk factors, the dose of low molecular weight heparin or unfractionated heparin can be reduced to prophylactic levels (40 mg enoxaparin once daily or 5000 IU dalteparin once daily; or 10,000 IU of unfractionated heparin twice daily) after 6 months. After delivery, treatment should continue for at least 6–12 weeks. Warfarin can be used after delivery. If the woman chooses to commence warfarin postpartum, this can be started on the second or third postnatal day. The INR should be checked on day 2, and subsequent warfarin doses titrated to maintain the INR between 2.0 and 3.0.[79] Heparin treatment should be continued until the INR is > 2.0 on 2 successive days.

LABOUR AND CAESAREAN DELIVERY IN THE WOMAN WITH GESTATIONAL VTE

The woman on anticoagulant treatment for VTE should be advised that once she is established in labour or thinks that she is in labour, she should not inject any further unfractionated heparin or low molecular weight heparin until she has been assessed by an obstetrician. If induction of labour is planned, the dose of heparin should be reduced to a thromboprophylactic level on the day before delivery. The treatment dose can be recommenced after delivery.

There has been concern about low molecular weight heparin and epidural haematoma because of postmarketing reports, largely from the USA, to the Food and Drug Administration. These events have mostly been in elderly women (median age 75 years) undergoing orthopaedic surgery. Additional factors such as concomitant use of non-steroidal anti-inflammatory drugs (which can enhance bleeding risk, particularly in the elderly) or multiple puncture attempts at spinal or epidural anaesthesia have also been implicated. The true incidence of epidural haematoma is impossible to determine because of lack of denominator data. In addition, practice in North America and Europe may differ, particularly with regard to the use of low molecular weight heparin. In Europe, enoxaparin is used in a dose of 40 mg daily, compared with 30 mg twice daily in North America. Such differences in patients and practice make it difficult to extrapolate the information in these reports to obstetric practice. A degree of caution must nonetheless be exercised in the concomitant use of low molecular weight heparin and neuraxial anaesthesia. In general terms, neuraxial anaesthesia is not used until at least 12 hours after the previous prophylactic dose of low molecular weight heparin. When a woman presents while on a therapeutic regimen of low molecular weight heparin, regional techniques should not be used for at least 24 hours after the last dose. Low molecular weight heparin should not be given for at least 3 hours after the epidural catheter has been removed, and the cannula should not be removed within 10–12 hours of the most recent injection.[80,81]

Individualized management plans are often required with regard to elective Caesarean delivery in women on anticoagulant treatment for VTE. However, in general terms, the woman should receive a thromboprophylactic dose of low molecular weight heparin on the day before delivery. On the day of delivery, the morning dose of low molecular weight heparin should be omitted. Graduated elastic compression stockings or mechanical methods can be used to provide intraoperative thromboprophylaxis. A thromboprophylactic dose of low molecular weight heparin should be given by 3 hours postoperatively and after removal of the epidural catheter if epidural anaesthesia is used. The treatment dose of low molecular weight heparin should be recommenced that evening. There is an increased risk of around 2% of wound haematoma following Caesarean delivery with both unfractionated heparin and low molecular weight heparin. Consideration should be given to the use of surgical drains (abdominal and rectus sheath drains). Skin closure with staples or interrupted sutures allows easier drainage of any haematoma.

A particular problem in obstetrics is the woman at high-risk of haemorrhage (e.g. high risk of major antepartum haemorrhage, progressive wound haematoma, suspected intra-abdominal bleeding, or postpartum haemorrhage) in whom heparin treatment is considered necessary because of VTE. She should be managed with intravenous, unfractionated heparin until the high risk of haemorrhage has resolved. Intravenous unfractionated heparin has a short duration of action, and anticoagulation will reverse shortly after cessation of the infusion should a haemorrhage occur.

REFERENCES

1. Department of Health, Welsh Office, Scottish Home and Health Department and Department of Health and Social Services Northern Ireland. Confidential Enquiries into Maternal Deaths in the United Kingdom 1994–1997. London: TSO, 1998.
2. Macklon NS, Greer IA. Venous thromboembolic disease in obstetrics and gynaecology: the Scottish experience. *Scott Med J* 1996;**41**:83–6.
3. Rutherford S, Montoro M, McGhee W, Strong T. Thromboembolic disease associated with pregnancy: an 11 year review [abstract]. *Am Obstet Gynecol* 1991;**164**(suppl):286.
4. McColl M, Ramsay JE, Tait RC, *et al.* Risk factors for pregnancy associated venous thromboembolism. *Thromb Haemost* 1997;**78**:1183–8.
5. McColl M, Ellison J, Greer IA, Tait RC, Walker ID. Prevalence of the post-thrombotic syndrome in young women with previous venous thromboembolism. *Br J Haematol* 2000;**108**:272–4.
6. Clarke P, Brennand J, Conkie JA, McCall F, Greer IA, Walker ID. Activated protein C sensitivity, protein C, protein S and coagulation in normal pregnancy. *Thromb Haemost* 1998;**79**:1166–70.
7. Greer IA. Haemostasis and thrombosis in

pregnancy. In: Bloom AL, Forbes CD, Thomas DP, Tuddenham EGD, eds. *Haemostasis and Thrombosis*. Edinburgh: Churchill Livingstone; 1994:987–1015.

8. Macklon NS, Greer IA, Bowman AW. An ultrasound study of gestational and postural changes in the deep venous system of the leg in pregnancy. *Br J Obstet Gynaecol* 1997;**104**:191–7.

9. Lindhagen A, Bergqvist A, Bergqvist D, Hallbook T. Late venous function in the leg after deep venous thrombosis occurring in relation to pregnancy. *Br J Obstet Gynaecol* 1986;**93**:348–52.

10. Den Heijer M, Koster T, Blom HJ *et al*. Hyperhomocysteinemia as a risk factor V for deep vein thrombosis. *N Engl J Med*;1998;**334**:759–62.

11. Greer IA. The challenge of thrombophilia in maternal–fetal medicine. *N Engl J Med* 2000;**342**:424–5.

12. Gerhardt A, Scharf RE, Beckman MW, *et al*. Prothrombin and factor V mutations in women with thrombosis during pregnancy and the puerperium. *N Engl J Med* 2000;**342**:374–80.

13. McColl MD, Ellison J, Reid F, *et al*. Prothrombin 20210GA, MTHFR C677T mutations in women with venous thromboembolism associated with pregnancy. *Br J Obstet Gynaecol* 2000;**107**:565–9.

14. Walker ID. Congenital thrombophilia. In: Greer IA, ed. *Baillière's Clinical Obstetrics and Gynaecology: Thromboembolic Disease in Obstetrics and Gynaecology*. London: Baillière Tindall; 1997:431–45.

15. Zoller B, Holm J, Dahlback B. Resistance to activated protein C due to a factor V gene mutation: the most common inherited risk factor of thrombosis. *Trends Cardiovasc Med* 1996;**6**:45–51.

16. Poort SR, Rosendaal FR, Reitsma PH, Bertina RM. A common genetic variation in the 3'-untranslated regions of the prothrombin gene is associated with elevated plasma prothrombin levels and an increase in venous thrombosis. *Blood* 1996;**88**:3698–703.

17. McColl MD, Walker ID, Greer IA. A mutation in the prothrombin gene contributing to venous thrombosis in pregnancy. *Br J Obstet Gynaecol* 1998;**105**:923–5.

18. Greer IA. Thrombosis in pregnancy: maternal and fetal issues. *Lancet* 1999;**353**:1258–65.

19. Rosendaal FR. Venous thrombosis: a multicausal disease. *Lancet* 1999;**353**:1167–73.

20. Conard J, Horellou MH, van Dreden P, Le Compte T, Samama M. Thrombosis in pregnancy and congenital deficiencies in AT III, protein C or protein S: study of 78 women. *Thromb Haemost* 1990;**63**:319–20.

21. Pabinger I, Study Group on Natural Inhibitors. Thrombotic risk in hereditary anti-thrombin III, protein C or protein S deficiency. *Arterioscler Thromb Vasc Biol* 1996;**16**:742–8.

22. de Stefano V, Leone G, Masterangela S, *et al*. Thrombosis during pregnancy and surgery in patients with congenital deficiency of anti-thrombin III, protein C and protein S. *Thromb Haemost* 1994;**71**:799–800.

23. Bokarewa MI, Bremme K, Blomback M. Arg 506–Gln mutation in factor V and risk of thrombosis during pregnancy. *Br J Haematol* 1996;**92**:473–8.

24. Ginsberg J, Greer IA, Hirsh J. Sixth ACCP consensus conference on antithrombotic therapy. Use of antithrombotic agents during pregnancy. *Chest* 2001;**119**(1 Suppl):122S–131S.

25. De Swiet M, Floyd E, Letsky E. Low risk of recurrent thromboembolism in pregnancy [letter]. *Br J Hosp Med* 1987;**38**:264.

26. Howell R, Fidler J, Letsky E, *et al*. The risk of antenatal subcutaneous heparin prophylaxis: a controlled trial. *Br J Obstet Gynaecol* 1983;**90**:1124–8.

27. Badaracco MA, Vessey M. Recurrent venous thromboembolic disease and use of oral contraceptives. *BMJ* 1974;**1**:215–17.

28. Tengborn L. Recurrent thromboembolism in pregnancy and puerperium: is there a need for thromboprophylaxis? *Am J Obstet Gynecol* 1989;**160**:90–4.

29. Brill-Edwards P, Ginsberg JS, for the Recurrence Of Clot In This Pregnancy (ROCIT) Study Group. Safety of withholding antepartum heparin in women with a previous episode of venous thromboembolism. *N Engl J Med* 2000;**343**:1439–44.

30. Hull RD, Raskob GF, Carter CJ. Serial IPG in pregnancy patients with clinically suspected DVT. Clinical validity of negative findings. *Ann Intern Med* 1990;**112**:663–7.

31. Hull RD, Hirsh J, Sackett D, *et al*. Diagnostic efficacy of IPG in suspected venous thrombosis: An alternative to venography. *N Engl J Med* 1977;**296**:1497–500.

32. Lensing AWA, Prandoni P, Brandjes D, *et al*. Detection of DVT by real-time B-mode ultrasonography. *N Engl J Med* 1989;**320**:342–5.

33. PIOPED Investigators. Value of the ventilation/perfusion scan in acute pulmonary embolism. Results of the prospective investigation of pulmonary embolism diagnosis (PIOPED). *JAMA* 1990;**263**:2753–9.

34. Hull RD, Hirsh J, Carter CJ, *et al*. Diagnostic value

of ventilation–perfusion lung scanning in patients with suspected pulmonary embolism. *Chest* 1985;**88**:819–28.

35. Macklon NS. Diagnosis of deep venous thrombosis and pulmonary embolism. In: Greer IA, ed. *Baillière's Clinical Obstetrics and Gynaecology: Thromboembolic Disease in Obstetrics and Gynaecology.* London: Baillière Tindall; 1997:463–77.

36. Wheeler HB, Hirsh J, Wells P, Anderson FA Jr. Diagnostic tests for deep vein thrombosis. Clinical usefulness depends on probability of disease. *Arch Intern Med* 1994;**154**:1921–8.

37. Wells PS, Anderson DR, Bormanis J, *et al.* Value of assessment of pretest probability of deep-vein thrombosis in clinical management. *Lancet* 1997;**350**:1795–8.

38. Thomson AJ, Greer IA. Non-haemorrhagic obstetric shock. In: Thompson W, Tamby Raja RL, eds. *Baillière's Clinical Obstetrics and Gynaecology: Emergencies in Obstetrics and Gynaecology.* London: Baillière Tindall; 2000;**14**:19–41.

39. Ginsberg JS, Hirsh J, Rainbow AJ, *et al.* Risks to the fetus of radiological procedures used in the diagnosis of materna/venous thromboembolic disease. *Thromb Haemost* 1989;**61**:189–96.

40. Bounameaux H. Factor V Leiden paradox: risk of deep-vein thrombosis but not of pulmonary embolism. *Lancet* 2000;**356**:182–3.

41. Bates SM, Ginsberg JS. Anticoagulants in pregnancy: fetal defects. In: Greer IA, ed. *Baillière's Clinical Obstetrics and Gynaecology: Thromboembolic Disease in Obstetrics and Gynaecology.* London: Baillière Tindall; 1997: 479–88.

42. Vitale N, De Feo M, De Santo LS, Pollice A, Tedesco N, Contrufo M. Dose-dependent fetal complications of warfarin in pregnant women with mechanical heart valves. *J Am Coll Cardiol* 1999;**33**:1642–5.

43. Letsky E. Peripartum prophylaxis of thromboembolism. In: Greer IA, ed. *Baillière's Clinical Obstetrics and Gynaecology: Thromboembolic Disease in Obstetrics and Gynaecology.* London: Baillière Tindall; 1997:523–43.

44. Flessa HC, Klapstrom AB, Glueck MJ, *et al.* Placental transport of heparin. *Am J Obstet Gynecol* 1965;**93**:570–3.

45. Forestier F, Daffos F, Capella-Pavlovsky M. Low molecular weight heparin (PK 10169) does not cross the placenta during the second trimester of pregnancy: study by direct fetal blood sampling under ultrasound. *Thromb Res* 1984;**34**:557–60.

46. Forestier F, Daffos F, Rainaut M, *et al.* Low molecular weight heparin (CY 216) does not cross the placenta during the third trimester of pregnancy. *Thromb Haemost* 1987;**57**:234.

47. Sanson BJ, Lensing AWA, Prins MH, *et al.* Safety of low-molecular-weight heparin in pregnancy: a systematic review. *Thromb Haemost* 1999;**81**:668–72.

48. Nelson-Piercy C. Hazards of heparin: allergy, heparin-induced thrombocytopenia and osteoporosis. In: Greer IA, ed. *Baillière's Clinical Obstetrics and Gynaecology: Thromboembolic Disease in Obstetrics and Gynaecology.* London: Baillière Tindall; 1997:489–509.

49. Macklon NS, Greer IA, Reid AW, Walker ID. Thrombocytopenia antithrombin deficiency and extensive thromboembolism in pregnancy: treatment with low molecular weight heparin. *Blood Coag Fibrinolysis* 1995;**6**:672–5.

50. Warkentin TE, Levine MN, Hirsh J, *et al.* Heparin induced thrombocytopenia in patients treated with low molecular weight heparin or unfractionated heparin. *N Engl J Med* 1995;**332**:1330–5.

51. Nelson-Piercy C, Letsky EA, de Swiet M. Low-molecular-weight heparin for obstetric thromboprophylaxis: experience of sixty-nine pregnancies in sixty-one women at high risk. *Am J Obstet Gynecol* 1997;**176**:1062–8.

52. Greer IA. Epidemiology, risk factors and prophylaxis of venous thromboembolism in obstetrics and gynaecology. In: Greer IA, ed. *Baillière's Clinical Obstetrics and Gynaecology: Thromboembolic Disease in Obstetrics and Gynaecology.* London: Baillière Tindall; 1997:403–30.

53. Ellison J, Walker ID, Greer IA. Antifactor Xa profiles in pregnant women receiving antenatal thromboprophylaxis with enoxaparin for prevention and treatment of thromboembolism in pregnancy. *Br J Obstet Gynaecol* 2000;**107**:1116–21.

54. Pettila V, Kaaja R, Leinonen P, Ekblad U, Kataja M, Ikkala E. Thromboprophylaxis with low-molecular-weight heparin 'dalteparin' in pregnancy. *Thromb Res* 1999;**96**:275–82.

55. Hunt BJ, Doughty HA, Majumdar G, *et al.* Thromboprophylaxis with low molecular weight heparin (Fragmin) in high risk pregnancies. *Thromb Haemost* 1997;**77**:39–43.

56. Blomback M, Bremme K, Hellgren M, Siegbahn A, Lindberg H. Thromboprophylaxis with low molecular mass heparin, 'Fragmin' (dalteparin), during pregnancy: longitudinal safety study. *Blood Coag Fibrinolysis* 1998;**9**:1–9.

57. Barbier P, Jongville AP, Autre TE. Coureau C.

Fetal risks with dextran during delivery. *Drug Saf* 1992;**7**:71–3.

58. Macklon NS, Greer IA. Technical note: compression stockings and posture: a comparative study of their effects on the proximal deep veins in the leg at rest. *Br J Radiol* 1995;**68**:515–18.

59. Lindoff-Last E, Willeke A, Thalhammer C, Nowak G, Bauersachs R. Hirudin treatment in a breastfeeding woman. *Lancet* 2000;**355**:467–8.

60. Clagett GP, Anderson FA, Geerts W, *et al.* Prevention of venous thromboembolism. *Chest* 1998;**114**(5 Suppl):521S–560S.

61. CLASP Collaborative Group. CLASP: a randomised trial of low dose aspirin for the prevention and treatment of pre-eclampsia among 9,364 pregnant women. *Lancet* 1994;**343**: 619–29.

62. Imperiale TF, Petrulis AS. A meta-analysis of low-dose aspirin for prevention of pregnancy-induced hypertensive disease. *JAMA* 1991;**266**: 260–4.

63. Hirsh J. Heparin. *N Engl J Med* 1991;**324**:1565–74.

64. Barritt DV, Jordan SC. Anticoagulant drugs in the treatment of pulmonary embolism: a controlled trial. *Lancet* 1960;**1**:1309–12.

65. Kanis JA. Heparin in the treatment of pulmonary thromboembolism. *Thromb Diath Haemorrhag* 1974;**32**:519–27.

66. Carson JL, Kelley MA, Duff A, *et al.* The clinical course of pulmonary embolism. *N Engl J Med* 1992;**326**:1240–5.

67. Hyers TM, Hull RD, Weg JG. Antithrombotic therapy for venous thromboembolic disease. *Chest* 1995; **108**(4 Suppl):335S–351S.

68. Dolovich L, Ginsberg JS. Low molecular weight heparin in the treatment of venous thromboembolism: an updated meta-analysis. *Vessels* 1997;**3**:4–11.

69. Gould MK, Dembitzer AD, Doyle RL, *et al.* Low molecular weight heparins compared with unfractionated heparin for treatment of acute deep venous thrombosis. A meta-analysis of randomized, controlled trials. *Ann Intern Med* 1999;**130**:800–9.

70. Simmoneau G, Sors H, Charbonnier B, *et al.* A comparison of low-molecular weight heparin with unfractionated heparin for acute pulmonary embolism. *N Engl J Med* 1997;**337**:663–9.

71. Thomson AJ, Walker ID, Greer IA. Low molecular weight heparin for the immediate management of thromboembolic disease in pregnancy. *Lancet* 1998;**352**:1904.

72. Lowe GDO. Treatment of venous thromboembolism. In: Greer IA, ed. *Baillière's Clinical Obstetrics and Gynaecology: Thromboembolic Disease in Obstetrics and Gynaecology.* London: Baillière Tindall; 1997:511–21.

73. Hirsh J, Raschke R, Warkentin TE, *et al.* Heparin: mechanism of action, pharmacokinetics, dosing considerations, monitoring, efficacy, and safety. *Chest* 1995;**108**(4 Suppl):258S–75S.

74. Hommes DW, Bura A, Mazzolai L *et al.* Subcutaneous heparin compared with continuous intravenous heparin administration in the initial treatment of deep venous thrombosis. A meta-analysis. *Ann Intern Med* 1992;**116**: 279–84.

75. Blomback M, Bremme K, Hellgren M, Lindberg H. A pharmacokinetic study of dalteparin (Fragmin) during late pregnancy. *Blood Coag Fibrinol* 1998;**9**:343–50.

76. Casele HL, Laifer SA, Woelkers DA, Venkataramanan R. Changes in the pharmacokinetics of the low molecular wight heparin enoxaparin sodium during pregnancy. *Am J Obstet Gynecol* 1999;**181**:1113–17.

77. Magnani HN. Heparin-induced thrombocytopenia (HIT): an overview of 230 patients treated with Orgaran (Org 10172). *Thromb Haemost* 1993;**70**:554–61.

78. Hull RD, Delmore T, Carter C, *et al.* Adjusted subcutaneous heparin versus warfarin sodium in the long-term treatment of venous thrombosis. *N Engl J Med* 1982;**306**:1676–81.

79. British Society for Haematology. Guidelines on oral anticoagulation: third edition. *Br J Haematol* 1998;**101**:374–87.

80. Checketts MR, Wildsmith JAW. Central nerve block and thromboprophylaxis: is there a problem? *Br J Anaesth* 1999;**82**:164–7.

81. Horlocker TT, Wedel DJ. Spinal and epidural blockade and perioperative low molecular weight heparin: smooth sailing on the Titanic. *Anesth Analg* 1998;**86**:1153–6.

14

Arterial thromboembolism in pregnancy

Isobel D Walker

INTRODUCTION

Arterial occlusion resulting from thrombosis or thromboembolism, although relatively uncommon in pregnancy, may have devastating consequences. The aetiology of arterial thrombosis, like that of venous thromboembolism, is multifactorial (Table 14.1). In the general population atherosclerotic plaque rupture and subsequent thrombus formation is the final common path that most frequently leads to coronary, cerebral or peripheral artery occlusion. However, although early atherosclerotic lesions are evident from adolescence, other mechanisms may play an important role in promoting thrombus formation and embolism in young patients. Altered blood flow or stasis in patients with cardiac arrhythmias, cardiac valve lesions or prosthetic heart valves may result in endothelial damage and platelet activation. Exposure of blood to foreign surfaces such as prostheses and grafts causes platelet activation and hypercoagulability, which, although more generally associated with enhancing the risk of venous thrombosis, may in some circumstances increase the risk of arterial occlusion.

Table 14.1 Causes of acute arterial occlusion	
Thrombosis	**Embolism**
Atherosclerosis	Cardiac source
Hypercoagulability	Prosthetic heart valve
Low or altered blood flow	Atrial fibrillation
Foreign surfaces (grafts)	Myocardial infarction
Trauma	Valvular disease
Accidental	Endocarditis
Iatrogenic	Arterial source
Drugs	Aneurysm
Ergot derivatives	Atherosclerosis
Cocaine	Paradoxical embolus

ANTICOAGULANT SAFETY IN PREGNANCY

The use of anticoagulants during pregnancy is problematic because of the potential adverse effects not only on the mother but also on her unborn child. The currently available antithrombotics include:

- coumarin derivatives;
- heparin and heparin-like compounds; and
- aspirin.

Around 2% of women anticoagulated during pregnancy suffer major bleeding complications.[1] In addition to the overall concerns of an increased risk of bleeding and an increased risk of premature delivery or pregnancy loss in women using an anticoagulant during pregnancy, there are problems specific to each type of anticoagulant drug.

Coumarin derivatives

A coumarin derivative such as warfarin is the long-term anticoagulant of choice in non-pregnant patients, but coumarins readily cross the placenta and may cause fetal bleeding or teratogenicity. Maternal coumarin ingestion between 6 and 12 weeks' gestation may result in developmental abnormalities of fetal cartilage and bone, with stippled epiphyses and nasal and limb hypoplasia.[2,3] The incidence of coumarin embryopathy is not known, and different series have reported widely varying ranges. In one survey no fetal abnormalities were recorded in the offspring of 46 women who took warfarin during the first trimester.[4] In contrast, in two separate studies warfarin embryopathy was reported in 30% of 37 pregnancies and in 12 of 18 infants born to mothers who took warfarin throughout pregnancy.[5,6]

Warfarin use later in pregnancy has been linked to abnormalities of the fetal central nervous system, including optic atrophy, microcephaly, spasticity, mental retardation and learning difficulty. These central nervous system abnormalities are thought to be the result of repeated cerebral microhaemorrhages and may not be evident at birth.[7] Warfarin-related bleeding in the central nervous system of the fetus probably occurs more frequently than severe abnormality resulting from teratogenicity.

Recently it has been suggested that the risk of fetal complications is dose-dependent. Of a total of 58 pregnancies in women anticoagulated with warfarin throughout pregnancy (33 taking 5 mg or less/day; 25 taking more than 5 mg/day) there were 27 fetal complications. Twenty-two were spontaneously aborted and one was stillborn; two cases of embryopathy and one with a ventricular septal defect were noted; one had intrauterine growth retardation. Twenty-two of these 27, including the two embryopathies and the ventricular septal defect, occurred in women taking more than 5 mg of warfarin daily.[8]

Heparins and heparin-like compounds

Unfractionated heparin, low molecular weight heparins and heparinoids do not cross the placental barrier.[9] Heparins are devoid of any known teratogenic risk and the fetus is not anticoagulated as a result of maternal heparin use. Early fears that heparin use was associated with a high fetal wastage rate have not been substantiated, and more recent studies suggest that fetal loss rates in women using heparins are similar to those in women not using anticoagulants.[1] Heparins are, however, inconvenient since they have to be administered parenterally. Heparins are associated with a risk of bone demineralization, with the risk of fracture in long-term treatment and the risk of heparin-induced thrombocytopenia. There is accumulating experience with the use of low molecular weight heparins and heparinoids during pregnancy. Low molecular weight heparins have a number of advantages over unfractionated heparin, including better bioavailability with a more predictable dose response and a longer plasma half-life. The risks of osteoporosis[10] and heparin-induced thrombocytopenia[11] seem to be lower in patients using low molecular weight heparins than in those using unfractionated heparin, and there is an increasing number of reports of safe long-term use of low molecular weight heparins in pregnant women.[12,13]

Aspirin

Aspirin used in pregnancy may cause bleeding in both the mother and fetus and, potentially, birth defects. However, the results of a large meta-analysis and of a large randomized trial have demonstrated that low-dose aspirin used in the second and third trimesters was not associated with adverse effects in mother or fetus.[14,15]

POTENTIAL CAUSES OF ARTERIAL THROMBOEMBOLISM

Hypercoagulability and the risk of arterial thromboembolism

Antiphospholipid syndrome
Antiphospholipids are autoantibodies with apparent specificity for negatively charged phospholipids. They are recognized causes not only of venous thromboembolism but also, less commonly, of arterial thrombosis. The antiphospholipid syndrome may be defined as the occurrence of thrombosis or recurrent pregnancy loss in association with persisting evidence of antiphospholipids detected either as a lupus inhibitor in functional clotting tests or as anticardiolipins on immunoassay. The antiphospholipid syndrome may be associated with other complications such as thrombocytopenia, infertility, intrauterine growth retardation and pre-eclampsia.

Antiphospholipids may be detected in apparently asymptomatic people. In one study, around 8% of healthy blood donors (40 out of 499) were found to have a positive functional test for lupus inhibitor and 0.6% (3 out of 499) had elevated levels of anticardiolipins.[16] In one large review, which included about 14,000 pregnant women, 5% of the women with normal pregnancies had evidence of antiphospholipids.[17]

The most common site of arterial thrombosis in the antiphospholipid syndrome is the cerebral circulation, but coronary, renal and mesenteric arteries may be involved. Single or multiple transient ischaemic attacks or strokes may occur as a result of arterial thrombi. Antiphospholipid syndrome should be suspected when a young patient presents with a cerebrovascular accident without other evident risk factors. Recurrence is common – in one study, 31% had recurrent ischaemic strokes.[18]

A potential association between antiphospholipids and an increased risk of myocardial infarction has been suggested but remains controversial.[19,20] Coronary artery disease has been reported in 2–16% of patients with systemic lupus erythematosus and can lead to myocardial infarction in young women.[21] Postpartum myocardial infarction has been described in a patient with antiphospholipid syndrome.[22]

Heritable thrombophilia and arterial thrombosis
There is no good evidence currently available to support the hypothesis that heritable thrombophilias increase the risk of arterial disease. A number of studies have reported no increased prevalence of the factor V Leiden mutation in patients with myocardial infarction or stroke.[23,24] There may, however, be an amplification of the risk of myocardial infarction in patients with factor V Leiden who have other coronary atherosclerosis risk factors. In a case control study of women aged 18–44 years, the factor V Leiden mutation was associated with a 2.4-fold increased risk of myocardial infarction but this risk was observed only in current cigarette smokers.[25]

The role of the prothrombin G20210A mutation in myocardial infarction risk is unclear. In one study of young women aged 18–44 years who had a history of myocardial infarction, the prothrombin variant was found in 5.1% compared with only 1.6% of the controls. The odds ratio for myocardial infarction was 4 but the risk appeared to be confined to women who had other cardiovascular risk factors.[26] A relationship between the prothrombin G20210A mutation and an increased risk of ischaemic stroke in young people has been suggested.[27] Other studies have, however, failed to confirm this association.[24]

Although a few case reports have suggested a link between inherited deficiency of antithrombin, protein C or protein S and a risk of arterial thrombosis, there is no convincing evidence.[28] Some small studies have suggested that deficiency of one of these natural anticoagulants may be associated with an increased risk of non-haemorrhagic stroke but larger studies have not supported this suggestion.[29–32]

Hyperhomocysteinaemia

Homocysteine is an intermediary metabolite in the conversion of methionine to cysteine. Hyperhomocysteinaemia results from a number of different mechanisms including genetic defects in the enzymes involved in homocysteine metabolism – deficiency in cystathione synthase activity or in methylene tetrahydrofolate reductase (MTHFR) activity, usually caused by homozygosity for a thermolabile variant of MTHFR. Non-genetic causes of hyperhomocysteinaemia include deficiency of vitamin B6 or vitamin B12 or folate, renal failure and liver disease.

There is clear evidence from many case control and cross-sectional studies that elevated plasma homocysteine is an independent risk factor for coronary, cerebral and peripheral vascular disease.[33] There is also evidence from a study that elevated homocysteine levels increase the risk of myocardial infarction in young women. Women with a history of myocardial infarction under the age of 45 years had higher homocysteine levels and lower plasma folate levels than normal controls.[34] In this study, homozygosity for the thermolabile variant of MTHFR correlated with increased homocysteine levels but did not relate directly to infarction risk. Homocysteine levels fall during normal pregnancy but hyperhomocysteinaemia and the thermolabile variant of MTHFR have been linked to obstetric complications such as pre-eclampsia, intrauterine growth retardation and placental abruption.[35,36]

Drugs and arterial occlusion

Ergot derivatives

Ergot derivatives used to control postpartum bleeding may cause coronary artery spasm and have been associated with myocardial infarction following delivery or abortion.[37,38]

Cocaine

Cocaine is the second most commonly used illicit drug in the USA (ranking after marijuana) and its use is increasing in most other Western countries. The most common presentations in cocaine users attending emergency care departments relate to the cardiovascular system. There is no evidence that pre-existing vascular disease is an essential prerequisite for the development of cocaine-related cardiovascular events. Cocaine-induced myocardial infarction may be the result of coronary artery spasm or thrombosis (or both). Coronary artery thrombi have been shown angiographically and at autopsy in patients who have had a cocaine-induced infarct.[39]

Pregnant cocaine users may be predisposed to myocardial ischaemia and infarction as a result of the normal haemodynamic changes associated with pregnancy. The incidence of cocaine-induced myocardial infarction in pregnancy is not known but cases have been reported and the problem may become more prevalent with the rising number of cocaine users.[40,41]

Prosthetic heart valves

Valvular heart disease may be the result of congenital abnormality, rheumatic heart disease or other acquired lesions such as aortic stenosis or mitral valve prolapse. Around 60% of prosthetic heart valves are mechanical valves that are made of carbon alloy and employ either a tilting disc or bileaflet design. The remainder is bioprostheses – usually heterografts of porcine or bovine origin or, less commonly, homografts that are preserved human aortic valves. Mechanical valves are thrombogenic and patients with these types of prostheses require long-term anticoagulant prophylaxis. Women with prosthetic heart valves requiring anticoagulation are at significant risk during pregnancy.

In the non-pregnant population the annual incidence of prosthetic valve thrombosis has been estimated to be between 0.1 and 5.7% – the higher rates being observed in patients with a mechanical mitral prosthesis or subtherapeutic anticoagulation (or both).[42] Systemic embolization (usually cerebrovascular) occurs in about

4% of non-anticoagulated patients with a mechanical prosthesis per year and in about 1% of those taking warfarin. Patients with a bioprosthesis can usually be spared long-term anticoagulation unless they have another indication for thromboprophylaxis (e.g. atrial fibrillation). Mechanical valves can usually be expected to last for 20–30 years. Bioprostheses, on the other hand, have a shorter lifespan and in the general population 30% of heterografts need to be replaced after 10–15 years. Structural failure of a bioprosthetic valve is usually the result of endocarditis or cusp tear and subsequent severe regurgitation. It occurs most commonly in prostheses in the mitral position and in younger patients. Bioprosthetic valves undergo accelerated deterioration during pregnancy.[43]

Valve replacement should, as far as possible, be avoided in young women of childbearing potential. Those with compensated valvular disease may be able to complete their family before surgery becomes essential. Those in whom surgery is essential should be counselled about the risks associated with the different types of prostheses particularly during pregnancy.

Efficacy and safety of anticoagulation in pregnant women with mechanical prosthetic heart valves

The vast majority of women with a mechanical heart valve prosthesis require anticoagulation throughout pregnancy. One widely quoted retrospective survey of outcomes in pregnant women with mechanical heart valves concluded that warfarin use throughout pregnancy was safe and not associated with embryopathy and that unfractionated heparin was associated with a greater risk of maternal bleeding and thromboembolism.[4]

In one study, 16 out of 108 pregnant women (14.8%) with mechanical heart valves suffered a thromboembolic accident – 13 out of 63 (20.6%) in the mitral position, two out of 44 (4.5%) in the aortic position and one in the pulmonary position. At the time of the event 12 patients were using unfractionated heparin and three were using an oral anticoagulant. One patient was not anticoagulated. No patient with a bioprosthetic

valve had a thromboembolic event. Seven of the 16 women who had a thromboembolic event were in atrial fibrillation. The other nine were in normal sinus rhythm.[44] This and other studies demonstrate that women with older types of mechanical valves (e.g. Starr–Edwards and Bjork–Shiley valves), particularly in the mitral position, and women with atrial fibrillation are at high thromboembolic risk, as are women with multiple prostheses and those who have a history of previous thromboembolism.

Recently, Chan *et al.* have reviewed the literature and reported on maternal and fetal outcomes in pregnant women with prosthetic heart valves included in six published cohort studies and 22 case series – a total of 1234 pregnancies in 976 women between 1966 and 1997.[45] Almost 50% of the women had cage and ball prostheses – only 7% had less thrombogenic and newer bileaflet valves. In two-thirds of the women, the prosthesis was in the mitral position. Three commonly used approaches to anticoagulation during pregnancy were identified:

- oral anticoagulants throughout pregnancy;
- replacing oral anticoagulants with unfractionated heparin from weeks 6–12; and
- use of unfractionated heparin throughout pregnancy.

In the first two regimens, heparin was usually substituted for oral anticoagulant close to term. The outcomes measured were maternal bleeding and thromboembolism and fetal complications, including pregnancy loss and embryopathy. In this review, fetal wastage rates were the same for all three management protocols. The use of warfarin throughout pregnancy was associated with a 6.4% incidence of embryopathy in the live births. Embryopathy was not observed in women using heparin throughout pregnancy or substituting heparin for warfarin between weeks 6 and 12.

Major maternal bleeding occurred in 31 of the 1234 pregnancies (2.5%). Twenty-five of these major bleeds occurred at the time of delivery. Thromboembolic complications occurred in 3.9% of the group that used oral anticoagulant throughout pregnancy, in 9.2% of the group that used an oral anticoagulant with heparin substitution from weeks 6–12, and in 33.3% of the group that used heparin throughout. In 29 of the 52 reported thromboembolic events heparin was the anticoagulant in current use. The overall maternal mortality rate was 2.9% – higher in the group that used heparin throughout (15.0%) than in the group that used an oral anticoagulant throughout (1.8%) or the group that used an oral anticoagulant with heparin substitution from weeks 6–12 (4.2%). Seventeen of the 25 deaths were due to thrombosis of the prosthesis or related complications and two were due to haemorrhage. This comprehensive review suggests that oral anticoagulants are more efficacious than unfractionated heparin for prophylaxis against thromboembolism in pregnant women with mechanical heart valves but coumarins are associated with the risk of embryopathy. Although substituting heparin for warfarin from weeks 6–12 avoids the risk of embryopathy, this regimen possibly exposes mother to an increased risk of thromboembolism during the period of substitution. This review clearly demonstrates that the use of low-dose heparin is inadequate, even for a short period.

Although the reported high rate of thromboembolism associated with unfractionated heparin use highlighted in the review by Chan *et al.*[45] and in the earlier reports may be explained by inadequate dosing or an inappropriately low target range, these reports do raise the question of whether patients with mechanical heart valves may be partially resistant to anticoagulation with unfractionated heparin.[4,44,45] Only a few case reports of low molecular weight heparin use in patients with prosthetic heart valves have been published; these include one report of the successful management of two pregnant women with prosthetic heart valves.[46,47] There are, however, also published reports of thromboses occurring on prosthetic valves in patients anticoagulated with a low molecular weight heparin.[48]

Management of pregnant women with prosthetic heart valves

Decisions about the most appropriate anticoagulation during pregnancy must be made on an individual patient basis after careful counselling of both the patient and her partner, ideally before conception and if possible over a period of time to allow the couple to understand as much as possible the potential adverse effects of each type of anticoagulant. Decisions should be based as far as possible on the relative risks of the various thromboprophylaxis regimens and on whether the patient is perceived to be at high or lower thromboembolic risk.

Women with older type mechanical prostheses (e.g. Starr–Edwards or Bjork–Shiley valves), women with a prosthesis in the mitral position, women with multiple prosthetic valves and women with atrial fibrillation may be regarded as being at high thromboembolic risk. On the other hand, women with newer, less thrombogenic mechanical valves (e.g. St Jude's or Duromedics valves), particularly in the aortic position, and providing that they are in normal sinus rhythm may be regarded as being at lower thromboembolic risk. With the information currently available it may be prudent to advise women in the high thromboembolic risk category to use an oral anticoagulant with an international normalized ratio target of 3.5 throughout pregnancy, although some may choose to substitute adjusted doses of unfractionated heparin (ideally by intravenous infusion and adjusted to put the activated partial thromboplastin time into the range usually recommended for the treatment of acute venous thromboembolism) or subcutaneous low molecular weight heparin (adjusted to put the plasma anti-factor Xa activity into the range usually recommended for the treatment of acute venous thromboembolism) between 6 and 12 weeks' gestation. Warfarin should be avoided close to term and unfractionated heparin or low molecular weight heparin substituted.

On the basis of one report that the risk of fetal complications with warfarin appear to be dose-related,[8] women with mechanical heart valves in the lower risk category may also choose to use warfarin throughout pregnancy or with substitution of heparin or low molecular weight heparin from 6–12 weeks if their daily warfarin requirement does not exceed 5 mg. Women in this lower thromboembolic risk category who require higher daily doses of warfarin (more than 5 mg) may wish to minimize the risk of fetal complications and may be prepared to rely on adjusted doses of unfractionated heparin or a low molecular weight heparin but they must be made aware that there is little published evidence to support the use of these regimens. Studies of the efficacy and safety of adjusted doses of low molecular weight heparins in pregnant women with prosthetic heart valves are urgently needed.

In general, women with bioprosthetic valves do not require anticoagulation, but anticoagulation may be necessary for other indications (e.g. atrial fibrillation).

ISCHAEMIC STROKE

There are three major types of ischaemic stroke and thrombosis plays a central role in all three:

- primary large vessel occlusion, which may be due to atherosclerosis, dissection or arteritis or an associated migraine condition;
- primary small vessel occlusive disease, which occurs in patients with arteritis, antiphospholipid syndrome or eclampsia; and
- embolic stroke, which may arise as a result of arterial thrombosis or 'paradoxically' following venous thrombosis in patients with, for example, a patent foramen ovale; most commonly, embolic stroke is cardiogenic – the result of atrial fibrillation, mural thrombus or prosthetic valve thrombosis.

There is no clear consensus about the incidence of stroke associated with pregnancy. Incidences of 4.3 non-haemorrhagic strokes and 4.3 haemorrhagic strokes per 100,000 deliveries have been recorded.[49] The rate of non-haemorrhagic stroke in this study was similar to that published in an earlier study, in which a frequency of 5 cases per 100,000 deliveries was calculated.[50] Recently, higher incidences have been reported in a retrospective analysis of patients with pregnancy or puerperal stroke admitted to one Canadian hospital during 1980–1997.[51] In this study, the overall incidence

of stroke was 26 per 100,000 deliveries – 18 infarcts and eight intracranial haemorrhages per 100,000 deliveries.

While it is generally accepted that pregnancy is associated with an increased risk of stroke, the magnitude of the risk remains unclear. In non-pregnant women of reproductive age, the overall incidence of stroke (haemorrhagic and non-haemorrhagic) has been reported as 10.7 per 100,000 woman–years.[52] In a population-based study, the risks of both cerebral infarction and intracerebral haemorrhage were shown to be increased in the puerperium but not during pregnancy itself. In this study, the overall increased risk of stroke associated with pregnancy and the puerperium was increased 2.4-fold.[53]

The early belief that the majority of thrombotic strokes associated with pregnancy were due to venous thrombosis has been challenged. Jaigobin and Silver identified 34 patients with pregnancy-associated stroke, 21 with infarctions and 13 with haemorrhages.[52] Of the patients with infarction, 13 had arterial infarctions and eight had venous infarctions (six confirmed by magnetic resonance imaging and two by angiography). This distribution is consistent with the preponderance of arterial occlusion in 60–80% of ischaemic strokes generally cited.[50,54]

The risk of thrombotic stroke is greater postpartum than during pregnancy itself. Six of the 13 arterial events and seven out of eight venous events in one study occurred in the puerperium.[51] In another study, 62% of pregnancy-associated cerebral infarctions occurred postpartum.[53] Compared with non-pregnant age-matched controls, the relative risk of antenatal cerebral infarction was 0.7 but postpartum the risk increased to 8.7.[53] The reasons for the greater risk postpartum are unclear.

In most studies the underlying aetiology has not been identified in the majority of patients. The most commonly identified causes of pregnancy-related cerebral infarction are eclampsia and pre-eclampsia. Other aetiologies not peculiar to pregnancy (e.g. cardiac emboli or paradoxical emboli and arterial dissection) may also cause ischaemic stroke in pregnancy and the puerperium

Cross *et al.* reported an immediate maternal mortality of 26% in thrombotic stroke,[50] but in more recent studies there were no deaths after arterial occlusions.[49,51]

Paradoxical embolization

A paradoxical embolus originates in the systemic venous circulation and enters the arterial circulation through a right-to-left shunt.[55] Lower limb or pelvic veins are the most common source. A patent foramen ovale is not uncommon. In one autopsy study, 34% of subjects under the age of 30 years and 25% aged 30–70 years had a patent foramen.[56] In patients under 55 years of age who had had a cryptogenic stroke (a stroke of undetermined origin), a patent foramen ovale was identified in 48%, compared with only 4% of the controls.[57] A right-to-left shunt that is sufficient to allow paradoxical embolization through a patent foramen ovale may develop in response to physiological mechanisms that transiently increase the volume and pressure difference between the right and left heart (e.g. a Valsalva manoeuvre as in straining to defaecate or during delivery).

HEART DISEASE

Although cardiac disease complicates only a small proportion of pregnancies, maternal cardiac disease is a major cause of maternal morbidity and mortality. Congenital heart defects accounted for between one-third and one-half of the maternal deaths due to cardiac disorders in the UK between 1985 and 1996.[58] Although decreasing in the indigenous populations in the developed world, rheumatic heart disease still predominates in Third World countries and in immigrant populations in the West. Women with prosthetic heart valves run significant risks during pregnancy. With the trend towards increasing maternal age, underlying medical conditions such as hypertension, diabetes and hypercholesterolaemia become significant contributors to the risk of cardiac disease complicating pregnancy.

Cardiocirculatory changes in normal pregnancy

Pregnancy is normally associated with major cardiocirculatory changes. These changes begin as early as 5–8 weeks' gestation, reach their maximum late in the second trimester and then remain relatively constant until delivery. Cardiac output increases by 30–50% as a result of increased blood volume, decreased systemic vascular resistance and increased maternal heart rate. The stress induced by this increased cardiac output, may cause some previously asymptomatic patients with underlying heart disease to decompensate in the later stages of pregnancy. During labour and delivery there are further changes in cardiac output, with increases up to 80% above the third trimester levels in some cases. Uterine contractions are associated with increased cardiac output, and the type of anaesthesia used has an important effect on the haemodynamic changes during labour – epidural anaesthesia is associated with peripheral vasodilation and a fall in blood pressure. In spite of the blood loss that occurs at delivery, cardiac output increases after delivery owing to 'autotransfusion' of blood from the uterus and relief of the vena caval obstruction. Caesarean section may result in even greater haemodynamic changes after delivery as the effects of anaesthesia and a possibly greater blood loss augment the changes normally associated with vaginal delivery.

Myocardial infarction

Acute myocardial infarction is rare in women of childbearing age and has been estimated to occur in only 10 per 100,000 women in association with pregnancy.[59,60] Risk factors include advanced maternal age, atherosclerosis, obesity, hypertension, cigarette smoking, stress, underlying cardiac disease and illicit drug use.

Acute myocardial infarction may occur at any stage of pregnancy and has been reported in patients aged 16–45 years. It most commonly involves the left anterior descending artery territory. Events usually occur in women over the age of 30 years in the peripartum or postpartum periods, but occasionally they occur in the third trimester.[61]

The cumulative reported maternal mortality rate for pregnancy-associated myocardial thrombosis has been quoted to be 21%, with higher rates peripartum and postpartum than antepartum. Most maternal deaths occur at the time of infarction or within 2 weeks of it. Fetal mortality in women with pregnancy-associated myocardial infarction is around 13%, most of the fetal deaths (62%) being associated with maternal death. About 40% of the women in whom coronary artery angiography or autopsy was performed had coronary atherosclerosis with or without intracoronary thrombosis, but 20–30% had definite or probable coronary thrombus without evidence of coronary atherosclerosis. In these patients coronary artery spasm, in some cases secondary to the injection of ergot derivatives and the hypercoagulability of pregnancy, seem the likely precipitants.[37,38] In one study atherosclerosis was found to be more common in women who had an antepartum event (58%) than in women who had a peripartum (12%) or postpartum (29%) myocardial infarction.[61] Normal coronary arteries were found in 29% of all pregnancy-associated myocardial infarctions and in 75% of those who had a peripartum event. In the immediate postpartum period, spontaneous coronary artery dissection was the leading cause of infarction (33%).[61]

Management of acute myocardial infarction in pregnancy

The management of acute myocardial infarction or angina associated with pregnancy should be guided by the same principles that are applied to their management in non-pregnant patients. However, certain unique considerations apply. There are no controlled studies of the efficacy and safety of thrombolytic therapy in pregnancy. Although teratogenicity does not appear to be a problem, there is a high risk of maternal haemorrhage – 8% in one study.[62] Information is limited because only a few cases have been described, but the risk of puerperal haemorrhage appears less than originally feared and seems to be confined to women treated with thrombolytic agents within 8 hours of delivery.[63–65]

Heparin is the anticoagulant of choice during pregnancy, and low-dose aspirin (81–120 mg/day) has been shown to be safe in pregnancy.[14] The fetus must be monitored carefully and early delivery planned if there is evidence of maternal or fetal deterioration. In the event of maternal cardiac arrest, the best prognosis for the fetus depends on delivery within 5 minutes. Delivery may also aid maternal resuscitation.

Intracardiac thrombosis and systemic embolization

Intraventricular mural thrombus occurs as a complication of acute myocardial infarction or chronic left ventricular aneurysm and with severe dysfunction of either ventricle. Once a mural thrombus has formed its surface provides a potent stimulus for further thrombus deposition. Without adequate anticoagulation about 30% of patients with anterior infarcts develop mural thrombi. Clinically silent emboli (usually visceral) are found in around 25–50% of patients who die of acute myocardial infarction. Clinically significant emboli are less common and are usually cerebral.

Atrial thrombosis occurs in patients with valvular heart disease or atrial fibrillation. Stasis and fibrin generation are probably the main components of the pathogenesis, but endocardial abnormalities and platelet activation contribute.

Valvular heart disease

Mitral stenosis is the most common valvular lesion of rheumatic origin found in women of childbearing age. In one study, mitral stenosis, mitral incompetence and aortic incompetence accounted respectively for 61%, 33% and 6% of pregnancies complicated by rheumatic heart disease.[66] The incidence of thromboembolism in mitral stenosis is reported to be around 1.5–4.5% per year. Most clinically significant events involve the cerebral circulation. The risk of embolization increases with age. The most significant risk factors are atrial fibrillation and previous thromboembolism. With the onset of atrial fibrillation the risk of embolism increases significantly, and about 75% of patients who have an embolus have evidence of chronic atrial fibrillation. As a result of the increase in left atrial pressure that occurs during pregnancy, previously asymptomatic patients with mitral stenosis may present with atrial fibrillation, and a stroke may be the first manifestation of 'occult' mitral stenosis.

Mitral and aortic incompetence of rheumatic origin are usually well tolerated during pregnancy. The risk of thromboembolism is somewhat lower in patients with mitral incompetence than in patients with mitral stenosis except when there is left atrial enlargement, which may result in atrial fibrillation and thrombus formation.

Patients with mitral stenosis, mitral incompetence or mixed lesions with atrial fibrillation require long-term anticoagulation, as do patients in sinus rhythm with atrial enlargement, patients with a reduced left ventricular ejection fraction, and patients who have a history of thromboembolism. Management during pregnancy involves restriction of activity, treatment of arrhythmias and judicious use of diuretics, beta-blockers and anticoagulants where appropriate.

Clinically apparent thromboembolism is much less common in patients with aortic valve disease than in patients with mitral disease, and it occurs most often in the presence of other predisposing factors such as atrial fibrillation or endocarditis. Routine thromboprophylaxis is not usually warranted in patients with aortic valve disease in the absence of other risk factors such as atrial fibrillation or concomitant mitral valve disease.

Mitral valve prolapse is the most common cause of mitral incompetence in pregnant women. In one study, 2% of the general population were found to have mitral valve prolapse with resultant severe mitral incompetence in 7% of these patients.[67] Mitral valve prolapse is usually asymptomatic but may occasionally be associated with serious symptoms, including transient or permanent cerebral ischaemic events. In general patients with mitral valve prolapse do not require long-term anticoagulation in the absence of other thromboembolic risk factors such as atrial fibrillation or left ventricular dysfunction or a history of previous transient ischaemic attack or stroke

PERIPHERAL ARTERIAL OCCLUSION

Peripheral arterial occlusion may be the result of thrombosis of a previously patent artery or embolism from a distant site. Eighty per cent of peripheral arterial emboli originate in the heart and travel to the extremities (usually the lower limbs). The majority of events occur in patients with severe underlying cardiac disease. Embolic sources include the left ventricle after myocardial infarction and atrial thrombi in patients with atrial fibrillation. In older patients, local thrombus formation in an artery is usually associated with significant atherosclerosis. In women of childbearing age, other mechanisms, including hypercoagulable states (e.g. the antiphospholipid syndrome) or the administration of ergot derivatives after delivery may be important.

Management of peripheral arterial occlusion in pregnancy

The management of peripheral artery occlusion remains challenging. Thrombectomy and grafting have in the past been the mainstay of therapy but thrombolysis and angioplasty are options for selected patients. Despite these newer options, mortality and morbidity remain significant and limb loss rates are high. Early diagnosis and intervention are essential.

REFERENCES

1. Ginsberg JS, Kowalchuk G, Hirsh J, *et al*. Heparin therapy during pregnancy. Risks to the fetus and mother. *Arch Intern Med* 1989;**149**: 2233–6.

2. Whitfield MF. Chondrodysplasia punctata after warfarin in early pregnancy. Case report and summary of the literature. *Arch Dis Child* 1980;**55**:139–42.

3. Zakzouk MS. The congenital warfarin syndrome. *J Laryngol Otolol* 1986;**100**:215–19.

4. Sbarouni E, Oakley CM. Outcome of pregnancy in women with valve prostheses. *Br Heart J* 1994;**71**:196–201.

5. Iturbe-Alessio I, Fonseca MC, Mutchinik O, *et al.* Risks of anticoagulant therapy in pregnant women with artificial heart valves. *N Engl J Med* 1986;**315**:1390–3.

6. Wong V, Cheng CH, Chan KC. Fetal and neonatal outcome of exposure to anticoagulants during pregnancy. *Am J Med Genet* 1993;**45**:17–21.

7. Beeley L. Adverse effects of drugs in later pregnancy. *Clin Obstet Gynaecol* 1986;**13**:197–214.

8. Vitale N, De Feo M, Salvatore De Santo L, *et al.* Dose-dependent fetal complications of warfarin in pregnant women with mechanical heart valves. *J Am Coll Cardiol* 1999;**33**:1636–41.

9. Forestier, F, Daffos F, Rainaut M, Toulemonde F. Low molecular weight heparin (CY 216) does not cross the placenta during the third trimester of pregnancy [letter]. *Thromb Haemost* 1987;**57**:234.

10. Monreal M, Lafoz E, Olive A, et al. Comparison of subcutaneous unfractionated heparin with a low molecular weight heparin (Fragmin) in patients with venous thromboembolism and contraindications for coumarin. *Thromb Haemost* 1994;**71**:7–11.

11. Warkentin, TE, Levine MN, Hirsh J, et al. Heparin induced thrombocytopenia in patients treated with low molecular weight heparin or unfractionated heparin. *N Engl J Med* 1995;**332**:1330–5.

12. Sanson BJ, Lensing AW, Prins MH, *et al.* Safety of low-molecular-weight heparin in pregnancy: a systematic review. *Thromb Haemost* 1999;**81**:668–72.

13. Ellison J, Walker ID, Greer IA. Antenatal use of enoxaparin for prevention and treatment of thromboembolism in pregnancy. *Br J Obstet Gynaecol* 2000;**107**:1116–21.

14. CLASP Collaborative Group. Low dose aspirin in pregnancy and early childhood development: follow up of the collaborative low dose aspirin study in pregnancy. *Br J Obstet Gynaecol* 1995;**102**:861–8.

15. Imperiale T, Petulis A. A meta-analysis of low dose aspirin for the prevention of pregnancy induced hypertension. *JAMA* 1991;**266**:260–4.

16. Shi W, Krilis, SA, Chong BH, *et al.* Prevalence of lupus anticoagulant in a healthy population: lack of correlation with anticardiolipin antibodies. *Aust NZ J Med* 1990;**20**:231–6.

17. Kutteh WH. Antiphospholipid antibodies and reproduction. *J Reproductive Immunol* 1997;**35**:151–71.

18. Levine SR, Brey RL. Neurological aspects of antiphospholipid antibody syndrome. *Lupus* 1996;**5**:347–53.

19. Raghavan C, Ditchfield J, Taylor RJ et al. Influence of anticardiolipin antibodies on immediate patient outcome after myocardial infarction. *J Clin Pathol* 1993;**46**:1113–15

20. Zuckerman E, Toubi E, Shiran A, *et al.* Anticardiolipin antibodies and acute myocardial infarction in non-SLE patients: a controlled prospective study. *Am J Med* 1996;**100**:381–6.

21. Manzi, S, Meilhan EN, Rairie JE, *et al.* Age specific incidence rates of myocardial infarction and angina in women with systemic lupus erythematosus. Comparison with the Framingham study. *Am J Epidemiol* 1997;**145**:408–15.

22. Thorp JM, Chescheir NC, Fann B. Postpartum myocardial infarction in a patient with antiphospholipid syndrome. *Am J Perinatol* 1994;**11**:1–3.

23. Demarmels Biasiutti F, Merlo C, Furlan M, *et al.* No association of APC resistance with myocardial infarction. *Blood Coagul Fibrinolysis* 1995;**6**:456–9.

24. Longstreth WT, Rosendaal FR, Siscovik DS, *et al.* Risk of stroke in young women and two prothrombotic mutations: factor V Leiden and prothrombin gene variant (G20210A). *Stroke* 1998;**29**:577–80.

25. Doggen C, Cats VM, Bertina RM, Rosendaal FR. Interaction of coagulation defects and cardiovascular risk factors: increased risk of myocardial infarction associated with factor V Leiden or prothrombin 20210A. *Circulation* 1998;**97**:1037–41.

26. Rosendaal FR, Siscovick DS, Schwartz SM, *et al.* A common prothrombin variant (20210 G to A) increases the risk of myocardial infarction in young women. *Blood* 1997;**9**:1747–50.

27. De Stefano V, Chiusolo P, Paciaroni K, *et al.* Prothrombin G20210A mutant genotype is a risk factor for cerebrovascular ischemic disease in young patients. *Blood* 1998;**91**:3562–5.

28. Coller B, Owen J, Jesty J, *et al.* Deficiency of plasma protein S, protein C or antithrombin III and arterial thrombosis. *Arteriosclerosis* 1987;**7**:456–62.

29. Camerlingo M, Finazzi G, Casto L, *et al.* Inherited protein C deficiency and nonhemorrhagic arterial stroke in young adults. *Neurology* 1991;**41**:1371–3.

30. Kohler J, Kasper J, Witt I, von Reutern GM. Ischemic stroke due to protein C deficiency. *Stroke* 1990;**21**:1077–80.

31. Munts AG, van Genderen PJ, Dippel DW, *et al.* Coagulation disorders in young adults with acute cerebral ischaemia. *J Neurol* 1998;**245**:21–5.

32. Douay X, Lucas C, Caron C, *et al.* Antithrombin, protein C and protein S levels in 127 consecutive young adults with ischemic stroke. *Acta Neurol Scand* 1998;**98**:124–7.

33. Christen WG, Ajani UA, Glynn RJ, Hennekens CH. Blood levels of homocysteine and increased risks of cardiovascular disease: causal or casual? *Arch Intern Med* 2000;**160**:422–34.

34. Schwartz SM, Siscovick DS, Malinow MR, *et al.* Myocardial infarction in young women in relation to plasma total homocysteine, folate and a common variant in methylenetetrahydrofolate reductase gene. *Circulation* 1997;**96**:412–17.

35. Walker MC, Smith GN, Perkins SL, *et al.* Changes in homocysteine levels during normal pregnancy. *Am J Obstet Gynecol* 1999;**180**:660–4.

36. Kupferminc MJ, Eldor A, Steinman N, *et al.* Increased frequency of genetic thrombophilia in women with complications of pregnancy. *N Engl J Med* 1999;**340**:9–13.

37. Liao J, Cockrill B, Yurchak P. Acute myocardial infarction after ergonovine administration for uterine bleeding. *Am J Cardiol* 1991;**68**:823–4.

38. Taylor GJ, Cohen B. Ergonovine-induced coronary artery spasm and myocardial infarction after normal delivery. *Obstet Gynecol* 1985;**66**:821–2.

39. Hollander JE, Hoffmann RS, Gennis P, *et al.* Prospective multicenter evaluation of cocaine-associated chest pain. Cocaine Associated Chest Pain (COCHPA) Study Group. *Acad Emerg Med* 1994;**1**:330–9.

40. Liu S, Forrester RM, Murphy GS, *et al.* Anaesthetic management of a parturient with myocardial infarction related to cocaine use. *Can J Anaesth* 1992;**39**:858–61.

41. Livingston J, Mabie B, Ramanathan J. Crack cocaine, myocardial infarction, and troponin I levels at the time of cesarean delivery. *Anesth Analg* 2000;**91**:913–15.

42. Cannegieter S, Rosendaal FR, Briet E. Thromboembolic and bleeding complications in patients with mechanical heart valve prostheses. *Circulation* 1994;**89**:635–41.

43. Badduke BR, Jamieson WR, Miyagishiama RT, *et al.* Pregnancy and childbearing in a population with biologic valvular prostheses. *J Thorac Cardiovasc Surg* 1991;**102**:179–86.

44. Hanania G, Thomas D, Michel PL, *et al.* Pregnancy and prosthetic heart valves; a French cooperative retrospective study of 155 cases. *Eur Heart J* 1994;**15**:1651–8.

45. Chan WS, Anand S, Ginsberg JS. Anticoagulation of pregnant women with mechanical heart valves. *Arch Intern Med* 2000;**160**:191–6.

46. Harenberg J, Huhle G, Piazolo L, *et al.* Long-term anticoagulation of outpatients with adverse events to oral anticoagulants using low-molecular-weight heparin. *Semin Thromb Hemost* 1997;**23**:167–72.

47. Lee L, Liauw P, Ng AI. Low molecular weight heparin for thromboprophylaxis during pregnancy in 2 patients with mechanical mitral valve replacement. *Thromb Haemost* 1996;**76**:628–30.

48. Lev-Ran O, Kramer A, Gurevitch J, *et al.* Low-molecular-weight heparin for prosthetic heart valves: treatment failure. *Ann Thorac Surg* 2000;**69**:264–6.

49. Sharshar T, Lamy C, and Mas J, Incidence and causes of stroke associated with pregnancy and puerperium; a study in public hospitals of Ile de France. *Stroke* 1995;**26**:930–6.

50. Cross J, Castro P, Jennett WB. Cerebral strokes associated with pregnancy and the puerperium. *BMJ* 1968;**3**:214–18.

51. Jaigobin C, Silver F. Stroke and pregnancy. *Stroke* 2000;**31**:2948–51.

52. Pettiti DB, Sidney S, Quesenberry CP, Bernstein A. Incidence of stroke and myocardial infarction in women of reproductive age. *Stroke* 1997;**28**:280–3.

53. Kittner SJ, Stern BJ, Feeser BR, *et al.* Pregnancy and the risk of stroke. *N Engl J Med* 1996;**335**:768–74.

54. Simolke GA, Cox SM, Cunningham FG. Cerebrovascular accidents complicating pregnancy and the puerperium. *Obstet Gynaecol* 1991;**78**:37–42.

55. Balli E, Alfieri A, del Citerna F. Direct evidence of a patent foramen ovale as a route for paradoxical embolism. *Br Heart J* 1995;**74**:470.

56. Hagen PT, Scholz DG, Edwards WD. Incidence and size of patent foramen ovale during the first 10 decades of life: an autopsy study of 965 normal hearts. *Mayo Clin Proc* 1984;**59**:17–20.

57. DiTullio M, Sacco RL, Gopal A, *et al.* Patent foramen ovale as a risk factor for cryptogenic stroke. *Ann Intern Med* 1992;**117**:461–5.

58. *Confidential Enquiries into Maternal Deaths. Why Mothers Die: Report on Confidential Enquiries into Maternal Deaths in the United Kingdom*

1994–1996. London: The Stationery Office Ltd; 1998.

59. Sullivan JM, Ramanathan KB. Management of medical problems in pregnancy – severe cardiac disease. *N Engl J Med* 1985;**313**:304–9.

60. Hankins GD, Wendel GD, Leveno KJ, Stoneham J. Myocardial infarction during pregnancy. A review. *Obstet Gynecol* 1985;**65**:139–46.

61. Roth A, Elkayam U. Acute myocardial infarction associated with pregnancy. *Ann Intern Med* 1996;**125**:751–62

62. Turrentine MA, Braems G, Ramirez MM. Use of thrombolytics for the treatment of thromboembolic disease during pregnancy. *Obstet Gynecol Surv* 1995;**50**:534–41.

63. Patterson DE, Raviola CA, D'Orazio EA, *et al.* Thrombolytic and endovascular treatment of peripartum iliac vein thrombosis: A case report. *J Vasc Surg* 1996;**24**:1030–3.

64. Roberts DH, Rodrigues EA, Ramsdale DR. Postpartum acute myocardial infarction successfully treated with intravenous streptokinase: a case report. *Angiology* 1993;**44**:570–3.

65. Cincotta RB, Davis SN, Gerraty RP, Thomson KR. Thrombolytic therapy for basilar artery thrombosis in the puerperium. *Am J Obstet Gynecol* 1995;**173**:967–9.

66. McFaul PB, Dornan JC, Lamki H, Boyle D. Pregnancy complicated by maternal heart disease. A review of 519 women. *Br J Obstet Gynaecol* 1988;**95**:861–7.

67. Freed LA, Levy D, Levine RA, *et al.* Prevalence and clinical outcome of mitral valve prolapse. *N Engl J Med* 1999;**341**:1–7.

15

Thrombotic thrombocytopenic purpura in pregnancy

Yossef Ezra and Amiram Eldor

INTRODUCTION

Thrombotic thrombocytopenic purpura (TTP) is a severe multisystem disorder characterized by low-grade fever, thrombocytopenia, microangiopathic hemolytic anemia (MAHA), fluctuating neurological symptoms and signs, and impaired renal function.[1,2] TTP usually affects young people in previously good health. Its presentation is variable, but most patients seek medical attention for fluctuating neurological abnormalities or hemorrhagic manifestations. Other presenting symptoms include malaise and weakness, abdominal pain, nausea and vomiting, and fever. The median age at diagnosis is 35 years, but TTP has been reported in all age groups. The male to female ratio is 2:3.[2–4]

There are four possible clinical courses of TTP:

- single-episode TTP;
- relapsing TTP;
- chronic TTP; and
- childhood or familial TTP.[5–7]

Although the majority of patients have only one episode of TTP, the higher survival rates resulting from new therapies has changed the course of the disease. About half of the patients now suffer from relapsing TTP, in which recurring episodes are separated by months or years of good health.[3,7–9] The Canadian Apheresis Group reported that 17 of 63 TTP patients have had one

or more recurrences, occurring 7 months to 8 years after the first episode. In all surviving patients the recurrence rate after 10 years was 36%.[10] Bell reported on 206 of 319 (64%) patients with TTP and hemolytic–uremic syndrome who experienced a relapse.[3] In 69% of these patients, the relapse occurred during the treatment period, while the others had a relapse 4–8 weeks after discontinuation of the plasma exchange therapy. The longest time interval between the first TTP episode and the relapse was 5 years. Of the 206 patients, 84% had only one episode of relapse while the others had between two and six relapses. Clinical deterioration was noted in only 3% of the patients. All other patients had only mild disease with some laboratory anomalies (mainly thrombocytopenia). In this study, no predicting factor for TTP relapse could be found.[3] A rare subgroup of patients had chronic relapsing TTP, characterized by very frequent episodes with abnormally large multimers of von Willebrand factor (vWF) in their plasma during remissions.[11] The childhood variant of TTP is even rarer and only a few cases have been reported.

Pregnancy is the precipitating factor in 10–25% of TTP episodes in women, and TTP has a tendency to recur in subsequent pregnancies.[12–15] Pregnancy may also be a precipitating condition for relapse in women with a history of TTP,[13] and the high prevalence of TTP during subsequent gestations suggests that pregnancy plays a permissive or provocative role in its development.[16] One study found that most pregnancy-associated TTP episodes develop during the antenatal period and only 11% occur during the postpartum period.[17] The mean maternal age is 23 years and the mean gestational age at onset of symptoms is 23 weeks.[17] In this study maternal mortality was as high as 68% in patients who did not receive plasma therapy, but in the treatment group there was no case of maternal fatality.[17] The overall perinatal mortality in TTP in pregnancy was high (80%).[17] The cause of fetal death is believed to be placental infarcts caused by the maternal disease.[18]

Ezra *et al.*[13] reported on five women who suffered at least one TTP episode during pregnancy. They had a total of 16 pregnancies, of which eight were complicated by TTP. Seven other TTP episodes in this group were not associated with pregnancy. Perinatal mortality occurred in 50% of the pregnancies associated with TTP. The absence of thrombocytopenia or anemia in these fetuses may indicate that the factor causing TTP in their mothers does not cross the placenta.[12,13] When complicated with only mild TTP, the pregnancy is more likely to result in a normal delivery than a pregnancy that is complicated by severe TTP. Pregnancy-associated TTP has been observed in sisters, suggesting the need for appropriate consultation of siblings of affected women.[16,19]

CLINICAL FEATURES

The widespread thrombotic process in TTP can affect almost any organ, and patients may suffer from visual defects, heart failure, conduction abnormalities, and abdominal pain. Interestingly, the pulmonary and hepatic microvasculature is spared.[20]

The main hematological finding in TTP is severe thrombocytopenia. The platelet count at presentation ranges from 8000 to 40 000 cells/μl, while the bone marrow shows an abundance of megakaryocytes, owing to peripheral destruction or sequestration of platelets.[2] Coagulation studies in TTP patients are normal or only mildly disturbed,[21,22] which helps to differentiate this condition from disseminated intravascular coagulation. Mildly prolonged prothrombin time and partial thromboplastin time occur in 8–20% of patients, and fibrinogen levels are usually normal. Mildly elevated fibrinogen degradation products have been reported in up to 70% of patients.[22] The hemoglobin at presentation averages 8–9 g/dl, with morphologic evidence of microangiopathic hemolysis. The peripheral blood smear shows abundance of schistocytes, reticulocytes, and occasional nucleated red blood cells. Serum levels of lactate dehydrogenase and indirect bilirubin are elevated, owing to the mechanical destruction of erythrocytes.[2]

Neurological manifestations may range from headache or subtle behavioral changes to frank motor and sensory deficits, seizures, and coma. Most of the neurological symptoms and signs are transient, and usually are completely reversible if the disease is treated early. However, some patients who recover from TTP have evidence of permanent neurological deficits.[5]

Proteinuria, microscopic hematuria, and azotemia characterize the renal involvement, but few patients need urgent dialysis. Furthermore, deterioration of TTP patients to chronic renal failure is rare.[4]

During an episode of TTP, patients may suffer from visual defects, heart failure, cardiac conduction abnormalities, and non-specific and poorly localized abdominal pain.[20]

A useful scoring system has been developed to characterize the severity of an individual TTP episode and to guide the intensity of therapy.[7] The score is based on four clinical and laboratory parameters: neurological findings, the degree of impaired renal function, platelet count, and hemoglobin value. Each parameter is marked on a scale of 0 to 2, a score of 0 meaning no disease and 8 reflecting severe TTP. The average severity score of patients who died was significantly higher than the average score of the surviving patients.[7] Moreover, the first episode of TTP in patients with relapsing disease was found to be milder than in patients who did not have a relapse.[7] Although a relapse of TTP can be fatal, most relapses were milder than the disease at presentation or in those who did not experience a relapse.[7]

PATHOGENESIS

The characteristic pathological feature of TTP is the formation of a hyaline thrombus composed mostly of platelets and vWF with small amounts of fibrinogen or fibrin.[2,23,24] The occluding thrombi are found in the capillaries and arterioles of all body tissues, but the most common sites are the brain, kidneys, pancreas, heart, adrenals, and skin.[25] Venules are normally not involved and there is minimal inflammatory reaction or none and obvious extracellular desquamation.[26] TTP is a syndrome with diverse causes, not all of which have been elucidated, and it probably has several pathogenic mechanisms. Pathological findings point to an interaction between the vascular endothelium and platelets, but it is still not known whether a primary endothelial cell injury with loss of its non-thrombogenic properties leads to enhanced platelet aggregation or whether platelet activation causes endothelial damage.

Several plasma factors that induce platelet clumping have been found in TTP patients, including a 37 kDa platelet agglutinating protein (PAP p37)[27] and a calcium-dependent cysteine protease (calpain A), which is probably cathepsin.[28–30] Kelton et al.[31] detected a platelet aggregating factor in the microparticle pellet of TTP sera; this factor could be immunodepleted using antibodies to calpain but not to cathepsin L.

Defective production of plasma vWF, which is mainly produced by the vascular endothelium, has been described in TTP patients. The plasma of patients in remission from chronic relapsing TTP contains unusually large vWF multimers (ULvWF), which disappear during relapses.[32,33] Patients with a single episode of TTP had vWF abnormalities during their acute disease, but not during remission. These abnormalities include either the presence of ULvWF multimers or a relative decrease in the largest plasma vWF forms. The ULvWF multimers consist of an increased number of mature vWF subunits; they are more efficient at binding under high fluid shear forces to the platelet receptors GPIb and GPIIb–IIIa and play an important role in triggering platelet aggregation in TTP.[34,35] Fresh frozen plasma contains proteolytic activity that reduces

the unusually large vWF multimers to the size ordinarily found in plasma.[36] This putative ULvWF-cleaving protease, together with a vWF metalloproteinase, depolymerize ULvWF by reducing the interdimeric disulfide bridges or by proteolytic degradation in the presence of fluid shear stress, and they are probably insufficient in TTP as a result of excessive release of ULvWF from perturbed endothelial cells.[33]

Furlan et al.[37] were the first to report on patients with reduced levels of the vWF-cleaving protease activity or its complete absence. Recently, this group has conducted a multicenter retrospective study of patients with familial or acquired TTP and hemolytic–uremic syndrome.[38] Complete protease deficiency was found in patients with familial TTP and in the majority of patients with non-familial TTP. The protease inhibitor was absent in familial cases whereas, in the majority of cases with acquired TTP, the protease deficiency was due to the presence of a neutralizing immunoglobulin G (IgG) antibody.[38] The inhibitor activity usually disappeared, at least temporarily, during remission.[39] In contrast, in hemolytic–uremic syndrome, which has many characteristic features of TTP, normal vWF-cleaving protease activity was observed in all the patients with familial or acquired disease, indicating a different pathogenesis of TTP and hemolytic–uremic syndrome.[39] Severely decreased or absent vWF-cleaving protease activity has been observed also by other investigators in classic TTP.[40–42]

Several autoantibodies that react with various endothelial components have been found in TTP patients. These autoantibodies include an anti-CD36 antibody, which is expressed on microvascular cells and platelets (glycoprotein IV),[11] an antibody to a cryptogenic 43 kDa antigenic target implying endothelial cell (EC) injury,[43] and antiphospholipid antibodies.[11,33] Plasma from TTP patients was found to suppress the synthesis of prostacyclin (prostaglandin (PG)I2), a potent inhibitor of platelet activation in the vessel wall.[44] PGI2 was also found to be degraded more rapidly in TTP plasma.[45] Plasma from acute TTP patients has been shown to induce apoptosis in cultured EC of microvascular origin but not in EC derived from large vessels.[20,46] Apoptosis is independent of tumor necrosis factor-α secretion or the presence of CD36 on microvascular ECs, but it was linked to the rapid induction of Fas (CD95) on these cells.

DIFFERENTIAL DIAGNOSIS OF TTP DURING PREGNANCY

The awareness to other conditions in pregnancy that may be associated with microangiopathy may be lifesaving, because of the significant difference in the treatment modalities and prognosis. The differential diagnosis includes:[47–49]

- hemolytic–uremic syndrome;
- pre-eclampsia and the HELLP (hemolysis, elevated liver enzymes, and low platelet count) syndrome;
- acute fatty liver of pregnancy;
- antiphospholipid syndrome; and
- exacerbation of systemic lupus erythematosus (SLE).

These different clinical conditions may resemble TTP; however, they differ in certain characteristic clinical and laboratory features (Table 15.1).

Pregnancy-related hemolytic–uremic syndrome usually occurs in the postpartum period and is characterized by severe acute renal failure, microangiopathic hemolytic anemia (MAHA), and thrombocytopenia, but neurological manifestations are rare.[17,47,48]

Patients with pre-eclampsia or HELLP syndrome may suffer from fever, seizures, microangiopathic anemia, and thrombocytopenia; however, the hematological manifestations are usually much milder than in TTP. A decline in plasma antithrombin III levels has been described in pre-eclampsia–HELLP syndrome but not in TTP, and this decline may help in differentiating these disorders.[17] The distinction between TTP and pre-eclampsia–HELLP syndrome is essential, since the treatment of TTP does not always necessitate termination of the pregnancy.[12,13] Hepatocellular damage may be found in pre-eclampsia and is usually absent in TTP and hemolytic–uremic syndrome. Postpartum thrombocytopenia with evidence of tissue ischemia that persists for more than a few days or a deterioration in renal or hematological function may also suggest the diagnosis of TTP or hemolytic–uremic syndrome.

The syndrome of acute fatty liver of pregnancy is a potentially fatal disease that usually occurs at the end of the third trimester of pregnancy, although it sometimes occurs at the 26–28 weeks' gestation. About 40% of the

Table 15.1 Differentiating clinical and laboratory features of conditions in pregnancy that may resemble TTP

	TTP	HUS	PET/HELLP	AFLP	SLE	APLA
MAHA	+++	+	+	+	+	±
Thrombocytopenia	+++	++	+++	+	+	+
DIC	±	±	+	+++	±	±
Hypertension	±	±	+++	±	±	±
Renal involvement	±	+++	+	±	++	±
CNS involvement	+++	±	+	+	+	+
Liver involvement	–	–	+	+++	–	–
Increased serum LDH	+++	+++	+	+++	+	+
Decreased ATIII	–	–	+	+	–	–
Decreased complement	–	–	±		+	+
vWF multimers	+	+	–	–	–	–

patients are nulliparous and 15% have twin gestation. Headache, nausea, vomiting, epigastric or right upper quadrant abdominal pain, and malaise are common presenting symptoms. Hypertension affects up to 50% of the patients and severe vaginal or gastrointestinal bleeding is a significant complication. Cholestatic impairment of liver function and hyperbilirubinemia are always present, with an increase of serum aminotransaminases. Hypoglycemia and hyperammonemia are typical, and hypofibrinogenemia, prolonged prothrombin time, and decreased levels of antithrombin III are common. Mortality is high as a result of hepatic encephalopathy, severe respiratory and renal failure, or cardiac arrest.[50–53]

Women with SLE may experience an exacerbation of their disease during pregnancy or postpartum, with features similar to those of TTP. These patients are also at increased risk of pre-eclampsia or HELLP syndrome. Low levels of serum complement (C3 and C4) may suggest an exacerbation of SLE, although this finding may also be present with pre-eclampsia. The presence of fragmented and nucleated red blood cells in the peripheral smear can differentiate between TTP and SLE. Normal complement levels are compatible with TTP.

Antiphospholipid syndrome may be associated with an increased risk of thrombosis, recurrent fetal loss, and severe pre-eclampsia.[54–57] However, patients with antiphospholipid syndrome may present with features of TTP or hemolytic–uremic syndrome.[58–60] These patients respond to corticosteroid therapy or plasmapheresis but not to termination of the pregnancy.

MANAGEMENT OF TTP DURING PREGNANCY

A TTP episode or relapse during pregnancy does not necessitate an emergency delivery unless the fetus is in distress. Unlike pre-eclampsia, termination of the pregnancy is not associated with a remission of the TTP.[14,15,17,47,48,61–63] Successful treatment modalities for an acute episode of TTP in pregnancy include plasma exchange, platelet inhibitor drugs, and corticosteroids.[12,13,62,63]

The benefit of plasma exchange is due to the removal from the patient's plasma of the injurious factor or an IgG antibody that blocks the vWF-cleaving protease, or to the infusion of a deficient factor (e.g. the vWF-cleaving protease) contained in the normal fresh frozen plasma (FFP). Initial therapy of TTP with plasma infusions (30 ml/kg per day) should be used only if plasma exchange is not readily available, since a response delay has been correlated with treatment failure.[64] The type of plasma used for exchange is important since it has been demonstrated that TTP patients that were refractory to plasma exchange with the usual FFP responded to the cryosupernatant fraction of the plasma.[65] This fraction does not contain the largest multimers of vWF, which sediment in the cryoprecipitate. Plasma exchange, with the replacement of one plasma volume per day (2–3 liters), should be offered immediately to all patients with a first episode of TTP or with a more severe relapse. Plasma exchanges should be continued until the platelet count is maintained above 150,000 cells/µl for 2–3 days; they should then be gradually replaced with plasma infusions until sustained remission is achieved. Plasma infusions alone may be considered for patients with a mild relapse of TTP (severity score less than 4). Bell[3] has recommended the administration of 65–140 ml of FFP/kg per exchange. The number of exchanges performed varies widely among medical centers and among patients. Some patients may recover after one plasma exchange, while others require prolonged therapy. Patients with severe TTP may require two daily plasma exchanges.[4] Some TTP patients have recovered from prolonged coma without neurological sequelae after receiving such an intensive plasma exchange.[66,67]

Platelet transfusions should not be administered to patients with TTP since they can lead to a rapid deterioration in the recipients condition.[4,7,26,68]

Corticosteroids are usually administered on the assumption that TTP is an autoimmune disorder. It has been difficult to assess the contribution made by corticosteroids, because they are usually given in conjunction with other therapeutic modalities. In a study of 108 patients with either TTP or hemolytic–uremic syndrome, 30 recovered after treatment with corticosteroids alone.[9] Patients with chronic relapsing TTP have been reported to respond to corticosteroids as a single agent,[69] and there is one report of a patient with severe TTP who responded to high-dose methylprednisolone alone.[70]

Corticosteroids have been recommended for all TTP patients in a dose equivalent to 1 mg/kg per day of prednisone, initially given parenterally and subsequently orally. The corticosteroids are tapered slowly once the patient is in remission. Bell[3] has recommended that all newly diagnosed patients who do not have neurological abnormalities may be treated with intravenous methylprednisolone (100 mg twice daily), which can later be replaced with prednisone. Kwaan and Soff[4] also recommend corticosteroids as the initial management of TTP. The recent discovery that the deficiency of ULvWF-cleaving protease in patients with non-familial TTP is mostly due to the presence of a neutralizing IgG antibody[38] provides a rationale for the use of corticosteroids in TTP.

Interestingly, intravenous immunoglobulin, which is operative in some immunological platelet disorders such as ITP, has shown conflicting results in TTP patients. Hematologic remission has been achieved in some patients,[71–73] while other reports have cast doubt on its efficacy.[74] The conflicting reports on IgG may be due to the diversity of TTP pathogenesis. Thus, this drug may be tried in patients who are refractory to the more conventional therapy. The doses used ranged from 250 mg to 1 g/kg per day for 1–5 days.

Platelet inhibitor drugs such as aspirin, dipyridamole, sulfinpyrazone, or dextran are currently used in many TTP patients.[75] In several case reports before the era of plasma therapy, recoveries were attributed to the addition of aspirin and dipyridamole to the therapeutic regimen.[76] On the other hand, some authors reported bleeding complications with no therapeutic benefit from these agents.[77] However, others continue to treat TTP patients with aspirin (100 mg/day) and dipyridamole (225 mg/day) without serious bleeding complications.[6] Two reports implied a role for ticlopidine in the treatment and prevention of TTP.[78,79] However, ticlopidine can precipitate TTP (as can clopidogrel, a related platelet inhibitor drug).[80,81]

Chemotherapy may have beneficial effect in TTP. Vincristine was found to be effective in patients refractory to plasma exchange, platelet inhibitor drugs, or corticosteroids.[81–84] One patient entered a complete remission after two cycles of CHOP (cyclophosphamide, adriamycin, vincristine, and prednisolone) chemotherapy.[85]

Splenectomy appears to have a beneficial effect in patients with refractory TTP or those with relapsing disease.[86,87] Splenectomy resulted in an 87% cure rate in 15 patients who were treated with corticosteroids and average molecular weight dextran – the highest cure rate reported before the plasma exchange era.[88] With the advent of plasma therapy, splenectomy remains an important therapeutic option for patients with resistance or dependence on plasma therapy.[6,89,90] Splenectomy has been indicated also for the prevention of TTP relapses.[7]

Women surviving an episode of TTP in pregnancy should be advised of the high risk of recurrence in successive pregnancies. It has been shown that prophylactic therapy with aspirin and dipyridamole was associated with a decrease in the incidence and severity of TTP relapses during pregnancy.[12,13] Ezra et al.[13] reported on five women who suffered at least one episode of TTP during pregnancy (total of 16 pregnancies, of which eight were complicated by TTP). Five of the 10 TTP relapses occurred while the patients were receiving prophylactic therapy with aspirin (100 mg/day) and dipyridamole (225 mg/day). One patient suffered two relapses while on prednisone 20 mg/day in addition to these antiplatelet agents, and she had to undergo splenectomy to prevent further relapses. However, the mean severity score of the five TTP relapses that occurred while the patients were receiving the prophylactic therapy was significantly lower than the mean severity score of the five relapses that occurred without prophylaxis. Prophylactic therapy also improved the pregnancy outcome. Moreover, of the seven pregnancies complicated by TTP before delivery, the three in which the mothers received prophylactic therapy were completed successfully to term, while the four in which no prophylaxis was given ended in intrauterine fetal demise.

Women with a history of TTP should be monitored closely during pregnancy. A weekly blood count is recommended in order to detect a relapse as early as possible. Awareness of any symptom or sign that might suggest a relapse is crucial. Prophylactic therapy with aspirin 100 mg/day and dipyridamole 225 mg/day should be given during the whole pregnancy. Additional therapeutic modalities such as corticosteroids and plasma may be considered when the risk of relapse is especially high.

There are some specific situations during pregnancy that should alert the physician to look for early signs of a relapse. Infections are the most common, reported in up to 40% of patients,[1,91,92] including *Shigella* spp., *Escherichia coli*, *Salmonella typhi*, *Campylobacter jejuni*, *Yersinia* spp., pneumococcus, *Legionella*, and *Mycoplasma*.[92,93] The authors have treated a patient who had eight relapses of TTP during bouts of streptococcal tonsillitis.[6] Specific viral infections that were associated with TTP include Coxsackie B virus, echovirus, influenza virus, Epstein–Barr virus, and herpes simplex virus.[93] The incidence of TTP in HIV patients is significantly higher than in the general population.[94–97]

In some patients, TTP is the first manifestation of HIV infection.[97] The clinical and laboratory manifestations of TTP in HIV patients are not different from those of other patients; however, additional symptoms may exist as a result of AIDS-related conditions (e.g. Kaposi sarcoma, cytomegalovirus infection). The use of penicillin may also be associated with TTP relapse.[4,81]

CONCLUSION

Much about TTP remains incompletely understood, especially during pregnancy. The inciting factors that may cause the disease in pregnancy (and their responsibility for the relapses associated with subsequent pregnancies) have not yet been identified. Directed research of the underlying etiology of TTP has revealed the role of endothelial injury and platelet activation, and has illustrated some functions of the ULvWF cleaving protease and its IgG inhibitor. These discoveries provide some explanation for the efficacy of plasma exchange, corticosteroids, and splenectomy in TTP. However, despite the dramatic improvement in the clinical outcome, TTP can recur and can be fatal. Thus, additional investigations are needed to disclose the etiology of TTP in pregnancy and to develop more effective therapies for patients who fail to respond or who relapse despite receiving all the available therapeutic modalities.

REFERENCES

1. Rose M, Rowe JM, Eldor A. The changing course of thrombotic thrombocytopenic purpura and modern therapy. *Blood Rev* 1993;**7**:94–103.
2. Bukowski R. Thrombotic thrombocytopenic purpura: A review. *Prog Hemost Thromb* 1982;**6**: 287–337.
3. Bell WR. Thrombotic thrombocytopenic purpura/hemolytic uremic syndrome relapse: frequency, pathogenesis, and meaning. *Semin Hematol* 1997;**34**:134–9.
4. Kwaan HC, Soff GA. Management of thrombotic thrombocytopenic purpura and hemolytic uremic syndrome. *Semin Hematol* 1997;**34**: 159–66.
5. Ben-Yehuda D, Rose M, Michaeli Y, Eldor A. Permanent neurological complications in patients with thrombotic thrombocytopenic purpura. *Am J Hematol* 1988;**29**:74–8.
6. Eldor A, Moser AM, Rose M *et al*. Thrombotic thrombocytopenic purpura: The Israeli experience. *Transfus Sci* 1992;**13**:53–7.
7. Rose M, Eldor A. High incidence of relapses in thrombotic thrombocytopenic purpura. Clinical study of 38 patients. *Am J Med* 1987;**83**:437–44.
8. Rock GA, Shumak KH, Buskard NA *et al*. Comparison of plasma exchange with plasma infusion in the treatment of thrombotic thrombocytopenic purpura. *N Engl J Med* 1991;**325**:393–7.

9. Bell WR, Braine HG, Ness PM, Kickler TS. Improved survival in thrombotic thrombocytopenic purpura-hemolytic uremic syndrome - clinical experience in 108 patients. *N Engl J Med* 1991;**325**:398–403.

10. Shumak KH, Rock GA, Nair RC. Late relapses in patients successfully treated for thrombotic thrombocytopenic purpura. Canadian Apheresis Group. *Ann Intern Med* 1995;**122**:569–72.

11. Moake JL. Thrombotic thrombocytopenic purpura and the hemolytic-uremic syndrome. In: *Hematology, Basic Principles and Practice*. (Hoffman R, Benz EJ, Shattil SJ, Furie B, Cohen HJ, eds). Churchill Livingstone, New York, 1991:1495–501.

12. Ezra Y, Mordel N, Sadovsky E *et al*. Successful pregnancies of two patients with thrombotic thrombocytopenic purpura. *Int J Gynaecol Obstet* 1989;**29**:359–63.

13. Ezra Y, Rose M, Eldor A. Therapy and prevention of thrombotic thrombocytopenic purpura during pregnancy: a clinical study of 16 pregnancies. *Am J Hematol* 1996;**51**:1–6.

14. Natelson EA, White D. Recurrent thrombotic thrombocytopenic purpura in early pregnancy: effect of uterine evacuation. *Obstet Gynecol* 1985;**66**(3 Suppl):54S-6S.

15. Lian EC-Y, Byrnes JJ, Harkness DR. Two successful pregnancies in a woman with chronic thrombotic thrombocytopenic purpura treated by plasma infusion. *Am J Hematol* 1984;**16**:287–91.

16. McCrae KR, Cines DB. Thrombotic microangiopathy during pregnancy. *Semin Hematol* 1997;**34**:148–58.

17. Weiner CP. Thrombotic microangiopathy in pregnancy and the postpartum period. *Semin Hematol* 1987;**24**:119–29.

18. Wurzel JM. TTP lesions in placenta but not fetus. *N Engl J Med* 1979;**301**:503–4.

19. Alqadah F, Zebeib MA, Awidi AS. Thrombotic thrombocytopenic purpura associated with pregnancy in two sisters. *Postgrad Med J* 1993;**69**:229–31.

20. Mitra D, Jaffe EA, Weksler B *et al*. Thrombotic thrombocytopenic purpura and sporadic hemolytic-uremic syndrome plasmas induce apoptosis in restricted lineages of human microvascular endothelial cells. *Blood* 1997;**89**:1224–34.

21. Jaffe EA, Nachman RL, Merskey C. Thrombotic thrombocytopenic purpura: coagulation parameters in twelve patients. *Blood* 1973;**42**:499–507.

22. Takahashi H, Tatewaki W, Nakamura T *et al*. Coagulation studies in thrombotic thrombo-cytopenic purpura, with special reference to von-Willebrand factor and protein S. *Am J Hematol* 1989;**30**:14–21.

23. Asada Y, Sumiyoshi A, Hayashi T *et al*. Immunohistochemistry of vascular lesions in thrombotic thrombocytopenic purpura with special reference to factor VIII related antigen. *Thromb Res* 1985;**38**:469–79.

24. Asada Y, Sumiyoshi A. Histopathology of thrombotic thrombocytopenic purpura. Nippon Rinsho 1993;**51**:159–62.

25. Berkowitz LR, Dalldorf FG, Blatt PM. Thrombotic thrombocytopenic purpura: A pathology review. *JAMA* 1979;**241**:1709–10.

26. Harkness DR, Byrnes JJ, Lian EC-Y *et al*. Hazard of platelet transfusion in thrombotic thrombocytopenic purpura. *JAMA* 1981;**246**:1931–3.

27. Siddiqui FA, Lian EC. Platelet-agglutinating protein p37 from a thrombotic thrombocytopenic purpura plasma forms a complex with human immunoglobulin G. *Blood* 1988;**71**:299–304.

28. Murphy WG, Moore JC, Kelton JG. Calcium-dependent cysteine protease activity in the sera of patients with thrombotic thrombocytopenic purpura. *Blood* 1987;**70**:1683–7.

29. Falanga A, Consonni R, Ruggenenti P, Barbui T. A cathepsin-like cysteine proteinase proaggregating activity in thrombotic thrombocytopenic purpura. *Br J Haematol* 1991;**79**:474–80.

30. Consonni R, Falanga A, Barbui T. Further characterization of platelet-aggregating cysteine proteinase activity in thrombotic thrombocytopenic purpura. *Br J Haematol* 1994;**87**: 321–4.

31. Kelton JG, Moore JC, Warkentin TE, Hayward CP. Isolation and characterization of cysteine proteinase in thrombotic thrombocytopenic purpura. *Br J Haematol* 1996;**93**:421–6.

32. Moake JL, Rudy CK, Troll JH *et al*. Unusually large plasma factor VIII: von Willebrand factor multimers in chronic relapsing thrombotic thrombocytopenic purpura. *N Engl J Med* 1982; **307**:1432–5.

33. Moake JL, Byrnes JJ. Thrombotic microangiopathies associated with drugs and bone marrow transplantation. *Hematol Oncol Clin North Am* 1996;**10**:485–97

34. Kelton JG, Moore JC, Murphy WG. Studies investigating platelet aggregation and release initiated by sera from patients with thrombotic thrombocytopenic purpura. *Blood* 1987;**69**:924–8.

35. Moore JC, Murphy WG, Kelton JG. Calpain proteolysis of von Willebrand factor enhances its binding to platelet membrane glycoprotein

IIb/IIIa: An explanation for platelet aggregation in thrombotic thrombocytopenic purpura. *Br J Haematol* 1990;**74**:457–64.

36. Frangos JA, Moake JL, Nolasco L, *et al.* Cryo-supernatant regulates accumulation of unusually large vWF multimers from endothelial cells. *Am J Physiol* 1989;**256**:H1635–44.

37. Furlan M, Robles R, Solenthaler M *et al.* Deficient activity of von Willebrand factor-cleaving protease in chronic relapsing thrombotic thrombocytopenic purpura. *Blood* 1997;**89**:3097–103.

38. Furlan M, Robles R, Galbusera M, *et al.* Von Willebrand factor-cleaving protease in thrombotic thrombocytopenic purpura and the hemolytic-uremic syndrome. *N Engl J Med* 1998;**339**:1578–84.

39. Furlan M, Robles R, Morselli B *et al.* Recovery and half-life of von Willebrand factor-cleaving protease after plasma therapy in patients with thrombotic thrombocytopenic purpura. *Thromb Haemost* 1999;**81**:8–13.

40. Tsai H-M, Lian EC. Antibodies to von Willebrand factor-cleaving protease in acute thrombotic thrombocytopenic purpura. *N Engl J Med* 1998;**339**:1585–94.

41. Gerritsen HE, Turecek PL, Schwarz HP *et al.* Assay of von Willebrand factor (vWF)-cleaving protease based on decreased collagen binding affinity of degraded vWF: a tool for the diagnosis of thrombotic thrombocytopenic purpura (TTP). *Thromb Haemost* 1999;**82**:1386–9.

42. Tsai HM, Rice L, Sarode R *et al.* Antibody inhibitors to von Willebrand factor metalloproteinase and increased binding of von Willebrand factor to platelets in ticlopidine-associated thrombotic thrombocytopenic purpura. *Ann Int Med* 2000;**132**:794–9.

43. Koenig DW, Barley-Maloney L, Daniel TO. A western blot assay detects autoantibodies to cryptic endothelial antigens in thrombotic microangiopathies. *J Clin Immunol* 1993;**13**:204–11.

44. Remuzzi G, Zoja C, Rossi EC. Prostacyclin in thrombotic microangiopathy. *Semin Hematol* 1987;**24**:110–18.

45. Chen YC, McLeod B, Hall ER, Wu KK. Accelerated prostacyclin degradation in thrombotic thrombocytopenic purpura. *Lancet* 1981;**2**:267–9.

46. Laurence J, Mitra D, Steiner M *et al.* Plasma from patients with idiopathic and human immunodeficiency virus-associated thrombotic thrombocytopenic purpura induces apoptosis in microvascular endothelial cells. *Blood* 1996;**87**:3245–54.

47. Kwaan HC. Thrombotic thrombocytopenic purpura and hemolytic uremic syndrome in pregnancy. *Clin Obstet Gynecol* 1985;**28**:101–6.

48. Miller JM, Pastorek JG. Thrombotic thrombocytopenic purpura and hemolytic uremic syndrome in pregnancy. *Clin Obstet Gynecol* 1991;**34**:64–71.

49. Sibai BM, Kustermann L, Velasco J. Current understanding of severe preeclampsia, pregnancy-associated hemolytic uremic syndrome, thrombotic thrombocytopenic purpura, hemolysis, elevated liver enzymes, and low platelet syndrome, and postpartum acute renal failure: Different clinical syndromes or just different names? *Curr Opin Nephrol Hypertens* 1994;**3**:436–45.

50. Usta IM, Barton JR, Amon EA *et al.* Acute fatty liver of pregnancy: an experience in the diagnosis and management of fourteen cases. *Am J Obstet Gynecol* 1994;**171**:1342–7.

51. Reyes H, Sandoval L, Wainstein A *et al.* Acute fatty liver of pregnancy: A clinical study of 12 episodes in 11 patients. *Gut* 1994;**35**:101–6.

52. Castro MA, Ouzounian JG, Colletti PM *et al.* Radiologic studies in acute fatty liver of pregnancy: A review of the literature and 19 new cases. *J Reprod Med* 1996;**41**:839–43.

53. Pereira SP, O'Donohue J, Wendon J, William R. Maternal and perinatal outcome in severe pregnancy-related liver disease. *Hepatology* 1997;**26**:1258–62.

54. Arnout J, Spitz B, VanAssche A *et al.* The antiphospholipid syndrome and pregnancy. *Hypert Pregn* 1995;**14**:147–78.

55. Friedman SA, Schiff E, Emeris JJ *et al.* Biochemical corroboration of endothelial involvement in severe preeclampsia. *Am J Obstet Gynecol* 1995;**172**:202–3.

56. Katano K, Aoki K, Sasa H *et al.* β2-Glycoprotein I-dependent anticardiolipin antibodies as a predictor of adverse pregnancy outcomes in healthy pregnant women. *Hum Reprod* 1996;**11**:509–12.

57. Pattison NS, Chamley LW, McKay EJ *et al.* Antiphospholipid antibodies in pregnancy: prevalence and clinical associations. *Br J Obstet Gynecol* 1993;**100**:909–13.

58. Hochfeld M, Druzin ML, Maia D *et al.* Pregnancy complicated by primary antiphospholipid syndrome. *Obstet Gynecol* 1994;**83**:804–5.

59. Kochenour NK, Branch DW, Rote NS, Scott JR. A new postpartum syndrome associated with antiphospholipid. *Obstet Gynecol* 1987;**69**:460–8.

60. Kniaz D, Eisenverg GM, Elrad H *et al.*

Postpartum hemolytic uremia syndrome associated with antiphospholipid antibodies. *Am J Nephrol* 1992:**12**:126–33.

61. Atlas M, Barkai G, Menczer J et al. Thrombotic thrombocytopenic purpura in pregnancy. *Br J Obstet Gynaecol* 1982;**89**:476–9.

62. Upshaw JD, Reidy TJ, Groshart K. Thrombotic thrombocytopenic purpura in pregnancy: response to plasma manipulations. *South Med J* 1985;**78**:677–80.

63. Ambrose A, Welham RT, Cefalo RC. Thrombotic thrombocytopenic purpura in early pregnancy. *Obstet Gynecol* 1985;**66**:267–72.

64. Pereira A, Mazzara R, Monteagudo J et al. Thrombotic thrombocytopenic purpura/hemolytic uremic syndrome: A multivariate analysis of factors predicting the response to plasma exchange. *Ann Hematol* 1995;**70**: 319–23.

65. Byrnes JJ, Moake JL, Klug P et al. Effectiveness of the cryosupernatant fraction of plasma in the treatment of refractory thrombotic thrombocytopenic purpura. *Am J Hematol* 1990;**34**:169–74.

66. Vianelli N, Sermasi G, D'Alessandro R et al. Prompt plasma-exchange treatment and coma reversibility in two patients with thrombotic thrombocytopenic purpura. *Haematologica* 1991; **76**:72–4.

67. Frankel AE, Rubenstein MD, Wall RT. Thrombotic thrombocytopenic purpura: Prolonged coma with recovery of neurologic function with intensive plasma exchange. *Am J Hematol* 1981;**10**:387–90.

68. Gordon LI, Kwaan HC, Rossi EC. Deleterious effects of platelet transfusions and recovery thrombocytosis in patients with thrombotic microangiopathy. *Semin Hematol* 1987;**24**:194–201

69. Petitt RM. Thrombotic thrombocytopenic purpura: a thirty five year review. *Semin Thromb Hemost* 1980;**6**:350–5.

70. Ozsoylu S. Intravenous high dose methylprednisolone for thrombotic thrombocytopenic purpura (letter). *Am J Hematol* 1988;**28**:128–9.

71. Viero P, Cortelazzo S, Buelli M et al. Thrombotic thrombocytopenic purpura and high-dose immunoglobulin treatment (letter). *Ann Intern Med* 1986;**104**:282.

72. Raniele DP, Opsahl JA, Kjellstrand CM. Should intravenous immunoglobulin G be first-line treatment for acute thrombotic thrombocytopenic purpura? Case report and review of the literature. *Am J Kidney Dis* 1991;**18**:264–8.

73. Chin D, Chyczij H, Etches W et al. Treatment of thrombotic thrombocytopenic purpura with intravenous gammaglobulin (letter). *Transfusion* 1987;**27**:115–6.

74. Centurioni R, Bobbio-Pallavicini E, Porta C et al. Treatment of thrombotic thrombocytopenic purpura with high-dose immunoglobulins: Results in 17 patients. Italian Cooperative Group for TTP. *Haematologica* 1995;**80**:325–31.

75. del Zoppo GJ. Antiplatelet therapy in thrombotic thrombocytopenic purpura. *Semin Hematol* 1987; **24**:130–9.

76. Myers TJ, Wakem CJ, Ball ED, Tremont SJ. Thrombotic thrombocytopenic purpura: combined treatment with plasmapheresis and antiplatelet agents. *Ann Intern Med* 1980;**92**:149–55.

77. Rosove MH, Ho WG, Goldfinger D. Ineffectiveness of aspirin and dipyridamole in the treatment of thrombotic thrombocytopenic purpura. *Ann Intern Med* 1982;**96**:27–33.

78. De Pasquale A, Venturoni L, Paterlini P et al. Possible usefulness of ticlopidine in combined treatment of thrombotic thrombocytopenic purpura. Report of one case. *Haematologica* 1986; **71**:53–5.

79. Vianelli N, Catani L, Belmonte MM et al. Ticlopidine in the treatment of thrombotic thrombocytopenic purpura: Report of two cases. *Haematologica* 1990;**75**:274–7.

80. Bennett CL, Connors JM, Carwile et al. Thrombotic thrombocytopenic purpura associated with clopidogrel. *N Engl J Med.* 2000;**342**: 1773–7.

81. Page Y, Tardy B, Zeni F et al. Thrombotic thrombocytopenic purpura related to ticlopidine. *Lancet* 1991;**337**:774–6.

82. Gutterman LA, Stevenson TD. Treatment of thrombotic thrombocytopenic purpura with vincristine. *JAMA* 1982;**247**:1433–6.

83. Welborn JL, Emrick P, Acevedo M. Rapid improvement of thrombotic thrombocytopenic purpura with vincristine and plasmapheresis. *Am J Hematol* 1990;**35**:18–21.

84. Levine M, Grunwald HW. Use of vincristine in refractory thrombotic thrombocytopenic purpura. *Acta Haematol* 1991;**85**:37–40.

85. Spiekermann K, Wormann B, Rumpf KW, Hiddemann W. Combination chemotherapy with CHOP for recurrent thrombotic thrombocytopenic purpura. *Br J Haematol* 1997;**97**:544–6.

86. Peterson J, Amare M, Henry JE, Bone RC. Splenectomy and antiplatelet agents in thrombotic thrombocytopenic purpura. *Am J Med Sci* 1979;**277**:75–80.

87. Rowe JM, Francis CW, Cyram EM, Marder VJ.

Thrombotic thrombocytopenic purpura: Recovery after splenectomy associated with persistence of abnormally large von Willebrand factor multimers. *Am J Hematol* 1985;**20**: 161–8.

88. Cuttner J. Thrombotic thrombocytopenic purpura: A ten-year experience. *Blood* 1980;**56**: 302–6.

89. Winslow GA, Nelson EW. Thrombotic thrombocytopenic purpura: indications for and results of splenectomy. *Am J Surg* 1995;**170**:558–61.

90. Hoffkes HG, Weber F, Uppenkamp M *et al.* Recovery by splenectomy in patients with relapsed thrombotic thrombocytopenic purpura and treatment failure to plasma exchange. *Semin Thromb Hemost* 1995;**21**:161–5.

91. Amorosi EL, Altmann JE. Thrombotic thrombocytopenic purpura: Report of 16 cases and review of the literature. *Medicine* 1966;**45**:139–59.

92. Kwaan HC. Miscellaneous secondary thrombotic microangiopathy. *Semin Hematol* 1987;**24**:141–7.

93. Keusch GT, Acheson DWK. Thrombotic thrombocytopenic purpura associated with Shiga Toxins. *Semin Hematol* 1997;**34**: 106–16.

94. Leaf AN, Laubenstein LJ, Raphael B *et al.* Thrombotic thrombocytopenic purpura associated with human imunodeficiency virus Type 1 (HIV-1) infection. *Ann Intern Med* 1988;**109**:194–7.

95. Nair JMG, Bellevue R, Bertoni M, Dosik H. Thrombotic thrombocytopenic purpura in patients with the acquired immunodeficiency syndrome (AIDS)-related complex. *Ann Intern Med* 1988;**109**:209–12.

96. Platanias LC, Paiusco D, Bernstein S, Murali MR. Thrombotic thrombocytopenic purpura as the first manifestation of human immunodeficiency virus infection. *Am J Med* 1989;**87**:699–700.

97. Hymes KB, Karpatkin S. Human immunodeficiency virus infection and thrombotic microangiopathy. *Semin Hematol* 1997;**34**:117–25.

16

Thrombophilia and fetal loss

Benjamin Brenner

INTRODUCTION

Successful outcome of pregnancy is dependent on the development of adequate placental circulation. Abnormalities of placental vasculature may result in a number of gestational pathologies, including first and second trimester miscarriages, intrauterine growth restriction (IUGR), intrauterine fetal death (IUFD), placental abruption, and pre-eclampsia.[1]

Inherited and acquired thrombophilia are the main causes of thrombosis in pregnant women.

A growing number of reports over the past few years have suggested that these disorders are also associated with an increased incidence of vascular pathologies resulting in poor gestational outcome (Table 16.1).[2]

This chapter reviews recent data about thrombophilia and vascular placental pathology resulting in fetal loss, and it discusses available therapeutic modalities for the prevention of placental vascular thrombosis in order to achieve successful gestational outcome.

Table 16.1 Placental vascular complications associated with thrombophilia

	Miscarriages	IUFD	Pre-eclampsia	Placental abruption
Antithrombin III deficiency	+ +	+ +	+	
Protein C deficiency	+	+ +	+	
Protein S deficiency	+	+ +	+	
Dysfibrinogenemia	+	+		
APC resistance	+ +	+ +	+ +	
Factor V Leiden	+ +	+ +	+ +	+ +
MTHFR C677T	+	+	+	+
Hyperhomocysteinemia	+	+	+ +	+ +
Factor II G20210A	+	+	+	+ +
Antiphospholipid syndrome	+ +	+ +	+ +	
Combined defects	+ +	+ +	+	

Degree of association: +: possible association; + +: established association.

RECURRENT FETAL LOSS

Recurrent fetal loss (RFL) is a common health problem, with three or more losses affecting 1–2% of women of reproductive age and two or more losses affecting up to 5%.[3,4] Although several etiologies have been implicated to play a role in RFL, including chromosomal translocations and inversions, anatomic alterations of the uterus, endocrinologic abnormalities and autoimmune disorders,[5,6] the majority of RFL remained unexplained until recently.

RFL is a well-established finding in certain acquired thrombophilic disorders such as antiphospholipid syndrome[7] and essential thrombocythemia.[8] The prevalence of venous thromboembolism (VTE) during gestation and the puerperium is increased in women with inherited thrombophilic states such as antithrombin III deficiency, protein C deficiency, or protein S deficiencies.[9,10]

A case control study of 60 women with these inherited thrombophilias documented an increased risk of RFL.[11] Forty-two out of 188 pregnancies (22%) in women with thrombophilia resulted in pregnancy loss, compared with 23 out of 202 (11%) in controls (odds ratio 2.0; 95% CI 1.2–3.3).[11] In addition, a high incidence of gestational abnormalities was reported in 15 women with dysfibrinogenemia associated with thrombosis. Of 64 pregnancies, 39% ended by miscarriage and 9% by IUFD.[12]

THROMBOPHILIC POLYMORPHISMS

Pregnancy is an acquired risk factor for VTE, with factor V Leiden and factor II G20210A mutations being the major causes for VTE in pregnant women.[13] However, most carriers will not develop clinical symptoms during gestations.[13] This indeed is also the case for RFL, which affects only a minority of women with factor V Leiden mutation.[14] Unlike factor V Leiden, methylene tetrahydrofolate reductase (MTHFR) C677T was not found to be a risk factor for gestational VTE or RFL.[15] However, studies of cohorts of women with RFL reveal a different picture. Three recent case control studies have evaluated the prevalence of factor V Leiden mutation in women with RFL (Table 16.2). Despite differences in ethnic Caucasian subpopulations and selection criteria for RFL, all three studies documented significantly increased prevalence of factor V Leiden mutation in women with RFL. Ridker et al. have studied women with RFL without an extensive etiological workup except for ruling out chromosomal abnormalities[16] and found a 2.3-fold increase in the prevalence of factor V Leiden.

In women with RFL of unknown cause, after exclusion of chromosomal abnormalities, infections, anatomic alterations, and endocrinological dysfunction, studies by Grandone et al.[17] and by the author's group[18] have suggested that evaluation for factor V Leiden mutation is highly warranted, since a significant proportion of women with RFL are carriers of the mutation. Nevertheless, other reports have not documented an association between factor V Leiden mutation and RFL.[19] Although Younis et al. have reported that activated protein C (APC) resistance and factor V Leiden mutation can be associated with first trimester RFL as well as second trimester RFL,[20] Roque et al. have documented that

---

Table 16.2 Factor V Leiden mutation in women with RFL

Study	Selection	Patients	Controls	Odds ratio	95% CI	p
Grandone et al.[17]	Yes	7/43 (16%)	5/118 (4%)	4.4	1.3–14.7	0.01
Ridker et al.[16]	No	9/113 (8%)	16/437 (3.7%)	2.3	1.0–5.2	0.05
Brenner.[18]	Yes	24/76 (32%)	11/106 (10%)	4.0	1.8–8.8	0.001

maternal thrombophilia is associated with second and third trimester pregnancy loss.[21] These differences probably result from differences in the populations studied – Roque et al. studied a cohort of pregnant women, whereas the author's group studied a cohort of women with a history of RFL.

In populations in which homozygosity for factor V Leiden is highly prevalent, a significant association of this state with RFL can also be demonstrated.[18] The risk of RFL is greater in homozygous carriers of factor V Leiden than in heterozygous carriers.[22] Sisters of thrombophilic women with factor V Leiden mutation are also at an increased risk of RFL.[23] Pregnant women with and without factor V Leiden exhibit substantial activation of coagulation, with higher D-dimer levels in those with factor V Leiden.[24] A study from Sweden documented that women who are primary aborters have a high frequency of factor V Leiden mutation – 10 out of 36 (28%) compared with two out of 69 (3%) in the control group (p = 0.0003).[25]

APC RESISTANCE IN PREGNANCY

A potential explanation for the association between RFL and APC resistance is that the APC sensitivity ratio falls progressively throughout normal pregnancy, either in correlation with changes in the levels of factor VIII, factor V and protein S[26] or without such a correlation.[27] Transient APC resistance can be documented during normal gestations even in women with a normal factor V genotype. APC sensitivity ratios may be further reduced during gestation in women with factor V Leiden mutation. Interestingly, APC resistance in the absence of factor V Leiden mutation has also been associated with pregnancy loss.[28,29] One potential explanation for this is presence of anti-β-2-glycoprotein-1 antibodies, which induce APC resistance.[30]

In view of the high prevalence of the three common thrombophilic mutations (factor V Leiden, factor II G20210A and MTHFR C677T) in the general population, the author's group has evaluated their prevalence in women with RFL.

At least one of these three mutations was found in 49% of women with RFL of unknown cause, compared with 23% in controls (odds ratio 3.2, 95% CI 1.7–6.1, p = 0.0002).[18]

Although this study demonstrated that factor II G20210A and MTHFR C677T as solitary defects are not associated with an increased risk of RFL compared with controls,[18] it cannot rule out the possibility that factor II G20210A mutation is a mild risk factor for certain types of RFL.[31] Indeed, in a recent study from Italy, Martinelli et al. have documented that both factor V Leiden mutation and factor II G20210A mutation are associated with IUFD.[32] Eleven of the 67 women with late loss (16%) and 13 of the 232 control women (6%) had either the factor V or the prothrombin mutation. The relative risks of late fetal loss in carriers of the factor V mutation was 3.2 (95% CI 1.0–10.9); in carriers of the prothrombin mutation it was 3.3 (95% CI 1.1–10.3). Thus, both the factor V mutation and the prothrombin mutation are associated with an approximate tripling of the risk of late fetal loss.

HYPERHOMOCYSTEINEMIA

An association of placental vascular complications and hyperhomocysteinemia is increasingly being reported. Hyperhomocysteinemia was documented in 26% of women with placental abruption, in 11% of the cases with IUFD, and in 38% of women delivering babies whose birth weight were below the fifth percentile, compared with an estimated 2–3% in the general control population.[33] Likewise, hyperhomocysteinemia was documented in 26 out of 84 women (31%) with previous placental infarcts or abruption, compared with four out of 46 (9%) in controls.[34] In addition, hyperhomocysteinemia was found in six out of 35 patients (17%) with recurrent abortions.[35]

In a recent meta-analysis, Nelen et al.[36] reviewed 10 case control studies that examined the association of RFL and hyperhomocysteinemia, and they reported a three- or four-fold increased risk, while in six studies the risk of homozygosity for MTHFR was only 1.4.

COMBINED THROMBOPHILIA

It is well established that combinations of inherited or acquired thrombophilic states increase the risk of thrombosis.[37,38] Likewise, combinations of thrombophilic states may further increase the risk of RFL. For example, coexistence of factor V Leiden and homozygous hyperhomocysteinemia[39] or a combination of factor V Leiden and familial antiphospholipid syndrome[40] were reported to result in thrombosis and RFL. It is therefore not surprising that the European Prospective Cohort on Thrombophilia (EPCOT) study documented the highest odds ratio for stillbirth (OR 14.3, 95% CI 2.4–86) in patients with combined thrombophilic defects.[41] In the author's recent study involving 76 women with RFL six (8%) had a combination of thrombophilic polymorphisms, compared with one out of 106 (0.9%) of controls ($p < 0.02$).[18] Factor II G20210A and homozygosity for MTHFR C677T both contribute to RFL when they present in combination with other thrombophilic defects.

In the recent study by Sang et al., at least one thrombophilic defect was found in 96 out of 145 women (66%) with RFL, compared with 41 out of 145 (28%) in controls (odds ratio 5.0, 95% CI 3.0–8.5, $p < 0.0001$).[42] Combined thrombophilic defects were documented in 31 out of 145 of women (21%) with pregnancy loss, compared with eight out of 145 (5.5%) in controls (odds ratio 5.0, 95% CI 2.0–11.5, $p < 0.0001$). Although the majority of pregnancy loss in the study group occurred at the first trimester, late pregnancy wastage occurred more frequently in women with thrombophilia (160 out of 429, 37%), compared with women without thrombophilia (39 out of 162, 24%, $p = 0.002$). APC resistance was the most common thrombophilic defect, documented in 39% of women with pregnancy loss, compared with only 3% of controls (odds ratio 18.0, 95% CI 7.0–53.6, $p < 0.0001$). APC resistance without factor V Leiden was documented in 18% of women with pregnancy loss, either as the only defect (9%) or in combination with other thrombophilias (9%). Although factor V Leiden was more common in women with pregnancy loss (25% versus 7.6%,

odds ratio 4.0, 95% CI 1.9–8.8, $p < 0.0001$), factor II G20210A and homozygosity for MTHFR C677T contributed to pregnancy loss only when associated with other thrombophilic defects.[42]

PLACENTAL PATHOLOGICAL FINDINGS

Mechanisms responsible for the association of inherited thrombophilia with RFL have not been elucidated. Pathological studies of placentae obtained from gestations terminated by fetal loss reveal thrombotic changes and infarcts. These can be observed in the maternal vessels in a large proportion of placentas in stillbirths.[43] However, these changes can also be found in a significant proportion of women with IUFD who do not have thrombophilia.[32,43,44]

Placental thrombotic changes can be located either in the fetal vessels or in the maternal vessels. A role for fetal–placental thrombosis has been suggested by studies that have demonstrated an association between the factor V genotype in miscarried fetuses and placental infarction.[45] However, support for the latter association is provided by findings of thrombotic changes on the maternal side and by the efficacy of low molecular weight heparin, which does not cross the placenta, in preventing fetal loss. In addition, the Nîmes Obstetricians and Haematologists (NOHA) 5 study demonstrated that the father's genotype did not contribute to stillbirth.[43]

As up to 65% of vascular gestational abnormalities can be accounted for by genetic thrombophilias,[18,46] the implication is to screen for these mutations in all women with vascular gestational abnormalities. Furthermore, this high prevalence of genetic thrombophilias, which is similar to the findings in women with pregnancy-related venous thromboembolism,[47] and the findings of thrombotic changes in the placentas of the majority of women with thrombophilia and stillbirth,[43] suggest that antithrombotic drugs may have a potential therapeutic benefit in women with gestational vascular complications.

THERAPEUTIC REGIMENS

Without therapeutic intervention (Table 16.3), only 20% of gestations in women with thrombophilia and RFL result in live birth.[18] Emerging data on therapy for women with inherited thrombophilia and pregnancy loss is mostly uncontrolled and include small series of patients treated mostly with low molecular weight heparin. The potential advantages of low molecular weight heparin over unfractionated heparin are a higher antithrombotic ratio (which means less bleeding for a better antithrombotic effect), a longer half-life with a potential need for only one injection a day, a smaller injected volume, and less heparin-induced thrombocytopenia. A recent collaborative study has demonstrated the safety of low molecular weight heparin during 486 gestations.[48] A successful outcome was reported in 83 out of 93 gestations (89%) in women with RFL and in all 28 gestations in women with pre-eclampsia in a previous pregnancy.[49] Administration of the low molecular weight heparin enoxaparin (20 mg/day) to women with primary early RFL and impaired fibrinolytic capacity resulted in normalization of impaired fibrinolysis, conception in 16 out of 20 (80%), and successful live birth in 13 out of 16 (81%).[49]

The author's group has treated 61 pregnancies in 50 women with thrombophilia who presented with RPL with enoxaparin throughout gestation and 4 weeks into the postpartum period. Enoxaparin dosage was 40 mg/day, except for patients with combined thrombophilia or in cases of abnormal Doppler velocimetry that suggested decreased placental perfusion, when the dosage was increased to 40 mg twice daily. In the case of previous thrombosis, therapy was continued for 6 weeks after delivery. Forty-six of the 61 pregnancies (75%) resulted in a live birth, compared with a success rate of only 20% in these 50 women in earlier gestations without antithrombotic therapy.[50] Although these preliminary results are very encouraging, the optimal dosage of low molecular weight heparin is not yet known. LIVE-ENOX is an ongoing multicenter prospective randomized trial comparing enoxaparin 40 mg once daily and 40 mg twice daily in 180 women with thrombophilia and RFL.

The role of aspirin, if any, in the setting of thrombophilia and vascular gestational abnormalities remains to be confirmed. In patients with antiphospholipid syndrome or in those with combined thrombophilia, aspirin is given along with low molecular

---

Table 16.3 Therapeutic modalities for prevention of fetal loss in thrombophilic patients

	Therapeutic modality				
	Folic acid	Corticosteroids	Aspirin	Heparin	Low molecular weight heparin
Hyperhomocysteinemia	++		+		+++
Antithrombin III deficiency	+			+++	+++
Protein C or Protein S deficiency	+			+++	+++
Factor V Leiden	+		+		+++
APC resistance	+		+		
Factor II mutation	+		+		
Antiphospholipid syndrome	+	+	++	+++	+++
Combined defects	+		+	+++	+++

Therapeutic benefit: +: Equivocal; ++: Substantial; +++: High

weight heparin. However, whether aspirin has an added benefit to heparin or low molecular weight heparin alone has not been evaluated.

FUTURE PERSPECTIVES

Future research in this field will most likely deal with four aspects. First, verification of the potential associations of the various genetic thrombophilias with gestational vascular pathologies is rapidly emerging (Table 16.4).

Secondly, 30–50% of vascular gestational pathologies currently cannot be accounted for by thrombophilia. Whether as yet unknown novel genetic or acquired thrombophilia will be found to play a role remains to be determined. Recent observations claim that polymorphisms of the thrombomodulin gene[51] and low levels of factor XII[52] may be associated with RFL. A high prevalence of increased levels of procoagulant microparticles was recently reported in women with RFL.[53] In view of the potential association of thrombophilia and RFL, the high prevalence of thrombophilia in Caucasian populations, the question of screening must be raised.

Thirdly, the pathogenetic mechanisms responsible for placental vascular pathologies in women with thrombophilia have not been fully elucidated. Furthermore, it is not yet known why only some women with thrombophilia express vascular gestational pathologies while others do not. It is possible that this may relate to local factors affecting coagulation, fibrinolysis and vascular tone at the level of placental vessels. Studies are being conducted to look at the local expression of tissue factor, tissue factor pathway inhibitor and thrombomodulin in placental trophoblasts from normal pregnancies and from women with gestational vascular pathologies.

Finally, the role of antithrombotic therapeutic modalities deserves prospective clinical trials, several of which are ongoing, to find ways of improving outcome for the large population of women who currently experience poor gestational outcome.

Table 16.4 Other inherited and acquired thrombophilic defects	
A. Inherited mutations and polymorphisms	Association with RFL
Thrombomodulin	Not evaluated
Tissue factor pathway inhibitor	Not evaluated
Endothelial protein C receptor	Not evaluated
B. Elevated coagulation levels	
Fibrinogen	Not evaluated
Factor II	Not evaluated
Factor VII	Not evaluated
Factor VIII	Not evaluated
Factor IX	Not evaluated
Factor XI	Not evaluated
C. Autoantibodies	
Anti-β-2-glycoprotein-1	Yes
Antiphosphotydil ethanolamine	Yes
Antiannexin V	Yes

REFERENCES

1. Salafia CM, Minior VK, Pezzullo JC, Popek EJ, Rosenkrantz TS, Vintzileos AM. Intrauterine growth restriction in infants of less than thirty-two weeks' gestation: associated placental pathologic features. *Am J Obstet Gynecol* 1995;**173**:1049–57.

2. Brenner B, Blumenfeld Z. Thrombophilia and fetal loss. *Blood Rev* 1997;**97**:551–4.

3. Cook CL, Pridham DD. Recurrent pregnancy loss. *Curr Opin Obstet Gynecol* 1995;**7**:357–66.

4. Clifford K, Rai R, Watson H, Regan L. An informative protocol for the investigation of recurrent miscarriage: preliminary experience of **500** consecutive cases. *Human Reprod* 1994;**9**:1328–32.

5. Hatasaka HH. Recurrent miscarriage: epidemiologic factors, definitions, and incidence. *Clin Obstet Gynecol* 1994;**37**:625–34.

6. Raziel A, Arieli S, Bukovsky I, Caspi E, Golan A. Investigation of the uterine cavity in recurrent aborters. *Fertil Steril* 1994;**62**:1080–2.

7. Triplett DA, Harris EN. Antiphospholipid antibodies and reproduction. *Am J Reprod Immunol* 1989;**21**:123–31.

8. Beressi AH, Tefferi A, Silverstein MN, Petitt RM, Hoagland WC. Outcome analysis of 34 pregnancies in women with essential thrombocythemia. *Arch Intern Med* 1995;**155**:1217–22.

9. Hellgren M, Tengborn L, Abildgaard U. Pregnancy in women with congenital antithrombin III deficiency: experience of treatment with heparin and antithrombin. *Gynecol Obstet Invest* 1982;**14**:127–41.

10. Conard J, Horellou MH, Van Dreden P, Lecompte T, Samama M. Thrombosis and pregnancy in congenital deficiencies in ATIII, protein C or protein S. *Thromb Haemost* 1990;**63**:319–20.

11. Sanson BJ, Friederich PW, Simioni P *et al*. The risk of abortion and stillbirth in antithrombin, protein C, and protein S-deficient women. *Thromb Haemost* 1996;**75**:387–8.

12. Haverkate F, Samama M. Familial dysfibrinogenemia and thrombophilia. Report on a study of the SSC Subcommittee on Fibrinogen. *Thromb Haemost* 1995;**73**:151–61.

13. Gerhardt A, Scharf RE, Beckmann MW *et al*. Prothrombin and factor V mutations in women with a history of thrombosis during pregnancy and the puerperium. *N Engl J Med* 2000;**342**:374–9.

14. Lindqvist PG, Svensson PJ, Masal K, Grennert L, Luterkort M, Bahlback B. Activated protein C resistance (FV:Q^{506}) and pregnancy. *Thromb Haemost* 1999;**81**:532–7.

15. Murphy RP, Donoghue C, Nallen RJ *et al*. Prospective evaluation of the risk conferred by factor V Leiden and thermolabile methylenetetrahydrofolate reductase polymorphisms in pregnancy. *Arterioscler Thromb Vasc Biol* 2000;**20**:266-70.

16. Rikder PM, Miletich JP, Buring JE *et al*. Factor V Leiden mutation as a risk factor for recurrent pregnancy loss. *Ann Intern Med* 1998;**128**:1000–3.

17. Grandone E, Margaglione M, Colaizzo D *et al*. Factor V Leiden is associated with repeated and recurrent unexplained fetal losses. *Thromb Haemost* 1997;**77**:822–4.

18. Brenner B, Sarig G, Weiner Z, Younis J, Blumenfeld Z, Lanir N. Thrombophilic polymorphisms in women with fetal loss. *Thromb Haemost* 1999;**82**:6–9.

19. Dizon-Townson DS, Kinney S, Branch DW, Ward K. The factor V Leiden mutation is not a common cause of recurrent miscarriage. *J Reprod Immunol* 1997;**34**:217–23.

20. Younis JS, Brenner B, Ohel G, Tal J, Lanir N, Ben-Ami M. Activated protein C resistance and factor V Leiden mutation can with first- as well as second-trimester recurrent pregnancy loss. *Am J Reprod Immunol* 2000;**43**:31–5.

21. Roque H, Paidas M, Rebarber A *et al*. Maternal thrombophilia is associated with second and third trimester fetal death [abstract]. *Am J Obstet Gynecol* 2001;**184**:S27, abstract 0060.

22. Meinardi JR, Middeldorp S, de Kam PJ *et al*. Increased risk for fetal loss in carriers of the factor V Leiden mutation. *Ann Intern Med* 1999;**130**:736–9.

23. Tormene D, Simioni P, Prandoni P *et al*. The risk of fetal loss in family member of probands with factor V Leiden mutation. *Thromb Haemost* 1999;**82**:1237–9.

24. Eichinger S, Weltermann A, Philipp K *et al*. Prospective evaluation of hemostatic system activation and thrombin potential in healthy pregnant women with and without factor V Leiden. *Thromb Haemost* 1999;**82**:1232–6.

25. Wramsby ML, Sten-Linder M, Bremme K. Primary habitual abortions are associated with high frequency of factor V Leiden mutation. *Fertil Steril* 2000,**74**:987–91.

26. Clark P, Brennand J, Conkie JA, McCall D, Greer IA, Walker ID. Activated protein C sensitivity, protein C, protein S and coagulation in normal pregnancy. *Thromb Haemost* 1998;**79**:1166–70.

27. Kjelberg U, Andersson NE, Rosen S, Tengborn L, Hellgren M. APC resistance and other

haemostatic variables during pregnancy and puerperium. *Thromb Haemost* 1999;**81**:527-31.

28. Tal J, Schliamser LM, Leibovitz Z, Ohel G, Attias D. A possible role for activated protein C resistance in patients with first and second trimester pregnancy failure. *Hum Reprod* 1999;**14**:1624–7.

29. Brenner B, Mandel H, Lanir N *et al*. Activated protein C resistance can be associated with recurrent fetal loss. *Br J Haematol* 1997;**97**:551–4.

30. Mercier E, Quere I, Mares P, Gris JC. Primary recurrent miscarriages: anti-β₂–glycoprotein I IgG antibodies induce an acquired activated protein C resistance that can be detected by the modified activated protein C resistance test. *Blood* 1998;**92**:2993-4.

31. Souza SS, Ferriani RA, Pontes AG, Zago MA, Franco RF. Factor V Leiden and factor II G20210A mutations in patients with recurrent abortion. *Hum Reprod* 1999;**14**:2448–50.

32. Martinelli I, Taioli E, Cetin I *et al*. Mutations in coagulation factors in women with unexplained late fetal loss. *N Engl J Med* 2000;**343**:1015–18.

33. de Vries JIP, Dekker GA, Huijgens PC, Jakobs C, Blomberg BM, van Geijn HP. Hyperhomocysteinaemia and protein S deficiency in complicated pregnancies. *Br J Obstet Gynaecol* 1997;**104**:1248–54.

34. Goddijn-Wessel TA, Wouters MG, van der Molen EF *et al*. Hyper-homocysteinemia: a risk factor for placental abruption or infarction. *Eur J Obstet Gynecol Rep Biol* 1996;**66**:23–9.

35. Coumans AB, Huijgens PC, Jakobs C *et al*. Haemostatic and metabolic abnormalities in women with unexplained recurrent abortion. *Hum Reprod* 1999;**14**:211–14.

36. Nelen WLDM, Blom HJ, Steegers EAP, den Heijer M, Eskes TKAB. Hyperhomocysteinemia and recurrent early pregnancy loss: a meta-analysis. *Fertil Steril* 2000,**74**:1196–9.

37. Zöller B, Berntsdotter A, Garcia de Frutos P, Dahlback B. Resistance to activated protein C as an additional genetic risk factor in hereditary deficiency of protein S. *Blood* 1995;**85**:3518–23.

38. Brenner B, Zivelin A, Lanir N, Greengard JS, Griffin JH, Seligsohn U. Venous thromboembolism associated with double heterozygosity for R506Q mutation of factor V and for T298M mutation of protein C in a large family of a previously described homozygous protein C deficient newborn with massive thrombosis. *Blood* 1996;**88**:877–80.

39. Mandel H, Brenner B, Berant M *et al*. Coexistence of hereditary homocysteinuria and factor V Leiden: effect on thrombosis. *N Engl J Med* 1996;**334**:763–8.

40. Brenner B, Vulfsons SL, Lanir N, Nahir M. Coexistence of familial antiphospholipid syndrome and factor V Leiden: impact on thrombotic diathesis. *Br J Haematol* 1996;**94**:166–7.

41. Preston FE, Rosendaal FR, Walker ID *et al*. Increased fetal loss in women with heritable thrombophilia. *Lancet* 1996;**348**:913–16.

42. Sarig G, Younis JS, Hoffman R *et al*. Thrombophilia is common in women with idiopathic pregnancy loss and is associated with late pregnancy wastage. *Fertil Steril* 2002;**77**: 342–7.

43. Gris JC, Quere I, Monpeyroux F *et al*. Case-control study of the frequency of thrombophilic disorders in couples with late feotal-loss and no thrombotic antecedent – the Nimes Obstetricians and Haematologists Study 5 (NOHA 5). *Thromb Haemost* 1999;**81**:891–9.

44. Mousa HA, Alfirevic Z. Do placental lesions reflect thrombophilia state in women with adverse pregnancy outcome? *Hum Reprod* 2000;**15**:1830–3.

45. Dizon-Townson DS, Meline L, Nelson LM, Varner M, War K. Fetal carriers of the factor V Leiden mutation are prone to miscarriage and placental infarction. *Am J Obstet Gynecol* 1997;**177**:402–5.

46. Kupferminc MJ, Eldor A, Steinman N *et al*. Increased frequency of genetic thrombophilias in women with complications of pregnancy. *N Engl J Med* 1999;**340**:9–13.

47. Grandone E, Margaglione M, Colaizzo D *et al*. Genetic susceptibility to pregnancy-related venous thromboembolism: roles of factor V Leiden, prothrombin G20210A, and methylenetetrahydrofolate reductase C677T mutations. *Am J Obstet Gynecol* 1998;**179**:1324–8.

48. Sanson BJ, Lensing AWA, Prins MH *et al*. Safety of low-molecular-weight heparin in pregnancy: a systematic review. *Thromb Haemost* 1999;**81**:668–72.

49. Gris JC, Neveu S, Tailland ML, Courtieu C, Mares P, Schved JF. Use of low-molecular weight heparin (enoxaparin) or of a phenformin-like substance (moroxydine chloride) in primary early recurrent aborters with an impaired fibrinolytic capacity. *Thromb Haemost* 1995;**73**:362–7.

50. Brenner B, Hoffman R, Blumenfeld Z, Weiner Z, Younis J. Gestational outcome in thrombophilic women with recurrent pregnancy loss treated by enoxaparin. *Thromb Haemost* 2000;**83**:693–97.

51. Nakabayashi M, Yamamoto S, Suzuki K. Analysis of thrombomodulin gene polymorphism in

women with severe early-onset preeclampsia. *Semin Thromb Hemost* 1999;**25**:473–9.

52. Yamada H, Kato EH, Ebina Y *et al*. Factor XII deficiency in women with recurrent miscarriage. *Gynecol Obstet Invest* 2000;**49**:80–3.

53. Laude I, Rongieres-Bertrand C, Boyer-Neumann C *et al*. Circulating procoagulant microparticles in women with unexplained pregnancy loss: a new insight. *Thromb Haemost* 2001;**85**:18–21.

17

Thrombophilia and gestational vascular complications

Michael J Kupferminc

INTRODUCTION

Pre-eclampsia, placental abruption, intrauterine growth retardation (IUGR) and intrauterine fetal death (IUFD) greatly contribute to maternal and fetal morbidity and mortality. Their causes are unknown, but all of them may be associated with abnormal placental vasculature and disturbances of hemostasis leading to inadequate maternal–fetal circulation.[1–7] Recent data from studies in pre-eclampsia suggest that endothelial dysfunction, vasoconstriction, placental ischemia and enhanced coagulation are associated with abnormal placental development, which may lead to inadequate maternal–fetal circulation and decreased placental perfusion.[8] In normal pregnancy, the trophoblasts invade the spiral arteries, which lose their muscular wall and become flaccid vessels that allow maximum blood flow to the placenta. The abnormal interaction between mother and fetal allograft in abnormal pregnancies leads to abnormal trophoblastic invasion of the spiral arteries, resulting in small, narrowed arteries. The subsequent vasculopathy and secondary thrombosis from hypercoagulability may result in inadequate perfusion of the intervillous space, pre-eclampsia, placental infarcts, IUGR, placental abruption and IUFD. In the case of pre-eclampsia, it is thought that, as pregnancy advances, the growing placenta becomes hypoxic and releases unknown substances that affect endothelial cells and begin the cascade of events that ultimately results in the clinically recognizable syndrome. The known thrombotic nature of the placental vascular lesions and the increased thrombotic risk associated with the existence of thrombophilias strongly suggest a cause–effect relationship between inherited and acquired thrombophilias and the above severe obstetric complications.

Many of the endothelial vascular changes associated with hyperhomocysteinemia can be found in pre-eclampsia.[1–5,8] As is discussed later, hyperhomocysteinemia has been associated with recurrent pregnancy loss,[9] placental infarction and abruption and stillbirth[10,11] as well as with severe pre-eclampsia.[12,13]

ANTIPHOSPHOLIPID SYNDROME AND PREGNANCY COMPLICATIONS

Antiphospholipid syndrome, an acquired autoimmune condition, is characterized by the presence of certain features and circulating antibodies. The most specific clinical features are thrombosis (both venous and arterial thrombosis), recurrent fetal loss (RFL) in the second and third trimester, and autoimmune thrombocytopenia.[14–16] Antiphospholipid syndrome is also associated with placental vascular thrombosis, decidual vasculopathy, intervillous fibrin deposition, and placental infarction.[7,17] These pathological changes in the placenta may result in abortion, IUGR, stillbirth, and early severe pre-eclampsia. In relation to fetal loss, positive test for anticardiolipin antibodies (aCL) or the presence of lupus anticoagulant (LAC) may be found in up to 20% of women with RFL.[18–23] It may present with either recurrent embryonic loss,[24] or fetal demise beyond 10 weeks' gestation.[25] Positive test for aCL or the presence of LAC is found in 10–15% of women with fetal death beyond 20 weeks of gestation.[26,27] The relation between antiphospholipid syndrome and pre-eclampsia has been shown in several studies.[27–33] In a series of more than 300 patients with severe pre-eclampsia reported by the Amsterdam group,[31] an overall incidence of 21% of detectable aCL (> 10 IgG phospholipid (GPL) units or IgM phospholipid (MPL) units) was found, with a 27.4% incidence in the group with delivery at less than 28 weeks' gestation and a 19.3% incidence in the group with delivery at more than 28 weeks' gestation. However, after considering the rate of nearly 20% of low positive immunoglobulin (Ig)G or IgM titers (< 15 GPL or MPL) in the control population of healthy female volunteers, the investigators concluded that 16% is a realistic estimate of the incidence of aCL-positive patients among those with a history of severe pre-eclampsia;[30] this is concordant with other studies.[29,32–34] It should be noted that several investigators found no correlation between antiphospholipid syndrome and pre-eclampsia.[35–37] However, most studies found an association between early-onset severe pre-eclampsia and a positive test for aCL antibodies, and testing in such patients may have therapeutic implications for future pregnancies.

Women with antiphospholipid syndrome are also at substantial risk of IUGR.[27,38–40] The rate of IUGR in women with antiphospholipid syndrome is around 30%. In one study, 24% of mothers delivered of IUGR infants had medium or high positive tests for aCL antibodies.[41]

Pre-eclampsia

The pathological findings observed in pre-eclampsia, IUGR, placental abruption, and IUFD, such as an increased number of villous infarcts, thrombosis of the spiral arteries, and endothelial dysfunction, raise the question of whether the associated hypercoagulability is a contributing factor in the pathophysiological process. Several studies have investigated the association between thrombophilias and pre-eclampsia. Dekker et al. tested women with severe pre-eclampsia at least 10 weeks postpartum for the presence of hyperhomocysteinemia, protein C deficiency, protein S deficiency, antithrombin III deficiency, activated protein C resistance (APC), LAC antibodies, and anti-aCL IgG and IgM. The results were compared with those of historical controls.[30] Of the women tested for coagulation disturbances, 24.7% had protein S deficiency, 16% had APC resistance, 17.7% had hyperhomocysteinemia, and 29.4% had IgG or IgM aCL antibodies. Dizon–Townson et al.,[42] Grandone et al.,[43] Nagy et al.[44] described a higher prevalence of factor V Leiden mutation in women with pre-eclampsia than in controls. In the study by Dizon–Townson et al.,[42] 158 women with severe pre-eclampsia were compared with 403 normotensive women, whereas in the study of Grandone et al. (in Italy), 96 women with pregnancy-induced hypertension (PIH) were compared with 129 healthy controls with a similar ethnic background.[43] Forty-five had pre-eclampsia, and 51 had non-proteinuric hypertension. Nagy et al. (in Hungary) described high prevalence of the factor V Leiden in 69 women with severe pre-eclampsia, compared with 71 healthy controls.[44] In the study by Lindoff et al., 50 women with pre-eclampsia were compared with 50 controls.[45] The APC ratios were significantly lower in women with pre-eclampsia, but the difference in factor V mutation was not significant.

Rajkovic et al. reported that homocysteine levels were doubled in 20 women with pre-eclampsia when compared with 20 healthy controls.[46] Levels of folate and vitamin B12 were similar between the groups. A significant increase in homozygosity for the C677T MTHFR mutation in pre-eclampsia was reported by Grandone et al.[43] and Shoda et al.[47] Shoda et al. tested 67 women with mild pre-eclampsia (by the criteria of the American College of Obstetricians and Gynecologists), and 98 pregnant control women, they found a 24% prevalence in women with pre-eclampsia compared with 11% in controls.[47] In several studies, however, an association between factor V Leiden and MTHFR mutations and pre-eclampsia was not found. O'Shaughnessy et al., in a prospective study performed in the East Anglian region of the UK, reported on 283 women with pre-eclampsia, who were compared with 100 age-matched normal women from the same maternity hospital and another 100 normotensive women from East Anglia, with regard to the frequency of the factor V and MTHFR mutations.[48] There was no difference in the frequency of factor V Leiden or MTHFR mutations compared with the pooled control group. Within this cohort, 149 were defined as having severe disease based only on delivery before 37 weeks' gestation, and 25 had HELLP syndrome, characterized by Hemolysis, Elevated Liver enzymes and Low Platelets. Also, no difference was found between these patients and controls in the frequency of the mutations. Powers et al. compared the prevalence of MTHFR mutation in 99 nulliparous women with pre-eclampsia, 24 women with transient hypertension of pregnancy, and 114 control women.[49] Seventy-one of the pre-eclamptic women had mild disease and 28 had severe disease. No differences were noted in homozygosity for the MTHFR mutation between the women with pre-eclampsia and the control women or between the women with severe pre-eclampsia and the control women. Folate concentrations were also similar between the groups. Krauss et al., in the only study that dealt specifically with HELLP syndrome, detected a higher incidence of APC resistance in 21 women who had HELLP syndrome, 6 months to 9 years after completion of pregnancy, compared with normal values obtained from 70 healthy non-pregnant women.[50] Four women had the factor V mutation, one woman had protein S deficiency, and one woman had protein C deficiency.

Kupferminc et al. conducted a comprehensive case control study in order to determine whether obstetric complications are associated with the genetic thrombophilic mutations.[34] One hundred and ten healthy women who had severe pre-eclampsia during pregnancy, IUGR below the fifth percentile for gestational age, severe placen-

tal abruption or IUFD before 23 weeks were enrolled in the study. The control group comprised 110 healthy patients who had had one or more normal pregnancies and who were matched for age and geographical origin. Thirty-four out of 110 patients had severe pre-eclampsia. Pre-eclampsia was characterized as severe because of blood pressure higher than 160/110 mmHg in most patients. The factor V Leiden mutation was found in 26% of patients, compared with 6.4% of the controls, whereas homozygosity for MTHFR was detected in 20.6% of the patients compared with 8.2% of the controls. The prothrombin mutation was twice as common in women with pre-eclampsia, but this was not a significant difference. Overall, 52.9% of patients with severe pre-eclampsia had a genetic thrombophilic mutation, compared with 17.3% of the controls. In addition, 14.7% study patients with another type of thrombophilia were found. Thus, the total prevalence of thrombophilias in the women with pre-eclampsia was 64.7%, compared with 18% in controls.

Women with pre-eclampsia and thrombophilia delivered at earlier gestational age and their neonates had lower birth weight than those of patients with pre-eclampsia but no thrombophilia. Half of the 44 patients with severe IUGR had a genetic thrombophilic mutation and 11.4% of the women were found to have other thrombophilias. Thus, the total prevalence of thrombophilias in IUGR was 61.4%. In placental abruption, an overall incidence of thrombophilic mutations of 60% was found, and other thrombophilias were found in another 10% of the women. In women with IUFD, the total prevalence of all thrombophilias was 50%.

Overall, 52% of patients with obstetric complications had a thrombophilic mutation and other thrombophilias were found in 13% of the women. Thus, the total prevalence of all thrombophilias detected was 65% compared with 18% in the controls. The women with obstetric complications also had a significantly higher incidence of combined thrombophilias than the controls. Of the 18 multiparous women in this group, 15 had had obstetric complications in a previous pregnancy. In 10 of these 15 multiparous women (67%), thrombophilia was found.

This indicates high rate of recurrence in these multiparous women with thrombophilias.

Following this study, van Pampus *et al.* described 345 women with a history of severe pre-eclampsia diagnosed before 34 weeks' gestation who were investigated postpartum for the presence of thrombophilias.[31] The control group consisted of 67 healthy women with a history of uncomplicated pregnancies. The women with pre-eclampsia were further divided according to whether the pre-eclampsia began before or after 28 weeks' gestation. In both these subgroups and in all the women taken as a single group, a higher prevalence of APC resistance was found compared with the control women, but the prevalence of the factor V Leiden was similar to that in the controls. Hyperhomocysteinemia was more prevalent in women with severe disease at less than 28 weeks' gestation.

Kupferminc *et al.* conducted another study on the association between severe pre-eclampsia and thrombophilias.[51] Sixty-three healthy women with severe pre-eclampsia made up the study group; 54 of them were nulliparous. Pre-eclampsia was characterized as severe because of blood pressure greater than 160/110 mmHg in 43 women, HELLP syndrome (in six women), thrombocytopenia (in six women), proteinuria in excess of 5 g per 24 hours (in six women) and eclampsia in two women. Each woman with severe pre-eclampsia was matched to two healthy control women who had had one or more normal pregnancies for their age and for the geographic origin of both parents, and all 189 women were tested for all thrombophilias. Again, factor V Leiden mutation was significantly more prevalent in women with severe pre-eclampsia, as was homozygosity for MTHFR. The prothrombin mutation was more than twice as prevalent in severe pre-eclampsia, but this difference was not significant. Overall, 56% of women with severe pre-eclampsia had a genetic thrombophilic mutation, compared with 19% in the control group. Other thrombophilias were found in 11% of women with severe pre-eclampsia, compared with 0.8% of the controls. Thus the incidence of all thrombophilias was 67% in severe pre-eclampsia, compared with 20% in the controls. Women with severe pre-eclampsia and

thrombophilia delivered earlier, and their neonates had a lower birth weight compared with the neonates of the women with pre-eclampsia but no thrombophilia. Moreover, more birth weights below the fifth percentile were seen in women with severe pre-eclampsia and thrombophilia. The incidence of combined thrombophilias was also more prevalent in those with severe pre-eclampsia. Thrombophilia was found in four of the seven multiparous study women (57%) who had had obstetric complications in a previous pregnancy.

Several more studies have emerged recently. Rigo *et al.* investigated 120 women with severe pre-eclampsia and 101 healthy women matched for age and parity.[52] Among the pre-eclamptic women, 18.3% were carriers of factor V Leiden, compared with 3% of the controls ($p < 0.001$). However, there was no difference in homozygosity for MTHFR. Among factor V Leiden-positive women, there was a statistically higher prevalence of HELLP syndrome than in factor V Leiden-negative women.

Mello *et al.* investigated the prevalence of thrombophilia in 46 women with pre-eclampsia and in 34 women with a history of fetal loss in the second and third trimester.[53] The frequency of APCR and factor V Leiden was significantly higher in women with pre-eclampsia (26.1%) or with a history of fetal loss (23%) than it was in the control group (3.8%). The prevalence of any single thrombophilia was 37% in women with a history of pre-eclampsia, 41.2% in those with a history of fetal loss, and 7.5% in the control group.

Lindqvist *et al.*, in a retrospective study, investigated the role of APC resistance and factor V Leiden in 2480 women, who were enrolled in early pregnancy.[54] The women were interviewed about their medical history, including VTE in relatives. The overall prevalence of APC resistance was 11% (270 out of 2480). The APC-resistant subgroup (270 patients) did not differ significantly from the non-APC-resistant subgroup (2210 patients) in terms of pregnancy complications but it was characterized by an eight-fold higher risk of VTE (three out of 270 versus three out of 2210), a lower rate of profuse intrapartum hemorrhage, and less intrapartum blood loss. Despite the high prevalence of APC resistance (11%) in this series of gravidae, its presence was unrelated to adverse pregnancy outcome apart from the eight-fold increased risk of VTE.

Vollset et al., in the Hodarland Homocysteine study, which is the largest performed to date, evaluated plasma homocysteine levels in 5883 women with 14,492 pregnancies.[55] When those in the upper quartile of plasma homocysteine levels were compared with those in the lower quartile, the adjusted risk for pre-eclampsia was found to be 1.32 (95% CI 0.98–1.77), the adjusted risk for prematurity was 1.38 (95% CI 1.09–1.75), that for very low birth weight was 2.01 (95% CI 1.23–3.27), and that for stillbirth was 2.03 (95% CI 0.98–4.21). Placental abruption had no correlation with the homocysteine quartile, but the adjusted odds ratio when homocysteine concentrations of more than 15 µmol/l were compared with lower concentrations was 3.13 (95% CI 1.63–6.03).

The differences between studies that have found an association between pre-eclampsia and thrombophilia and those that have not may be related to different populations studied, the study design used and the type of pre-eclampsia. For example, the factor V Leiden mutation is highly prevalent among the Caucasian population, the prevalence being 10–15% in Sweden, 4–8% in central Europe, and 2% in southern Europe, with some exceptions. In the USA, a prevalence of 5% is reported. The mutation is almost non-existent in Asia, Japan, Africa and South America. This stresses the need for meticulous matching in studies that compare the mutation prevalence in women who have had obstetric complications such as pre-eclampsia or IUGR with women who have had normal pregnancies. Pre-eclampsia is a multigenetic disease, and there are important differences in prognosis and management between late, mild pre-eclampsia and early-onset, severe disease. Most studies suggest that there is an association between thrombophilias and the development of severe pre-eclampsia but not mild pre-eclampsia. In the presence of a maternal hypercoagulable state, the low-pressure intervillous blood flow may trigger fibrin deposition in the placenta and cause placental infarcts, which may

cause the development of early, severe disease. This also could be the explanation for the observations that the women with pre-eclampsia and thrombophilia had higher rates of IUGR and also delivered at an earlier gestational age than women with pre-eclampsia but without thrombophilia.[51]

Placental abruption or placental infarction

van der Molen et al. investigated coagulation inhibitors and abnormalities of the homocysteine metabolism as risk factors for placental vasculopathy.[10] They compared non-pregnant women with a history of placental vasculopathy (defined as placental abruption or placental infarction) with non-pregnant women matched for age and occupation. Placental infarction was defined as villous necrosis combined with a stillborn baby or IUGR less than the tenth percentile. Twenty-two of the 101 patients also had hypertension during pregnancy. Protein C activity was significantly lower in the study group, and homozygotes for the MTHFR mutation and carriers of the factor V Leiden were significantly more common in the study group. The median homocysteine levels, APC resistance ratio, protein S level and antithrombin level III were not different between the groups. However, a significant odds ratio for homocysteine concentrations above 14.4 µmol/l was found; this was the 80th percentile of the controls. Moreover, a combination of risk factors (e.g. homocysteine above 14.4 µmol/l and protein S deficiency) resulted in a significant odds ratio. Thus, the thrombotic risk factors for placental vasculopathy are decreased levels of APC resistance and protein C, elevated homocysteine levels, and the MTHFR mutation (or a combination of these factors).

Wiener–Megnagi et al. studied 27 women who had placental abruption and 29 control subjects matched for age, parity, and ethnic origin.[56] Sixty-three percent of the patients had an activated protein C ratio ≤ 2.5, compared with 17% of the control subjects (odds ratio 8.16, $p = 0.00125$). Only participants with APC resistance ≤ 2.5 underwent DNA analysis. Eight out of 15 patients tested (29.6%) were found to have the factor V Leiden (five were heterozygous and three were homozygous); there was one heterozygote (3.4%) among the control subjects who were tested.

Goddjin-Wessel *et al.* found hyperhomocysteinemia in 31% of women with abruption infarction, compared with 9% of controls ($p < 0.05$).[57] Kupferminc *et al.* found a 70% incidence in thrombophilia in women with placental abruption.[34] Sixty percent of the women had thrombophilic mutations and 10% had antithrombin III deficiency or antiphospholipid syndrome. Twenty women had placental abruption; among these, three also had mild pre-eclampsia and seven had antepartum or postpartum hypertension; eleven of this group's neonates were below the 10th percentile for gestational age. In this study, which was the first to examine the prothrombin mutation in women with pregnancy complications, the odds ratio for this mutation in women with abruptio placenta was 8.9 (95% CI 1.8–43.6), whereas the odds ratio for factor V Leiden in these women was 4.9 (95% CI 1.4–17.4) and the odds ratio for MTHFR mutation was 2 (CI 0.5–8.1).

IUGR

Few studies have reported the association of IUGR and thrombophilia. de Vries *et al.* studied thrombophilias in 62 women with obstetric complications but the study did not have a control group.[58] Thirty-one women had placental abruption, 18 had IUFD, and 13 had IUGR. Most prominent in women with IUGR was the high incidence of hyperhomocysteinemia (38%), protein S deficiency (23%) and factor V Leiden mutation (12.5%).

Kupferminc *et al.* found that women with severe IUGR had a higher prevalence of homozygosity for MTHFR and a higher prevalence of the prothrombin mutation.[34] The factor V Leiden mutation was twice as common in the study group but this difference was not significant. The prevalence of all thrombophilias in the women with IUGR was 61.4%.

Recently, Kupferminc *et al.*, in another study, tested the prothrombin mutation in 222 patients with severe pre-eclampsia (55 patients), mild pre-eclampsia (25 patients), IUGR defined as birthright below the 10th percentile (72 patients), severe placental abruption (27 patients), unexplained stillbirth later than 23 weeks' gestation (16 patients), second trimester fetal loss (7 patients) and three or more consecutive first trimester losses (20 patients).[59] The control group comprised 156 healthy women who had had at least one normal pregnancy. Twenty-eight women in the study group (13%) were found to be heterozygous carriers of the 20210 variant of the prothrombin gene, compared with five (3.2%) of the control group (odds ratio 2.9, 95% CI 1.3–6.5, $p = 0.001$). Compared with the control women, the prothrombin gene mutation was significantly more prevalent in women with IUGR, placental abruption, and second trimester loss, but it was not significantly more prevalent in women with mild or severe pre-eclampsia, stillbirth and habitual abortion. The 28 women in the study group who were carriers of the prothrombin mutation had 62 pregnancies, of which only seven (11.3%) were normal. Within the study group, of the nine multiparous carriers of the mutation, six (66%) had had complications in previous pregnancies, compared with 27 out of 112 (24%) multiparous women without the mutation in the study group ($p = 0.01$).

Other thrombophilias and pregnancy complications

Recently, the role of genetic hypofibrinolysis was also investigated for an association with obstetric complications.[60] Inherited hypofibrinolytic mutations are also associated with miscarriage,[61] prematurity, IUFD, IUGR, pre-eclampsia, and placental abruption.[62] Genetic abnormalities in fibrinolysis have been described in the plasminogen activator inhibitor (PAI-1) gene, which acts as a fast-acting inhibitor of tissue plasminogen activator activity and is the major circulating inhibitor of fibrinolysis.[61–63] The PAI-1 gene contains several polymorphic loci, including a 4G/5G insertion–deletion.[64] PAI-1 levels in 4G/4G subjects are approximately 25% higher than in 5G/5G subjects; the 4G/4G mutation is associated with increased risk of thrombosis.[61,63,64]

Glueck *et al.* compared 94 women who had had obstetric complications with 95 matched controls who had had normal pregnancies.[60] Women with obstetric complications were more likely than controls to be 4G/4G homozygotes (32% versus 19%, odds ratio 2.0, 95% CI 1.02–3.9). Factor V Leiden was much more common in the patients who had PAI-1 4G/4G than in the 18 4G/4G controls (33% versus 0%, Fisher's $p = 0.008$). Therefore women with severe pre-eclampsia, placental abruption, severe IUGR, and IUFD have an increased incidence of the hypofibrinolytic 4G/4G mutation of the PAI-1 gene, which is frequently associated with factor V Leiden, further predisposing them to thrombosis.

This finding is in agreement with previous findings.[61,62] Factor V Leiden-induced thrombosis in the placental bed with subsequent hypoxia might enhance expression of PAI-1 as an important mechanism suppressing fibrinolysis under conditions of low oxygen tension.[65] In a previous study the 4G/4G mutation was positively and independently associated with adverse pregnancy outcomes, including prematurity, miscarriage, stillbirth, IUGR, eclampsia, and placental abruption.[62] The 4G/4G homozygosity of the PAI-1 gene is often associated with venous or arterial thrombosis (or both).[61,63,64,66] High levels of PAI activity (the PAI-1 gene product) can contribute to the initiation of placental damage and to thrombotic complications that occur in pre-eclampsia.[67,68] High levels of PAI activity also contribute to miscarriage in early pregnancy.[61,69,70] Gris *et al.* reported high PAI activity in 616 patients with unexplained early recurrent miscarriages of unknown origin.[71,72] They speculated that impaired plasmin-dependent proteolysis in women might favor miscarriage by inhibiting early placental circulation or by limiting trophoblast development (or both). Recently, Yamada *et al.* reported on similar results of the association between 4G/5G polymorphism of the PAI-1 gene and severe pre-eclampsia.[73]

PLACENTAL FINDINGS ASSOCIATED WITH THROMBOPHILIAS AND PREGNANCY COMPLICATIONS

Kupferminc *et al.* described placental findings in women who had severe complications during pregnancy and were carriers of thrombophilias, and compared them to women with severe complications during pregnancy but who had no thrombophilias.[74] Sixty-eight women with singleton pregnancies who had severe pre-eclampsia, IUGR, placental abruption, or IUFD comprised the study population. They were evaluated after delivery for the occurrence of mutations of factor V Leiden, MTHFR, and the prothrombin gene, and for deficiencies of protein S, protein C, and antithrombin III. All were negative for the antiphospholipid antibodies. Thirty-two women carried a thrombophilia and 36 women did not. All placentas were evaluated by a single pathologist who was blinded for the results of thrombophilic assessment. Each placenta was examined for villous infarcts, fibrinoid necrosis of decidual vessels, vessel thrombosis, evidence of placental abruption, syncytiotrophoblast knotting, perivillous fibrin deposition, and absent physiological changes of the spiral arteries. The parameters were graded according to severity. There was no difference between the groups in the maternal age, parity, type of pregnancy complication, and fetal–placental weight ratio. The gestational age at delivery, the birth weight and the placental weight were significantly lower in the 32 women with thrombophilias than in the 36 women without thrombophilias. There were no differences between the two groups in the parameters of thrombosis, placental abruption, syncytiotrophoblast knotting, perivillous fibrin deposition or the degree of physiological change in the spiral arteries. However, the number of women with villous infarcts was significantly higher among those with thrombophilia (72% versus 39%, $p < 0.01$), as was the number of women with multiple infarcts ($p < 0.05$). The incidence of placentas with fibrinoid necrosis of decidual vessels was also significantly higher in women with thrombophilias ($p < 0.05$). The study concluded that the placentas of women with severe complications and thrombophilia have an increased rate of infarctions compared with the placentas of women with similar complications but no thrombophilia. This increased rate may reflect a higher degree of vascular damage in women with thrombophilia.

However, in a recent study with a very similar design, which also examined the relationship between placental histology and thrombophilia in women with severe complications, no specific histological pattern could be identified when thrombophilia-positive and thrombophilia-negative groups were compared.[75]

Arias et al. evaluated 13 women with thrombotic lesions of the placenta.[76] All the women had had obstetric complications such as pre-eclampsia, preterm labor, IUGR or stillbirth. In 10 of the 13 women (77%) inherited thrombophilias were found; seven were heterozygous for factor V Leiden and three had protein S deficiency. The most prominent placental lesions were fetal stem vessel thrombosis, infarcts, hypoplasia, spiral artery thrombosis, and perivillous fibrin deposition.

SCREENING FOR THROMBOPHILIA

Who should be screened for thrombophilia? Although at the moment our knowledge of the optimal treatment during pregnancy is limited, the data suggest that certain risk groups should be screened for thrombophilia, including pregnant women with a personal or family of thromboembolism. Testing should also be performed for women with a history of recurrent first trimester loss, second trimester loss, IUFD, severe pre-eclampsia, IUGR or placental abruption.

MANAGEMENT OF WOMEN WITH THROMBOPHILIA AND OBSTETRIC COMPLICATIONS

Are women with pregnancy complications or placental thrombosis and thrombophilias candidates for antithrombotic therapy as those with venous and arterial thrombosis? There are no controlled trials to guide us how to manage women with thrombophilia and previous placental thrombosis or severe pregnancy complications. However, some data presented above suggest a high recurrence rate of complications in future pregnancies in women who have had pregnancy complications and are

carriers of thrombophilia.[34,51,59] In these studies, in relatively small groups of women, high recurrence rates of 50–60% were shown.[34,51,59] Nevertheless, it is not known how we should treat these women with pregnancy complications or placental thrombosis associated with thrombophilias in subsequent pregnancies.

In women with thrombophilia and no history of thromboembolism but with a history of severe pre-eclampsia, fetal loss or other severe complications, antithrombotic therapy seems reasonable, although data are limited. The combination of aspirin and heparin or low molecular weight heparin is effective in recurrent fetal loss in antiphospholipid syndrome, and it could be considered for women with inherited thrombophilias and a history of severe pre-eclampsia, IUGR, placental abruption, or fetal loss, although no controlled studies are currently available.

Riyazi et al. evaluated treatment with low molecular weight heparin combined with aspirin in pregnant women with thrombophilia and a history of pre-eclampsia or IUGR.[77] A total of 276 patients with a history of pre-eclampsia or fetal growth restriction were tested for the presence of coagulation abnormalities and aCL antibodies. Ninety patients with pre-eclampsia and 15 patients with isolated fetal growth restriction had haemostatic abnormalities. Twenty-six patients with coagulation abnormalities – protein S deficiency, APC resistance, or elevated aCL antibodies (≥ 15 GPL or MPL) – had a subsequent pregnancy and were treated with low molecular weight heparin plus aspirin. Their pregnancy outcome was compared with all the patients from the same cohort who had a subsequent pregnancy without abnormalities and who had received aspirin (19 patients). There was no difference in birth weight between the groups; however, when 18 patients out of 26 with single coagulation abnormalities (excluding those with multiple thrombophilias) were considered, the birth weights were found to be significantly higher ($p = 0.019$) than the birth weights of the neonates of the 19 patients with no abnormality. The other eight patients had combined thrombophilia and may have required higher doses. Two perinatal deaths occurred in the aspirin group. In this preliminary study, low molecular weight heparin appears to have a favorable effect on the pregnancy outcome of women with a history of pre-eclampsia or IUGR plus documented thrombophilia.

Leeda et al. studied the effects of folate and vitamin B6 supplementation on women with hyperhomocysteinemia and a history of pre-eclampsia or IUGR.[78] A total of 207 consecutive patients with a history of pre-eclampsia or IUGR were tested for hyperhomocysteinemia. Thirty-seven were found to be positive and were treated with folate and vitamin B6, and 27 had a second methionine loading test after vitamin supplementation. Fourteen patients became pregnant again while receiving vitamins and aspirin. All patients who underwent a methionine loading test after vitamin supplementation had a completely normalized methionine loading test. Of the 14 pregnancies in women receiving vitamins and aspirin, seven were complicated by pre-eclampsia. Birth weights were 2867 ± 648 g, compared with 1088 ± 570 g in the previous pregnancies ($p < 0.001$). Thus, vitamin B6 and folate correct the methionine loading test in patients with hyperhomocysteinemia. Vitamin supplementation in patients with a history of pre-eclampsia or fetal growth restriction and hyperhomocysteinemia appears to be favorable effect on birth weight but not the rate of pre-eclampsia.

Kupferminc et al. conducted the largest treatment study with low molecular weight heparin.[79] The study group comprised 33 consecutive women who had had one of four severe pregnancy complications in their last pregnancy: severe pre-eclampsia (12 patients), severe placental abruption (5 patients), severe IUGR (11 patients), or IUFD after 23 weeks' gestation (5 patients). In all the women, thrombophilias (mutations of factor V Leiden, MTHFR, prothrombin mutation or protein S deficiency) were detected several months after delivery. In the subsequent pregnancies, all women received low molecular weight heparin (enoxaparin 40 mg/day), which was started at 8–12 weeks' gestation and continued until 6 weeks postpartum. The patients also received aspirin 100 g/day from 8–12 weeks' gestation until 37–38 weeks' gestation. Twenty women were primiparous and the 13 women who were multiparous had had 34 pregnancies, of which only three (8.8%) had been normal. The mean gestational age at delivery in the untreated pregnancies was 32.1 ± 5.0 weeks, compared with 37.6 ± 2.3 weeks in the ensuing pregnancies, which were treated with combined low molecular weight heparin and aspirin ($p < 0.0001$). The mean birth weight of the infants in the untreated pregnancies was 1175 ± 590 g, compared with 2719 ± 526 g in the treated pregnancies ($p < 0.0001$). Pregnancy complications occurred in only three (9.1%) of the treated women. One patient had mild pre-eclampsia, oligohydramnios, and late decelerations and was delivered of a 960 g neonate at 30 weeks' gestation. The other two patients had IUGR. Their neonates were born at week 35 (1300 g) and at week 33 (1070 g). All the neonates survived with no major morbidities.

The results of this study suggest that low molecular weight heparin may be effective in preventing recurrence of late pregnancy complications in women with a history of gestational vascular complications. However, double blind controlled randomized trials are needed to establish the efficacy of low molecular weight heparin in the prevention of recurrence of pregnancy complications in this population.

REFERENCES

1. Roberts JM, Taylor RN, Musici TJ, Rodgers GM, Hubel CA, McLaughlin MK. Pre-eclampsia: an endothelial cell disorder. *Am J Obstet Gynecol* 1989;**161**:1200–4.
2. Salafia CM, Pezzulo JC, Lopez-Zeno JA, Minior VK, Vintzileos AM. Placental pathologic features of preterm pre-eclampsia. *Am J Obstet Gynecol* 1995;**173**:1079–1105.
3. Shanklin DR, Sibai BM. Ultrastructural aspects of pre-eclampsia. *Am J Obstet Gynecol* 1989;**161**:735–41.
4. Khong TY, Pearce JM, Robertson WB. Acute atherosis in pre-eclampsia: maternal determination and

fetal outcome in the presence of the lesion. *Am J Obstet Gynecol* 1987;**157**:360–3.

5. Salafia CM, Minior VK, Pezzulo JC, Popek EJ, Rosenkrantz TS, Vintzileos AM. Intrauterine growth restriction in infants of less than thirty-two weeks' gestation: associated placental pathologic features. *Am J Obstet Gynecol* 1995;**173**:1049–57.

6. Green JR. Placenta previa and abruptio placentae. In: Creasy RK, Resnik R, eds. *Maternal Fetal Medicine: Principles and Practice*. Philadelphia: WB Saunders; 1994:609–19.

7. Infante-Rievard C, David M, Gauthier R, Ribard GE. Lupus anticoagulants, anticardiolipin antibodies and fetal loss. *N Engl J Med* 1991;**325**:1063–6.

8. Dekker GA, Sibai BM. Etiology and pathophysiology of pre-eclampsia: current concepts. AJOG Review. *Am J Obstet Gynecol* 1998;**179**:1359–75.

9. Wouters MG, Boers GH, Blom HJ *et al.* Hyperhomocysteinemia: a risk factor in women with unexplained recurrent early pregnancy loss. *Fertil Steril* 1993;**60**:820–5.

10. van der Molen EF, Verbruggen B, Novakova I, Eskes TK, Monnens LA, Blom HJ. Hyperhomocysteinemia and other thrombotic risk factors in women with placental vasculopathy. *Br J Obstet Gynaecol* 2000;**107**:785–91.

11. de Vries JI, Dekker GA, Huijgens PC, Jakobs C, Blomberg BM, van Geijn HP. Hyperhomocystinemia and protein S deficiency in complicated pregnancies. *Br J Obstet Gynaecol* 1997;**104**:1248–54.

12. Dekker GA, de Vries JI, Doelitzsch PM, *et al.* Underlying disorders associated with severe early-onset pre-eclampsia. *Am J Obstet Gynecol* 1995;**173**:1042–8.

13. Van Pampus MG, Dekker GA, Wolf H, *et al.* High prevalence of hemostatic abnormalities in women with a history of pre-eclampsia. *Am J Obstet Gynecol* 1999;**180**:1146–50.

14. Alarcon-Segovia D, Delete M, Oria CV, *et al.* Antiphospholipid antibodies and the antiphospholipid syndrome in systemic lupus erythematosus: a prospective analysis of 500 consecutive patients. *Medicine* 1989;**68**:353–65.

15. Asherson RA, Khamashta MA, Ordi-Ros J, *et al.* The 'primary' anti-phospholipid syndrome: major clinical and serological features. *Medicine* 1989;**68**:366–74.

16. Harris EN. Syndrome of the black swan. *Br J Rheumatol* 1987;**26**:324–6.

17. Rand JH, Xiao-Xuan W, Andree HAM, *et al.* Pregnancy loss in the antiphospholid-antibody syndrome: a possible thrombogenic mechanism. *N Engl J Med* 1997;**337**:154–60.

18. Branch DW, Silver RM, Pierangeli S, van Leeuwen I, Harris EN. Antiphospholipid antibodies other than lupus anticoagulant and anticardiolipin antibodies in women with recurrent pregnancy loss, fertile controls, and antiphospholipid syndrome. *Obstet Gynecol* 1997;**89**:549–55.

19. MacLean MA, Cumming GP, McCall F, Walker ID, Wallter JJ. The prevalence of lupus anticoagulant and anticardiolipin antibodies in women with a history of first trimester miscarriages. *Br J Obstet Gynaecol* 1994;**101**:103–10.

20. Out HJ, Bruinse HW, Christiaens GCML, *et al.* Prevalence of antiphospholipid antibodies in patients with fetal loss. *Ann Rheum Dis* 1991;**50**:553–7.

21. Parazzini F, Acaia B, Faden D, Lovotti M, Marelli G. Cortelazzo S. Antiphospholipid antibodies and recurrent abortion. *Obstet Gynecol* 1991;**77**:854–8.

22. Petri M, Golbus M, Anderson R, Whiting-O'Keefe Q, Corash L, Hellmann D. Antinuclear antibody, lupus anticoagulant, and anticardiolipin antibody in women with idiopathic habitual abortion. A controlled prospective study of forty-four women. *Arthritis Rheum* 1987;**30**:601–6.

23. Yetman DL, Kutteh WH. Antiphospholipid antibody panels and recurrent pregnancy loss: prevalence of anticardiolipin antibodies compared with other antiphospholipid antibodies. *Fertil Steril* 1996;**66**:540–6.

24. Rai RS, Clifford K, Cohen H, Regan L. High prospective fetal loss rate in untreated pregnancies of women with recurrent miscarriage and antiphospholipid antibodies. *Hum Reprod* 1995;**10**:3301–4.

25. Oshiro BT, Silver RM, Scott JR, Yu H, Branch DW. Antiphospholipid antibodies and fetal death. *Obstet Gynecol* 1996;**87**:489–93.

26. Bocciolone L, Meroni P, Parazrini F *et al.* Antiphospholipid antibodies and risk of intrauterine late fetal death. *Acta Obstet Gynecol Scand* 1994;**73**:389–92.

27. Branch DW, Silver RM, Blackwell JL, Reading JC, Scott JR. Outcome of treated pregnancies in women with antiphospholipid syndrome: an update of the Utah experience. *Obstet Gynecol* 1992;**80**:614–20.

28. Scott RAH. Anti-cardiolipin antibodies and pre-eclampsia. *Br J Obstet Gynaecol* 1987;**94**:604–5.

29. Branch DW, Andres R, Digre KB, Rote NS, Scott JR. The association of antiphospholipid antibodies

with severe pre-eclampsia. *Obstet Gynecol* 1989;**73**:541–5.

30. Dekker GA, de Vries JIP, Doelitzsch PM *et al.* Underlying disorders associated with severe early-onset pre-eclampsia. *Am J Obstet Gynecol* 1995;**173**:1042–8.

31. van Pampus MG, Dekker GA, Wolf H, *et al.* High prevalence of hemostatic abnormalities in women with a history of severe pre-eclampsia. *Am J Obstet Gynecol* 1999;**180**:1146–50.

32. Pattison NS, Chamley LW, McKay W, Liggins GC, Butler WS. Antiphospholipid antibodies in pregnancy: prevalence and clinical associations. *Br J Obstet Gynaecol* 1993;**100**:909–13.

33. Yasuda M, Takakuwa K, Tokunaga A, Tanaka K. Prospective studies of the association between anticardiolipin antibody and outcome of pregnancy. *Obstet Gynecol* 1995;**86**:555–9.

34. Kupferminc MJ, Eldor A, Steinman N *et al.* Increased frequency of the genetic thrombophilia in women with complications of pregnancy. *N Engl J Med* 1999;**340**:9–13.

35. Rajah SB, Moodley J, Pudifin D, Duursma J. Anticardiolipin antibodies in hypertensive emergencies. *Clin Exp Hypertens Pregnancy* 1990;**B9**:267–71.

36. Out HJ, Bruinse HW, Christiaens GCML, *et al.* A prospective, controlled multicenter study on the obstetric risks of pregnant women with antiphospholipid antibodies. *Am J Obstet Gynecol* 1992;**167**:26–32.

37. Lynch A, Marlar R, Murphy J, *et al.* Antiphospholipid antibodies in predicting adverse pregnancy outcome. A prospective study. *Ann Intern Med* 1994;**120**:470–5.

38. Branch DW, Scott JR, Kochenour NK, Hershgold E. Obstetric complications associated with lupus anticoagulant. *N Engl J Med* 1985;**313**:1322–6.

39. Caruso A, De Carolis S, Ferrazzani S, Valesini G, Caforio L, Manusco S. Pregnancy outcome in relation to uterine artery flow velocity waveforms and clinical characteristics in women with antiphospholipid syndrome. *Obstet Gynecol* 1993;**82**:970–6.

40. Lima F, Khamashta MA, Buchanan NMM, Kerslake S, Hunt BI, Hughes GRV. A study of sixty pregnancies in patients with the antiphospholipid syndrome. *Clin Exp Rheumatol* 1996;**14**:131–6.

41. Polzin WJ, Kopelman JN, Robinson RD, Read JA. Brady K. The association of antiphospholipid antibodies with pregnancy complicated by fetal growth restriction. *Obstet Gynecol* 1991;**78**:1108–11.

42. Dizon-Townson DS, Nelson LM, Easton K, Ward K. The factor V Leiden mutation may predispose women to severe pre-eclampsia. *Am J Obstet Gynecol* 1996;**175**:902–5.

43. Grandone E, Margaglione M, Colaizzo D, *et al.* Factor V Leiden, C > T MTHFR polymorphism and genetic susceptibility to pre-eclampsia. *Thromb Haemost* 1997;**77**:1052–4.

44. Nagy B, Tóth T, Rigó JJR, Karádi I, Romics L, Papp Z. Detection of factor V Leiden in severe pre-eclamptic Hungarian women. *Clin Genet* 1998;**53**:478–81.

45. Lindoff C, Ingemarsson I, Martinsson G, Segelmark M, Thysell H, Astedt B. Pre-eclampsia is associated with reduced response to activated protein C. *Am J Obstet Gynecol* 1997;**176**:457–60.

46. Rajkovic A, Catlano PM, Malinow MR. Elevated homocysteine levels with pre-eclampsia. *Obstet Gynecol* 1997;**90**:168–71.

47. Sohda S, Arinami T, Hamada HM, Yamada N, Hamaguchi H, Kubo T. Methylenetetrahydrofolate reductase polymorphism and pre-eclampsia. *J Med Genet* 1997;**34**:525–6.

48. O'Shaughnessy KM, Fu B. Ferraro F, Lewis I, Downing S, Morris NH. Factor V Leiden and thermolabile methylenetetrahydrofolate reductase gene variants in an East Anglian pre-eclampsia cohort. *Hypertension* 1999;**33**:1338–41.

49. Powers RW, Minich LA, Lykins DL, Ness RB, Crombleholme WR, Roberts JM. Methylenetetrahydrofolate reductase polymorphism, folate, and susceptibility to pre-eclampsia. *J Soc Gynecol Invest* 1999;**6**:74–9.

50. Krauss T, Augustin HG, Osmers R, Meden H, Unterhalt M, Kuhn W. Activated protein C resistance and factor V Leiden in patients with hemolysis, elevated liver enzymes, low platelets syndrome. *Obstet Gynecol* 1998;**92**:457–60.

51. Kupferminc MJ, Fait G, Many A, Gordon D, Eldor A, Lessing JB. Severe pre-eclampsia and high frequency of genetic thrombophilic mutations. *Obstet Gynecol* 2000;**96**:45–9.

52. Rigo J Jr, Nagy B, Fintor L, *et al.* Maternal and neonatal outcome of preeclamptic pregnancies: the potential roles of factor V Leiden mutation and 5,10 methylenetetrahydrofolate reductase. *Hypertens Pregnancy* 2000;**19**:163–72.

53. Mello G, Parretti E, Martini E *et al.* Usefulness of screening for congenital or acquired hemostatic abnormalities in women with previous complicated pregnancies. *Haemostasis* 1999;**29**:197–203.

54. Lindqvist PG, Svensson PJ, Marsaal K, Grennert

L, Luterkort M, Dahlback B. Activated protein C resistance (FV:Q506) and pregnancy. *Thromb Haemost* 1999;**81**:532–7.

55. Vollset SE, Refsum H, Irgens LM *et al.* Plasma total homocysteine, pregnancy complications, and adverse pregnancy outcomes: the Hordaland Homocysteine study. *Am J Clin Nutr* 2000;**71**: 962–8.

56. Wiener-Megnagi Z, Ben-Shlomo I, Goldberg Y, Shalev E. Resistance to activated protein C and the Leiden mutation: high prevalence in patients with abruptio placentae. *Am J Obstet Gynecol* 1998;**179**:1565–7.

57. Goddijn-Wessel TA, Wouters MG, van de Molen EF, *et al.* Hyperhomocystinemia: a risk factor for placental abruption or infarction. *Eur J Obstet Gynecol Reprod Biol* 1996;**66**:23–9.

58. de Vries JI, Dekker GA, Huijgens PC, Jakobs C, Blomberg BM, van Geijn HP. Hyperhomo-cystinemia and protein S deficiency in compli-cated pregnancies. *Br J Obstet Gynaecol* 1997; **104**:1248–54.

59. Kupferminc MJ, Peri H, Zwang E, Yaron Y, Wolman I, Eldor A. High prevalence of the prothrombin gene mutation in women with intrauterine growth retardation, abruptio placen-tae and second trimester loss. *Acta Obstet Gynecol Scand* 2000;**11**:963–7.

60. Glueck CJ, Kupferminc MJ, Fontaine RN, Wang P, Weksler BB, Eldor A. Increased frequency of the hypofibrinolytic 4G/4G polymorphism of the plasminogen activator inhibitor-1 (PAI-1) gene in women with obstetric complications. *Obstet Gynecol* 2001;**97**:44–8.

61. Glueck CJ, Wang P, Fontaine RN, Sieve-Smith L, Tracy T, Moore SK. Plasminogen activator inhibitor activity: an independent risk factor for the high miscarriage rate during pregnancy in women with polycystic ovary syndrome. *Metabolism* 1999;**48**:1589–95.

62. Glueck CJ, Phillips H, Cameron D, *et al.* The 4G/4G polymorphism of the hypofibrinolytic PAI-1 gene: an independent risk factor for serious pregnancy complications. *Metabolism* 2000;**49**: 845–52.

63. Eriksson P, Kallin B, van't Hooft FM, Bavenholm P, Hamsten A. Allele-specific increase in basal transcription of the plasminogen-activator inhibitor 1 gene is associated with myocardial infarction. *Proc Natl Acad Sci USA* 1995;**92**:1851–5.

64. Glueck CJ, Fontaine RN, Gruppo R, *et al.* The plasminogen activator inhibitor-1 gene, hypofib-rinolysis, and osteonecrosis. *Clin Orthop* 1999; **366**:133–46.

65. Pinsky DJ, Liao H, Lawson CA, *et al.* Coordinated induction of plasminogen activator inhibitor-1 (PAI-1) and inhibition of plasminogen activator gene expression by hypoxia promotes pulmonary vascular fibrin deposition. *J Clin Invest* 1998;**102**:919–28.

66. Glueck CJ, Bell H, Vadlamani L, *et al.* Heritable thrombophilia and hypofibrinolysis. Possible causes of retinal vein occlusion. *Arch Ophthalmol* 1999;**117**:43–9.

67. Estelles A, Grancha S, Gilabert J, *et al.* Abnormal expression of plasminogen activator inhibitors in patients with gestationa trophoblastic disease. *Am J Pathol* 1996;**149**:1229–39.

68. Halligan A, Bonnar J, Sheppard B, Darling M, Walshe J. Haemostatic, fibrinolytic, and endothelial variables in normal pregnancies and pre-eclampsia. *Br J Obstet Gynaecol* 1994;**101**: 488–92.

69. Estelles A, Gilabert J, Keeton M, *et al.* Altered expression of plasminogen activator inhibitor type 1 in placentas from pregnant women with pre-eclampsia and/or intrauterine fetal growth retardation. *Blood Coagul Fibrinolysis* 1995;**6**: 703–8.

70. Estelles A, Gilabert J, Aznar J, Loskutoff DJ, Schleef RR. Changes in plasma levels of type 1 and 2 plasminogen activator inhibitors in normal pregnancy and in patients with severe pre-eclampsia. *J Obstet Gynaecol Res* 1996;**22**:9–16.

71. Gris JC, Ripart-Neveu S, Maugard C, *et al.* Respective evaluation of the prevalence of haemostasis abnormalities in unexplained primary early recurrent miscarriages. The Nimes Obstetricians and Haematologists (NOHA) study. *Thromb Haemost* 1997;**77**:1096–103.

72. Gris JC, Neuveu S, Mares P, Biron C, Hedon B, Schved JF. Plasma fibrinolytic activators and their inhibitors in women suffering from early recurrent abortion of unknown etiology. *J Lab Clin Med* 1993;**122**:606–15.

73. Yamada N, Arinami T, Yamakawa-Kobayashi K, *et al.* The 4G/5G polymorphism of the plasminogen activator inhibitor-1 gene is associated with severe pre-eclampsia. *J Hum Genet* 2000;**45**:138b–141b.

74. Many A, Schreiber L, Rosner S *et al.* Pathologic features of the placenta in women with severe pregnancy complications and thrombophilia. *Obstet Gynecol* 2001;**98**:1041–4.

75. Mousa HA, Alfirevic Z. Do placental lesions reflect thrombophilia state in women with adverse pregnancy outcome? *Hum Reprod* 2000;**15**:1830–3.

76. Arias F, Romero R, Joist H, Kraus FT. Thrombophilia: a mechanism of disease in women with adverse pregnancy outcome and thrombotic lesions in the placenta. *J Matern Fetal Med* 1998;**7**:277–86.

77. Riyazi N, Leeda, M, de Vries JI, Huijgens PC, van Geijn HP, Dekker GA. Low-molecular-weight heparin combined with aspirin in pregnant women with thrombophilia and a history of preeclampsia or fetal growth restriction: a preliminary study. *Eur J Obstet Gynecol Reprod Biol* 1998;**80**:49–54.

78. Leeda M, Riyazi N, de Vries JI, Jakobs C, van Geijn HP, Dekker GA. Effects of folic acid and vitamin B6 supplementation on women with hyperhomocysteinemia and a history of pre-eclampsia or fetal growth restriction. *Am J Obstet Gynecol* 1998;**179**:135–9.

79. Kupferminc MJ, Fait G, Many A, *et al*. Low molecular weight heparin for the prevention of obstetric complications in women with thrombophilias. *Hypertens Pregnancy* 2001;**20**:35–44.

18

Disseminated intravascular coagulation in pregnancy and amniotic fluid embolism

Shmuel Gillis

DISSEMINATED INTRAVASCULAR COAGULATION

INTRODUCTION

Disseminated intravascular coagulation (DIC) is a distinct clinical syndrome, characterized by widespread activation of the coagulation cascade, leading to intravascular formation of fibrin and thrombotic occlusion of small and medium-sized vessels; in parallel, consumption and depletion of platelets and coagulation proteins, coupled with activation of the fibrinolytic system, may result in severe bleeding (Figure 18.1).[1] In most obstetric patients, as in many other cases, the bleeding manifestations predominate.[2,3]

The most common clinical condition associated with DIC is infection, most commonly Gram-negative or Gram-positive sepsis.[1,3,4]

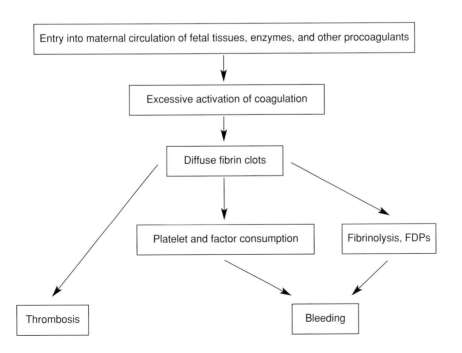

Figure 18.1
Pathophysiology of pregnancy-associated DIC.

Although severe bacterial infection with DIC may also occur during pregnancy and the puerperium, DIC is associated with several conditions unique to the obstetric patient, including placental abruption, pre-eclampsia and eclampsia, induced abortion, acute fatty liver of pregnancy and prolonged intrauterine fetal demise.[2,3] Amniotic fluid embolism is discussed separately in this chapter. Obstetric complications were the cause of DIC in 18 patients out of a total of 464 patients (3.9%) with DIC reported in two large series.[5,6] Since the pathophysiology of DIC in these disorders has many similarities, a brief discussion of the mechanisms of DIC precedes a more detailed review of the relevant clinical syndromes.

PATHOPHYSIOLOGY

The mechanism common to all events that trigger DIC is excessive widespread activation of the coagulation system. For example, leakage of thromboplastin-like material into the maternal systemic circulation is the likely cause of DIC in most obstetric disorders. Other mechanisms include the release of fat, phospholipids and tissue factor into the circulation that may follow extensive trauma.[1] In patients with infection, bacterial endotoxin or exotoxin is responsible for activating the coagulation cascade.[1,4]

Excessive activation of coagulation results in increased thrombin formation, leading to fibrin deposition in the microvasculature.[1,3] Substantial microvascular thrombosis may cause end-organ damage, primarily in the cardiac, pulmonary, renal, hepatic and central nervous systems.[7] Thrombin also indirectly causes thrombosis by inducing release from monocytes of tumor necrosis factor and interleukin-1,[8] as well as by inducing release from endothelial cells of thrombomodulin, E-selectin and endothelin.[8–10] Endothelin induces vasoconstriction and vasospasm leading to more vascular thrombosis.[10]

However, the major clinical manifestations of DIC are hemorrhagic. Several mechanisms are involved. First, excessive fibrin generation results in severe depletion of both clotting factors and platelets. In parallel, there is activation of the fibrinolytic system, generating plasmin. Plasmin cleaves both fibrin clots and fibrinogen into fibrin(ogen) degradation products (FDPs).[11] FDPs further impair hemostasis by combining with circulating fibrin monomers before polymerization, leading to the formation of soluble fibrin polymers.[7]

CLINICAL MANIFESTATIONS

The clinical manifestations of DIC are a combination of those of the underlying disease and both hemorrhagic and thrombotic complications. The most common presentation is hemorrhage, occurring in 64–77% of patients[5,6] and including spontaneous bruising, petechiae, mucosal oozing and prolonged bleeding at venepuncture sites.[3] In an appropriate clinical setting, bleeding from multiple sites should immediately suggest DIC. Thrombotic manifestations are usually clinically less obvious[7] and may include acute renal failure, generalized cortical and brain stem dysfunction leading to impaired consciousness and coma, as well as hypoxia and progressive respiratory failure.[3] However, microvascular thrombosis may lead to failure of any organ.[7]

LABORATORY DIAGNOSIS

A laboratory diagnosis of DIC can usually be made by a combination of several simple tests. The prothrombin time and activated partial thromboplastin times are abnormal, owing to factor consumption, in 70% and 50% of patients respectively.[5] Similarly, the fibrinogen concentrations are low in approximately 50–60% of patients with DIC,[3,5] but even values in the normal range should be interpreted with caution since levels are typically increased in pregnancy.[2] Thrombocytopenia, which is occasionally severe, is an almost universal finding in DIC.[3,5,6] Examination of a peripheral blood smear will confirm the thrombocytopenia, and usually shows schistocytes, as evidence of a microangiopathic hemolytic anemia.[1,3]

The most specific tests are those of fibrin and FDPs, with elevated concentrations being found in at least 85% of patients.[3,5] The D-dimer assay, which measures a specific degradation product of cross-linked fibrin, was abnormal in 94% of DIC patients in one study.[11] More specialized laboratory tests that are useful in the diagnosis of DIC include the measurement of soluble fibrin monomers, prothrombin activation fragment F1+2, thrombin–antithrombin (TAT) complexes and plasmin–antiplasmin (PAP) complexes.[1,12] In a recent study, the combination of soluble fibrin monomers, TAT and PAP complexes had the highest sensitivity and specificity for diagnosing DIC.[12] However, these tests are not generally available and they are usually not essential in general clinical practice.[1,3] Others have found that the combination of FDP and D-dimer have the highest specificity and sensitivity.[13]

SPECIFIC PREGNANCY-RELATED SYNDROMES

Placental abruption

The incidence of placental abruption varies depending on the diagnostic criteria used, but it ranges from approximately one in 75 to one in 225 deliveries.[2,14] It is associated with intrauterine growth retardation and with an increased risk of major fetal malformations.[15] Important maternal risk factors include increasing age, smoking, hypertension, thrombophilia, and lack of education. Among women at least 18 years of age, completion of high school has been found to be associated with a reduced risk.[15–18] One study showed that with each additional half pack of cigarettes smoked daily, the incidence increased by approximately 20%.[15] Parity was a risk factor in some studies,[17] but not in others.[15]

The diagnosis of placental abruption is usually based on vaginal bleeding, a tender, hypertonic uterus with a retroplacental clot or depression of the underlying placental tissue.[2,19] However, not all of these signs are invariably present, and their absence does not exclude the diagnosis.[14]

The coagulopathy is initiated by the release of placental enzymes or tissue into the systemic maternal coagulation.[7] The degree of placental separation correlates with the extent of DIC.[1]

Severe clotting disorders are associated with significant separation of the placenta – significant enough to result in fetal demise.[2,19] In one study, DIC developed in five out of 16 women (29.6%) with placental abruption complicated by fetal death, but in none of 38 cases in which the fetus survived.[19]

Pre-eclampsia and eclampsia

Pre-eclampsia is estimated to complicate 3–5% of all pregnancies in the USA. Although the etiology remains unknown, it is now thought to be primarily a disease that involves damage to the vascular endothelium,[20] such damage then allowing activation of procoagulant proteins and platelets.[7] Usually occurring in the third trimester, eclampsia is characterized by hypertension, sodium retention with edema, proteinuria and hyper-reflexia.[21] Eclampsia with convulsions occurs in approximately four or five cases per 10,000 live births; it is associated with a maternal mortality rate of 0.5–14% and a perinatal mortality rate of up to 25–50%.[20]

Clinically relevant consumptive coagulopathy is uncommon even in severe pre-eclampsia and eclampsia. In one study, DIC was reported in 7.3% of patients with severe pre-eclampsia;[22] in another, FDPs were elevated in 3% of women with eclampsia.[23] However, increased levels of markers of intravascular coagulation and fibrinolysis have been reported in most patients with pre-eclampsia in the absence of clinical DIC.[24]

A distinct complication of pre-eclampsia and eclampsia is the HELLP syndrome, characterized by Hemolysis, Elevated Liver enzymes and Low Platelets.[22,25] The HELLP syndrome occurs in 8.5–19% of patients with pre-eclampsia or eclampsia, and it is associated with serious maternal morbidity and mortality. In a series of 442 pregnancies with HELLP, the maternal mortality rate was 1.1%, and significant morbidity included placental abruption (16%), acute renal failure (7.7%) and pulmonary edema (6%).[25] DIC has been reported in 8–21% of women with the HELLP syndrome.[25–27] Between 25 and 55% of patients require blood product support.[25,26] A recent report suggests that HELLP developing before 28 weeks' gestation is not associated with an increased risk of adverse fetal or maternal outcome in comparison with the outcomes in women with severe pre-eclampsia without the the HELLP syndrome.[27]

Induced abortion

DIC caused by intra-amniotic injection of hypertonic saline was first described in 1972. Although clinically apparent DIC occurred in only one patient, decreased fibrinogen and platelets and elevated FDPs were observed in all 12 patients studied prospectively.[28] This finding was confirmed by a review of more than 16,000 induced abortions, which showed that coagulopathy developed in two out of 304 women (0.66%) undergoing hypertonic saline or urea instillation, compared with one out of 13,272 women (0.008%) undergoing suction curettage; this corresponds to a relative risk of 87. Abortion induced by dilatation and evacuation carried an intermediate risk.[29]

DIC may also be secondary to complications of abortion, both spontaneous and induced, including infection and massive blood loss. A summary of 62 spontaneous abortion-related deaths in the USA over a 10-year period (1981–1991) reported that DIC was an associated condition in 48% of the deaths.[30]

Acute fatty liver of pregnancy

Acute fatty liver (or acute yellow atrophy) is a rare, potentially fatal disorder of unknown etiology that affects women in the latter part of pregnancy.[31] It is estimated to occur in one in 6700–15,000 pregnancies.[21,31] It is characterized by a prodrome of non-specific symptoms, followed by jaundice, profound hepatic failure with encephalopathy or coma, coagulopathy and frequently hypoglycemia.[31] Although laboratory evidence of DIC is commonly reported,[31,32] it is extremely difficult to distinguish between the coagulopathy of liver failure and DIC. Factor VIII levels, which are often elevated in liver disease and reduced in DIC, have not been reported in patients with this syndrome. A markedly decreased antithrombin III level secondary to severe liver disease

(average level 11%, normal range 80–100%) may contribute to thrombotic complications.[31]

Intrauterine fetal demise

In 1959, Pritchard reported that significant hypofibrinogenemia develops in approximately 25% of women with a fetal death retained for more than 4 weeks.[33] If the woman retains a dead fetus *in utero* for longer than 5 weeks, the incidence of DIC approaches 50%.[7] DIC is caused by the release of necrotic fetal tissue into the maternal circulation activating the coagulation system.[2,7] In this syndrome, the DIC is usually low-grade and compensated,[7] and most women deliver within a month and do not manifest a coagulopathy.[2] Reports of this syndrome are rare in the recent literature, suggesting that improved prenatal care and monitoring have virtually eliminated prolonged fetal demise as a cause of clinically relevant DIC.

Coagulopathy has also been reported with the demise of one or more fetuses in women with multifetal gestations. In the largest series reported, 100 selective termination procedures were performed by transabdominal injection of potassium chloride into the heart or umbilical vein of an anomalous fetus in multifetal pregnancies. Laboratory evidence of DIC was found in three women; however, there were no cases of clinical DIC.[34] In a similar report that examined 28 cases, including 19 in which fetal loss was spontaneous, there were no signs of DIC in any of the mothers.[35]

MANAGEMENT

Management of pregnancy-associated DIC is summarized in Table 18.1.

Treatment of the underlying disorder

DIC is a syndrome, not a disease, and therefore the cornerstone of the management of DIC is the treatment of the underlying disorder.[1–3] In pregnancy-related conditions, this usually means immediate termination of pregnancy.

In placental abruption, the majority of women can deliver vaginally, preferably without an

Table 18.1 Pregnancy-associated DIC: principles of management
Treat basic disease
Consider rapid delivery of fetus and placenta
Control hypertension (in pre-eclampsia)
Antibiotics (if infectious etiology)
Maintain and restore blood volume
Intravenous crystalloid fluids
Packed red blood cells (as indicated)
Correct coagulopathy (except in emergency, based on clotting tests)
Fresh frozen plasma
Cryoprecipitate
Platelets
Other and experimental therapy
Heparin (only if thrombotic manifestations predominate)
Antithrombin III concentrates (if available)
Tranexamic acid (in uncontrolled, life-threatening bleeding)

episiotomy.[2] Caesarean delivery is usually reserved for rapid delivery of a live stressed fetus remote from immediate vaginal delivery and in cases of uncontrolled hemorrhage.[36] Contrary to common belief, optimal treatment may start to normalize coagulation even before the uterus has been emptied.[19] An interesting report describes a patient who developed DIC at 19 weeks' gestation, presumably as the result of placental abruption, that resolved spontaneously with conservative management.[37]

Treatment of pre-eclampsia includes controlling hypertension, administering magnesium sulfate for seizure prophylaxis, and careful assessment of the mother and fetus. In general, mild cases may be managed expectantly until term or evidence of fetal maturity. Uncontrolled hypertension, thrombocytopenia, elevated liver or renal function tests, and fetal distress are all indications for expedited delivery.[20] The decision whether to induce labor with vaginal delivery or proceed with primary Caesarean

section depends both on the clinical condition of the mother and fetus and on whether the cervical examination is favorable for induction.[20] The HELLP syndrome is usually an indication for prompt delivery, often by Caesarean section.[31] High doses of corticosteroids (> 24 mg/day of dexamethasone) administered antepartum may improve platelet count, reduce liver enzymes, and possibly improve outcome in these patients.[38]

Therapy for acute fatty liver of pregnancy is early delivery, and general supportive care for hepatic failure and its complications. Similarly, in cases of fetal demise in a singleton pregnancy, evacuation of the uterine content should be undertaken promptly.[36]

Replacement of blood components

The most common clinical manifestation of DIC is hemorrhage.[5,6] Intravenous fluids and packed red blood cells should be administered as necessary to maintain blood volume, especially in women with active bleeding. Aggressive correction of impaired coagulation is imperative. This usually requires the administration of fresh frozen plasma, cryoprecipitate and platelets. Except in life-threatening circumstances, a 'shotgun' approach is discouraged. Rather, the decision as to which blood components should be administered is based on the concentration of platelets and fibrinogen and the prothrombin and activated partial thromboplastin times.[3] These tests should be repeated after administration of blood products to monitor the response.

Heparin

The logic for administering heparin in DIC is its ability to halt further activation of the coagulation system and intravascular thrombosis. However, heparin has not been shown in controlled trials to have a beneficial effect.[1] Most authors recommend restricting its use to those patients with DIC who have overt thrombotic manifestations.[3] Even those who recommend heparin use in patients with DIC state that it is not usually required in pregnancy-related DIC.[7] An exception is DIC caused by intrauterine fetal demise in which the maternal circulation is intact.[2] If heparin is used, it should be given with extreme caution and at a low dose in order to minimize the risk of exacerbating any hemorrhagic predisposition.[3] Low molecular weight heparin has been used in some patients with DIC,[7,39] but there are no reports of its use in pregnancy-associated DIC.

Antifibrinolytic therapy

Antifibrinolytic agents such as epsilon aminocaproic acid and tranexamic acid are generally considered to be contraindicated in DIC because of the risk of increased end-organ damage from microvascular thrombosis.[3] However, in rare instances when uncontrolled life-threatening bleeding continues despite maximum treatment with blood components, they may be useful.[3,7] Tranexamic acid can be administered intravenously at a dose of 1 g every 6 hours.

Concentrates of natural inhibitors

Antithrombin III is a natural anticoagulant that is synthesized in the liver and plays a major role in the regulation of hemostasis by inhibiting thrombin and many other activated factors, including factors Xa, IXa, XIa, XIIa kallikrein and plasmin.[40] In DIC, antithrombin III is consumed, and its level is reduced. In animal models, antithrombin III treatment has shown promising results.[41] The experience with antithrombin III concentrate in patients with DIC is difficult to interpret because of variability in study design, the small number of patients evaluated, the diverse inclusion criteria, the variable pretreatment levels of antithrombin III, and the differences in response criteria.[40] Nevertheless, a meta-analysis of all trials demonstrated a statistically significant reduction in mortality (odds ratio 0.59, 95% CI 0.39–0.87).[41] It is still unclear which patients with DIC will benefit the most from antithrombin III treatment, but values below 50% can be considered worthy of correction.

The other major natural anticoagulant pathway is the protein C system. Protein C

levels are significantly depressed in DIC, and clinical observations suggest that this change is associated with a fatal outcome.[41] In a recent uncontrolled study, activated protein C concentrate was administered to 16 patients with placental abruption and DIC. All patients recovered, and coagulation parameters improved within 24 hours;[42] however, controlled trials are required.

Novel therapies

Gabexate mesylate is a synthetic inhibitor of serine proteases, including thrombin and plasmin. It is widely used in Japan for DIC on the basis of the results of a non-randomized study.[3] Unfortunately, a recent randomized study of patients with mild DIC failed to demonstrate any effect of this agent on the DIC severity score or the mortality rate.[43]

A logical anticoagulant to use in DIC is one that is directed against tissue factor activity.[41] Tissue factor pathway inhibitor (TFPI) is an endogenous inhibitor of thrombin generation. It acts by forming an inhibitory quaternary complex with tissue factor, factor VIIa and factor Xa. Several phase I and phase II studies suggest that TFPI may be useful in improving outcome of severe sepsis. A large phase III trial is under way.[44] Recombinant NAPc2 is derived from a family of nematode anticoagulants that were originally isolated from hematophagous hookworm nematodes. It also inhibits the tissue factor–factor VIIa–factor Xa complex, and it is currently evaluated in clinical trials, including a study in DIC patients.[41]

Dithiocarbamates are agents that inhibit the NF-κ-B pathway, a key transcriptional mechanism in the induction of tissue factor. Preliminary data suggest that they ameliorate the effects of endotoxin in an animal model of DIC.[45]

AMNIOTIC FLUID EMBOLISM

Amniotic fluid embolism (AFE) is an unexpected and rare complication of pregnancy. It often presents with sudden maternal dyspnea, followed by cardiovascular collapse, DIC, and even maternal and fetal death.[7] First described by Meyer in 1926,[46] AFE became an established clinical entity in 1941 with a report by Steiner and Lushbaugh.[47] They described in detail the clinical histories and postmortem examinations of eight women and showed that these patients formed a distinct group with a typical constellation of clinical symptoms. By intravenously injecting human amniotic fluid or meconium into dogs or rabbits they were able to reproduce the pathological changes found in the women's lungs, thus demonstrating the pathophysiological basis for AFE.

EPIDEMIOLOGY

Steiner and Lushabugh estimated the incidence of AFE as one in 8000 deliveries,[47] whereas a recent population-based study in California reported 53 cases among 1,094,248 deliveries for a frequency of one in 20,646 deliveries.[48] Although uncommon, AFE accounted for 26 of the 254 maternal deaths (10.2%) directly related to pregnancy reported in the UK between 1991 and 1996.[49] Similarly, several studies in the USA have shown that AFE represented 9–10% of all maternal deaths.[50,51] The largest series of AFE are either population-based studies, autopsy series, or national registries. The most detailed analysis comes from the US national registry initiated in 1988 and reported in 1995.[52] A UK registry has also been set up.[53] In the US national registry, the syndrome occurred during labor in 70% of patients, whereas 19% were reported during Caesarean section and 11% after vaginal delivery.[52] AFE has also been reported after second trimester abortions,[52] in uncomplicated second trimester pregnancies,[54] and up to 48 hours postpartum.[55]

RISK FACTORS

Several risk factors are associated with the development of AFE. Older age has been reported in some series,[48,50,54,56] but not in the US national registry.[52] Similarly the US national registry shows no association with race and parity, although other series show an increased

risk in multiparous[48,50,54] white[48] women. Older reports associated AFE with long and hard labor and the use of oxytocin.[50,57] However, more recent series find no such relationships.[52,54]

A clear risk factor is rupture (spontaneous or artificial) of the fetal membranes.[52,54] Indeed, 13% of the patients in the US national registry exhibited a striking temporal relationship between artificial rupture of the membranes and acute cardiovascular collapse.[52]

PATHOPHYSIOLOGY

Although our understanding of the pathophysiology of AFE is incomplete, three distinct mechanisms are probably involved:

- maternal exposure to fetal tissue;
- pulmonary insult;
- coagulopathy.

Maternal exposure to fetal tissue

Entry of amniotic fluid into the uterine circulation and subsequently into the systemic maternal circulation is considered a prerequisite for AFE. However, several detailed postmortem examinations failed to clearly define the portals of entry.[50,56] It has been postulated that the fetal head obstructs the intracervical canal, blocking drainage and generating retrograde hydrostatic pressure, which leads to the injection of amniotic fluid into the open cervical veins.[57]

However, not every transfer of fetal tissue to the maternal blood stream results in AFE. For example, squamous cells (presumably of fetal origin) commonly occur in the maternal pulmonary circulation apparently without causing physiological derangement.[58]

Pulmonary insult

It was originally thought that the major insult in AFE is a mechanical obstruction of the pulmonary circulation by the amniotic fluid and its contents, leading to acute right heart failure, increased pulmonary artery pressure, and subsequent decreased left ventricular filling.[54] However, animal studies suggest that humoral mechanisms may play a role in the pathogenesis of the cardiovascular collapse seen in AFE. Work by Kitzmiller and Lucas suggests the importance of prostaglandin F2, which is detectable in amniotic fluid only during labor.[59] They reproduced clinical manifestations in cats after systemic injection of prostaglandin F2 and amniotic fluid from women in labor, whereas the same effects were not found when the animals were injected with amniotic fluid from women who were not in labor. More recent work has focused on the expression of endothelin-1, a potent vasoconstrictor the presence of which in amniotic fluid may explain the initial pulmonary hypertension.[60] On the basis of his analysis of the data in the US national registry, Clark noted that the pathophysiological events in patients with AFE were more consistent with septic and anaphylactic shock than with an embolic process, and he proposed changing the term AFE to 'anaphylactoid syndrome of pregnancy'.[52]

The results of hemodynamic studies in patients with AFE have been conflicting. Some have suggested that left ventricular dysfunction is the primary mechanism, with increased pulmonary capillary wedge pressure.[61,62] However, a recent report of early transesophageal echocardiography found severe pulmonary hypertension without initial left ventricular dysfunction.[63]

Coagulopathy

The procoagulant properties of amniotic fluid have been known for more than 50 years.[64] Yaffe et al. have shown that amniotic fluid has thromboplastin activity, which increases with the progression of pregnancy.[65] Furthermore, addition of antibodies against tissue factor virtually eliminated amniotic fluid clotting in a functional assay, suggesting that tissue factor is responsible for nearly all the procoagulant activity of amniotic fluid.[66] Excess tissue factor in the maternal vascular system presumably activates the clotting cascade, leading to DIC. This is consistent with thromboelastographic data, which show that amniotic fluid significantly increases clot initiation and propagation of

whole blood.[67] Interestingly, no evidence of enhanced fibrinolysis was noted, consistent with other data showing increased activity of plasminogen activator inhibitors and decreased tissue-type plasminogen activator levels in amniotic fluid compared with plasma levels in pregnant women.[68] Animal studies have shown that when amniotic fluid is contaminated with meconium, the coagulopathy is significantly more severe.[69]

CLINICAL FEATURES

The most common presenting features reported in three large series include dyspnea with cyanosis (in 50–83% of patients), severe (and otherwise unexplained) hypotension (in 27–100%), and convulsions or other signs of central nervous system irritability (in 10–48%).[50,52,54] All mothers undelivered at the time of the AFE experienced fetal bradycardia or the abrupt onset of severe variable decelerations, leading within minutes to bradycardia.[52] In the national registry, 87% of the patients experienced cardiac arrest, and an additional 9% a serious dysrythmia, in almost all cases within 1 hour of the onset of symptoms.[52]

Clinical and laboratory evidence of a coagulopathy were present in 37–75% of patients;[50,52,54] however the hemorrhagic tendency was one of the presenting features in only 12% of the cases,[50,54] typically developing only in patients who survive the initial pulmonary insult.

Pulmonary edema or adult respiratory distress syndrome has been reported in 24–93% of patients.[52,54] However, this is usually a secondary complication of prolonged shock, over-vigorous fluid and blood product replacement therapy,[54] and possibly a direct depressant effect of amniotic fluid on the myocardium.[7] Hemodynamic monitoring has rarely been performed within 2 hours after the onset of symptoms.[52,61,63]

Fever was not a typical manifestation, and bronchospasm was a rare symptom, being mentioned as a feature in only 1–11% of patients.[52,54] Furthermore, urticarial rashes or other cutaneous manifestations, except for purpura, were also absent. Taken together, these clinical observations are inconsistent with a recent theory that considered AFE to be an anaphylactoid syndrome of pregnancy.[52]

LABORATORY FINDINGS

Only limited data are available on patients in the immediate period after the onset of AFE. Arterial blood gases were performed in 17 patients in the US national registry within 30 minutes of the acute event; all were receiving an inspired oxygen tension of 100%. In 11 patients, the oxygen partial pressure was < 30 mmHg, reflecting profound intrapulmonary shunting. In five patients (presumably survivors) the hypoxia corrected within 15–60 minutes.[52] Laboratory assessment of the coagulopathy reveals prolonged prothrombin and partial thromboplastin times, increased fibrin degradation products or D-dimer, and marked hypofibrinogenemia and thrombocytopenia in the vast majority of patients who survive to be tested.[52]

DIAGNOSIS

The diagnosis of AFE is based on the clinical presentation and supportive laboratory studies (Table 18.2). There is no single diagnostic test that is pathognomonic for AFE. The presence of squamous cells in the maternal pulmonary vasculature has been considered diagnostic.[56] However, squamous cells have been identified in the maternal pulmonary arterial circulation, by aspirating blood from a pulmonary artery catheter, in a variety of pregnant and non-pregnant patients.[58] Conversely, in the US national registry cohort, fetal elements were detected by histological examination of distal port pulmonary artery catheter blood in only four of the eight cases studied.[52] More recently, studies have used the monoclonal antibody TKH-2 to identify fetal mucin in the maternal pulmonary vasculature.[70,71] However, the accuracy of this method has been determined only in an autopsy study.[71] Others have suggested determining the maternal plasma concentrations of zinc coproporphyrin I, a characteristic component of meconium. The plasma levels were significantly higher in four

Table 18.2 AFE: entry criteria of US registry
Acute hypotension or cardiac arrest
Acute hypoxia or dyspnea, cyanosis or respiratory arrest
Coagulopathy, defined as laboratory evidence of intravascular consumption, fibrinolysis or severe clinical hemorrhage*
Onset of the above during labor, Caesarean section, or dilatation and evacuation, or within 30 minutes postpartum
Absence of any other significant confounding condition or potential explanation for the signs and symptoms observed

Adapted from Clark *et al.*[52]

*Patients meeting all other criteria who died before coagulopathy could be assessed were also eligible

women with AFE than in women after a normal delivery.[72] However, this test requires high-performance liquid chromatography followed by fluorometry and is not widely available, and results are unlikely to be available during the acute episode or to be useful for clinical management.

MANAGEMENT

Initial care is mainly supportive. All patients should receive oxygen at a high concentration (100%), and most patients require endotracheal intubation and mechanical ventilation.[7,73] Hypotension should be treated with an isotonic crystalloid solution. Patients with persistent hypotension despite adequate volume expansion should be treated with inotropic agents such as dopamine or dobutamine.[55,73] In patients who survive the initial hypotensive phase, fluid therapy needs to be carefully monitored to ensure optimal blood pressure and to prevent or blunt pulmonary edema and the adult respiratory distress syndrome.[73] Monitoring usually requires the insertion of a central venous line, or preferably a pulmonary artery catheter that can measure pulmonary capillary wedge pressures.[7,55,73]

Almost all patients who survive the initial insult go on to develop a coagulopathy with active bleeding. Large quantities of fresh frozen plasma, cryoprecipitate, platelets, and packed red blood cells are usually required. Initial treatment should be empiric, with further therapy guided by the results of clotting tests. Some have advocated using heparin,[54] low molecular weight heparin, or antithrombin concentrates.[7] However, as in any case of DIC, the use of heparin is controversial,[55] and this author reserves the use of heparin in DIC for those cases in which a thrombotic tendency predominates.

Oxytocin should be administered to induce uterine contraction and prevent further bleeding from the placental site and uterus.[7] If the fetus is still undelivered, immediate Caesarean delivery has been recommended.[73]

Many other therapies, all either untested or based on isolated case reports, have been proposed. Clark *et al.*, considering an 'anaphylactoid' basis for AFE, have suggested giving hydrocortisone 500 mg intravenously every 6 hours until the patient improves or dies.[52] Selective pulmonary vasodilators may reverse the pulmonary hypertension without worsening the systemic hypotension. The successful use of aerosolized prostacyclin has been reported in one case,[74] and others have proposed trying inhaled nitric oxide.[75] More aggressive approaches include either extracorporeal membrane oxygenation and intra-aortic balloon counterpulsation,[76] or cardiopulmonary bypass and pulmonary artery thromboembolectomy.[77]

PROGNOSIS

AFE is commonly fatal for both the mother and the child. The maternal mortality rate in a summary of 272 cases before 1979 was 86%.[54] The US national registry analysis reported a mortality rate of 61%,[52] whereas a recent population-based series claimed a mortality rate of 26.4%.[48] A large Chinese series reported a mortality rate of 89%; however, four of the last seven patients (57%) survived.[78] Among survivors the morbidity is high, with the US national registry finding only 15% of patients surviving neurologically intact.[52] Fetal death has been reported in 21–66% of AFE,[50,52,56] and severe fetal distress with subsequent neurological impairment is common in these babies.[50,52]

SUMMARY

DIC is a syndrome that may complicate several obstetric conditions, including placental abruption, pre-eclampsia, and AFE. Excessive activation of the coagulation system leads to diffuse fibrin clots, depletion of platelets and clotting factors, and activation of the fibrinolytic system. Hemorrhagic manifestations usually predominate. Prompt recognition, treatment of the underlying disease, maintenance blood volume, and replacement as indicated of clotting factors usually results in a successful outcome.

REFERENCES

1. Levi M, ten Cate H. Disseminated intravascular coagulation. *N Engl J Med* 1999;**341**:586–92.
2. Richey ME, Gilstrap LC, Ramin SM, *et al.* Management of disseminated intravascular coagulopathy. *Clin Obstet Gynecol* 1995;**38**:514–20.
3. Baglin T. Disseminated intravascular coagulation: Diagnosis and treatment. *BMJ* 1996;**312**:683–7.
4. Bone RC. Gram-positive organisms and sepsis. *Arch Intern Med* 1994;**154**:26–34.
5. Spero JA, Lewis JH, Hasiba U. Disseminated intravascular coagulation: findings in 346 patients. *Thromb Haemost* 1980;**43**:28–33.
6. Siegal T, Seligsohn U, Aghai E, Modan M. Clinical and laboratory aspects of disseminated intravascular coagulation (DIC): a study of 118 cases. *Thromb Haemost* 1978;**39**:122–34.
7. Bick RL. Syndromes of disseminated intravascular coagulation in obstetrics, pregnancy and gynecology. *Hematol Oncol Clin North Am* 2000;**14**:999–1044.
8. Gando S, Kameue T, Nanzaki S, Nakanishi Y. Cytokines, soluble thrombomodulin and disseminated intravascular coagulation in patients with systemic inflammatory response syndrome. *Thromb Res* 1995;**80**:519–26.

9. Okajima K, Uchiba M, Murakami K, *et al*. Plasma levels of soluble E-selectin in patients with disseminated intravascular coagulation. *Am J Hematol* 1997;**54**:219–24.

10. Ishibashi M, Ito N, Fujita M, *et al*. Endothelin-1 as an aggravating factor of disseminated intravascular coagulation associated with malignant neoplasms. *Cancer* 1994;**73**:191–5.

11. Bick RL, Baker WF. Diagnostic efficacy of the D-dimer assay in disseminated intravascular coagulation. *Thromb Res* 1992;**65**:785–90.

12. Wada H, Gabazza E, Nakasaki T, *et al*. Diagnosis of disseminated intravascular coagulation by hemostatic molecular markers. *Semin Thromb Hemost* 2000;**26**:17–21.

13. Yu M, Nardella A, Pechet L. Screening tests of disseminated intravascular coagulation. *Crit Care Med* 2000;**28**:1777–80.

14. Baron F, Hill WC. Placenta previa, placenta abruptio. *Clin Obstet Gynecol* 1998;**41**:527–32.

15. Raymond EG, Mills JL. Placental abruption: maternal risk factors and associated fetal conditions. *Acta Obstet Gynecol Scand* 1993;**72**:633–9.

16. Avanth CV, Smulian JC, Vintzileos AM. Incidence of placental abruption in relation to cigarette smoking and hypertensive disorders during pregnancy: a meta-analysis of observational studies. *Obstet Gynecol* 1999;**93**:622–8.

17. Pritchard JA, Cunningham G, Pritchard SA, Mason RA. On reducing the frequency of severe abruptio placentae. *Am J Obstet Gynecol* 1991;**165**:1345–51.

18. Brenner B. Inherited thrombophilia and fetal loss. *Curr Opin Hematol* 2000;**5**:290–5.

19. Twaalfhoven FCM, van Roosmalen J, Briet E, Gravenhorst JB. Conservative management of placental abruption complicated by severe clotting disorders. *Eur J Obstet Gynecol Reprod Biol* 1992;**46**:25–30.

20. Repke JT, Robinson JN. The prevention and management of pre-eclampsia and eclampsia. *Int J Gynecol Obstet* 1998;**62**:1–9.

21. Schorr-Lesnick B, Lebovics E, Dworkin B, Rosenthal WS. Liver diseases unique to pregnancy. *Am J Gastroenterol* 1991;**86**:659–70.

22. Sibai BM, Spinnato JA, Watson DL, *et al*. Pregnancy outcome in 303 cases with severe pre-eclampsia. *Obstet Gynecol* 1984;**64**:319–25.

23. Pritchard JA, Cunningham DG, Mason RA. Coagulation changes in eclampsia: Their frequency and pathogenesis. *Am J Obstet Gynecol* 1976;**124**:855–9.

24. Schjetlein R, Haugen G, Wisloff F. Markers of intravascular coagulation and fibrinolysis in pre-eclampsia: Association with intrauterine growth retardation. *Acta Obstet Gynecol Scand* 1997;**76**:541–6.

25. Sibai BM, Ramadan MK, Usta I, *et al*. Maternal morbidity and mortality in 442 pregnancies with hemolysis, elevated liver enzymes and low platelets (HELLP syndrome). *Am J Obstet Gynecol* 1993;**169**:1000–6.

26. Haddad B, Barton JR, Livingston JC, *et al*. Risk factors for adverse maternal outcomes among women with HELLP (hemolysis, elevated liver enzymes, and low platelet count) syndrome. *Am J Obstet Gynecol* 2000;**183**:444–8.

27. Haddad B, Barton JR, Livingston JC, *et al*. HELLP (hemolysis, elevated liver enzymes, and low platelet count) syndrome versus severe pre-eclampsia: onset at ≤ 28.0 weeks' gestation. *Am J Obstet Gynecol* 2000;**183**:1475–9.

28. Spivak JL, Spangler DB, Bell WR. Defibrinogenation after intra-amniotic injection of hypertonic saline. *N Engl J Med* 1972;**287**:321–3.

29. Kafrissen ME, Barke MW, Workman P, *et al*. Coagulopathy and induced abortion methods: Rates and relative risks. *Am J Obstet Gynecol* 1983;**147**:344–5.

30. Saraiya M, Green CA, Berg CJ, *et al*. Spontaneous abortion-related deaths among women in the United States: 1981–1991. *Obstet Gynecol* 1999;**94**:172–6.

31. Castro MA, Goodwin TM, Shaw KJ, *et al*. Disseminated intravascular coagulation and antithrombin III depression in acute fatty liver of pregnancy. *Am J Obstet Gynecol* 1996;**174**:211–16.

32. Castro MA, Fassett MJ, Reynolds TB, *et al*. Reversible peripartum liver failure: a new perspective on the diagnosis, treatment, and cause of acute fatty liver of pregnancy, based on 28 consecutive cases. *Am J Obstet Gynecol* 1999;**181**:389–95.

33. Pritchard JA. Fetal death in utero. *Obstet Gynecol* 1959;**14**:573–7.

34. Berkowitz RL, Stone JL, Eddelman KA. One hundred consecutive cases of selective termination of an abnormal fetus in a multifetal gestation. *Obstet Gynecol* 1997;**90**:606–10.

35. Petersen IR, Nyholm HC. Multiple pregnancies with single intrauterine demise: description of 28 pregnancies. *Acta Obstet Gynecol Scand* 1999;**78**:202–6.

36. Lurie S, Feinstein M, Mamet Y. Disseminated intravascular coagulopathy in pregnancy: thorough comprehension of etiology and management reduces obstetrician's stress. *Arch Gynecol Obstet* 2000;**263**:126–30.

37. Marinoff DN, Honegger, MM, Girard JB. Spontaneous resolution of disseminated intravascular coagulopathy in the second trimester. *Am J Obstet Gynecol* 1999;**181**:759–60.

38. O'Brien JM, Milligan DA, Barton JR. Impact of high-dose corticosteroid therapy for patients with HELLP (hemolysis, elevated liver enzymes, and low platelet count) syndrome. *Am J Obstet Gynecol* 2000;**183**:921–4.

39. Gillis S, Dann EJ, Eldor A. Low molecular weight heparin in the prophylaxis and treatment of disseminated intravascular coagulation of acute promyelocytic leukemia. *Eur J Hematol* 1995;**54**:59–60.

40. Bucur SZ, Levy JH, Despotis GJ, et al. Use of antithrombin III concentrate in congenital and acquired deficiency states. *Transfusion* 1998;**38**:481–98.

41. Levi M, de Jonge E, van der Poll T, ten Cate H. Novel approaches to the management of disseminated intravascular coagulation. *Crit Care Med* 2000;**28(suppl 9)**:S20–S24.

42. Kobayashi T, Terao T, Maki M, et al. Activated Protein C is effective for disseminated intravascular coagulation associated with placental abruption. *Thromb Haemost* 1999;**82**:1363.

43. Nishiyama T, Matsukawa T, Hanaoka K. Is protease inhibitor a choice for the treatment of pre- or mild disseminated intravascular coagulation? *Crit Care Med* 2000;**28**:1419–22.

44. Abraham E. Tissue factor inhibition and clinical trial results of tissue factor pathway inhibitor in sepsis. *Crit Care Med* 2000;**28(suppl 9)**:S31–S33.

45. Drollinger AG, Netser JC, Rodgers GM. Dithiocarbamates ameliorate the effects of endotoxin in a rabbit model of disseminated intravascular coagulation. *Semin Thromb Hemost* 1999;**25**:429–33.

46. Meyer JR. Embolis pulmonary caseosa. *Braz J Med Biol Res* 1926;**1**:301–3.

47. Steiner PE, Lushbaugh CC. Maternal pulmonary embolism by amniotic fluid. *JAMA* 1941;**117**:1245–54.

48. Gilbert WM, Danielsen B. Amniotic fluid embolism: decreased mortality in a population-based study. *Obstet Gynecol* 1999;**93**:973–7.

49. de Swiet M. Maternal mortality: confidential enquiries into maternal deaths in the United Kingdom. *Am J Obstet Gynecol* 2000;**182**:760–6.

50. Petersen EP, Taylor HB. Amniotic fluid embolism: an analysis of 40 cases. *Obstet Gynecol* 1970;**35**:787–93.

51. Dorfman SF. Maternal mortality in New York City, 1981–1983. *Obstet Gynecol* 1990;**76**:317–23.

52. Clark SL, Hankins GDV, Dudley DA, et al. Amniotic fluid embolism: analysis of the national registry. *Am J Obstet Gynecol* 1995;**172**:1158–69.

53. Tuffnell DJ, Johnson H. Amniotic fluid embolism: the UK register. *Hosp Med* 2000;**15**:163–72.

54. Morgan M. Amniotic fluid embolism. *Anaesthesia* 1979;**34**:20–32.

55. Clark SL. New concepts of amniotic fluid embolism: a review. *Obstet Gynecol Surv* 1990;**45**:360–8.

56. Liban E, Raz S. A clinicopathological study of fourteen cases of amniotic fluid embolism. *Am J Clin Pathol* 1969;**51**:477–86.

57. Reid DE, Weiner AE, Roby CC. I. Intravascular clotting and afibrinogenemia, the presumptive lethal factors in the syndrome of amniotic fluid embolism. *Am J Obstet Gynecol* 1953;**66**:465–74.

58. Clark SL, Pavlova Z, Greenspoon J, et al. Squamous cells in the maternal pulmonary circulation. *Am J Obstet Gynecol* 1986;**154**:104–6.

59. Kitzmiller JL, Lucas WE. Studies on a model of amniotic fluid embolism. *Obstet Gynecol* 1972;**39**:626–7.

60. Khong TY. Expression of endothelin-1 in amniotic fluid embolism and possible pathophysiological mechanism. *Br J Obstet Gynaecol* 1998;**105**:802–4.

61. Clark SL, Cotton DB, Gonik B et al. Central hemodynamic alterations in amniotic fluid embolism. *Am J Obstet Gynecol* 1988;**158**:1124–6.

62. Gregory MG, Clayton EM. Amniotic fluid embolism. *Obstet Gynecol* 1973;**42**:236–44.

63. Schechtman M, Ziser A, Markovits R, Rozenberg B. Amniotic fluid embolism: Early findings of transesophageal echocardiography. *Anesth Analg* 1999;**89**:1456–8.

65. Weiner AE, Reid DE, Roby CC. The hemostatic activity of amniotic fluid. *Science* 1949;**110**:190–1.

65. Yaffe H, Hay-Am E, Sadovsky E. Thromboplastic activity of amniotic fluid in term and postmature gestations. *Obstet Gynecol* 1980;**57**:490–2.

66. Lockwood CJ, Bach R, Guha A, et al. Amniotic fluid contains tissue factor, a potent initiator of coagulation. *Am J Obstet Gynecol* 1991;**165**:1335–41.

67. Liu EHC, Shailaja S, Koh SCL, Lee TL. An assessment of the effects on coagulation of midtrimester and final-trimester amniotic fluid on whole blood by thromboelastograph analysis. *Anesth Analg* 2000;**90**:333–6.

68. Estelles A, Gilabert J, Andres C, et al. Plasminogen activator inhibitors type 1 and type 2 and plasminogen activators in amniotic fluid during pregnancy. *Thromb Haemost* 1990;**64**:281–5.

69. Petroianu GA, Altmannsberger SHG, Maleck WH, *et al.* Meconium and amniotic fluid embolism: effects on coagulation in pregnant mini-pigs. *Crit Care Med* 1999;**27**:348–55.

70. Kobayashi H, Hidekazu O, Terao T. A simple, non-invasive, sensitive method for diagnosis of amniotic fluid embolism by monoclonal antibody TKH-2 that recognizes NeuAcα2-6GalNac. *Am J Obstet Gynecol* 1993;**168**:848–53.

71. Kobayashi H, Ooi H, Hayakawa H, *et al.* Histological diagnosis of amniotic fluid embolism by monoclonal antibody TKH-2 that recognizes NeuAc alpha 2-6Gal Nac epitope. *Hum Pathol* 1997;**28**:428–33.

72. Kanayama N, Yamazaki T, Naruse H, *et al.* Determining zinc coproporphyrin in maternal plasma – a new method for diagnosing amniotic fluid embolism. *Clin Chem* 1992;**38**:526–9.

73. Locksmith GJ. Amniotic fluid embolism. *Obstet Gynecol Clin North Am* 1999;**26**:435–44.

74. Van Heerden PV, Webb SA, Hee G, *et al.* Inhaled aerosolized prostacyclin as a selective pulmonary vasodilator for the treatment of severe hypoxaemia. *Anaesth Intensive Care* 1996;**24**:87–90.

75. Tanus-Santos JE, Moreno H. Inhaled nitric oxide and amniotic fluid embolism. *Anesth Analg* 1999;**88**:691.

76. Hsieh YY, Chang CC, Li PC, *et al.* Successful application of extracorporeal membrane oxygenation and intra-aortic counterpulsation as lifesaving therapy for a patient with amniotic fluid embolism. *Am J Obstet Gynecol* 2000;**183**:496–7.

77. Esposito RA, Grossi EA, Coppa G, *et al.* Successful treatment of postpartum shock caused by amniotic fluid embolism with cardiopulmonary bypass and pulmonary thromboembolectomy. *Am J Obstet Gynecol* 1990;**163**:572–4.

78. Weiwen Y. Study of the diagnosis and management of amniotic fluid embolism: 38 cases of analysis. *Obstet Gynecol* 2000;**95(suppl 4)**:38S (Abst).

19

Inherited bleeding disorders in women

Rezan A Kadir and Christine A Lee

INTRODUCTION

Hereditary deficiency of each of the 12 coagulation factors has been reported. von Willebrand's disease, haemophilia A (factor VIII deficiency) and haemophilia B (factor IX deficiency) account for 82.6% of all patients registered on the UK Haemophilia Centre Doctors' Organisation registry in 1997, and factor XI deficiency account for another 4.9%. Other rarer coagulation defects (deficiencies of fibrinogen, prothrombin, factor V, factor VII, factor X, factor XII and factor XIII, combined factor deficiency and platelet defects) account for the remaining 12.5%. Factor XI deficiency is the most common genetic disorder among Ashkenazi Jews, and the frequency of heterozygous status is reported to be 8% in this population.[1]

von Willebrand's disease is the most common inherited bleeding disorder and appears clinically to be a disease of women since they are more likely to be symptomatic than men. This was reported by Dr Erik von Willebrand in 1926, when he first described the disease.[2] Among 66 members of the bleeder family from Fölgö on the Åland Islands in the Gulf of Bothnia who were examined in this study, there were 23 bleeders, 16 of whom were female (Figure 19.1). Among the female members, five deaths from bleeding occurred, including the index case (Hjördis), who died of uncontrollable menstrual loss at the age of 13. A disproportionate number of females to males to males has also been reported by other investigators.[3,4]

Because of the sex-linked mode of inheritance, haemophilia A and B affects males predominantly, females being carriers. Most of these carrier females have factor VIII and factor IX levels within the normal range since they have only one affected X chromosome. Thus they are unlikely to experience major bleeding problems, although studies have shown them to be at risk of bruising and prolonged bleeding after trauma and following surgery and delivery.[5] Similarly, women with factor XI deficiency (whether severe or partial) do not generally suffer from spontaneous bleeding, but they may do so after haemostatic challenges.

Women are exposed more to haemostatic challenges during their life than men, owing to monthly menstruation and to childbirth, which can render mild forms of bleeding disorders symptomatic, although objective assessment of blood loss in these situations may be difficult.[6–8]

PREVALENCE AND PATHOGENESIS

von Willebrand's disease

von Willebrand's disease is far more common than was previously suspected, and it is the most common inherited bleeding abnormality, affecting 0.8–1.3% of women.[9,10] However, the exact frequency of von Willebrand's disease in the general population is difficult to determine because of variable penetrance and expressivity of von Willebrand's disease mutations,[11] the interindividual and intraindividual variability,[12] and temporal variability.[11,13]

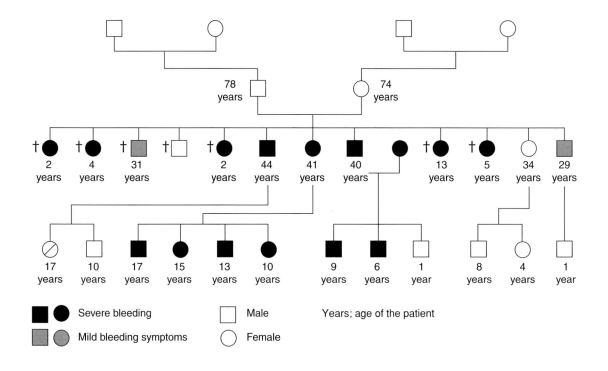

Figure 19.1 Pedigree of a bleeder family from Följö.

von Willebrand's disease exhibits significant phenotypic heterogeneity. Two main categories of patients can be identified, distinguished on the basis of whether the main pathogenetic factor is a quantitative defect (in types 1 and 3 or a qualitative defect (in type 2) of von Willebrand's factor.

Type 1 is the most common form, accounting for approximately 70% of all cases; it is characterized by equally low plasma levels of von Willebrand factor (usually 5–40 IU/dl) and factor VIII activity. This is caused by decreased synthesis of normally functioning von Willebrand factor. Since von Willebrand factor serves as a carrier protein for factor VIII, this will result in reduced levels of factor VIII.

Type 2 von Willebrand's disease results from a qualitative abnormality of von Willebrand factor that results, in most cases, in abnormal multimeric structure of the molecule and hence defective interaction among platelets, von Willebrand factor and vessel walls. The plasma concentration of von Willebrand factor, as well as factor VIII activity, may be only modestly

reduced, or may even be normal. Type 2 accounts for about 20% of all von Willebrand's disease.[14] It is phenotypically very heterogeneous and has been recently reclassified into four main subtypes (subtypes 2A, 2B, 2N, 2M),[15] The bleeding disorder is mild to moderate in the majority of cases (types 2A and 2B), but it can be of variable severity in types 2N and 2M.

Type 3 von Willebrand's disease is rare, with a prevalence of 0.1–5.3 per million depending on country.[16,17] It results from deletions in the von Willebrand factor gene. It is characterized by a marked reduction of plasma and platelet levels of von Willebrand factor, with severe bleeding. von Willebrand factor antigen and activity (vWF:Ag and vWF:Ac) are usually undetectable even with very sensitive assays, and factor VIII levels are also markedly reduced, typically to less than 10 IU/dl.

The prevalence of haemophilia A is between one and two per 10 000 in the UK.[18] However, the prevalence of carrier women is unknown. A wide range of factor VIII values (range 22–116 IU/dl, mean 54 IU/dl) has been reported[19] as a result of random inactivation of one of the X chromosomes. A small number of haemophilia carriers may have very low factor levels,[20] owing to extreme lyonization, homozygosity for haemophilia gene[21] coincidence of carriership and Turner's syndrome, and other chromosomal abnormalities[22,23] or coinheritance of a variant von Willebrand factor allele. Bleeding tendency is minimal and limited to post-traumatic states, especially in those with low factor levels below 50 IU/dl.

Factor XI deficiency

Factor XI deficiency is a rare bleeding disorder with an autosomal mode of inheritance. Factor levels are severely reduced (to >15 IU/dl) in homozygotes and partially deficient or low normal in heterozygotes.[24] Factor XI deficiency is particularly common in Ashkenazi Jews; however, the disorder has been described in all racial groups. In the UK, there were 694 patients on the Haemophilia Centre Directors' national register in 1997 and a significant number of them have no known Jewish roots. Bleeding tendency in factor XI deficiency is mild and is mostly related to trauma or surgery. There is a poor correlation between factor XI level and bleeding tendency in patients with factor XI deficiency.[24,25] Some patients with severe deficiency may not bleed at all following trauma, while some heterozygotes have excessive bleeding after challenge. The bleeding tendency may also vary in the same patient following haemostatic challenge.[1] This is dependent on the patient's genotype, the site of surgical intervention and the presence of additional coagulation factor defects, most commonly von Willebrand's disease.

GENETICS OF INHERITED BLEEDING DISORDERS

von Willebrand's disease

The von Willebrand factor gene is located on the short arm of chromosome 12 at 12p12-pter.[26] Specific mutations in the von Willebrand factor gene have recently been identified in a significant number of patients with von Willebrand's disease (mainly type 2 disease). However, the molecular basis of type 1 disease, the most common type of von Willebrand's disease, is still unknown in most cases. The mode of inheritance of type 1 von Willebrand's disease is autosomal dominant. Type 2 disease is also transmitted as an autosomal dominant except type 2N, which is a recessively inherited disorder. Type 3 von Willebrand's disease is an autosomal-recessive disorder, and affected people are either homozygotes or compound heterozygotes. If a child with type 3 disease has already been born in the family, the risk of a subsequent child being affected is 25%.

Haemophilia

Haemophilia A and B are X-linked recessive bleeding disorders, and in each pregnancy in a carrier there is a 50% probability that a male fetus will be affected and that a female fetus will be a carrier. The genes for factor VIII and factor IX are located near the tip of the long arm of the X chromosome (Xq2.8). Many genetic defects have been identified in haemophilic families, including gene rearrangements, deletions and point mutations.[27]

Factor XI deficiency

The inheritance of factor XI deficiency is autosomal, with severe deficiency in homozygotes and partial deficiency in heterozygotes.[24] The factor XI gene is located on chromosome 4 q34–35.[28] Several genetic mutations that cause factor XI deficiency have been reported.[29–32] In Ashkenazi Jews, factor deficiency is caused by a type II mutation (a stop codon in exon 5) and a type III mutation (a single base change in exon 9) in most kindreds.[1,33,34] However, identification of mutations in non-Jews is in progress.

MENSTRUATION AND BLEEDING DISORDERS

Menorrhagia in women with inherited bleeding disorders

Menorrhagia is defined as a menstrual blood loss of 80 ml or more per period. It is seen in 5% of

Menstrual pictorial chart and scoring system

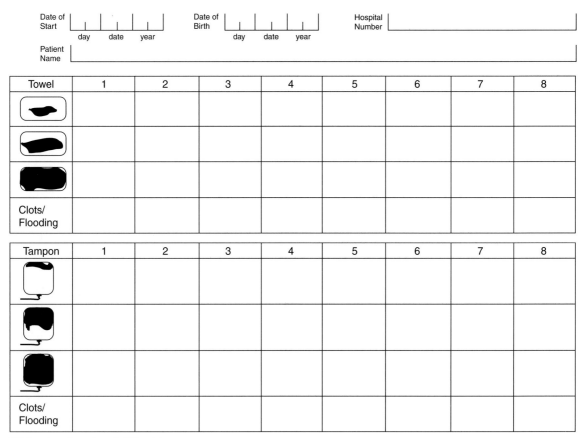

(Clots: size of a coin = 1p/50p etc)

Scoring System

Towels		
1 point	for each lightly stained towel	
5 points	for each moderately soiled towel	
20 points	if the towel is completely saturated with blood	
Tampons		
1 point	for each lightly stained tampon	
5 points	for each moderately soiled tampon	
10 points	if the tampon is completely saturated with blood	
Clots		
1 point	for small clots (size of 1p coin)	
5 points	for large clots (size of 50p coin)	

Figure 19.2 Pictorial blood assessment chart and the scoring system. Reproduced by kind permission of Blackwell Science from Higham et al.[85]

women of reproductive age, and 12% of gynae-cological referrals are because of this problem. In clinical practice, assessment of menstrual blood loss is usually subjective and relies on the description provided by the patient. Unfortunately, this is an inaccurate method since there is a lack of correlation between the patient's impression and the objective assessment of actual volume of blood loss. Most techniques used to quantify menstrual blood loss require laboratory facilities and are costly; therefore they have never become established as part of routine practice. Using a special scoring system, a simple pictorial chart (Figure 19.2) for objective assessment of menstrual loss has been put together.[35] Compared to the alkaline haematin method, this chart has been shown to have a reasonable accuracy for the assessment of menstrual blood loss and the diagnosis of menorrhagia, and it has proved to be useful in clinical practice.

Menorrhagia is a common bleeding symptom in women with bleeding disorders. It may be the first bleeding symptom. It usually begins at menarche and can be the presenting symptom. Ragni *et al.*[36] reported menorrhagia as the most common bleeding symptom in their study, occurring in 93% of 38 women with type 1 von Willebrand's disease, as well as the most common initial symptom, occurring in 53% of the women. In a large series of 116 women, objectively confirmed menorrhagia (using a pictorial blood assessment chart) in patients with von Willebrand's disease, carriers of haemophilia and factor XI deficiency occurred in 73%, 57% and 59% of the patients, respectively; these figures compare with 29% in an aged-matched control group (Figure 19.3).[37] In the same study, the duration of menstrual bleeding was 5 days in 83% of the patients and 8 days in 25%. (In the general population, the length of a menstrual period varies from 2 to 8 days, with a mean of 5 days.) There was bleeding through protection, flooding at night and passage of clots in 64%, 57% and 68% of the patients, respectively.

No relationship has been found between the number of the days of menstruation and the total menstrual blood loss in the general population.[7] In contrast, a strong relationship has been found in women with inherited bleeding disorders, which indicates that these women bleed

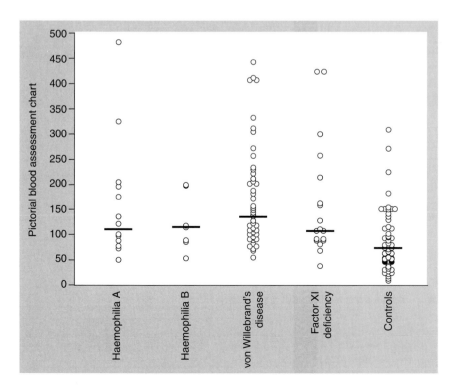

Figure 19.3 Menstrual scores in women who are carriers of haemophilia von Willebrand's disease or factor XI deficiency and in controls. The horizontal lines represent median values. Reproduced by kind permission of Blackwell Science from Kadir *et al.*[82]

Table 19.1 Other bleeding symptoms and symptom scores in women with menorrhagia

	Total – number (%)	Group A – no bleeding disorder – number (%)	Group B – von Willebrand's disease – number (%)	p (comparison between group A and group B)	Group C – factor XI deficiency – number (%)	p (comparison between group A and group C)
Number of patients	150	123	20		6	
Bruising	88 (58.7)	66 (53.7)	16 (80)	0.05	4 (66.7)	0.69
Nose bleeding	22 (14.7)	17 (13.8)	5 (25)	0.20	0	1.00
Gum bleeding	54 (36)	41 (33.3)	9 (45)	0.45	1 (16.7)	0.66
Bleeding after tooth extraction	13 out of 98 (13.3)	6 out of 81 (7.4)	6 out of 13 (46.2)	0.001	1 out of 3 (33.3)	0.23
Postoperative bleeding	18 out of 109 (16.5)	7 out of 90 (7.8)	8 out of 13 (61.5)	< 0.001	3 out of 5 (60)	0.008
Postpartum bleeding	29 out of 97 (29.9)	17 out of 80 (21.3)	8 out of 13 (61.5)	0.005	3 out of 3 (100)	0.01
Number of other bleeding symptoms other than menorrhagia						
Median (range)	1 (0–5)	1 (0–5)	2 (1–5)	< 0.001	1.5 (0–4)	0.26
0	40 (26.7)	39 (31.7)	0		1 (16.7)	
1–2	78 (52)	65 (52.9)	11 (55)		3 (50)	
3–4	28 (18.7)	17 (13.8)	7 (35)		2 (33.3)	
5–6	4 (2.7)	2 (1.6)	2 (10)	< 0.001	0	0.41

Reproduced from Kadir et al.[95] by kind permission of the Lancet.

heavily throughout their menstrual period.

Heavy menstruation has also been reported in women with the less common and rare bleeding disorders, including deficiencies of prothrombin, fibrinogen, factor V, factor VII and factor X.[38–41] Factor XIII is important in the final stage of haemostasis since it helps polymerization and cross-linkage of fibrin, and deficiencies of this factor have also been associated with menorrhagia.[40]

Frequency of inherited bleeding disorders in women with menorrhagia

Acute adolescent menorrhagia requiring urgent medical intervention has long been recognized as being associated with undiagnosed underlying bleeding disorders. A primary coagulation disorder was found in almost 20% of 59 adolescents with such menorrhagia,[42] and screening for von Willebrand's disease and platelet disorders has been recommended in these patients.[43,44] However, the prevalence of bleeding disorders in older women with menorrhagia has been underestimated and has not been extensively investigated. In addition, screening for bleeding disorders has not been a part of the clinical investigations of menorrhagia. However, the high frequency of bleeding disorders, especially von Willebrand's disease, in women with menorrhagia has been shown in several studies.[45–49] The reported prevalences (ranging from 16% to 26%) strongly suggest that evaluation for bleeding disorders should be recommended.

In a study in our centre, in 150 women with menorrhagia, 26 were found to have inherited bleeding disorder. The incidence of bleeding after tooth extraction, postpartum and postoperative bleeding, and the number of bleeding symptoms other than menorrhagia were significantly higher in the group with bleeding disorders (Table 19.1).

Obtaining a careful medical history is very important when assessing women complaining of menorrhagia, since certain predictive factors may suggest a high probability of a bleeding disorder in the aetiology of menorrhagia. These factors include a history of long-standing menorrhagia (specifically menorrhagia since menarche) and a history of bleeding after tooth extraction, postoperatively or postpartum. However, the clinical severity of inherited bleeding disorders varies considerably, and menorrhagia may be the only clinical manifestation. Therefore, testing for these disorders, especially von Willebrand's disease, should be performed in women with menorrhagia without any obvious pelvic pathology before embarking on any invasive procedures. Diagnosis of inherited bleeding disorders in these women has several advantages. It enhances rapid and effective treatment of menorrhagia, thereby avoiding unnecessary surgical interventions. In six out of seven women (86%) who had a hysterectomy for menorrhagia in a series of 38 women with type 1 von Willebrand's disease, the diagnosis of von Willebrand's disease was not known pre-operatively.[36] Moreover, if any surgical procedure were to become necessary, the risk of haemorrhage can be prevented by appropriate prophylactic treatment when indicated. Lastly, it has genetic implications and may affect the management of future pregnancies.

The menstrual cycle and the use of oral contraception are associated with variations in coagulation markers (Figure 19.4).[12] Therefore, when testing for mild bleeding disorders in women, especially type 1 von Willebrand's disease, it is advisable that blood should be drawn during

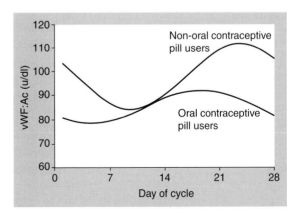

Figure 19.4 Changes in von Willebrand factor activity (vWF:Ac) during menstrual cycle for oral contraceptive pill users and non-users. Reproduced by kind permission of FK Schattauer Verlagsgesellschall mbH from Kadir et al.[12]

the early follicular phase, no later than day 7 of the cycle.[50] It is also advisable to avoid any planned surgical intervention during this phase in patients with mild von Willebrand's disease since factor VIII and von Willebrand factor activities are at their nadir.[45,50]

Quality of life during menstruation

In addition to its medical implications, menorrhagia has been shown to have a negative effect on the quality of life in patients with inherited bleeding disorders.[51] Over one-third of these women cut down on the time spent on their work or other activities and accomplish less than they would like, and over one-half experienced moderate to very severe dysmenorrhea.[51]

In women with inherited bleeding disorders, menstruation is usually excessive from menarche and, because of the genetic nature of the disease, sisters may also have heavy menstruation. Therefore, these women might consider that it is normal to have heavy menstruation and might not seek medical advice and thus are not aware of treatment options. Hence, it is recommended that women with inherited bleeding disorders should be asked regularly about their periods and an objective assessment of menstrual loss should be performed using a pictorial blood assessment chart in those who complain of excessive blood loss. Those with a normal score on objective assessment can be reassured, for those with heavy loss, appropriate investigations, treatment and referral to a gynaecologist should be arranged.

In addition, clinicians should also be aware that menorrhagia is a common and a major problem in women with inherited bleeding disorders and that it can be the presenting symptom. Liaison between haematologists and gynaecologists helps early detection, appropriate management and improvement of quality of life of these patients.

Management of menorrhagia

Menorrhagia in women with inherited bleeding disorders is usually due to their clotting factor deficiency. However, each individual patient should be appropriately assessed and local causes should be excluded, especially the possibility of malignancy in older women. The treatment is then usually medical; the options are tranexamic acid, combined oral contraceptive compounds, or (more recently) intranasal desmopressin spray. Cyclical progestogens are widely used in the treatment of dysfunctional uterine bleeding despite there being limited evidence to support this. They are effective only in women with anovulatory dysfunctional uterine bleeding. However, most women with dysfunctional uterine bleeding show no evidence of hormonal imbalance and have regular ovulatory cycles.[7,52] This treatment modality may be used as a second choice in patients with bleeding disorders who do not respond to the first-choice treatments or when the first-choice treatments are contraindicated. Other medical treatments, including danazol and gonadotropin releasing hormone agonists, are used with reasonable efficacy in the treatment of menorrhagia in general. However, experience about their effectiveness in women with inherited bleeding disorders is lacking in the literature. In addition, the side effects and risks associated with a long-term hypo-oestrogenic state make them unacceptable for long-term use.

Non-steroidal anti-inflammatory drugs are used successfully to reduce menstrual blood loss in women with primary menorrhagia (i.e. dysfunctional uterine bleeding).[52,53] However, in patients with underlying bleeding disorders they are ineffective and may increase the menstrual blood loss.[53] It has been demonstrated that although the production of prostacyclin (a vasodilator and an antiaggregation agent) and thromboxane A2 (a vasoconstrictor and a proaggregation agent) are normal in the endometrium of patients with primary menorrhagia, the balance is shifted to a relative thromboxane deficiency.[53] Non-steroidal anti-inflammatory drugs are non-selective (i.e. they suppress the production of both prostacyclin and thromboxane A2). However, it has been shown that this may not necessarily be true in the uterine vasculature.[54] In addition, in normal people, inhibition of prostaglandin production in the uterine vasculature outweighs the antiaggregatory effects of these drugs on platelet function. These features explain the otherwise paradoxical clinical success of non-steroidal anti-inflammatory drugs in the treatment of primary menorrhagia.

Antifibrinolytic agents have a beneficial role in the management of menorrhagia because fibrinolytic activity increases during menstruation.[55,56] Dockeray et al. found a significant reduction in plasminogen activator activity and plasmin activity in the menstrual fluid with tranexamic acid.[57] It has also been shown that tranexamic acid significantly reduces endometrial tissue plasminogen activator activity and antigen[58] and that it reduces menstrual blood loss in patients with menorrhagia in general[52,58] as well as in patients with inherited bleeding disorders.[59] Bonnar and Sheppard randomized 76 women to one of three treatments: ethamsylate (a general haemostatic agent), mefenamic acid (a prostaglandin synthetase inhibitor) and the fibrinolytic agent, tranexamic acid at a dose of 1 g every 6 hours.[52] Menstrual loss measured by the spectrophotometric method in three control menstrual periods and three menstrual periods during treatment showed that there was no reduction in menstrual blood loss with ethamsylate, a 20% reduction with mefenamic acid and a 54% reduction with tranexamic acid. The bioavailability of tranexamic acid is only about 35%,[60] which necessitates frequent administration of high doses (at least 1 g four times daily), this may reduce patient compliance. However, there is a recent report of the successful use of single high-dose antifibrinolytic therapy (tranexamic acid at a dose of 4 g orally once daily) in three patients with either type 2A or type 2B von Willebrand's disease.[61] Antifibrinolytic therapy is safe and far less expensive than other treatment modalities and is certainly worth trying as a first-line treatment especially in patients with menorrhagia who are not responsive to desmopression (i.e. patients with type 2 or 3 von Willebrand's disease, before a concentrate that contains von Willebrand factor is used.

Combined oral contraceptives increase factor VIII activity and von Willebrand factor activity,[61a–63] as well as controlling the menstrual cycle. They are therefore effective and are currently the most commonly used treatment of menorrhagia in patients with inherited bleeding disorders. However, the response has been reported to be variable and unpredictable in von Willebrand's disease.[63,64] Interestingly, in a survey of patients with type 2 or type 3 von Willebrand's disease, by 88% of 25 women treated with oral contraceptives stated that the treatment was effective.[65] On the other hand, in patients with type I von Willebrand's disease, a standard dose of oral contraceptives was effective in only 24%, while high-dose contraceptive therapy was effective in only 37%.[66]

Occasionally, a girl with von Willebrand's disease presents at menarche or shortly afterwards with marked, sometimes life-threatening, menorrhagia. In these cases, collaboration between the gynaecologist and haemophilia specialist is essential. Hormonal treatment such as norethisterone (10 mg three times a day) together with desmopressin on von Willebrand factor-containing concentrates is usually required. Once control of bleeding is achieved, a combined oral contraceptive is prescribed.

Home therapy for menorrhagia with desmopressin is now possible with the advent of intranasal formulations[67–69] and subcutaneous forms.[70,71] Desmopressin administered intranasally as a spray has been shown to increase plasma levels of factor VIII and von Willebrand factor in patients with mild haemophilia A or type 1 von Willebrand's disease.[67,72] It is effective when used prophylactically for minor procedures or for the treatment of bleeding episodes in these patients. It has been shown by several investigators to be effective (based on women's subjective assessment) in the management of menorrhagia.[68,70,73] Recently, in a small randomized placebo-controlled trial, the effect of desmopressin nasal sprays on menstrual blood loss in patients with menorrhagia was objectively evaluated using a pictorial blood assessment chart.[74] Desmopressin treatment was safe and resulted in a decrease in menstrual scores, but there was no differences when compared with placebo spray. Further larger randomized trials are required. At present, there is no consensus about the optimal frequency and duration of treatment. Desmopressin nasal spray is given during the first 2–3 days of menstruation based on the fact that 90% of all menstrual flow is in the first 3 days.[75] However, women with inherited bleeding disorders bleed heavily throughout their period.[37]

Hormone-releasing intrauterine systems, originally developed for use as contraceptives, have now been shown to be highly effective in reducing menstrual loss in premenopausal women. The system currently licensed in the UK for contraception is the levonorgestrel intrauterine system, Mirena. In a study by Andersson and Rybo, menstrual loss was significantly reduced in women with dysfunctional menorrhagia (menstrual blood loss of 80 ml or more per period).[76] After 3 months treatment with the levonorgestrel intrauterine system, there was an 85% reduction in menstrual loss and after 12 months there was a 97% reduction (as measured by extraction of blood), and there was also a significant increase in serum ferritin in the first year of use. This system is now increasingly used on a 'named patient basis' for non-contraceptive indications, and the recent Government-funded Effective Health Care Bulletin (The Management of Menorrhagia) stated that data from Scandinavia pointed to the effectiveness of this device as a first-line treatment for menorrhagia. Data about use and effectiveness of this device in menorrhagia caused by bleeding disorders are lacking from the literature. Owing to the high local level of progestagens, the use of these hormone-releasing systems is associated with suppression of endometrial growth and spiral arterioles as well as capillary thrombosis. In addition, it has also been shown that there is no effect on endometrial factor VIII activity, which is reduced by ordinary coils.[77] Therefore, it is reasonable to believe that they will be as effective in reducing menstrual blood loss in women with bleeding disorders as in those with dysfunctional menorrhagia. This needs to be confirmed by appropriate studies.

GYNAECOLOGICAL SURGERY

Surgical intervention is sometimes required in patients who are unresponsive to medical treatment. Surgical procedures, even relatively minor operations such as hysteroscopy or diagnostic curettage,[37] can be complicated by haemorrhage in patients with inherited bleeding disorders. Therefore, good liaison between the local haematologist and the surgical and anaesthetic team is essential. Patients' factor levels should be checked preoperatively and adequate cover provided. The treatment may need to be continued postoperatively, sometimes for up to 10 days, to reduce the development of secondary haematomas. Any surgical intervention should be carried out by a senior gynaecologist, the technique with the least risk of bleeding should be chosen, bleeding vessels should be ligated and not cauterized since oozing can occur after surgery, and the use of surgical drains should be considered. Endometrial ablative techniques are increasingly used for management of menorrhagia that does not respond to medical treatment. These procedures, in particular endometrial resection, are associated with a risk of bleeding complications. It is therefore sensible to choose thermal or laser ablation in these patients.

It is also important to remember that excessive bleeding may be surgical rather than a result of a failure of adequate replacement therapy. Postoperative monitoring is continued depending on the nature of the operation and the patient's factor levels. In contrast, unexplained operative and postoperative bleeding that does not respond to general measures should alert the gynaecologist to the possibility of bleeding disorders as causative factor.

OTHER GYNAECOLOGICAL PROBLEMS

In addition to heavy and prolonged menstruation, women with inherited bleeding disorders my suffer from intermenstrual bleeding, dysmenorrhea[37,78] and sexual problems including pain, bleeding and/or bruising during sexual intercourse.[79]

Acute abdomen due to haemoperitoneum caused by spontaneous rupture of a corpus luteum is a rare but recognized complication in women with inherited bleeding disorders, especially those with severe deficiency such as type 3 von Willebrand's disease.[37,80,81] It is important to recognize this clinical situation and if possible to avoid or delay surgical intervention until adequate haemostasis is achieved.

Prevention with long-term combined oral contraceptive therapy has been recommended for women with severe deficiency.

REFERENCES

1. Seligsohn U. Factor XI deficiency [review]. *Thromb Haemost* 1993;**70**:68–71.
2. von Willebrand EA. Hereditäre pseudohaemophilie. *Finnska Iaekaellsk Handl* 1926;**68**: 87–112.
3. Sramek A, Eikenboom JC, Briet E, Vandenbroucke JP, Rosendaal FR. Usefulness of patient interview in bleeding disorders. *Arch Intern Med* 1995;**155**:1409–15.
4. Federici AB, Mannucci PM. Actual management of von Willebrand disease: first report on 880 cases of the Italian registry of vWD [abstract]. *Blood* 1997;**90**:33.
5. Mauser Bunschoten EP, van Houwelingen JC, Sjamsoedin Visser EJ. Bleeding symptoms in carriers of haemophilia A and B. *Thromb Haemost* 1988;**59**:349–52.
6. Hallberg L, Hogdahl AM, Nilsson L, Rybo G. Menstrual blood loss and iron deficiency. *Acta Med Scand* 1966;**180**:639–50.
7. Haynes PJ, Hodgson H, Anderson AB, Turnbull AC. Measurement of menstrual blood loss in patients complaining of menorrhagia. *Br J Obstet Gynaecol* 1977;**84**:763–8.
8. Fraser IS, McCarron G, Markham, R, Resta T, Watts A. Measured menstrual blood loss in women with menorrhagia associated with pelvic disease or coagulation disorder. *Obstet Gynecol* 1986;**68**:630–3.
9. Rodeghiero F, Castaman G, Dini E. Epidemiological investigation of the prevalence of von Willebrand's disease. *Blood* 1987;**69**:454–9.
10. Werner EJ, Broxson EH, Tucker EL, Giroux DS, Shults J, Abshire TC. Prevalence of von Willebrand's disease in children: a muliethnic study. *J Pediatr* 1993;**123**:893–8.
11. Bloom AL. von Willebrand factor: clinical features of inherited and acquired disorders [review]. *Mayo Clin Proc* 1991;**66**:743–51.
12. Kadir RA, Economides DL, Sabin CA, Owens D, Lee CA. Variations in coagulation factors in women: effect of age, ethnicity, menstrual cycle and combined oral contraceptive. *Thromb Haemost* 1999;**82**:1456–61.
13. Triplett DA. Laboratory diagnosis of von Willebrand's disease [review]. *Mayo Clin Proc* 1991;**66**:832–40.
14. Ruggeri ZM. Structure and function of von Willebrand factor: relationship to von Willebrand's disease [review]. *Mayo Clin Proc* 1991;**66**:847–61.
15. Sadler JE. A revised classification of von Willebrand disease. For the Subcommittee on von Willebrand Factor of the Scientific and Standardization Committee of the International Society on Thrombosis and Haemostasis. *Thromb Haemost* 1994;**71**:520–5.
16. Weiss HJ, Ball AP, Mannucci PM. Incidence of severe von Willebrand's disease [letter]. *N Engl J Med* 1982;**307**:127.
17. Berliner S, Horowitz I, Martinowitz U, Brenner B, Seligshon U. Dental surgery in patients with severe factor XI deficiency without plasma replacement. *Blood Coagul Fibrinolysis* 1992;**3**:465–8.
18. Forbes CD. Clinical aspects of haemophilias. In: Ratnoff OD, Forbes CD, eds, *Disorders of Haemostasis*. Grune & Stratton: New York; 1984:177–239.
19. Rizza CR, Rhymes IL, Austen DE, Kernoff PB, Aroni SA. Detection of carriers of haemophilia: a 'blind' study. *Br J Haematol* 1975;**30**:447–56.
20. Lusher JM, McMillan CW. Severe factor VIII and factor IX deficiency in females. *Am J Med* 1978;**65**:637–48.
21. Graham JB, Barrow ES, Roberts HR, *et al.* Dominant inheritance of hemophilia A in three generations of women. *Blood* 1975;**46**:175–88.
22. Mori PG, Pasino M, Vadal CR, Bisogni MC, Tonini GP, Scarabicchi S. Haemophilia 'A' in a 46,X,i(Xq) female. *Br J Haematol* 1979;**43**:143–7.
23. Neuschatz J, Necheles TF. Hemophilia B in a phenotypically normal girl with XX (ring) XO mosaicism. *Acta Haematol* 1973;**49**:108–13.
24. Bolton-Maggs PH, Young Wan-Yin B, McCraw AH, Slack J, Kernoff PB. Inheritance and bleeding in factor XI deficiency. *Br J Haematol* 1988;**69**: 521–8.
25. Collins PW, Goldman E, Lilley P, Pasi KJ, Lee CA. Clinical experience of factor XI deficiency: the role of fresh frozen plasma and factor XI concentrate. *Haemophilia* 1995;**1**:227–31.
26. Ginsburg D, Handin RI, Bonthron DT *et al.* Human von Willebrand factor (vWF): isolation of

complementary DNA (cDNA) clones and chromosomal localisation. *Science* 1985;**228**: 1501–6.

27. Miller CH. Genetics of haemophilia and von Willebrand's disease. In: Hilgartner MW, ed. *Haemophilia in the Child and Adult.* New York: Masson; 1982:29–62.

28. Kato A, Asakai R, Davie EW, Aoki N. Factor XI gene (F11) is located on the distal end of the long arm of human chromosome 4. *Cytogenet Cell Genet* 1989;**52**:77–8.

29. Asakai R, Chung DW, Ratnoff OD, Davie EW. Factor XI (plasma thromboplastin antecedent) deficiency in Ashkenazi Jews is a bleeding disorder that can result from three types of point mutations. *Proc Natl Acad Sci USA* 1989;**86**:7667–71.

30. Imanak Y, McVey JH, Nishimura T, *et al.* Identification and characterisation of mutations in factor XI gene of non-Jewish factor XI-deficient patients. *Thromb Haemost* 1993;**69**:752.

31. Peretz U, Zivelin A, Usher S, Eichel R, Seligsohn U. Identification of a new mutation in factor XI gene of an Ashkenazi-Jew with severe factor XI deficiency. *Blood* 1993;**82(suppl 1)**:66.

32. Pugh RE, McVey JH, Tuddenham EG, Hancock JF. Six point mutations that cause factor XI deficiency. *Blood* 1995;**85**:1509–16.

33. Asakai R, Gung DW, Davie EW, Seligsohn U. Factor XI deficiency in Ashkenazi Jews in Israel. *N Engl J Med* 1991;**325**:153–8.

34. Hancock JF, Wieland K, Pugh RE, *et al.* A molecular genetic study of factor XI deficiency. *Blood* 1991;**77**:1942–8.

35. Highham JM, O'Brien PM, Shaw RW. Assessment of menstrual blood loss using a pictorial chart. *Br J Obstet Gynaecol* 1990;**97**:734–9.

36. Ragni MV, Bontempo FA, Cortese Hassett A. von Willebrand disease and bleeding in women. *Haemophilia* 1999;**5**:313–17.

37. Kadir RA, Economides DL, Sabin CA, Pollard D, Lee CA. Assessment of menstrual blood loss and gynaecological problems in patients with inherited bleeding disorders. *Haemophilia* 1999;**5**:40–8.

38. Silwer J. von Willebrand's disease in Sweden. *Acta Paediatr Scand Suppl* 1973;**238**:1–159.

39. Mariani G, Mazzucconi MG. Factor VII congenital deficiency. Clinical picture and classification of the variants [review]. *Haemostasis* 1983;**13**:169–77.

40. Roberts HR, Lozier JN. Other clotting factor deficiencies. In: Hoffman R, Benz EJ, Shattil SJ, Furie B, Cohen HJ, eds. *Hematology: Basic Principles and Practice.* Edinburgh: Churchill Livingstone; 1991:1332–43.

41. Peyvandi F, Mannucci PM, Asti D, Abdoullahi M, DiRocco N. Clinical manifestations in 28 Italian and Iranian patients with severe factor VII deficiency. *Haemophilia* 1997;**3**:242–6.

42. Claessens EA, Cowell CA. Acute adolescent menorrhagia. *Am J Obstet Gynecol* 1981;**139**: 277–80.

43. Claessens EA, Cowell CA. Dysfunctional uterine bleeding in the adolescent. *Pediatr Clin North Am* 1981;**28**:369–78.

44. Ward CL. Hemorrhaging at menarche: a case report. *J Fam Pract* 1992;**34**:351–4.

45. Edlund M, Blomback M, von Schoultz B, Andersson O. On the value of menorrhagia as a predictor for coagulation disorders. *Am J Hematol* 1996;**53**:234–8.

46. Kadir RA, Economides DL, Sabin CA, Owens D, Lee CA. Frequency of inherited bleeding disorders in women with menorrhagia. *Lancet* 1998;**351**:485–9.

47. Baindur S, Shetty S, Pathare AV, Salvi V, Ghosh K, Mohanty D. Screening for von Willbrand disease in patients with menorrhagia [abstract]. *Haemophilia* 2000;**6**:240.

48. Kouides P, Phatak P, Sham R, Braggin C, Tara M, Cox C. The prevelance of subnormal von Willebrand factor levels in menorrhagia patients in Rochester, NY: final analysis [abstract]. *Haemophilia* 2000;**6**:244.

49. Krause M, Aygören-Pürsun E, Ehrenforth S, *et al.* Coagulation disorders in women with menorrhagia [abstract]. *Haemophilia* 2000;**6**:245.

50. Blombäck M, Eneroth P, Landgren BM, Lagerstrom M, Anderson O. On the intraindividual and gender variability of haemostatic components. *Thromb Haemost* 1992;**67**:70–5.

51. Kadir RA, Sabin CA, Pollard D, Lee CA, Economides DL. Quality of life during menstruation in patients with inherited bleeding disorders. *Haemophilia* 1998;**4**:836–41.

52. Bonnar J, Sheppard BL. Treatment of menorrhagia during menstruation: randomised controlled trial of ethamsylate, mefenamic acid, and tranexamic acid. *BMJ* 1996;**313**:579–82.

53. Mäkäräinen L, Ylikorkala O. Primary and myoma-associated menorrhagia: role of prostaglandins and effects of ibuprofen. *Br J Obstet Gynaecol* 1986;**93**:974–8.

54. Powell AM, Chan WY. Differential effects of ibuprofen and naproxen sodium on menstrual prostaglandin release and on prostaglandin production in the rat uterine homogenate. *Prostaglandins Leukot Med* 1984;**13**:129–37.

55. Cederblad G, Han L, Korsan-Bengsten K, Pehrsson NG, Rybo G. Variations in blood coagulation, fibrinolysis, platelet function and various plasma proteins during the menstrual cycle. *Haemostasis* 1977;**6**:294–302.

56. Hahn L, Cederblad G, Rybo G, Pehrsson NG, Bengtsen KK. Blood coagulation, fibrinolysis and plasma proteins in women with normal and with excessive menstrual blood loss. *Br J Obstet Gynaecol* 1976;**83**:974–80.

57. Dockeray CJ, Sheppard BL, Daly L, Bonnar J. The fibrinolytic enzyme system in normal menstruation and excessive uterine bleeding and the effect of tranexamic acid. *Eur J Obstet Gynecol Reprod Biol* 1987;**24**:309–18.

58. Gleeson NC, Buggy F, Sheppard BL, Bonnar J. The effect of tranexamic acid on measured menstrual loss and endometrial fibrinolytic enzymes in dysfunctional uterine bleeding. *Acta Obstet Gynecol Scand* 1994;**73**:274–7.

59. Bonnar J, Guillebaud J, Kasonde JM, Sheppard BL. Clinical applications of fibrinolytic inhibition in gynaecology [review]. *J Clin Pathol Suppl (R Coll Pathol)* 1980;**14**:55–9.

60. Pilbrant X, Schannong M, Vessman J. Pharmacokinetics and bioavailability of tranexamic acid. *Eur J Clin Pharmacol* 1981;**20**:65–72.

61. Ong YL, Hull DR, Mayne EE. Menorrhagia in von Willebrand disease successfully treated with single daily dose tranexamic acid. *Haemophilia* 1998;**4**:63–5.

61a. Schiffman S, Rapaport SI. Increased factor 8 levels in suspected carriers of hemophilia A taking contraceptives by mouth. *N Engl J Med* 1966;**275**:599.

62. Glueck HI, Flessa HC. Control of hemorrhage in von Wilebrand's disease and a haemophiliac carrier with norethynordrelmestranol. *Thromb Res* 1972;**1**:253–66.

63. Alperin JB. Estrogens and surgery in women with von Willebrand's disease. *Am J Med* 1982;**73**:367–71.

64. Mannucci PM. Treatment of von Willebrand's disease [review]. *J Intern Med Suppl* 1997;**740**: 129–32.

65. Foster PA. The reproductive health of women with von Willebrand Disease unresponsive to DDAVP: results of an international survey. On behalf of the Subcommittee on von Willebrand Factor of the Scientific and Standardization Committee of the ISTH. *Thromb Haemost* 1995;**74**:784–90.

66. Kouides P, Burkhart P, Phatak P. Type 1 von Willebrand disease causes significant obstetric–gynaecological morbidity [abstract]. *Blood* 1997;**90**:131.

67. Rose EH, Aledort LM. Nasal spray desmopressin (DDAVP) for mild hemophilia A and von Willebrand disease. *Ann Intern Med* 1991;**114**: 563–8.

68. Lethagen S, Ragnarson TG. Self-treatment with desmopressin intranasal spray in patients with bleeding disorders: effect on bleeding symptoms and socioeconomic factors. *Ann Hematol* 1993;**66**:257–60.

69. Seremetis SV, Aledort LM. Desmopressin nasal spray for hemophilia A and type I von Willebrand disease [letter]. *Ann Intern Med* 1997;**126**:744–5.

70. Rodeghiero F, Castaman G, Mannucci PM. Prospective multicenter study on subcutaneous concentrated desmopressin for home treatment of patients with von Willebrand disease and mild or moderate hemophilia A. *Thromb Haemost* 1996;**76**:692–6.

71. Mannucci PM. Desmopressin (DDAVP) in the treatment of bleeding disorders: the first 20 years [review]. *Blood* 1997;**90**:2515–21.

72. Lethagen S, Harris AS, Nilsson IM. Intranasal desmopressin (DDAVP) by spray in mild hemophilia A and von Willebrand's type I. *Blut* 1990;**60**:187–91.

73. Kobrinsky N, Goldsmith J. Efficacy of stimate (desmopressin acetate) nasal spray, 1.5 mg/ml, for the treatment of menorrhagia in women with inherited bleeding disorders [abstract]. *Blood* 1997;**90**:3186.

74. Kadir RA, Lee CA, Pollard D, Economides DL. DDAVP nasal spray for treatment of menorrhagia in women with inherited bleeding disorders: a randomised placebo controlled cross-over study. *Haemophilia* (submitted for publication).

75. Janssen CA, Scholten PC, Heintz AP. A simple visual assessment technique to discriminate between menorrhagia and normal menstrual blood loss. *Obstet Gynecol* 1995;**85**:977–82.

76. Andersson JK, Rybo G. Levonorgestrel-releasing intrauterine device in the treatment of menorrhagia. *Br J Obstet Gynaecol* 1990;**97**:690–4.

77. Zhu P, Hongzhi L, Wenliang S. Observation of the activity of factor VIII in the endometrium of women pre- and post-insertion of three types of IUDs. *Contraception* 1991;**44**:367–87.

78. Forrest H. Young women with von Willbrand disease associated with dysmenorrhea [abstract]. *Haemophilia* 2000;**6**:242.

79. Wysocki DK. Psychosexual and gynaecological

aspects of women with bleeding disorders. [abstract]. *Haemophilia* 2000;**6**:247.

80. Greer IA, Lowe GD, Walker JJ, Forbes CD. Haemorrhagic problems in obstetrics and gynaecology in patients with congenital coagulopathies. *Br J Obstet Gynaecol* 1991;**98**:909–18.

81. Gomez A, Lucia JF, Perella M, Aguilar C. Haemoperitoneum caused by haemorrhagic corpus luteum in a patient with type 3 von Willebrand's disease. *Haemophilia* 1998;**4**:60–2.

20

Pregnancy in women with inherited bleeding disorders

Paul LF Giangrande

HAEMOPHILIA

Haemophilia A is a congenital disorder of coagulation, characterized by deficiency of factor VIII in the blood. Deficiency of factor IX results in an identical clinical condition known as haemophilia B (also known as Christmas disease). Haemophilia is encountered in all racial groups, with an incidence of approximately one in 10,000 males. The clinical picture is dependent on the degree of deficiency of the coagulation factor in the blood: severe haemophilia is associated with a level of less than 1% of normal. The hallmark of severe haemophilia is recurrent and spontaneous bleeding into joints, principally the knees, elbows and ankles. Repeated bleeding into joints can, in the absence of treatment, result in disabling arthritis at an early age. Bleeding into muscles and soft tissues is also frequently seen.

Advances in the treatment of haemophilia have led to improvements in both the longevity and quality of life of patients with even severe haemophilia. As patients live longer and integrate fully into society, it is anticipated that the number of patients with severe haemophilia in the developed world will increase significantly, since the daughters of haemophiliacs are obligate carriers of the condition. Obstetricians will thus be faced more frequently than in the past with the problem of management of pregnancy in known or possible carriers of this condition.

Carriers of haemophilia

The genes for both factor VIII and IX are located on the X chromosome and thus the inheritance is sex-linked and recessive, like colour blindness. However, one-third of cases arise in families with no previous family history, and reflect new mutations. The daughters of men with haemophilia are obligate carriers of the condition, and such women have a 50:50 chance of passing on the clinical condition to a son and a 50:50 chance of passing the carrier state to a daughter. The severity of haemophilia within a given family remains constant. If a woman has relatives with only very mild haemophilia, then she may be reassured that there is no risk of transmitting a severe form of the disease.

Most female carriers of haemophilia have levels of factor VIII (or IX) within the normal range, but a significant proportion have a modest reduction in the baseline level. The baseline level is seldom lower than 20% of the normal level and should thus certainly suffice to protect against significant bleeding problems in day-to-day life. However, female carriers with low levels of factor VIII (or IX) are at risk of bleeding in the setting of surgery or other invasive procedures (e.g. dental extractions, biopsies). In such circumstances, haemostatic support may be required, and the choice of product depends both on the factor level and on the nature of the procedure. Recombinant coagulation factor concentrates should be considered to be the products of choice.

There is no need to carry out special genetic tests in daughters of men with haemophilia to determine their carrier status, but the status of other women in the extended family may not be so clear. A woman who has an affected uncle, for example, may or may not be a carrier. A common and difficult problem is a pregnant woman with a vague history of a bleeding disorder in a distant relative. Carrier testing can take some weeks to perform and it may seem logical to initiate carrier testing to determine carrier status as soon as possible in girls with a family history of the condition, since this would facilitate management of pregnancy in the case of an early and unexpected pregnancy. However, testing of young children ignores the ethical and legal rights of children, since testing cannot be considered to have been obtained with the informed consent of the individual child concerned. These issues must be discussed openly with the family. Once the carrier status has been determined and DNA markers have been identified, it is then possible to offer antenatal diagnosis of haemophilia to pregnant women.

Antenatal diagnosis of haemophilia

As a general rule, antenatal diagnosis of haemophilia is offered only when a termination of the pregnancy is being contemplated if an affected fetus were to be identified. It is certainly not necessary to determine the status of a male fetus for purposes of pregnancy management. Women will require counselling about haemophilia before they make this important decision about termination. The general experience has been that only a minority of women subsequently take up the offer of antenatal diagnosis with a view to termination if an affected fetus is identified.[1,2] This may well reflect the fact that many women with affected relatives recognize the tremendous advances in treatment in recent years, such as the use of recombinant products, which have resulted in an essentially normal life for the younger generation of haemophiliacs. Chorion villus sampling or biopsy is the principal method used for antenatal

diagnosis of haemophilia. It offers the major advantage over amniocentesis of permitting diagnosis during the first trimester, although it should not be carried out before 11 weeks' gestation since earlier biopsy may be associated with a risk of subsequent fetal limb abnormalities.[3,4] The sample of chorionic villus is obtained by either the transabdominal or transvaginal route, under ultrasound guidance; the sample is then subjected to DNA analysis. It is possible that in the not-too-distant future, non-invasive antenatal diagnostic procedures may become available in which fetal DNA can be extracted from fetal normoblasts in the maternal circulation.[5]

Fetal blood sampling is carried out when it has not been possible to establish the status of the fetus, either because DNA-based studies were not possible or because they were carried out but were not informative. In this technique, fetal blood is taken from fetal umbilical vessels under ultrasound guidance. The procedure is not available in all hospitals and requires considerable expertise to perform. It is usually carried out at a minimum of 18 weeks' gestation. Approximately 1 ml of blood is required for assay of coagulation factor levels. The levels of factor VIII and factor IX in a normal fetus at around 19 weeks' gestation are significantly lower than that in an adult, at approximately 40 iu/dl and 10 iu/dl respectively.[6,7] It is therefore essential to ensure that the blood is wholly fetal and not contaminated with maternal blood, which could result in diagnostic error through spurious elevation of the factor level, for example by measuring the mean corpuscular volume (MCV) or fetal haemoglobin contents. The fetal MCV is typically at least 120 fl at this stage of pregnancy, while that of the mother is around 90 fl. However, the Kleihauer technique based on demonstrating resistance of fetal haemoglobin to acid elution is more reliable, but it takes longer to carry out.[8] The factor assay results should never be communicated without results of such additional tests to confirm fetal origin of the sample.

All invasive methods used for antenatal diagnosis may cause fetal–maternal haemorrhage, and anti-D immunoglobulin should be given if the mother is Rh-D negative. These procedures are likely to be carried out early in a pregnancy, when the factor VIII level has not risen significantly, and so some form of haemostatic support may be required to prevent maternal bleeding.

Management of delivery in carriers of haemophilia

Ultrasound examination to determine fetal sex during pregnancy is strongly recommended, since this may influence decisions in the management of delivery. Even if the mother does not wish to know the result, it is important that this information should be available to the obstetrician at the time of delivery. The levels of factor VIII and von Willebrand's factor rise during normal pregnancy, particularly during the third trimester, when levels of factor VIII may rise to double that of the normal baseline value. By contrast, factor IX levels do not rise significantly in pregnancy and thus carriers of haemophilia B with a low baseline factor IX level are more likely to require haemostatic support to cover delivery, particularly for a Caesarean delivery. Treatment with coagulation factor concentrate is only rarely required during pregnancy in carriers of haemophilia A. Coagulation factor concentrate was not required in any of 117 pregnancies in carriers of haemophilia in a retrospective study from Sweden, although four mothers required a blood transfusion after delivery.[9] In another study from a London Hospital, factor VIII was given during pregnancy in only one of 48 pregnancies although desmopressin was given to another woman after delivery.[1] If treatment is required in carriers of either haemophilia A or B, recombinant (genetically engineered) products should be regarded as the products of choice. Plasma-derived products, including those subjected to dual inactivation processes, have the potential to transmit parvovirus. Although parvovirus does not normally cause a serious infection in a non-immunocompromised adult, infection of the fetus may result in hydrops fetalis and fetal death.[10] Desmopressin is of potential value in these cases, since it can boost the plasma levels of von Willebrand's factor and

factor VIII in the blood.[11] However, the manufacturers advise that it should only be used with caution during pregnancy (see below for a more detailed discussion). Desmopressin may be used after delivery, when the umbilical cord has been clamped. It does not pass into breast milk in significant amounts, and so it may be given to breastfeeding mothers. It does not boost the level of factor IX in the blood and is thus of no value in carriers of haemophilia B.

After delivery, a small volume (0.5–1.0 ml) of citrated cord blood should be obtained for coagulation factor assay. Because of the risk of bleeding, intramuscular injection of vitamin K should be withheld (or given orally) until the result of the factor assay is known.

There is no need to administer coagulation factor concentrates to a haemophilic neonate after a normal vaginal delivery unless there is evidence of bleeding (e.g. a cephalohaematoma), but it is advisable to give recombinant concentrate if instruments have been used to assist delivery or if delivery was considered traumatic to the fetus. Although the risk of intracranial bleeding after a normal vaginal delivery is very low,[12] consideration should be given to performing an ultrasound scan of the brain to exclude this possibility.

In the past, Caesarean section was often carried out when there was any doubt about whether a fetus was haemophilic. However, vaginal delivery is safe even when the fetus is known to have haemophilia, assuming that there are no obstetric contraindications.[9] However, vacuum extraction should be avoided since it is associated with a high risk of cephalohaematoma or intracranial bleeding. Application of fetal scalp electrodes to monitor fetal heart rate is also best avoided, particularly since there are external monitors that can be used as an alternative.

It is helpful for the obstetrician to know the sex of the fetus at the time of delivery, even if the status with regard to haemophilia is uncertain.

The principal points relating to management of delivery may be summarized as follows:

- good liaison is essential between the haemophilia centre and the obstetricians, who may be based in a different hospital;

- baseline levels of factor VIII or factor IX should be checked at booking in, and in the third trimester (ideally at around 34 weeks' gestation);
- fetal sex should be determined by ultrasound, and the results should be available to the obstetrician at the time of delivery;
- Caesarean delivery is not routinely indicated because of possible haemophilia;
- epidural anaesthesia is permitted if the factor level is more than 40 iu/dl;
- avoid the use of fetal scalp electrodes for monitoring during delivery;
- avoid vacuum extraction;
- check the cord factor level after birth;
- withhold intramuscular vitamin K until the result of factor assays are known;
- give recombinant products to the baby if forceps have been applied (but not routinely otherwise);
- special observations after delivery may be warranted, including ultrasound examination of the head to exclude the possibility of intracranial bleeding; and
- be aware of the risk of delayed postpartum haemorrhage in carriers; it is wise to check the factor level a few days after delivery; desmopressin may be useful after delivery.

VON WILLEBRAND'S DISEASE

von Willebrand factor is a protein that is encoded on chromosome 12 and synthesized in endothelial cells.[13] It binds to collagen and to platelets through the platelet glycoprotein Ib receptor and is essential for platelet adhesion to endothelial cells. It also binds circulating factor VIII non-covalently and protects it from degradation and uptake into endothelial cells. Deficiency of von Willebrand factor typically results in easy bruising, prolonged bleeding from cuts and scratches, epistaxis and menorrhagia.

Much of what has been said above about pregnancy in women who are carriers of haemophilia also applies to women with von Willebrand's disease. It is important to establish both the type and plasma levels of factor VIII and von Willebrand factor for the management of pregnant women with von Willebrand's

disease. The level of von Willebrand factor usually rises to within the normal range by the third trimester, and haemostatic support is rarely needed. The level of von Willebrand factor may not rise significantly during the first trimester or even during the second trimester, and therefore an early miscarriage may be accompanied by significant bleeding. Type 2B von Willebrand's disease may be associated with a mild and progressive thrombocytopenia during pregnancy, and indeed this may lead to the first identification of the disorder. The von Willebrand factor level in severe (type 3) von Willebrand's disease does not rise significantly in pregnancy. Approximately 80% of all cases of von Willebrand's disease are of the type 1 variety, characterized by low plasma levels of von Willebrand factor but qualitatively normal multimers.

A concentrate of recombinant von Willebrand factor is not yet available, but desmopressin is of potential value in these cases, since this chemical can boost the plasma levels of von Willebrand factor and factor VIII in the blood.[11] However, the manufacturers advise that it should only be used with caution during pregnancy. Although desmopressin is theoretically a V2 agonist devoid of action on smooth muscle, there are case reports of premature labour and hyponatraemia associated with seizures that appear to have been precipitated by intravenous infusion to pregnant women with von Willebrand's disease.[14] However, growing but as yet unpublished positive experience with desmopressin in pregnancy suggests that such adverse events are very rare, and desmopressin should not be regarded as contraindicated in pregnancy. As a general rule, desmopressin is of no value in the other types of von Willebrand's disease.

Normal vaginal delivery and epidural anaesthesia can usually be allowed with a factor VIII level (often used as a surrogate marker for von Willebrand factor levels) of >40 iu/dl, and Caesarean delivery can usually be allowed with a factor VIII level of >50 iu/dl. If haemostatic support is required for any reason, plasma-derived concentrates that contain von Willebrand factor are required; high-purity products containing factor VIII alone are of no value. Cryoprecipitate also contains von Willebrand factor, but it cannot be subjected to virucidal treatment (e.g. heat-treatment) and so it is not used to treat von Willebrand's disease in developed countries.

Several studies have documented a significantly increased risk of both primary and secondary postpartum haemorrhage in women with von Willebrand's disease, and this risk appears to be higher than in carriers of haemophilia.[15–17] From these studies the risk appears to be relatively higher in women with type 2 von Willebrand's disease than in women with the more common type 1 disease. It is thus prudent to check the von Willebrand factor level in all women with von Willebrand's disease a few days after delivery, and an infusion of desmopressin may be indicated if the level falls significantly soon after delivery. Desmopressin does not pass in significant quantities into breast milk and is therefore safe for breastfeeding mothers.

Antenatal diagnosis of von Willebrand's disease is not usually required or requested because the bleeding tendency is relatively mild. von Willebrand's disease is inherited as an autosomal-dominant condition, and thus children of either sex may inherit the condition. Severe (type 3) von Willebrand's disease may be readily diagnosed after birth from an umbilical cord blood sample. However, it is almost impossible to diagnose the much more common and milder forms of von Willebrand's disease in a neonate, since the level of von Willebrand factor rises significantly during birth and an apparently normal result may thus mask a mild form of the disease. Testing is therefore best deferred for some months unless surgery or some other invasive procedure is necessary in the interim period. The expression of von Willebrand factor is also affected by the blood group (people with blood group O have the lowest levels and those with blood group AB have the highest levels), and this can result in variable penetrance of the phenotype in a given family (in contrast with haemophilia, where the phenotype (or severity) of the haemophilia remains constant within a given kindred).

OTHER CONGENITAL BLEEDING DISORDERS

Women with congenital deficiencies of other coagulation factors may occasionally be encountered.[18]

Afibrinogenaemia may be associated with menorrhagia, recurrent abortions and postpartum haemorrhage. However, regular replacement treatment with infusions of fibrinogen concentrate (aiming for a trough fibrinogen level of 1 g/l) may result in a successful outcome.[19]

Deficiency of factor XI is associated with a bleeding tendency but the correlation between the plasma level of factor XI and the severity of haemorrhagic manifestations is poor. Levels of 15 iu/dl or less are very likely to be associated with a bleeding tendency, but postoperative bleeding may be seen in patients with only modest deficiency (levels of 50–70 iu/dl). Factor XI deficiency is particularly common amongst Ashkenazi Jews, but it has also been reported in other ethnic groups. Menorrhagia is a frequent problem in women with factor XI deficiency.

The level of factor XI does not rise during pregnancy, in contrast to many other coagulation factors. In view of the unpredictable nature of the bleeding tendency and the poor correlation with the plasma level of factor XI, labour and delivery should be managed with caution in a centre where fresh frozen plasma can be given promptly if required. In one study of 28 pregnancies in 11 women with factor XI deficiency, the incidence of primary postpartum haemorrhage was 16%.[17] Prophylactic infusion of plasma may be required (e.g. to cover a Caesarean delivery). Cryoprecipitate does not contain factor XI but a lyophilized plasma-derived concentrate of factor XI is available, which has the advantage of having been subjected to a virucidal treatment, such as heat treatment. However, this advantage should be balanced against the apparent thrombogenicity of the concentrate, and this material is probably best reserved for severely factor XI-deficient women, and the postinfusion level of factor XI should be monitored and maintained below 100 iu/dl.[20]

Factor XIII enhances the stability of fibrin clots by forging covalent bonds between adjacent strands of monomeric fibrin. Congenital deficiency of this protein is very rare but is associated with a very serious bleeding tendency as well as poor wound healing. Early reports in the literature suggested that women with factor XIII deficiency are prone to infertility and recurrent miscarriages.[21] However, a programme of regular prophylaxis with regular, monthly infusions of factor XIII concentrates is now usually initiated as soon as the condition is diagnosed in childhood, and so this problem does not arise. Continued monthly infusions of factor XIII concentrate, aiming for a trough level of not less than 1.5%, is likely to result in a successful outcome in pregnancy.[21]

REFERENCES

1. Kadir RA, Economides DL, Braithwaite J et al. The obstetric experience of carriers of haemophilia. *Br J Obstet Gynaecol* 1997;**104**: 803–10.
2. Tedgård U, Ljung R, Mcneil TF. Reproductive choices of haemophilia carriers. *Br J Haematol* 1999;**106**:421–6.
3. Firth HV, Boyd PA, Chamberlain P et al. Severe limb abnormalities after chorion villus sampling at 56–66 days' gestation. *Lancet* 1991;**337**:762–3.
4. Firth HV, Boyd PA, Chamberlain PF et al. Analysis of limb reduction defects in babies exposed to chorionic villus sampling. *Lancet* 1994;**343**:1069–71.
5. Cheung M-C, Goldberg JD, Kan YW. Prenatal diagnosis of sickle cell anaemia and thalassaemia by analysis of fetal blood cells in maternal blood. *Nat Genet* 1996;**14**:264–8.
6. Forestier F, Daffos F, Rainaut M et al. Vitamin dependent proteins in fetal hemostasis at mid trimester pregnancy. *Thromb Haemost* 1985;**53**: 401–3.
7. Forestier F, Daffos F, Galactéros F et al. Hematological values of 163 normal fetuses between 18 and 30 weeks of gestation. *Pediatr Res* 1986;**20**:342–6.
8. Lewis SM, Bain BJ, Bates I (eds), *Practical Haematology* 9th edn. New York: Churchill Livingstone; 2001:275–6.
9. Ljung R, Lidgren AC, Petrini P, Tengborn L. Normal vaginal delivery is to be recommended for haemophilia carrier gravidae. *Acta Paediatr* 1994;**83**:609–11.
10. Tolfvenstam T, Papadogiannakis N, Norbeck O et al. Risk of adverse outcomes of pregnancy after human parvovirus B19 infection in intrauterine fetal death. *Lancet* 2001;**357**:1494–7.
11. Mannucci PM. Desmopressin (DDAVP) in the treatment of bleeding disorders: the first 20 years. *Blood* 1997;**90**:2515–21.
12. Yoffe G, Buchanan GR. Intracranial hemorrhage in newborn and young infants with hemophilia. *J Pediatr* 1988;**113**:333–6.
13. Gianelli F. Genetics of blood coagulation and haemostasis. In: Rizza C, Lowe G (eds), *Haemophilia and Other Inherited Bleeding Disorders*. London: WB Saunders; 1997:43–86.
14. Chediak JR, Alban G, Maxey B. von Willebrand's disease and pregnancy: management during delivery and outcome of offspring. *Am J Obstet Gynecol* 1986;**155**:618–24.
15. Ramsahoye BH, Davies SV, Dasani H, Pearson JF et al. Obstetric management of von Willebrand's disease: a report of 24 cases and a review of the literature. *Haemophilia* 1995;**1**:140–4.
16. Greer IA, Lowe GDO, Walker JJ, Forbes CD. Haemorrhagic problems in obstetrics and gynaecology in patients with congenital coagulopathies. *Br J Obstet Gynaecol* 1991;**98**:909–18.
17. Kadir RA, Lee CA, Sabin CA et al. Pregnancy in women with von Willebrand's disease or factor XI deficiency. *Br J Obstet Gynaecol* 1998;**105**:314–21.
18. Giangrande PLF. Other inherited disorders of blood coagulation. In: Rizza C, Lowe G (eds), *Haemophilia and Other Inherited Bleeding Disorders*. London: WB Saunders; 1997:291–307.
19. Grech H, Majumdar G, Lawrie AS, Savidge GF. Pregnancy in congenital afibrinogenaemia: report of a successful case and review of the literature. *Br J Haematol* 1991;**78**:571–82.
20. Richards EM, Makris MM, Cooper P, Preston FE. In vivo coagulation activation following infusion of highly purified factor XI concentrate. *Br J Haematol* 1997;**96**:293–7.
21. Burrows RF, Ray JG, Burrows EA. Bleeding risk and reproductive capacity among patients with factor XIII deficiency: a case presentation and review of the literature. *Obstet Gynecol Surv* 2000;**55**:103–8.

21

Gestational thrombocytopenia: immune thrombocytopenic purpura in pregnancy

Regine Ahner and James B Bussel

DEFINITION OF THROMBOCYTOPENIA IN PREGNANCY

Pregnancy causes a range of physiological and psychological changes, which may influence the woman's life significantly. In order to fulfil the needs of the growing fetus, the body functions adapt in various ways. One of the major changes occurs in the fluid system – the plasma volume increases up to 40%, and, although erythropoiesis increases at the same time, it cannot keep up with the fluid amount, which ultimately leads to physiological hydremia. The limit for anemia is therefore much lower than in a non-pregnant woman (11 g/dl).

Other than the relative decrease in the number of erythrocytes, it had been thought that the platelet count remains stable throughout pregnancy. The normal range of the platelet count in non-pregnant people is 150,000–400,000 cells/μl, defining thrombocytopenia usually as a platelet count under 150,000 cells/μl. This value represents the 2.5th percentile of the distribution in a healthy population of men and non-pregnant women. (Mild thrombocytopenia may be defined as 100,000–150,000 cells/μl, moderate thrombocytopenia as 50,000–100,000 cells/μl, and severe thrombocytopenia as less than 50,000 cells/ml.

However, in recent prospective studies on pregnant women, a left shift of the whole distribution of platelet counts at term, with a 2.5th percentile of 116,000 cells/μl, respectively 123,000 cells/μl has been documented.[1,2] Verdy et al. showed in their study that the platelet count falls by about 10% during an uncomplicated pregnancy, with the decline being greatest in the last trimester.[3] In the light of these results it should be asked whether lowering the threshold of what is considered to be a normal platelet count during pregnancy would be appropriate. To alter the threshold from 150,000 to 100,000 cells/μl in otherwise healthy pregnant women would not only lower the number of diagnoses of thrombocytopenia but also avoid unnecessary interventions.[1,4] The fear is that recognition of thrombocytopenia as the first sign of significant pathology (e.g. pre-eclampsia, thrombotic thrombocytopenic purpura (TTP), idiopathic thrombocytopenic purpura (ITP) could be delayed.

DIFFERENTIAL DIAGNOSIS OF THROMBOCYTOPENIA IN PREGNANCY

Thrombocytopenia is the most common hemostatic abnormality during pregnancy. Platelets counts of less than 150,000 have been observed in 7–15% of unselected pregnancies, although severe maternal thrombocytopenia is rare, occurring in fewer than 0.1% of pregnancies.[1,5–7] An antepartum diagnosis of maternal thrombocytopenia has become more common because platelet counts are now included in routine automated full blood cell counts at least twice during routine prenatal screening (i.e. at the first prenatal visit and again at 7–8 months of gestation).[4]

However, the increased recognition of maternal thrombocytopenia has not clarified the obstetric management in all cases. Whenever thrombocytopenia is discovered during pregnancy, certain of the maternal hematological and obstetric conditions that are associated with high maternal and perinatal mortality must be considered initially and, if possible, ruled out. Although the majority of thrombocytopenic pregnant women are healthy, it is important to select those who are at risk and require treatment (Figure 21.1).

The occurrence of thrombocytopenia in pregnant women may derive from the effects of diverse processes, either physiological or pathological. Thrombocytopenia is due to either increased platelet destruction or decreased platelet production; increased sequestration of platelets appears to be infrequent. Increased platelet destruction may be caused by immuno-

logical destruction, abnormal platelet activation, or platelet consumption. Decreased platelet production may be associated with leukemia, aplastic anemia, or folate deficiency. Thrombocytopenia may be an isolated finding or part of a systemic process. By far the most common cause of thrombocytopenia during pregnancy is gestational thrombocytopenia (in more than 70% of cases); Fig. 21.2 shows causes of maternal thrombocytopenia in pregnancy. The major causes of thrombocytopenia during pregnancy are discussed in this chapter.

Pre-eclampsia

Pre-eclampsia is a relatively common cause of thrombocytopenia during pregnancy and is usually defined by the triad of hypertension, proteinuria and edema. In approximately 20–50% of pre-eclamptic patients, platelet counts are decreased, usually to a mild degree.[8–10] The pathophysiological abnormalities of pre-eclampsia

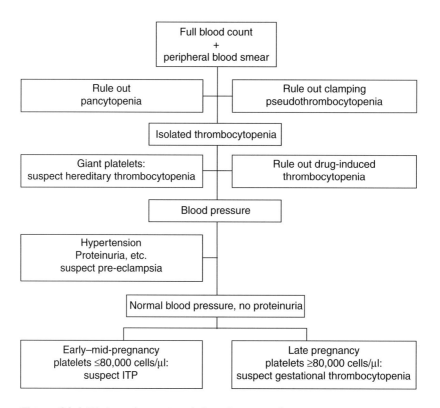

Figure 21.1 Work-up for maternal thrombocytopenia

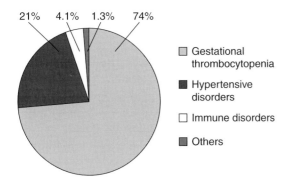

21%   4.1%   1.3%   74%

☐ Gestational thrombocytopenia

■ Hypertensive disorders

☐ Immune disorders

■ Others

Adapted from Burrows and Kelton;[6] it represents 1027 thrombocytopenic episodes complicating 15,471 pregnancies.

Figure 21.2 Causes of thrombocytopenia in pregnancy

include inadequate maternal vascular response to placentation, endothelial dysfunction, generalized vasospasm, activation of platelets, and abnormal hemostasis.

Thrombocytopenia is probably due to platelet consumption at the microvascular level, where platelets adhere to damaged vascular endothelium.[11] In some cases, microangiopathic hemolytic anemia and elevated liver function tests are associated with thrombocytopenia in patients with pre-eclampsia, known as HELLP syndrome (characterized by Hemolysis, Elevated Liver enzymes, and Low Platelets). This syndrome is a group of clinical and pathological manifestations resulting from an insult that leads to platelet activation and microvascular damage. Some investigators believe that disseminated intravascular coagulopathy (DIC) is the primary process in HELLP syndrome.[12] The thrombocytopenia, at worst, is usually moderate, and platelet counts rarely decrease to levels below 20,000 cells/μl.

Infection

The most common causes of thrombocytopenia in non-pregnant patients are infections. Thrombocytopenia can occur in infections caused by viruses (e.g. HIV, cytomegalovirus, Epstein– Barr virus), mycoplasma, bacteria, mycobacteria, rickettsiae, or protozoal parasites

(e.g. malaria). In most cases the mechanism is decreased platelet production, although almost any infection can instigate ITP and can result in non-immune increased platelet consumption.

HIV is a special case. In HIV infection, thrombocytopenia is relatively frequent and resembles that seen in classical ITP (see below). In addition to immune-mediated thrombocytopenia, other mechanisms include infection of marrow stromal cells that facilitate hemopoiesis.[13]

Systemic lupus erythematosus

Systemic lupus erythematosus (SLE) is a chronic autoimmune disease of unknown etiology that affects many of the body's organs. SLE complicates one in 2000–5000 pregnancies, with a five-fold increase in prevalence among African–American women. Patients generally present with intermittent unexplained pyrexia, butterfly rash, malaise, arthralgias, myositis, serositis, nephritis, or neurological abnormalities.

A positive antinuclear antibody is found in 98% of SLE patients, but it is also found in 3–5% of normal women. The diagnosis of SLE is established when four or more of the criteria published by the American Rheumatism Association are present.[14] Hematological abnormalities include hemolytic anemia, lymphopenia, and thrombocytopenia. Management of thrombocytopenia is similar to that of ITP.

Thrombotic thrombocytopenic purpura–hemolytic–uremic syndrome

The central feature in the pathogenesis of the thrombotic thrombocytopenic purpura–hemolytic–uremic syndrome (TTP–HUS) is endothelial-cell damage.[15] The diagnosis of TTP–HUS is made by the presence of five cardinal features:

• thrombocytopenia;
• hemolytic anemia;
• renal abnormalities;
• neurological abnormalities.

A very high lactate dehydrogenase level as well as distinctive arteriolar hyaline thrombi on histopathology are characteristic.[16] Ever since effective plasma exchange treatment has been available, mortality has been lowered from 90% to 20%.

However, not all of the five diagnostic criteria have to be present; thrombocytopenia and microangiopathic hemolytic anemia alone need to be considered as a likely diagnosis. The distinction between TTP–HUS and other diseases that are accompanied by symptoms of acute thrombocytopenia and anemia (e.g. viral, bacterial, or rickettsial sepsis) is unclear in many cases.[17,18] Recent studies have shown that TTP is associated with the absence, usually caused by an autoantibody, of the von Willebrand factor protease. HUS is not so well defined clinically. Pathophysiologically, epidemic HUS is a result of infection by a micro-organism, usually *Escherichia coli*, that contains a plasmid for the shiga-like toxin. The injection of the toxin causes renal vascular damage. Overall hemolytic thrombocytopenia results from many causes and can be associated with a variety of clinical disorders.[19]

Hematological malignancies

Hematological malignancies or myelopthisic processes (e.g. acute leukemia) may also lead to the development of thrombocytopenia in the pregnant woman. These disorders are rarely associated with isolated thrombocytopenia and can usually be excluded by examination of the peripheral blood film.[20]

Disseminated intravascular coagulation

DIC is caused by a widespread activation of the coagulation sequence. Formation of microthrombi can cause infarcts, while massive consumption of platelets, fibrin, and coagulation factors cause uncontrolled bleeding. In obstetrics, DIC is seen in association in placental abruption, dead fetus syndrome, amniotic embolism, Gram-negative sepsis, and sever pre-eclampsia or eclampsia. The diagnosis of DIC is supported by a prolonged prothrombin time (PT) and activated partial thromboplastin time

(APTT), decreased fibrinogen and platelet counts, and evidence on smear of a microangiopathic hematolytic anemia. Not all of these features are found in all cases.

Congenital thrombocytopenia

A congenital thrombocytopenia should be considered in patients who have persistent thrombocytopenia.[21] Most hereditary thrombocytopenias are apparent in infancy, although some are symptomless and not detected until later in life. Diagnostic features include those diagnostic of ITP:

- an isolated thrombocytopenia; and
- no findings in physical examination other than those consistent with bleeding.

Familial thrombocytopenia should be suspected in the presence of:

- a stable platelet count for a prolonged period of time;
- macro- or microthrombocytopenia more consistent than that seen in ITP;
- characteristic abnormalities on smear (i.e. Dohle bodies in the neutrophils of patients with May–Hegglin syndrome);
- characteristic systemic features of certain symptoms hearing and renal abnormalities in Alport's syndrome; and
- a family history of thrombocytopenia (perhaps the most important feature).

Most of these features are autosomal dominant traits, such as the May–Hegglin anomaly and type 2B von Willebrand's disease. Others are X-linked, such as Wiskott–Aldrich syndrome.

It is important to distinguish these disorders from ITP to avoid inappropriate treatment.[19] Failure to respond, even transiently, to treatments for ITP (e.g. intravenous immunoglobulin (IVIG)) is helpful in the diagnosis.

Drug-induced thrombocytopenia

In patients with unexpected, isolated thrombocytopenia, a drug-induced mechanism must be considered. Commonly reported drugs are quinine and quinidine, rifampin (rifampicin), and trimethoprim–sulphamethoxazole.

A suspicion of drug-induced thrombocytopenia is confirmed by recovery from thrombocytopenia after the suspected drug is withdrawn, which usually occurs within 5–7 days.[22] Rarely, if the thrombocytopenia is a result of marrow suppression, recovery may take up to 2 months.

Another drug that may be used during pregnancy is heparin. Heparin-induced thrombocytopenia or heparin-induced thrombocytopenia with thrombosis (HITT) is a difficult diagnosis to make because it may present with additional thrombosis appearing to be a failure of heparin therapy rather than a result of it. Fortunately, in severe cases, thrombocytopenia helps to establish the diagnosis. In addition to discontinuing the heparin, alternative anticoagulants need to be provided in the setting of HITT. Either a non-cross-reactive heparinoid (danaparoid) or a direct thrombin inhibitor such as hirudin are the treatments of choice. Warfarin should not be started until the patient is well anticoagulated and the HITT is clinically resolved. Testing is available, but debate continues as to the optimal approach.

Pseudothrombocytopenia

Last but not least, pseudothrombocytopenia must always be considered. Large studies have shown that falsely low platelet counts occur in about one person in 1000, irrespective of the presence or absence of any disease. In most cases, the pseudothrombocytopenia platelet agglutination is caused by the anticoagulant edetic acid, which is used for routine blood counts. Therefore, a diagnosis of thrombocytopenia should always be confirmed by examination of the peripheral blood smear,[19] which will reveal clumps of platelets.

GESTATIONAL THROMBOCYTOPENIA

Gestational or incidental thrombocytopenia is the most common cause of thrombocytopenia in pregnancy, occurring in 60–70 per 1000 live births.[6] Burrows and Kelton first reported patients with this disorder when these patients were confused with pregnant women who had ITP.[4] In contrast to many of the previously discussed etiologies of thrombocytopenia, gestational thrombocytopenia appears to be benign and to pose no significant risk to the mother or fetus. Women with gestational thrombocytopenia are healthy and not at risk of bleeding complications. It has been defined as a mild thrombocytopenia (usually with a platelet count of more than 80,000 cells/µl) that is associated with fetal thrombocytopenia.[23] Platelet counts typically return to normal within 6–12 weeks after delivery.[4] This would be approximately the same time as that required for other hemostatic factors that are altered during normal pregnancy to return to normal.[24] In general, gestational thrombocytopenia is assumed to be secondary to an increased platelet consumption within the placental circulation or to hormonal inhibition of megakaryocytopoiesis (or to both).[25]

It is often difficult to distinguish between gestational thrombocytopenia and ITP because there is no specific test available to make a definitive diagnosis.[26] Table 21.1 describes differences between gestational thrombocytopenia and ITP. Concentrations of antibodies against platelets are increased in both ITP and gestational thrombocytopenia.[27] The key factors in the diagnosis of gestational thrombocytopenia remain, therefore, a healthy-appearing pregnant woman with no prior history of thrombocytopenia (unless in a previous pregnancy) and with a platelet count that never decreases to below 70,000–100,000 cells/µl. Until the platelet count returns to normal after delivery, one cannot be certain that apparent gestational thrombocytopenia is not really the onset of ITP in which the mild decrease in platelet count is incidentally discovered in a routine blood count.[28]

IDIOPATHIC THROMBOCYTOPENIC PURPURA

ITP is an autoimmune disorder in which platelets sensitized to autoantibodies are destroyed by the reticuloendothelial system. In most patients with ITP there is evidence of immunoglobulin antibodies that blind to

Table 21.1 Comparison of clinical characteristics and laboratory findings of gestational thrombocytopenia and ITP in pregnancy

Thrombocytopenia		Gestational thrombocytopenia	ITP
History of maternal thrombocytopenia in a previous pregnancy		—	+
Maternal platelet count	< 50,000 cells/μl	—	+
	> 50,000 cells/μl	+	—
Antiplatelet antibody in mother's plasma		+	++
Fetal or neonatal thrombocytopenia		—	(+)
Normal maternal platelet count 6–8 weeks postpartum		+	—

platelet surface antigens;[29,30] these are typically carried on platelet glycoproteins IIb and IIIa and to a lesser extent on glycoproteins Ib and IX.[31] Platelets from patients with thrombocytopenia resulting from other causes may display similar abnormalities because of the lack of specificity of the diagnostic test.[32,33]

Acute ITP is a self-limited disorder that usually occurs in childhood. The chronic form usually presents in the second to third decade of life with clinical symptoms such as petechiae, ecchymosis, epistaxis, menorrhagia, or other bleeding. There is a female-to-male ratio of 3:1, and ITP may affect as many as one or two per 1000 live births.[34,35] There are no pathognomonic signs, symptoms or specific laboratory tests for ITP, a diagnosis that is based mainly on exclusion criteria. Four findings have been traditionally associated with the condition:[10]

- isolated thrombocytopenia (platelet count less than 100,000 cells/μl with or without accompanying megathrombocytes but with no blasts on the peripheral smear) and a normal hemoglobin and leukocyte count;
- normal or increased numbers of megakaryocytes as determined by examination of the bone marrow (if performed);
- exclusion of other systemic disorders or drugs that are known to be associated with thrombocytopenia; and

- absence of hepatosplenomegaly and lymphadenopathy.

However, with the recent introduction of platelet glycoprotein-specific antigen capture assays, the diagnosis of ITP by serological tests may be improved.[31]

ITP affects both mother and fetus but it is typically benign for both. There have been no reported maternal mortalities from ITP *per se* in more than 20 years. Mothers with ITP may experience disease exacerbation during pregnancy but many do not. This remains to be better studied. It is generally thought (though similarly unsubstantiated) that if ITP alters during the pregnancy, it will revert to its pre-pregnancy state after delivery.[34] Although the management of ITP depends on the severity of the disease, in general the threshold for treatment of pregnant women is not different from that for non-pregnant patients with ITP.

Women who are asymptomatic and whose platelet count is greater than 30,000 cells/μl should be managed expectantly in the absence of bleeding. A platelet count at least once a month is recommended.[21,31,36] Kelton proposed that mothers with ITP do not need to maintain a platelet count higher than 30,000 cells/μl,[37] as did Silver.[38] Procedures such as amniocentesis or delivery are considered safer if the platelet count is > 50,000 cells/μl. Obstetric anesthesiologists may require platelet counts > 70,000–80,000 cells/µl to place an epidural catheter. The requirement for an epidural anesthetic is the reason to treat a patient with mild ITP.

Treatment of the thrombocytopenic mother is usually possible with prednisone or IVIG.[23,39–41] The first-line treatment is glucocorticoid administration, most commonly prednisone in a dosage of 1 mg/kg per day. An increase in platelet counts to more than 50,000 cells/µl usually occurs within 3–7 days, and the count reaches a maximum within 2–3 weeks. To avoid a relapse, patients are continued on oral corticosteroids, the dosage of which should be gradually reduced. With a platelet count of less than 10,000 cells/µl or in cases refractory to steroids, IVIG therapy is indicated. The usual dose is 400–1000 mg/kg per day for 1–3 days. A response can be expected in almost all patients within 1–3 days. Drawbacks to IVIG include its expense and the need to repeat dosing every 2–4 weeks.[36]

An approach currently implemented at the authors' center (which works in most cases) is to combine a single infusion of IVIG (1000 mg/kg) with prednisone 20 mg/day. This daily dose of prednisone has substantially less toxicity than higher doses. IVIG increases the platelet count immediately and allows the prednisone time to take effect and maintain an adequate platelet count.[34]

Potential adverse effects of corticosteroids include gestational diabetes, psychological disturbances, osteoporosis, acne, and weight gain. The side effects of IVIG include headache, nausea, aseptic meningitis and fever.

Studies are ongoing at the authors' center into the use of intravenous RhD immunoglobulin (anti-D) to treat ITP during pregnancy. It is acutely effective in almost all cases and appears to be safe for the fetus and newborn. Since it costs approximately half the amount of an equivalent dose of IVIG and can be infused in 3 minutes, it has important advantages over IVIG. Recipients must, however, be RH-positive and not splenectomized.

Management of ITP during gestation with IVIG or corticosteroids is almost always feasible until after delivery.[20] In the very rare pregnant woman known to have ITP who is resistant to both corticosteroid and IVIG therapy, splenectomy may be considered. Reported efficacy rates achieving a stable increased platelet count have varied from 50% to 80%.[42,43] Splenectomy is traditionally avoided in the first trimester, when it may increase the risk of premature labor, and in the third trimester, because to technical difficulties.[31,44,45] Recent reports advocate that, owing to improved surgical techniques and advances in the care of premature infants, the gestational age when surgery could be performed might be less important than previously expressed, but it should virtually never be required intrapartum.[46]

Therapy with immunosuppressive drugs, such as vincristine and cyclophosphamide, are relatively contraindicated in pregnancy because of the potential of adverse effects on the fetus.[36] The renal transplantation data about azathioprine suggest it can be used in pregnancy. Platelet transfusions should be only used a temporary measure to control life-threatening hemorrhage. Platelet transfusions to prevent maternal bleeding during labor and delivery are considered unnecessary for women with platelet counts greater than 20,000–30,000 cells/µl who do not have bleeding symptoms.[23]

Because of placental transfer of maternal IgG antiplatelet antibodies, the fetus is at risk of developing thrombocytopenia. The primary risk of the fetal thrombocytopenia is significant hemorrhage, especially peripartum intracranial hemorrhage. Severe thrombocytopenia in neonates born to mothers with ITP is relatively common. A review of studies from 1980 to 1990 concluded that 10% of infants born to mothers with ITP have a platelet count of less than 50,000 cells/µl and 4% have a platelet count of less than 20,000 cells/µl.[44] A recent analysis of the literature in the decade 1990–2000 confirms these data;[31] moderate neonatal thrombocytopenia occurred in 9% of infants and severe neonatal thrombocytopenia occurred in 4% of the infants. Minor neonatal complications (such as petechiae, cephalohematoma, hematuria, mild gastrointestinal bleeding, and umbilical bleeding) occurred in 3% of the infants, and major complications (such as intracranial hemorrhage, gastrointestinal bleeding, and bloody pericardial effusion), occurred in 1%.

Although there is broad agreement in the literature about the incidence and severity of neonatal thrombocytopenia, many questions about the management of ITP in pregnancy have not yet been answered. The most important question is whether there is a way to predict severe fetal thrombocytopenia, and, if so, what would be the appropriate mode of delivery in such a thrombocytopenic fetus.

Non-invasive methods of predicting the fetal platelet count are still very limited and, most of the time, unsuccessful. There is poor correlation between the maternal and the neonatal platelet count.[6,20] This is supported by reports of discordant platelet counts in two sets of twins.[47,48] Several so far unproven speculations hypothesize a link between the mother's history and treatment of her ITP and the neonatal platelet count – one study suggests that a pregnancy in which the mother has a platelet count of less than 50,000 cells/µl is at greater risk of fetal thrombocytopenia, while another hypothesis is that, if maternal ITP first develops during the relevant pregnancy, there is less risk of neonatal thrombocytopenia than if the ITP pre-existed the pregnancy.[49] Some investigators report that women who have undergone splenectomy are at greater risk of neonatal thrombocytopenia,[50,51] but others did not find this correlation.[52] Neither has the level of maternal platelet-associated IgG proved to be predictive of neonatal thrombocytopenia. Although some investigators have seen a positive association,[49] others have not.[35,48,50,52] The strongest predictor of severe neonatal thrombocytopenia for the time being is the history of a previously affected infant.[46,49] In one series of 34 mothers with ITP, no second child had a platelet count of less than 100,000 cells/µl when the first sibling had a platelet count greater than 100,000 cells/µl.[47]

Presently the only way to determine the fetal platelet count is by invasive testing, which involves fetal scalp sampling or percutaneous umbilical blood sampling.

Fetal scalp sampling is the collection of a small amount of fetal blood via a small scalp incision. The patient must be in labor with ruptured membranes and the fetal head must be engaged in the pelvis. Unfortunately, platelet clumping can lead to falsely low platelet results and unnecessary emergency Caesarean deliveries in unexperienced hands.[53] There are techniques to avoid this problem, but they require an institutional commitment to make them work.[54]

The most accurate method of determining the fetal platelet count is to perform percutaneous umbilical blood sampling. The technique, however is difficult and requires skilled staff, normally based in a tertiary center. The procedure can be complicated by fetal distress requiring emergency Caesarean delivery, and has also been associated with fetal bleeding and fetal death. In a recent review of 278 cases of percutaneous umbilical blood sampling, a 2% complication rate (including fetal bradycardia and hematomas requiring emergency Caesarean delivery) was calculated.[31]

However, one has to keep in mind that successful prediction of the neonatal platelet count is necessary only if it is justified to modify the antenatal treatment in order to increase the fetal platelet count or the route of delivery. Although there is enough material in the literature to demonstrate effective therapy in mothers suffering from ITP, there is no proof, so far, that any therapy can increase the fetal platelet count.[38]

The most controversial aspect in the treatment of pregnant women with ITP remains, therefore, the mode of delivery for the infant, who is potentially thrombocytopenic and at risk of bleeding.[24] In a decision analysis by Stamilio and Macones, three strategies of selecting the delivery method in women with ITP were compared – fetal platelet testing with either percutaneous umbilical blood sampling at term or fetal scalp sampling, with decisions about the mode of delivery based on the platelet count, and no testing of fetal platelets with the mode of delivery determined by standard obstetric care.[55] The goal of each strategy was to minimize the number of severely thrombocytopenic neonates (i.e. those with platelet counts < 50,000 cells/µl) delivered vaginally, while maintaining an acceptable rate of Caesarean deliveries. Neither percutaneous umbilical blood sampling nor fetal scalp sampling resulted in any cases of severely thrombocytopenic neonates delivered vaginally, but the former method of sampling showed a much lower overall rate of Caesarean delivery (36.6% versus 69.1%). Compared with the non-testing strategy, percutaneous umbilical blood sampling was associated with a lower number of severely thrombocytopenic neonates delivered vaginally (0 versus 82 per 1000) although there was a moderate increase in the rate of Caesarean deliveries (1.9 Caesarean deliveries to prevent vaginal delivery of one severely thrombocy-topenic neonate).

However, the only potential benefit influenced by delivery mode is a reduction of the incidence of neonatal intracranial hemorrhage. Several investigators have advocated Caesarean delivery to prevent intracranial hemorrhage.[56] Other investigators have questioned the influence of the mode of delivery on neonatal outcome at all.[6,57] However, there are as yet no series large enough to assess the connection between mode of delivery and intracranial hemorrhage in thrombocytopenic infants born to mothers with ITP.[48]

In an analysis of the literature between 1970 and 1990, 474 infants of mothers with ITP were reported, and the overall rate of intracranial hemorrhage in neonates with moderate or severe thrombocytopenia was 3%. No significant association was found between the rate of intracranial hemorrhage and the mode of delivery for moderately or severely thrombocy-topenic neonates together (weighted odds ratio 1.69, 95% CI 0.14–44.6) or for those with severe thrombocytopenia (crude odds ratio 1.38, 95% CI 0.07–84.67).[48] In a recent review of 601 infants of mothers with ITP, severe neonatal thrombo-cytopenia was reported in 72 (12%), with infants being born almost equally commonly by sponta-neous vaginal delivery or Caesarean delivery. Six infants had an intracranial hemorrhage, of whom two had been delivered by Caesarean section. Four of these six infants had severe neonatal thrombocytopenia.[50] Hence, there is little evidence to support the common belief that a vaginal delivery is harmful to the fetus. However, there is no good evidence against it either.

After weighing the risk of percutaneous umbilical blood sampling at term and the poten-tial neonatal risk of hemorrhage in ITP, many patients and physicians would choose not to undergo fetal platelet testing at all. In a survey of perinatologists in the USA in which questions were asked about the management of ITP in pregnancy with respect to mode of delivery, the results were controversial.[58] Approximately two-thirds of perinatologists would allow a trial of labor without a procedure to determine fetal platelet count. Most physicians surveyed did not consider Caesarean delivery to be protective against intracranial hemorrhage.[58]

Neonates born to mothers with ITP can, during the first week of life, either develop thrombocytopenia or experience further deterio-ration of thrombocytopenia noted at birth.[23,59] In a study of 61 neonates born to 50 women with ITP, the platelet count decreased in two-thirds of the infants, reaching a nadir by day 6.[5] This correlates better with the neonatal risk than with the obstetric risk.[52] The effect of breastfeeding on the neonatal platelet count seems to be negligible, although IgG antibodies (especially IgG4) are transmitted in breast milk. Only one study in which a correlation between breastfeeding and late thrombocytopenia could not be established was found in the literature.[60] It is the authors' practice to allow breastfeeding in women with ITP but to monitor the neonatal platelet count for 1–3 weeks.

THE RISK OF NEONATAL THROMBOCYTOPENIA

Most infants in whom thrombocytopenia develops are ill and premature and have other disorders that could contribute to the thrombo-cytopenia, including DIC, bacteremia, or respi-ratory distress. In these sick infants, the frequency of thrombocytopenia is as high as 15%, and it is most severe several days after delivery.[58] In a retrospective study of 5194 fetal blood samples obtained from the umbilical cord, 245 fetuses had thrombocytopenia.[62] Fetal thrombocytopenia was attributed to infec-tious diseases (toxoplasmosis, rubella, and cytomegalovirus) in 29% of the patients, to immune-mediated platelet destruction in 18%, to congenital chromosomal abnormalities in 17%, to unknown causes in 11%, and to a variety of disorders in 25%. Asphyxia during birth is another risk factor for thrombocytopenia.[62] In the severely thrombocytopenic fetus (i.e. those with a platelet count < 50,000 cells/µl), the primary entities were PLA incompatibility, cytomegalovirus infection and rubella.

However, severe thrombocytopenia in an otherwise healthy neonate is an uncommon (but important) clinical finding.[20,63] Intracranial hemorrhage, the most severe side effect of fetal or neonatal thrombocytopenia, may cause lifelong residual neurological defects or even death. Methods to recognize infants at risk as early as possible, as well as methods to recognize maternal characteristics that could predict neonatal thrombocytopenia, are therefore most warranted. In a cross-sectional study that included 15,471 mothers and 15,932 new-born infants, platelet counts were determined.[6] The incidence of infants with a cord blood platelet count below 50,000 cells/µl was 0.12% (95% CI 0.07–0.19%). The only severely affected neonates (i.e. those with a platelet count < 20,000 cells/µl) were born to mothers with antiplatelet allo-antibodies. The disorders that cause thrombocytopenia in mothers (such as gestational thrombocytopenia, SLE and the hypertensive disorders of pregnancy) did not cause moderate-to-severe fetal or neonatal thrombocytopenia in their infants.

NEONATAL ALLOIMMUNE THROMBOCYTOPENIA

Other than in ITP, the maternal platelet count is normal in neonatal alloimmune thrombocytopenia (AIT) (Table 21.2). AIT affects approximately one in 1000–2000 live births and is a serious, potentially life-threatening disorder.[39,47] The pathophysiological process is similar to that of erythroblastosis fetalis (Rh disease), except that maternal IgG alloantibodies are directed against paternally derived fetal platelet antigens. A rapidly increasing number of human platelet alloantigen systems (HPA-1-15) have been established as being associated with AIT;[64,65] the most frequent cause of severe AIT is still the HPA-1a or PLA-1 antigen.[39] AIT occurs when the antiplatelet antibodies of a sensitized PIA-1-negative mother cross the placenta and cause thrombocytopenia in a PLA-1-positive fetus. Fetal thrombocytopenia caused by HPA-1 sensitization tends to be severe and can occur early in gestation. In a cohort study that looked at 107 fetuses with AIT (97 with HPA-1a incompatibility) *in utero* before they received any therapy, 50% had initial platelet counts of less than 20,000 cells/µl; many of these fetus with low platelet counts were determined before 26 weeks' gestation.[39]

Unlike erythroblastosis fetalis, which occurs in second or subsequent pregnancies in response to alloimmunization of the mother by fetal red blood cells, AIT cases usually occur during first pregnancies,[34] and the diagnosis is made after

Table 21.2 Characteristics of ITP and AIT

	ITP	AIT
Normal maternal platelet count	No	Yes
Early, severe fetal thrombocytopenia	No	Yes
Anticipation of possible neonatal thrombocytopenia in affected pregnancy	Yes	No
Antenatal fetal intracranial hemorrhage	Not documented	Yes
Rate of neonatal intracranial hemorrhage	1%	20%
Severity of disorder in subsequent affected infant	Similar	More severe
Antenatal therapy of fetal thrombocytopenia	No	Yes

birth. The neonates are either born with evidence of profound thrombocytopenia or develop symptomatic thrombocytopenia within hours after birth. Bleeding, such as petechiae and ecchymoses, may be the first sign. The most serious complication is intracranial hemorrhage, which occurs in 10–20% of infants,[66,67] of whom 25–50% have intracranial hemorrhage *in utero*.[68] The recurrence rate of AIT in subsequent pregnancies is as high as 85–90%.[69] If the father is heterozygous (PlA-1/PlA-2), the recurrence rate is 50%, whereas if the father is homozygous for PlA-1, the recurrence rate is virtually 100%. The degree of thrombocytopenia in subsequent infants is at least as severe as in the preceeding affected sibling, often worse.[39]

Unfortunately, other than documenting intracranial hemorrhage in an older affected sibling, there is no non-invasive way of identifying fetuses at risk of intracranial hemorrhage.[39] The first step is to evaluate the history of having delivered infants with otherwise unexplained bleeding or thrombocytopenia. The platelet type and the zygosity of both parents should be determined. In cases of paternal heterozygosity, amniocentesis allows identification of the platelet antigen genotype of the fetus.[70] If the fetus does not have the incompatible platelet antigen, the fetus will be unaffected. In cases in which the amniocentesis demonstrates the fetus to have platelet–antigen incompatibility and in cases of paternal homozygosity, cordocentesis should be performed to determine the initial fetal platelet count.[39] Fetuses with severe thrombocytopenia seem to be at increased risk of hemorrhage during cordocentesis,[71] to minimize this risk, transfusion of maternal platelets is recommended at the time of procedure.[67]

The primary goal of obstetric management is to prevent intracranial hemorrhage in the fetus. Various treatment protocols have been described in the literature.[72–75] The authors have presented data on 107 cases treated by the administration to the mother of IVIG with or without a glucocorticoid.[67,76,77] In these 107 fetuses, the mean platelet count increased by more than 50,000 cells/μl on the basis of a comparison of the platelet count at the initial cordocentesis with the platelet count at birth or of a comparison of the platelet count at birth of the treated fetus with an older affected (and untreated) sibling. Treatment very likely prevents intracranial hemorrhage, because only one fetus had an intracranial hemorrhage.

REFERENCES

1. Boehlen F, Hohlfeld P, Extermann P, *et al*. Platelet count at term pregnancy: a reappraisal of the threshold. *Obstet Gynecol* 2000;**95**:29–33.

2. Sainio S, Kekomaki R, Riikonen S, Teramo K. Maternal thrombocytopenia at term: a population-based study. *Acta Obstet Gynecol Scand* 2000;**79**:744–9.

3. Verdy E, Uzan S. Groupe de travail sur les thrombopénies maternelles et foetales: plaquettes en cours de grossesse. Etiologie et moyens du diagnostic d'une thrombopénie maternelle. In: *Première Journée parisienne obstetrico-pediatrique*. Paris: Doin; 1993:49–53.

4. Burrows RF, Kelton JG. Incidentally detected thrombocytopenia in healthy mothers and their infants. *N Engl J Med* 1988;**319**:142–5.

5. Burrows RF, Kelton JG. Thrombocytopenia at delivery: a prospective survey of 6715 deliveries. *Am J Obstet Gynecol* 1990;**162**:731–4.

6. Burrows RF, Kelton JG. Fetal thrombocytopenia and its relation to maternal thrombocytopenia. *N Engl J Med* 1993;**329**:1463–6.

7. Verdy E, Bessous V, Dreyfus M, *et al*. Longitudinal analysis of platelet count and volume in normal pregnancy. *Thromb Haemost* 1997;**77**:806–7.

8. Katz V, Thorp J, Rozas L, Bowes W. The natural history of thrombocytopenia associated with preeclampsia. *Am J Obstet Gynecol* 1990;**163**:1142–3.

9. Burrows RF, Hunter DJ, Andrew M, Kelton JG. A prospective study investigating the mechanism of thrombocytopenia in preeclampsia. *Obstet Gynecol* 1987;**70**:334–8.

10. Gibson B, Hunter D, Neame PB, Kelton JG. Thrombocytopenia in pre-eclampsia and eclampsia. *Semin Thromb Hemost* 1982;**8**:234–47.

11. Pritchard JA, Cunningham FG, Mason RA. Coagulation changes in eclampsia: their

frequency and pathogenesis. *Am J Obstet Gynecol* 1976;**124**:855–9.

12. Vandam PA, Renier M, Backelandt M, *et al.* Disseminated intravascular coagulation and the syndrome of hemolysis, elevated liver enzymes, and low platelets in severe preeclampsia. *Obstet Gynecol* 1989;**73**:97–102.

13. Bahner I, Kearns K, Couthino S, *et al.* Infection of human marrow stroma by human immunodeficiency virus-1 (HIV-1) is both required and sufficient for HIV-1 induced hematopoietic suppression in vitro: demonstration by gene modification of primary human stroma. *Blood* 1997;**90**:1787–98.

14. Tan EM, Cohen AS, Fries JF, *et al.* The 1982 revised criteria for the classification of systemic lupus erythematosus. *Arthritis Rheum* 1982;**25**:1271–7.

15. Dang CT, Magid MS, Weksler B, *et al.* Enhanced endothelial cell apoptosis in splenic tissues of patients with thrombotic thrombocytopenic purpura. *Blood* 1999;**93**:1264–70.

16. Amorosi EL, Ultman JE. Thrombotic thrombocytopenic purpura: report of 16 cases and review of the literature. *Medicine* 1966;**45**:139–59.

17. George NJ, Gilcher RO, Smith JW, *et al.* Thrombotic thrombocytopenic purpura: hemolytic uremic syndrome: diagnosis and management. *J Clin Apheresis* 1998;**13**:120–5.

18. McCrae KR, Cines DB. Thrombotic microangiopathy during pregnancy. *Semin Hematol* 1997;**34**:148–58.

19. George J. Platelets. *Lancet* 2000;**355**:1531–9.

20. McCrae KR, Samuels P, Schreiber AD. Pregnancy-associated thrombocytopenia: pathogenesis and management. *Blood* 1992;**80**:2697–714.

21. Najean Y, Lecompte T. Hereditary thrombocytopenias in childhood. *Semin Thromb Hemost* 1995;**21**:294–304.

22. George JN, Raskob GE, Shah SR, *et al.* Drug-induced thrombocytopenia: a systemic review of published case reports. *Ann Intern Med* 1998;**129**:886–90.

23. George JN, Woolf SH, Raskob GE, *et al.* Idiopathic thrombocytopenic purpura: a practice guideline developed by explicit methods for the American Society of Hematology. *Blood* 1996;**88**:3–40.

24. Shehata N, Burrows R, Kelton GG. Gestational thrombocytopenia. *Clin Obstet Gynecol* 1999;**42**:327–34.

25. Ajzenberg N, Dreyfus M, Kaplan C, Yvart J, Weill B, Tchernia G. Pregnancy-associated thrombocy-

topenia revisited: assessment and follow-up of 50 cases. *Blood* 1998;**92**:4573–80.

26. Rouse DJ, Owen J, Goldenberg RL. Routine maternal platelet count: an assessment of a technologically driven screening practice. *Am J Obstet Gynecol* 1998;**179**:573–6.

27. Lescale KB, Eddleman KA, Cines DB, *et al.* Antiplatelet antibody testing in thrombocytopenic pregnant women. *Am J Obstet Gynecol* 1996;**174**:1014–18.

28. Schwartz KA. Gestational thrombocytopenia and immune thrombocytopenias in pregnancy. *Hemat Oncol Clin* 2000;**14**:1101–16.

29. McMillan R. Chronic idiopathic thrombocytopenic purpura. *N Engl J Med* 1981;**304**:1135–47.

30. Kelton JG, Gibbons S. Autoimmune platelet destruction: Idiopathic thrombocytopenic purpura. *Semin Thromb Hemost* 1982;**8**:83–104.

31. Gill KK, Kelton JG. Management of idiopathic thrombocytopenic purpura in pregnancy. *Semin Hematol* 2000;**37**:275–89.

32. Kelton JG, Powers PJ, Carter CJ. A prospective study of the usefulness of measurement of platelet-associated IgG for the diagnosis of idiopathic thrombocytopenic purpura. *Blood* 1982;**60**:1050–3.

33. Mueller-Eckhardt C, Mueller-Eckhardt G, Kayser W, *et al.* Platelet-associated IgG, platelet survival and platelet sequestration in thrombocytopenic states. *Br J Haematol* 1982;**52**:49–58.

34. Bussel JB. Immune thrombocytopenia in pregnancy: autoimmune and alloimmune. *J Reprod Immun* 1997;**37**:35–61.

35. Sainio S, Joutsi L, Karvenpaa AL, *et al.* Idiopathic thrombocytopenic purpura in pregnancy. *Acta Obstet Gynecol Scand* 1998;**77**:272–7.

36. Johnson JR, Samuels P. Review of autoimmune thrombocytopenia: pathogenesis, diagnosis and management in pregnancy. *Clin Obstet Gynecol* 1999;**42**:317–26.

37. Kelton JG. Management of the pregnant patient with idiopathic thrombocytopenic purpura. *Ann Intern Med* 1983;**99**:796–800.

38. Silver RM. Maternal thrombocytopenia in pregnancy: time for a reassessment. *Am J Obstet Gynecol* 1995;**173**:479–82.

39. Bussel JB, Zabusky MR, Berkowitz RL, *et al.* Fetal alloimmune thrombocytopenia. *N Engl J Med* 1997;**337**:22–6.

40. Bussel JB, Pham LC. Intravenous treatment with gamma globulin in adults with immune thrombocytopenic purpura: review of the literature. *Vox Sang* 1987;**52**:206–11.

41. Christiaens GC, Nieuwenhuis HK, von dem Borne AE, *et al*. Idiopathic thrombocytopenic purpura in pregnancy: a randomized trial on the effect of antenatal low dose corticosteroids on neonatal platelet count. *Br J Obstet Gynaecol* 1990;**97**:893–8.

42. Stasi R, Stipa E, Masi M, *et al*. Long-term observation of 208 adult with chronic idiopathic thrombocytopenic purpura. *Am J Med* 1995;**98**:436–42.

43. Schiavotto C, Rodeghiero F. Twenty years' experience with treatment of idiopathic thrombocytopenic purpura in a single department: results in 490 cases. *Haematologica* 1993;**78**:22–8.

44. Burrows RF, Kelton JG. Pregnancy in patients with idiopathic thrombocytopenic purpura: assessing the risk of the infant at delivery. *Obstet Gynecol Surv* 1993;**48**:781–8.

45. Bell WR. Hematological abnormalities in pregnancy. *Med Clin North Am* 1977:**61**:165–96.

46. Gottlieb P, Axelsson O, Bakos O, Rastad J. Splenectomy during pregnancy: an option in the treatment of autoimmune thrombocytopenic purpura. *Br J Obstet Gynaecol* 1999;**106**:373–5.

47. Williams LM, Hackett G, Rennie J, *et al*. The natural history of fetomaternal alloimmunization to the platelet-specific antigen HPA-1a (PlA1, ZW a) as determined by antenatal screening. *Blood* 1998;**92**:2280–7.

48. Cook RL, Miller RC, Katz VL, Cefalo RC. Immune thrombocytopenic purpura in pregnancy: a reappraisal of management. *Obstet Gynecol* 1991;**78**:578–83.

49. Samuels P, Bussel JB, Braitman LE, *et al*. Estimation of the risk of thrombocytopenia in the offspring of pregnant women with presumed immune thrombocytopenic purpura. *N Engl J Med* 1990;**323**:229–35.

50. Payne SD, Resnik R, Moore TR, *et al*. Maternal characteristics and risks of severe neonatal thrombocytopenia and intracranial hemorrhage in pregnancies complicated by autoimmune thrombocytopenia. *Am J Obstet Gynecol* 1997;**177**:149–55.

51. Yamada H, Fujimoto S. Perinatal management of idiopathic thrombocytopenic purpura in pregnancy: risk factors for passive immune thrombocytopenia. *Ann Hematol* 1998;**76**:211–14.

52. Burrows RF, Kelton JG. Low fetal risks in pregnancies associated with idiopathic thrombocytopenic purpura. *Am J Obstet Gynecol* 1990;**163**:1147–50.

53. Christiaens GCL, Helmerhorst FM. Validity of intrapartum diagnosis of fetal thrombocytopenia. *Am J Obstet Gynecol* 1987;**157**:864–5.

54. Adams DM, Bussel JB, Druzin ML. Accurate intrapartum estimation of fetal platelet count by fetal scalp samples smear. *Am J Perinatol* 1994;**11**:42–5.

55. Stamilio DM, Macones GA. Selection of delivery method in pregnancies complicated by autoimmune thrombocytopenia: a decision analysis. *Obstet Gynecol* 1999;**94**:41–7.

56. al-Mofada SM, Osman ME, Kides E, al-Momen AK, al Herbish AS, al-Mobaireek K. Risk of thrombocytopenia in the infants of mothers with idiopathic thrombocytopenia. *Am J Perinatol* 1994;**11**:423–6.

57. Laros RK, Kagan R. Route of delivery for patients with immune thrombocytopenic purpura. *Am J Obstet Gynecol* 1984;**148**:901–8.

58. Peleg D, Hunter SK. Perinatal management of women with immune thrombocytopenic purpura: survey of United States perinatologists. *Am J Obstet Gynecol* 1999;**180**:645–9.

59. Kelton JG, Inwood MJ, Barr RM, et al. The prenatal prediction of thrombocytopenia in infants of mothers with clinically diagnosed immune thrombocytopenia. *Am J Obstet Gynecol* 1982;**144**:449–54.

60. Andrew M, Castle V, Saigal S, *et al*. Clinical impact of neonatal thrombocytopenia. *J Pediatr* 1987;**110**:457–64.

61. Hohlfeld P, Forestier F, Kaplan C, *et al*. Fetal thrombocytopenia: a retrospective survey of 5194 fetal blood samplings. *Blood* 1994;**84**:1851–6.

62. Castle V, Andrew M, Kelton J, *et al*. Frequency and mechanism of neonatal thrombocytopenia. *J Pediatr* 1986;**108**:749–55.

63. Bussel JB, Schreiber AD. Immune thrombocytopenic purpura, neonatal alloimmune thrombocytopenia and post-transfusion purpura. In: Hoff R, Benz EJ, Shattil SJ, Furie B, Cohen HJ, eds. *Hematology: Basic Principles and Practice*. New York: Churchill Livingstone; 1991:1485–94.

64. Santoso S, Kiefel V. Human platelet-specific alloantigens: update. *Vox Sang* 1998;**74**:249–53.

65. Kekomaeki S, Partanen J, Kekomaeki R. Platelet alloantigens HPA-1, -2, -3, -5, and 6b in Finns. *Transfus Med* 1995;**5**:193–8.

66. Mueller-Eckhardt C, Kiefel V, Grubert A, *et al*. 348 cases of suspected neonatal alloimmune thrombocytopenia. *Lancet* 1989;**1**:363–6.

67. Bussel JB, Berkowitz RL, Lynch L, *et al*. Antenatal management of alloimmune thrombocytopenia with intravenous gamma-globulin: a randomized trial of the addition of low-dose steroid to intravenous gamma-globulin. *Am J Obstet Gynecol* 1996;**174**:1414–23.

68. Herman JH, Jumbelic MI, Ancona RJ, Kickler TS. In utero cerebral hemorrhage in alloimmune thrombocytopenia. *Am J Pediatr Hematol Oncol* 1986;**8**:312–17.

69. Newman PJ, Derbes RS, Aster RH. The human platelet alloantigens, P1A1 and P1A2, are associated with a leucine33/proline33 amino acid polymorphism in membrane glycoprotein IIIA, and are distinguishable by DNA typing. *J Clin Invest* 1989;**83**:1778–81.

70. Bussel JB, Neonatal immune thrombocytopenia study group. Neonatal alloimmune thrombocytopenia: a prospective case accumulation study. *Pediatr Res* 1988;**23**:337A.

71. McFarland JG, Aster RH, Bussel JB, *et al.* Prenatal diagnosis of neonatal alloimmune thrombocytopenia using allele-specific oligonucleotide probes. *Blood* 1991;**78**:2276–82.

72. Bussel JB, Skupski DW, McFarland JG. Fetal alloimmune thrombocytopenia: consensus and controversy. *J Matern Fetal Med* 1996;**5**:281–92.

73. Sainio S, Teramo K, Kekomaki R. Prenatal treatment of severe fetomaternal alloimmune thrombocytopenia. *Transfus Med* 1999;**9**:321–30.

74. Silver RM, Porter TF, Branch DW, Esplin MS, Scott JR. Neonatal alloimmune thrombocytopenia: antenatal management. *Am J Obstet Gynecol* 2000;**182**:1233–8.

75. Lynch L, Bussel JB, McFarland JG, Chitkara U, Berkowitz RL. Antenatal treatment of alloimmune thrombocytopenia. *Obstet Gynecol* 1992;**80**: 67–71.

76. Bussel JB, Berkowitz RL, McFarland JG, Lynch L, Chitkara U. Antenatal treatment of neonatal alloimmune thrombocytopenia. *N Engl J Med* 1988;**319**:1374–8.

77. Kaplan C, Murphy MF, Kroll H, Waters AH. Feto-maternal alloimmune thrombocytopenia: antenatal therapy with IVIgG and steroids – more questions than answers. *Br J Haematol* 1998;**100**: 62–5.

22

Fetal and neonatal alloimmune thrombocytopenia

Cécile Kaplan

INTRODUCTION

Fetal–neonatal alloimmune thrombocytopenia (NAIT) results from maternal alloimmunization during pregnancy against fetal platelet antigen inherited from the father that the mother lacks.[1] NAIT is considered to be the counterpart of Rh haemolytic disease of the newborn. In contrast to haemolytic disease of the newborn, NAIT may affect the first child. Alloimmune thrombocytopenia is a transient passive disease in an otherwise healthy infant but there is a risk of intracerebral haemorrhage during the whole severe thrombocytopenic period and, therefore, of neurological damage or death. The risk of life-threatening haemorrhage necessitates a prompt diagnosis and effective therapy. Over the past few years remarkable progress has led to a better understanding of the natural history of NAIT, and this has led in turn to more precise diagnosis of the condition, the development of antenatal diagnosis and therapy, and better management of high-risk groups, which is still evolving.

PATHOGENESIS

Alloimmune thrombocytopenia results from platelet destruction caused by specific alloantibodies. The incidence of NAIT has been estimated by prospective studies to be 1 per 800 or 1000 live births.[2,3] The precise mechanism of maternal sensitization to the fetal platelet antigens is unknown; it seems, however, to be somehow different from the mechanism that leads to haemolytic disease of the newborn because, in NAIT, the first fetus can be affected.

During an affected pregnancy, the mother, who lacks a specific platelet antigen, becomes immunized against a fetal antigen inherited from the father. The IgG maternal antiplatelet antibodies can cross the placenta and they recognize fetal platelets as targets. This can occur from the 14th week of pregnancy. Platelets appear in the fetal circulation from 5 weeks' gestation,[4] and the fetal platelet alloantigens are fully expressed as early as 18 weeks' gestation.[5,6] It has been shown that maternal antiplatelet antibodies can be detected as early as 16 weeks' gestation in a primipara primigravida woman.[3] Thrombocytopenia (defined as a platelet count below 150×10^9 cells/litre) can occur very early during pregnancy. Severe thrombocytopenia may lead to intracerebral haemorrhage. Although the true incidence of such complications is unknown, fetal death in utero and significant neonatal morbidity and mortality have been reported in different series up to 20–30% of affected cases. After birth, the duration of thrombocytopenia depends on the rate of removal of the maternal antiplatelet antibody from the neonatal circulation. Usually, the thrombocytopenia disappears within 1–3 weeks.

Table 22.1 Specific platelet alloantigens implicated in NAIT

Systems	Antigens	Glycoproteins	Amino acid substitution
HPA-1 (=Zw=PlᴬA)	HPA-1a	IIIa	Leu_{33}
	HPA-1b		Pro_{33}
HPA-2 (Ko)	HPA-2a	Ibα	Thr_{145}
	HPA-2b		Met_{145}
HPA-3 (=Bak=Lek)	HPA-3a	IIb	Ile_{843}
	HPA-3b		Ser_{843}
HPA-4 (=Yuk=Pen)	HPA-4a	IIIa	Arg_{143}
	HPA-4b		Gln_{143}
HPA-5 (=Br=Hc=Zav)	HPA-5a	Ia	Glu_{505}
	HPA-5b		Lys_{505}
HPA-6w (=Ca=Tu)	HPA-6wb	IIIa	Gln_{489}
			Arg_{489}
HPA-7w (=Mo)	HPA-7wb	IIIa	Ala_{407}
			Pro_{407}
HPA-8w (=Sr)	HPA-8wb	IIIa	Cys_{636}
			Arg_{636}
HPA-9w (Max)	HPA-9wb	IIb	Met_{837}
			Val_{837}
HPA-10w (=La)	HPA-10wb	IIIa	Gln_{62}
			Arg_{62}
HPA-11w (=Gro)	HPA-11wb	IIIa	His_{633}
			Arg_{633}
HPA-12w (=Iy)	HPA-12wb	GPIbβ	Glu_{15}
			Gly_{15}
HPA-13w (=Sit)	HPA-13bw	GPIa	Met_{799}
			Thr_{799}

Although platelets express HLA class I and ABH blood groups antigens at their surface, NAIT is mainly due to alloantibodies against platelet-specific alloantigens. Prospective study analysis showed that HLA antibodies did not cause thrombocytopenia,[7,8] but another report discusses this possibility, especially in low birth-weight infants when thrombocytopenia was associated with neutropenia.[9] It has also been reported that rare cases of neonatal alloimmune thrombocytopenia can be observed in infants whose mothers were treated by allogenic leuko-cyte immunization for unexplained recurrent abortions.[10] Casual observations suggest that NAIT is sometimes due to ABO incompatibility, although the particular features of these cases have not been well established.

The so-called platelet-specific alloantigens, defined conventionally by their exclusive presence on the megakaryocyte lineage, have a phenotype frequency that depends on ethnic group. There is now evidence that some of these antigens are also expressed on other cell types, such as the endothelial cells or long-term

FETAL AND NEONATAL ALLOIMMUNE THROMBOCYTOPENIA **299**

activated lymphocytes.[11] The wider distribution of platelet antigens may play a role in the pathophysiology of alloimmune thrombocytopenia, especially in the central nervous system where brain damage, such as porencephaly, can result either from haemorrhage or ischaemia. Alterations of the vascular endothelium may also lead to intracerebral thrombosis.

Since the first reports of platelet-specific alloantigens,[1,12] improvement in platelet immunology methods has led to the description of a number of new platelet alloantigenic systems. To avoid confusion concerning the assignation of a name, the working party on platelet serology proposed a new nomenclature in 1990.[13] Platelet-specific antigen systems are called HPA (human platelet antigen), numbered chronologically in order of the date of publication, the allelic antigens designated alphabetically in order of frequency in the population, 'a' for the high frequency, 'b' for the low frequency.[13] Progress in molecular biology has led to the identification of the polymorphisms responsible for several of the platelet allotypes (Table 22.1),[14–21] and a new nomenclature is under discussion in an attempt to incorporate the molecular genetic basis.[22] However, the working party nomenclature is still in use in laboratories, clinical departments and blood transfusion centres. Among the platelet-specific alloantigens, HPA-1a antigen (Pl[A1], Zw[a]) is by far the most common antigen implicated in NAIT in Caucasians,[23] followed (at much lower frequency) by HPA 5b.[24] In Asians, NAIT is essentially linked with the HPA-4 system.

Retrospective and prospective studies draw attention to the importance of immunogenetic factors in platelet alloimmunization. The HLA class II DRB3*0101allele may be implicated in anti-HPA-1a immunization[25,26] whereas anti-HPA-5b alloimmunization has been reported to be associated with a cluster of HLA DR molecules that share a particular polymorphic amino acid sequence at position 69–70 of the DRβ1 chain.[27] A better understanding of the immune response to platelet alloantigens would allow for a better definition – and thus appropriate management – of pregnant women at high risk.

CLINICAL ASPECTS

Fetal thrombocytopenia

A retrospective survey of 5194 fetal blood samplings has shown that the fetal thrombocytopenia that results from maternal alloimmunization is the most severe among various disorders, including chromosomal malformations, infections and maternal autoimmune

---

Table 22.2 Main other causes of neonatal thrombocytopenia

Immune destruction	Maternal autoimmunity: lupus, autoimmune idiopathic thrombocytopenia. Maternal drugs
Infection	Bacterial or viral infections
Disseminated intravascular coagulation	
Platelet consumption	Hemangioma
Megakaryocytopoiesis impairment	Association with absent radii (thrombocytopenia–absent radius syndrome)
	Sex-linked Wiskott–Aldrich syndrome
	Bone marrow metastasis
	Congenital leukaemia
	Down regulation of megakaryocytopoiesis during the course of Rhesus haemolytic disease or chronic hypoxia

thrombocytopenia. It has thus been suggested that a study of alloimmunization is warranted when an isolated incidental thrombocytopenia is discovered, even if another cause appears to be present, if the thrombocytopenia is more severe than expected for that aetiology.[28]

Severe thrombocytopenia can occur very early during gestation; *in utero* intracerebral haemorrhage with a reported frequency of 10% of cases has been observed whatever platelet alloantigens are implicated[23,29] occurring sometimes before 20 weeks' gestation.[30–32] When serial platelet counts are available, the platelet count is found to fall as gestation progresses[33] and there is no spontaneous correction of thrombocytopenia.

In utero intracerebral haemorrhage can be diagnosed by ultrasonography and magnetic resonance imaging. Reports have suggested Doppler flow velocimetry and colour Doppler imaging as additional tools in detecting fetal intracerebral haemorrhage.[34] In NAIT, intracerebral haemorrhages are most commonly intraparenchymal, although they may also be intraventricular. Intraventricular haemorrhage may result in arachnoiditis, with or without cerebrospinal fluid obstruction leading to hydrocephalus. Porencephalic cysts resulting either from ischaemic or haemorrhagic lesions have been described.[29,35,36] In fact, with any type of intracerebral haemorrhage, NAIT should be considered among other aetiological factors.

As the recurrence of NAIT is estimated to be over 90% in subsequent pregnancies, with an incompatible fetus at least as severely affected as the previous one, management of these high-risk pregnant women must be done in referral centres. Considerable advances have been made to prevent fetal bleeding and to avoid birth trauma.

Neonatal thrombocytopenia

The usual presentation of NAIT is that of a healthy mother giving birth to a full-term neonate that exhibits widespread purpura at birth or a few hours afterwards. Otherwise the infant is well, with no clinical signs of infection (e.g. hepatosplenomegaly) or malformation (e.g.

haemangioma, absence of radii). Reported series of neonates affected with alloimmune thrombocytopenia involve essentially anti-HPA-1a immunization, the most frequent cause of NAIT in Caucasians; therefore the following data focus on HPA-1a incompatibility. Visceral haemorrhages, such as gastrointestinal bleeding or haematuria, are less common than purpura or haematoma (6–30% of cases versus 65–90%). The most serious complication is intracerebral haemorrhage (10–30% of cases), which leads to death in up to 10% of the reported cases and to neurological sequelae in 20%.[23,37] Intracerebral haemorrhages have been reported in NAIT whichever platelet antigen is implicated, and they may be present at birth or occur as long as the newborn is severely thrombocytopenic.

In a series of 30 cases of anti-HPA-3a immunization, haemorrhagic symptoms due to a severe neonatal thrombocytopenia were observed in 90% of the cases, and intracerebral haemorrhages in 24%.[38] However NAIT linked to HPA-5b incompatibility seems to be less severe than HPA-1a NAIT:[24] in a retrospective study of 39 cases of anti-HPA-5b incompatibility, 59% of the infants did not exhibit haemorrhagic symptoms at birth and 8% had an intracerebral haemorrhage. The risk of life-threatening haemorrhage necessitates prompt diagnosis and effective therapy. Conversely, the infant may be symptomless with thrombocytopenia discovered incidentally, even in case of HPA-1a alloimmunization.

Therefore, unexpected or unexplained neonatal thrombocytopenia or severe early-onset thrombocytopenia in both pre-term and full-term babies should raise the possibility of NAIT and guide investigations accordingly.

In summary, then, the diagnosis of alloimmunization is initially made on clinical grounds. Other known aetiologies of neonatal thrombocytopenia (Table 22.2) should be considered and excluded by a careful examination of the affected neonate.[37] The maternal history should be taken into account to eliminate drug ingestion during pregnancy, maternal autoimmune thrombocytopenia or familial thrombocytopenia. However, one must be aware that NAIT may also be associated with other causes of neonatal thrombocytopenia, especially with maternal autoimmune thrombocytopenic purpura.[2] If the infant is not a first-born child, attention should be paid to previous siblings during the neonatal period; a history of thrombocytopenia in previous children is a strong argument for the diagnosis.

LABORATORY DIAGNOSIS

The first step in the laboratory diagnosis of NAIT is confirmation of the isolated thrombocytopenia. The platelet count is variable, usually low at birth ($< 50 \times 10^9$ cell/litre). In HPA-1a incompatibility, the lowest platelet count is usually observed on the first day of postnatal life, whereas it is usually reached on the third day in anti HPA-5a NAIT. Whatever the platelet counts, a platelet count below 150×10^9 cell/litre necessitates controls by phase microscopy. In any case, smear examination, microsampling, coagulation assessment and repeated platelet counts are mandatory. Anaemia is seen only when secondary to bleeding.

Platelet immunological investigations must be performed in a laboratory well versed in this technology. The testing involves the detection of circulating maternal antibody, identification of the offending platelet antigen and determination of the platelet phenotype of both parents. Highly sensitive, specific and reproducible serological biochemical and molecular biological assays must be available. Testing for the identification of the maternal antibody and platelet phenotyping include assays such as flow cytometry, radioactive test ('radioactive platelet Coombs test') and different enzyme-linked immunoassay (ELISA) techniques; some of these are commercially available. These tests are usually combined with an antigen-capture ELISA, such as the monoclonal antibody-specific immobilization of platelet antigen (MAIPA-test), the immunobead assay or the modified antigen-capture enzyme-linked immunosorbent assay,[39] which allow detection of weak antibodies or mixtures of antibodies. Since the molecular polymorphisms determining the alloantigen differences have been elucidated, genotyping is widely used. Analyses are done with DNA amplification by polymerase chain reaction (PCR) and restriction fragment length polymorphism, allele specific oligonucleotide hybridization, sequence-specific primers or single-strand conformational polymorphism methods.[40] Fetal genotyping can be performed either on chorionic villi or on amniotic cells if necessary.

The diagnosis is straightforward when a parental antigen incompatibility and a corresponding maternal antibody are present. If the father is heterozygous for the antigen in question or if the paternity is uncertain, the infant's platelet typing should be performed to confirm the diagnosis. It can be equivocal in the absence of maternal antibody – 30% of HPA-1b/1b women have no detectable antibody at the time of delivery. The author has observed that antibody kinetics are highly variable among pregnant women, and anti-platelet-specific antibodies can last for many years after pregnancy without apparent exposure or they can disappear at the end of pregnancy.

If an antigen incompatibility is determined but no antibody detected at the first screening, the parents and child should be tested again later, especially when improved methods of detection become available or early in the next pregnancy to confirm the diagnosis and the best management. Another issue is the implication of a new, rare or private antigen leading to extend testing with other techniques such as Western blotting, immunoprecipitation and DNA sequencing. Knowledge of the ethnic origin of the family is essential because it has been shown that phenotype frequencies of the platelet antigens differ among ethnic groups.

If there are difficulties in confirming the diagnosis, therapy should not be delayed, especially when there is a risk of life-threatening haemorrhage and there are sufficient grounds for the diagnosis.

MANAGEMENT AND OUTCOME
Unexpected neonatal thrombocytopenia

Until there is a prospective screening programme for detecting maternal immunization, and thus possibly fetal thrombocytopenia, most cases of NAIT will continue to be unexpected. Throughout the severe thrombocytopenic period, the infant is at risk of haemorrhage. The potential hazards of death or disabling neurological sequelae following intracerebral haemorrhage call for rapid and effective therapy. The optimal management should be initiated depending upon the clinical situation, even without confirmation by platelet immunological testing.

Infant with haemorrhages or platelet counts below 30 × 10⁹ platelets/litre during the first 24 hours of life

The treatment of choice is the transfusion of platelets that will not be destroyed by the maternal antibodies present in the infant's circulation, and the mother is the best donor. After maternal transfusion, the infant's platelet count usually increases promptly, which itself argues in favour of alloimmunization. The maternal platelets must be washed to remove the antiplatelet antibody and irradiated to prevent graft-versus-host disease. However, maternal transfusion may be delayed or not possible depending on the mother's physical condition and the results of predonation screening. If this is so, considering that HPA-1a incompatibility is the most frequent cause of NAIT, blood banks can provide HPA1b/1b donor platelets.

Once the results of platelet immunological testing are known, members of the family can be phenotyped, especially when antigens other than HPA-1a are implicated, to find donor platelets.

In cases where compatible platelets are not available or their delivery is delayed, the management is a matter of debate:

- random platelet transfusion is controversial since it may result in a transient response or worsening thrombocytopenia.
- an exchange-transfusion may be considered; this will partly remove the circulating antibody[41] and can be followed by transfusion of matched platelets.

In this setting, intravenous immunoglobulin G (IVIgG) (1 g/kg per day for 2 days) can be considered to raise the platelet count, but not for the treatment of actual haemorrhage because the effect is delayed for 12–18 hours after injection.[42]

There is no evidence that corticosteroid therapy is of help in such a situation.

Infant without haemorrhage and a platelet count above 30 × 10⁹ platelets/litre

In this situation, close clinical and ultrasound monitoring of the infant is required. A platelet transfusion is not usually necessary, the platelet counts will increase rapidly. However IVIgG (1 g/kg/day for 2 days) has been considered to raise the platelet count.

Outcome

The outcome depends of the severity of thrombocytopenia at birth and on the promptitude of diagnosis and treatment. A report suggests that NAIT is still underdiagnosed and that delay in providing effective therapy occurs.[43] The effect of breastfeeding on the outcome has not been fully addressed although one report suggests that there is no deleterious effect.[44]

Retrospective studies report a mortality of 10% and a rate of 20% of neurological sequelae in series of anti-HPA-1a NAIT.[23,45]

In any case of NAIT, the platelet count should be closely monitored and cranial and abdominal ultrasounds are required. It is mandatory to monitor all infants with NAIT for at least 2 years after birth for evidence of neurological impairment due to clinically silent intracerebral haemorrhage unless a nuclear magnetic resonance imaging scan has been performed.

Management of subsequent pregnancies

Owing to the rate of recurrence and the high risk of more severe clinical manifestations, especially intracerebral haemorrhage, the management of at-risk pregnancies is exacting. The principal aim of antenatal therapy is to prevent periods of significant thrombocytopenia in order to minimize the risk of significant haemorrhage. This requires prompt diagnosis and treatment before serious morbidity occurs. The major objective of antenatal management remains sensitive prenatal diagnosis that restricts therapeutic interventions to affected fetuses.

With regard to the subsequent pregnancies, up to now there has been no means of predicting the fetal status without invasive procedures. The infant will be affected only if there is incompatibility for the offending antigen with the immunized mother. Therefore if the father is heterozygous or if the paternity is uncertain, fetal genotyping should be performed (see above). In the majority of cases, any subsequently affected fetus will be more severely thrombocytopenic than the previously affected sibling. Nevertheless, there are anecdotal cases of an incompatible fetus not being affected at all, even though it followed two or three previous siblings with severe NAIT, including intracerebral haemorrhage.[46]

Controversy exists about the prediction of fetal thromcytopenia by monitoring the maternal antiplatelet antibody level or titre:

- in the author's experience, serial monitoring of maternal antiplatelet antibodies seems not to be reliable for predicting fetal thrombocytopenia in anti-HPA-1a NAIT,[33] since 15–20% of the women with affected fetuses had no detectable circulating antibodies, moreover, when antibody was present, there was no correlation between the antibody level, the IgG subclass, and the severity of the fetal thrombocytopenia;[47]
- according to some authors, pregnancies most at risk are those in which the mother has a high level of antibody;[48,49]
- A high titre of anti-HPA-5b may be associated with a higher risk of neonatal thrombocytopenia,[50] but most pregnant women with anti-HPA-5b antibody do not go onto deliver a thrombocytopenic child.[51]

The reported frequency of spontaneous intracerebral haemorrhage *in utero* is about 10%, although the exact incidence, the most likely time of occurrence and the rate of recurrence are not known. Reports have mentioned that some families seem to be particularly at risk, especially those in which intracerebral haemorrhage occurred early during pregnancy.

These observations suggest that predicting fetal thrombocytopenia (and intracerebral haemorrhage) is still impossible and we may have to consider other possibilities. In this respect, preliminary results of one *in vitro* study of a few cases suggested that the inhibition of colony-forming unit megakaryocyte cultures in the presence of maternal anti-HPA-1a antibody seemed to correlate with the severity of thrombocytopenia.[52]

Taking into account these data, the only means of detecting and assessing the severity of fetal thrombocytopenia is to perform percutaneous umbilical blood sampling (PUBS). The risk of fetal bleeding and possible exsanguination from the puncture site on the cord is an important consideration.[53,54] The risk of the procedure itself varies depending on the skill of the operator,[55] and PUBS must be done at referral centres experienced in this technique: in these circumstances the risk is of the order of 1% or less. Fetal and neonatal losses related to PUBS have been reported in pregnancies affected with alloimmune thrombocytopenia and studied at various centres. Compared with a control group of fetuses with fetomaternal alloimmune thrombocytopenia that underwent PUBS without any complications, the analysis showed that an increased bleeding tendency was a feature of this group of cases, as suggested by severe thrombocytopenia and a history of intracerebral haemorrhage in previous siblings. Thus, severe thrombocytopenia may cause prolonged bleeding at the cord puncture site, with streaming visible by ultrasonography. Moreover, alloantibodies may interfere with platelet function, resulting in a Glanzmann thrombasthenia-like state. In this latter condition, fetal exsanguination after PUBS has been documented. However, since the affected fetus is an obligatory heterozygote for the platelet antigen target of the maternal alloantibody, it is difficult to understand how 50% inhibition of the platelet function by the antibody could lead to such a severe state. It has also been postulated that alteration of the endothelial cells by the alloantibody may modify primary haemostasis. These documented cases of severe complications have led some teams to transfuse platelets routinely and immediately after PUBS when severe thrombocytopenia is expected.[53]

Fetal platelet counts are very reliable, provided that strict control is maintained in assessing the purity of the fetal blood sample.[56]

Significant contamination by amniotic fluid and maternal blood should be searched for. The normal value for fetal platelet counts is $245 \pm 65 \times 10^9$ platelets/litre. There is no significant variation with gestational age.

The optimal antenatal therapy to reverse fetal thrombocytopenia is still a matter of debate.[46,54] Pharmacological studies are particularly difficult in fetal medicine, and access to fetal blood is limited since cordocentesis cannot easily be repeated.

The differences in outcome that have been documented may result from different treatment protocols or from the evaluation of the results. This evaluation is complex, especially since the published reports are not based on comparative methodology or randomized controlled trials. Such trials are difficult to carry out in a single centre, because of the low incidence of the condition, the risk of fetal damage and ethical issues, including the legal relationship between the mother and her fetus.

At present, alternatives include maternal injection of IVIgG with or without corticosteroids or weekly intrauterine platelet transfusions with antigen-negative platelets.

Maternal injection of intravenous immunoglobulins was considered after the observation that it was helpful in the therapy of the neonate with alloimmune thrombocytopenia. The inhibitory effect of IVIgG may be the result of competition with the maternal antibody for placental Fcγ receptors involved in the endocytotic uptake of IgG. *In vitro* experiments with an isolated perfused lobule of human placenta showed that IVIgG clearly inhibited the transfer of specific maternal anti-HPA-1a alloantibody to the fetal circulation. This effect was observed with the different batches tested.[57] However, it is important to point out that these experiments were conducted with full-term placentas, which have been shown to have maximal capacity for active IgG transfer. The timing of IgG therapy during gestation could, therefore, be another important factor. An adequate dose of IVIgG has been considered to be important. It seems that doses lower than 1 g/kg per week fail to produce an increase in platelet counts. IVIgG might increase the catabolism of maternal antiplatelet antibody by saturating a specialized intracellular Fc receptor (FcRn)[58] and modifying the maternal and fetal immune responses.

The addition of corticosteroids may play a supplementary role by modulating the maternal immune response.

Weekly *in utero* platelet transfusions involve repeated PUBS with the risk of the procedure itself and the risk of fetal exposure to multiple donors. The main issues in the preparation of platelet concentrates for fetal transfusions are compatibility with maternal antibodies, adequate dosage without volume overload, and avoidance of transfusion-transmitted infections and transfusion-associated graft-versus-host disease.[59,60] Platelet concentrates (concentration of platelet to a count of $2500–4000 \times 10^9$ platelets/litre) should be prepared by plateletpheresis of compatible donors. The mother is the most convenient donor for a single transfusion but this is not practicable for repeated transfusions, and panels of selected donors should be established. This may be a logistical problem, especially if the antibody specificity is other than HPA-1a. Fetal haemolysis caused by transfusion of high-titre anti-A, anti-B antibodies should be avoided by testing donors for these high-titre antibodies. Maternal anti-HLA antibodies may occasionally be responsible for shortened survival of platelets transfused to the fetus, in which case the platelets should be prepared from the mother or HLA-matched HPA-compatible donors.[61]

Repeated transfusions may increase the mother's sensitization, as has been described for red blood cells. Finally, it is not known if frequent transfusion alters fetal thrombopoiesis and thus enhances the thrombocytopenia by a central effect.

Maternal injection of immunoglobulins with or without corticosteroids has been reported to be effective, increasing the platelet counts and protecting from intracerebral haemorrhage.[37,62,63] However, intracerebral haemorrhage has been documented during this therapy,[64] and IVIg has not been found to be useful in other studies.[61,65] Low-dose corticosteroids have been given to a limited number of mothers, but the resulting rise in fetal platelet counts is variable.[66] Thus, definite recommendations cannot be provided.

A large prospective randomized trial of the addition of low-dose corticosteroids to IVIg has been published.[67] None of the 54 fetuses developed an intracerebral haemorrhage. Among the fetuses, 62–85% responded to the therapy and low-dose corticosteroids (dexamethasone 1.5 mg/day) did not add to the effect of IVIgG.

In the first European multicentre study, a satisfactory response to maternal treatment with IVIgG was observed in 26% of cases ($n = 27$). However, in 41% of cases treated with IVIg there was no significant change in the fetal platelet count and absence of silent or overt intracerebral haemorrhage during pregnancy and delivery. The significance of this observation is uncertain. It may indicate a stabilization of thrombocytopenia and hence a beneficial effect of therapy, or it may be the natural course of the platelet count in a low-risk pregnancy which was not influenced by therapy. Among the therapy failures, there were proportionally more severely affected siblings (i.e. those suffering intracerebral haemorrhage or death). The study therefore concluded that intracerebral haemorrhage or thrombocytopenia less than 20×10^9 platelets/litre during the first 24 hours of life in the previous sibling are parameters to be included in the definition of the most severe cases.[46]

The most important question about antenatal therapy is whether the most severe cases will respond or not. The current multicentre protocol in the USA allocates cases to different groups according to the estimated risk of intracerebral haemorrhage:[68]

- an extremely high-risk group with antenatal intracerebral haemorrhage documented in a previous sibling before 28 weeks' gestation: maternal therapy with prednisone (1 mg/kg per day) and IVIg (1 g/kg per week) from 12 weeks' gestation, first PUBS is performed at 20 weeks' gestation;
- a very high-risk group with a previous sibling having had an antenatal intracerebral haemorrhage at 28–36 weeks' gestation: maternal therapy with IVIgG (1 g/kg per week) from 12 weeks' gestation, with first PUBS is performed at 20 weeks' gestation;

- a high-risk group with either a previous sibling with a perinatal intracerebral haemorrhage or an initial platelet count ≤ 20 × 10⁹ platelets/litre: the first PUBS is performed before maternal therapy with IVIgG alone or IVIgG plus prednisone; and
- a standard risk group with no history of intracerebral haemorrhage in a previous sibling and an initial platelet count > 20 × 10⁹ platelets/litre: the first PUBS is performed before maternal therapy with IVIgG (1 g/kg per week) or prednisolone 0.5 mg/kg per day.

There is an ongoing European multicentre study with three different antenatal managements: maternal therapy with IVIgG, or regular *in utero* platelet transfusions or a single *in utero* platelet transfusion before delivery. The first results of this study have shown that the incidence of intracerebral haemorrhage in the study group is less than the incidence in the previous siblings, but complications from repeated *in utero* transfusion may occur.

Based on the author's data the following approach is recommended. High-risk pregnant women must be followed in a referral centre. In the case of an incompatible fetus, fetal blood sampling should be performed in order to determine the fetal platelet count at around 20–22 weeks' gestation. If the fetus is thrombocytopenic (platelet count < 150 × 10⁹ platelets/litre), maternal therapy with IVIgG (1 g/kg per week) should be considered. To assess the therapy efficacy, a second fetal blood sampling should be performed at around 34 weeks' gestation. Corticosteroids could be added in case of therapy failure. For delivery, there are two options: Caesarean delivery without control of the fetal platelet count or the approach to be decided following the results of a third fetal blood sampling. In this latter case, vaginal delivery is allowed if the fetal platelet count is > 50 × 10⁹ platelets/litre after maternal therapy or after *in utero* platelet transfusion. Weekly *in utero* platelet transfusion are not recommended since they seem to be too invasive, but in very severe cases in which the other therapeutic regimens fail, weekly *in utero* platelet transfusions may offer the only possibility of reversing the fetal thrombocytopenia. In any case, at-risk pregnant women must be advised to avoid vigorous exercise, trauma and ingestion of drugs that interfere with platelet function (e.g. aspirin, different antibiotics).

It is mandatory to monitor all affected infants for at least 2 years after birth (see below). After prenatal treatment with maternal infusions of high-dose immunoglobulins, the development of immunocompetence in the child must also be assessed.

ROUTINE ANTENATAL SCREENING

Because NAIT frequently affects first pregnancies and is diagnosed after birth when bleeding has occurred, the question of routine screening has been raised. A prospective study was conducted in France over 35 months to compare the medical outcomes and the costs of two screening strategies for HPA-1a-linked NAIT.[3] A total of 2066 primiparas and 6081 neonates were included. Primiparous women were screened once for the HPA-1 phenotype at the time of their first clinic visit. When a woman was found to be HPA-1b/1b, the father was phenotyped. In case of incompatibility, the mother was screened twice during pregnancy for the identification of antiplatelet alloantibodies. HLA typing was done but was not found to add any valuable information. The prevalence of anti-HPA-1a maternal immunization was 2 per 1000 and the prevalence of fetal or neonatal alloimmune thrombocytopenia was 1 per 1000. Until procedures are found to predict which immunized women will have thrombocytopenic infants, maternal screening has a low sensitivity. Identifying only thrombocytopenic newborns at birth (platelet count determined on cord blood sampling) increases the sensitivity but misses babies who have had an intracerebral haemorrhage *in utero* and should have been treated. The trade-offs between the primiparous strategy and the neonatal strategy could be assessed in terms of cost-effectiveness. Analysis indicates that screening for NAIT is not more expensive than programme already in operation and that screening neonates was more cost-effective than screening primiparous women. Moreover, the neonatal strategy detected

platelet disorders and asymptomatic thrombocytopenia that would otherwise have been unnoticed. The major failure of the neonatal strategy is that it cannot prevent fetal death or disability during the course of the index pregnancy. When screening mothers, one must consider the availability of therapy, the risk of fetal loss resulting from PUBS and the possibility of increasing maternal alloimmunization during the puncture. Therefore, PUBS is not recommended in high-risk women in the absence of detectable antibody. In any case, for high-risk women the best management of delivery can be planned.

The major limitations concerning antenatal screening are the absence of parameters to predict which fetuses would be thrombocytopenic, and since optimal antenatal therapy is controversial, which ones need to be treated and what should be done. A recent evaluation of antenatal screening has been performed in the UK, and the conclusions were similar.[69]

In conclusion, at present HPA-1a screening is not offered to all pregnant women because antenatal interventions have not been proven entirely effective and feasible.

Another important issue is the detection of high-risk women among the sisters of an HPA-1b/1b mother who has delivered an affected infant. Information should be given to the family and platelet typing should be performed. If a sister is found to be HPA-1b/1b, the husband is typed and, in the case of antigen incompatibility, screening is performed once every 2–3 months during pregnancy for anti-platelet alloantibodies. PUBS and antenatal therapy are proposed only when alloantibodies are detectable. This strategy has allowed delivery of affected infants without haemorrhagic complications.

CONCLUSION

Antenatal management is still evolving. As there is no predictive parameter for the response to therapy, randomized and collaborative studies are necessary to establish the best strategy for management of fetuses at risk. It will only be after the efficacy of antenatal management has been established that routine screening can be considered as a public health issue.

REFERENCES

1. Shulman NR, Marder VJ, Hiller MC, Collier EM. Platelet and leukocyte isoantigens and their antibodies. Serologic, physiologic and clinical studies. In: Moor CV, Brown EB, eds. *Progress in Hematology*. New York: Grune and Stratton; 1964:222–304.
2. Dreyfus M, Kaplan C, Verdy E, *et al*. Frequency of immune thrombocytopenia in newborns: a prospective study. *Blood* 1997;**89**:4402–6.
3. Durand-Zaleski I, Schlegel N, Blum-Boisgard C, *et al*. Screening primiparous women and newborns for fetal/neonatal alloimmune thrombocytopenia: a prospective comparison of effectiveness and costs. *Am J Perinatol* 1996;**13**:423–31.
4. Hann IM. Development of blood in the fetus. In: Hann IM, Gibson BES, Letsky E, eds. *Fetal and Neonatal Haematology*. London: Baillière Tindall; 1991:1–28.
5. Kaplan C, Patereau C, Reznikoff-Etievant MF, *et al*. Antenatal PLA1 typing and detection of GP IIb-IIIa complex. *Br J Haematol* 1985;**60**:586–8.
6. Gruel Y, Boizard B, Daffos F, *et al*. Determination of platelet antigens and glycoproteins in the human fetus. *Blood* 1986;**68**:488–92.
7. Skacel PO, Contreras M. Neonatal alloimmune thrombocytopenia. *Blood Rev* 1989;**3**:174–9.
8. Sharon R, Amar A. Maternal anti-HLA antibodies and neonatal thrombocytopenia. *Lancet* 1981;**1**:313.
9. Koyama N, Ohama Y, Kaneko K, *et al*. Association of neonatal thrombocytopenia and maternal anti-HLA antibodies. *Acta Paediatr Jpn* 1991;**33**:71–6.
10. Tanaka T, Umesaki N, Nishio J, *et al*. Neonatal thrombocytopenia induced by maternal anti-HLA antibodies: a potential side effect of allogenic leukocyte immunization for unexplained recurrent aborters. *J Reprod Immunol* 2000;**46**:51–7.
11. von dem Borne AEGKr, Kuijpers RWAM. Platelet antigens, new aspects. In: Kaplan-Gouet C, Schlegel N, Salmon C, McGregor J, eds. *Platelet Immunology: Fundamental and Clinical Aspects*. Paris: John Libbey; 1991:219–40.
12. van Loghem JJ, Dorfmeijer H, van der Hart M, Schreuder F. Serological and genetical studies on a platelet antigen (Zw). *Vox Sang* 1959;**4**:161–9.
13. von dem Borne AEGKR, Decary F. Nomenclature of platelet specific antigens. *Br J Haematol* 1990;**74**:2039–240.
14. Newman PJ, Derbes RS, Aster RH. The human platelet alloantigens, PlA1 and PlA2, are associated with a leucine33/proline33 amino acid polymorphism in membrane glycoprotein IIIa, and are distinguishable by DNA typing. *J Clin Invest* 1989;**83**:1778–81.
15. Lyman S, Aster RH, Visentin GP, Newman PJ. Polymorphism of human platelet membrane glycoprotein IIb associated with the Baka/Bakb alloantigen system. *Blood* 1990;**75**:2343–8.
16. Wang L, Juji T, Shibata Y, Kuwata S, Tokunaga K. Sequence variation of human platelet membrane glycoprotein IIIa associated with the Yukᵃ/Yukᵇ alloantigen system. *Proc Jpn Acad* 1991;**67**:102–6.
17. Kuijpers RW, Faber NM, Cuijpers HT, *et al*. NH2-terminal globular domain of human platelet glycoprotein alpha has a methionine 145/threonine145 amino acid polymorphism which is associated with HPA-2 (Ko) alloantigens. *J Clin Invest* 1992;**89**:381–4.
18. Kuijpers RWAM, Simsek S, Faber NM, *et al*. Single point mutation in human glycoprotein IIIa is associated with a new platelet-specific alloantigen (Mo) involved in neonatal alloimmune thrombocytopenia. *Blood* 1993;**81**:70–6.
19. Kalb R, Santoso S, Unkelbach K, *et al*. Localization of the Br polymorphism on a 144 bp exon of the GPIa gene and its application in platelet DNA typing. *Thromb Haemost* 1994;**71**:651–4.
20. Santoso S, Kalb R, Kroll H, *et al*. A point mutation leads to an unpaired cysteine residue and a molecular weight polymorphism of a functional platelet beta3 integrin subunit. The Sra alloantigen system of GPIIIa. *J Biol Chem* 1994;**269**:8439–44.
21. Peyruchaud O, Bourre F, Morel-Kopp MC, *et al*. HPA-10wb (Laa): genetic determination of a new platelet specific alloantigen on glycoprotein IIIa and its expression in cos-7 cells. *Blood* 1997;**89**:2422–8.
22. Santoso S, Kiefel V. Human platelet-specific alloantigens: update. *Vox Sang* 1998;**74**:249–53.
23. Mueller-Eckhardt C, Kiefel V, Grubert A, *et al*. 348 cases of suspected neonatal allo-immune thrombocytopenia. *Lancet* 1989;**i**:363–6.
24. Kaplan C, Morel-Kopp MC, Kroll H, *et al*. HPA-5b (Bra) neonatal alloimmune thrombocytopenia: clinical and immunological analysis of 39 cases. *Br J Haematol* 1991;**78**:425–9.
25. Valentin N, Vergracht A, Bignon JD, *et al*. HLA DRw52a is involved in alloimmunisation against Pl-A1 antigen. *Hum Immunol* 1990;**27**:73–79.
26. Decary F, L'Abbé D, Tremblay L, Chartrand P. The immune response to the HPA-1a antigen:

association with HLA-DRw52a. *Transfus Medicine* 1991;**1**:55–62.

27. Semana G, Zazoun T, Alizadeh M, *et al.* Genetic susceptibility and anti-human platelet antigen 5b alloimmunization. Role of HLA class II and TAP genes. *Hum Immunol* 1996;**46**:114–19.

28. Hohlfeld P, Forestier F, Kaplan C, *et al.* Fetal thrombocytopenia: a retrospective survey of 5,194 fetal blood samplings. *Blood* 1994;**84**: 1851–6.

29. Friedman JM, Aster RH. Neonatal alloimmune thrombocytopenic purpura and congenital porencephaly in two siblings associated with a 'new' maternal antiplatelet antibody. *Blood* 1985;**65**:1412–15.

30. de Vries LS, Connell J, Bydder GM, *et al.* Recurrent intracranial haemorrhages in utero in an infant with alloimmune thrombocytopenia. Case report. *Br J Obstet Gynaecol* 1988;**95**:299–302.

31. Giovangrandi Y, Daffos F, Kaplan C, *et al.* Very early haemorrhage in alloimmune thrombocytopenia. *Lancet* 1990;**336**:310.

32. Waters AH, Murphy M, Hambley H, Nicolaides K. Management of alloimmune thrombocytopenia in the fetus and neonate. In: Nance S, ed. *Clinical and Basic Science: Aspects of Immunohematology.* Arlington, VA, USA: American Association of Blood Banks: 1991:155–77.

33. Kaplan C, Daffos F, Forestier F, *et al.* Management of alloimmune thrombocytopenia: antenatal diagnosis and in utero transfusion of maternal platelets. *Blood* 1988;**72**:340–3.

34. Sherer DM, Anyaegbunam A, Onyeije C. Antepartum fetal intracranial hemorrhage, predisposing factors and prenatal sonography: a review. *Am J Perinatol* 1998;**15**:431–41.

35. Burrows RF, Caco CC, Kelton JG. Neonatal alloimmune thrombocytopenia: spontaneous in utero intracranial hemorrhage. *Am J Hematol* 1988;**28**:98–102.

36. Govaert P, Bridger J, Wigglesworth J. Nature of the brain lesion in fetal alloimmune thrombocytopenia. *Dev Med Child Neurol* 1995;**37**:485–95.

37. Kaplan C, Morel-Kopp MC, Clemenceau S, *et al.* Fetal and neonatal alloimmune thrombocytopenia: current trends in diagnosis and therapy. *Transfus Med* 1992;**2**:265–71.

38. Glade-Bender J, McFarland J, Kaplan G, *et al.* Anti HPA-3a induces severe neonatal alloimmune thrombocytopenia. *J Pediat* 2001;**138**:862–7.

39. Kaplan C. Evaluation of serological platelet antibody assays. *Vox Sang* 1998;**74 (suppl 2)**:355–8.

40. Kroll H, Kiefel V, Santoso S. Clinical aspects and typing of platelet alloantigens. *Vox Sang* 1998;**74 (suppl 2)**:345–54.

41. Bussel JB, Kaplan C, McFarland JG, and the Working Party on Neonatal Immune Thrombocytopenia of the Neonatal Hemostasis Subcommittee of the Scientific and Standardization Committee of the ISTH. Recommendations for the evaluation and treatment of neonatal autoimmune and alloimmune thrombocytopenia. *Thromb Haemost* 1991;**65**:631–4.

42. Massey GV, McWilliams NB, Mueller DG, Napolitano A, Maurer HM. Intravenous immunoglobulin in treatment of neonatal isoimmune thrombocytopenia. *J Pediatr* 1987;**111**: 133–5.

43. Murphy MF, Verjee S, Greaves M. Inadequacies in the postnatal management of fetomaternal alloimmune thrombocytopenia (FMAIT). *Br J Haematol* 1999;**105**:123–6.

44. Reese J, Raghuveer TS, Dennington PM, Barfield CP. Breast feeding in neonatal alloimmune thrombocytopenia. *J Paediatr Child Health* 1994;**30**:447–9.

45. Kaplan C, Daffos F, Forestier F, *et al.* Current trends in neonatal alloimmune thrombocytopenia: diagnosis and therapy. In: Kaplan-Gouet C, Schlegel N, Salmon C, McGregor J, eds. *Platelet Immunology: Fundamental and Clinical Aspects*, vol 206. Paris: John Libbey; 1991:267–78.

46. Kaplan C, Murphy MF, Kroll H. Waters AH. Feto-maternal alloimmune thrombocytopenia: antenatal therapy with IvIgG and steroids: more questions than answers. *Br J Haematol* 1998;**100**: 62–65.

47. Proulx C, Filion M, Goldman M, *et al.* Analysis of immunoglobulin class, IgG subclass and titre of HPA-1a antibodies in alloimmunized mothers giving birth to babies with or without neonatal alloimmune thrombocytopenia. *Br J Haematol* 1994;**87**:813–17.

48. Williamson LM, Hackett G, Rennie J, *et al.* The natural history of fetomaternal alloimmunization to the platelet-specific antigen HPA-1a (PLA1, Zwa) as determined by antenatal screening. *Blood* 1998;**92**:2280–7.

49. Jaegtvik S, Husebekk A, Aune B, *et al.* Neonatal alloimmune thrombocytopenia due to anti HPA-1a antibodies: the level of maternal antibodies predicts the severe thrombocytopenia in the newborn. *Br J Obstet Gynaecol* 2000;**107**:691–4.

50. Ohto H, Yamaguchi T, Takeuchi C, *et al.* Anti-HPA-5b-induced neonatal alloimmune thrombocytopenia: antibody titre as a predictor. *Br J Haematol* 2000;**110**:223–7.

51. Panzer S, Auerbach L, Cechova E, *et al*. Maternal alloimmunization against fetal platelet antigens: a prospective study. *Br J Haematol* 1995;**90**: 655–60.

52. Warwick RM, Vaughan J, Murray N, *et al*. In vitro culture of colony forming unit-megakaryocyte (CFU-MK) in fetal alloimmune thrombocytopenia. *Br J Haematol* 1994;**88**:874–7.

53. Paidas MJ, Berkowitz RL, Lynch L, *et al*. Alloimmune thrombocytopenia: fetal and neonatal losses related to cordocentesis. *Am J Gynecol* 1995;**172**:475–9.

54. Silver RM, Porter TF, Branch DW, *et al*. Neonatal alloimmune thrombocytopenia: antenatal management. *Am J Gynecol* 2000;**182**:1233–8.

55. Ghidini A, Sepulveda W, Lockwood CJ, Romero R. Complications of fetal blood sampling. *Am J Gynecol* 1993;**168**:1339.

56. Daffos F, Capella-Pavlosky M, Forestier F. Fetal blood sampling during pregnancy with use of a needle guided by ultrasound: a study of 606 consecutive cases. *Am J Gynecol* 1985;**153**: 655–60.

57. Morgan CL, Cannell GR, Addison RS, Minchinton RM. The effect of intravenous immunoglobulin on placental transfer of a platelet-specific antibody: anti-Pl[A1]. *Transfus Med* 1991;**1**:209–16.

58. Yu Z, Lennon VA. Mechanism of intravenous immune globulin therapy in antibody-mediated autoimmune diseases. *N Engl J Med* 2001;**340**:227–8.

59. Murphy MF, Pullon HWH, Metcalf P, *et al*. Management of fetal alloimmune thrombocytopenia by weekly in utero platelet transfusions. *Vox Sang* 1990;**58**:45–9.

60. Murphy MF, Waters AH, Doughty HA, *et al*. Antenatal management of fetomaternal alloimmune thrombocytopenia: report of 15 affected pregnancies. *Transfus Med* 1994;**4**:281–92.

61. Murphy MF, Metcalfe P, Waters AH, *et al*. Antenatal amanagement of severe feto-maternal alloimmune thrombocytopenia: HLA incompatibility may affect responses to fetal platelet transfusions. *Blood* 1993;**81**:2174–9.

62. Bussel JB, Berkowitz RL, McFarland JG, *et al*. Antenatal treatment of neonatal alloimmune thrombocytopenia. *N Engl J Med* 1988;**319**:1374–8.

63. Lynch L, Bussel JB, McFarland JG, *et al*. Antenatal treatment of alloimmune thrombocytopenia. *Obstet Gynecol* 1992;**80**:67–71.

64. Kroll H, Kiefel V, Giers G, *et al*. Maternal intravenous immunoglobulin treatment does not prevent intracranial haemorrhage in fetal alloimmune thrombocytopenia. *Transfus Med* 1994;**4**: 293–6.

65. Mir N, Samson D, House MJ, Kovar IZ. Failure of antenatal high-dose immunoglobulin to improve fetal platelet count in neonatal allo-immune thrombocytopenia. *Vox Sang* 1988;**55**:188–9.

66. Daffos F, Forestier F, Kaplan C. Prenatal treatment of fetal alloimmune thrombocytopenia. *Lancet* 1988;**ii**:910.

67. Bussel JB, Berkowitz RL, Lynch L, *et al*. Antenatal management of alloimmune thrombocytopenia with intravenous gamma-globulin: a randomized trial of the addition of low-dose steroid to intravenous gamma-globulin. *Am J Gynecol* 1996;**174**: 1414–23.

68. Bussel J, Kaplan C. The fetal and neonatal consequences of maternal alloimmune thrombocytopenia. In: Michiels JJ, ed. *Acquired Disorders of Haemostasis: Pathophysiology, Clinical Practice and Basic Research*, vol 11. London: Baillière Tindall; 1998:391–408.

69. Murphy MF, Williamson LM. Antenatal screening for fetomaternal alloimmune thrombocytopenia: an evaluation using the criteria of the UK national screening committee. *Br J Haematol* 2000;**111**:726–32.

23

Development of hemostasis in the fetus

Marilyn J Manco-Johnson

INTRODUCTION

Hematologists, neonatologists, and obstetricians have long been fascinated with the development of the fetal hemostatic system, which this chapter reviews. First, it should be noted that hemostasis is functionally intact in well full-term infants, and clinical presentation of excessive bleeding or clotting in a healthy infant is rare. However, the sick infant, especially the sick preterm infant, is uniquely prone to overt signs of paradoxical bleeding and clotting, often simultaneously. Histological signs of hemorrhage and thrombosis are routinely found on autopsies of babies who have died from any cause.

Secondly, all global screening tests of coagulation are prolonged in the plasma of healthy infants compared with adult values in the absence of bleeding.[1,2] Values in stable preterm infants are more prolonged compared with results in full-term infants.[1,3–5] In contrast, global tests of whole blood coagulation reproducibly show the hemostatic competence of neonatal blood to be equal to, if not superior to, that of adult blood.[6–8]

Thirdly, assays of specific hemostatic proteins have determined that plasma concentrations of various coagulation proteins mature at different rates.[1–3] The normal adult range may be achieved as early as midgestation for certain proteins and as late as several months after birth for others. Thus, the fetus demonstrates a unique balance in levels of specific coagulation proteins in the maintenance of hemostasis.

EARLIEST EVIDENCE OF THE FETAL HEMOSTATIC SYSTEM

A search for the earliest evidence of coagulation protein production was begun over 30 years ago.[9] Fibrinogen was found in the liver by 5 weeks' gestation.[9] Using immunohistochemical staining, von Willebrand factor (vWF) was consistently detected in endothelial cells of the placenta from 4 weeks onwards, with successive detection in fetal bone marrow and tissues over the next 4 weeks.[10,11] Newer techniques in molecular biology have facilitated the determination of expression profiles of active genes by collection of sequences with a 3'-directed DNA library that mirrors the composition of the messenger RNA (mRNA) population. Such studies have demonstrated that synthesis of coagulation proteins is among the most active in the fetus after production of plasma proteins such as albumin.[12] A methodology termed differential display reverse transcriptase–polymerase chain reaction has shown that approximately 99% of hepatic genes expressed during development are not transcriptionally regulated, but are most likely controlled at the level of translation.[13]

Hassan *et al.* demonstrated that by 5 weeks' gestation mRNA and intracellular proteins for coagulation factors VII, VIII, IX, X, fibrinogen, protein C, and antithrombin could be detected in hepatic cells of human embryos.[14] Between 5 and 10 weeks of fetal development most coagulation mRNAs increased from 30% to 50% of the normal adult level.[14] Exceptions in this study included factor IX, which increased only from 2% to 10% of adult abundance of mRNA, and factor X, which consistently showed 100% adult abundance of mRNA. Soluble liver protein of factors VII and X per gram of tissue were 100% relative to normal adult between 5 and 10 weeks, whereas plasma concentrations from 6 to 8 weeks were 40%. In comparison, soluble liver and plasma factor IX levels were both 10% of adult levels. These data were interpreted to suggest that factor X is preferentially activated by complexes of factor VII with tissue factor rather than factor IXa–factor VIIIa–phospholipid during human embryonic and early fetal life.

DEVELOPMENT OF PLASMA CONCENTRATIONS OF COAGULATION PROTEINS

Determination of fetal plasma concentrations of various coagulation proteins is hampered by technical difficulty in accessing fetal blood. Most results reported for the first half of gestation have been determined on samples obtained after abortion.[15–22] In these early studies, it was demonstrated that the blood of fetuses does not clot before 10–11 weeks' gestation. Thereafter, the whole blood clotting time rapidly becomes equal to or shorter than that of the normal adult.[16] Fibrinolytic activity is also detectable by 10–11 weeks' gestation and thereafter is similar to adult values or even greater (indicating shorter lysis times).[16] Bleyer et al. reported a significant correlation between whole blood clotting and clot lysis[16] based on an analysis of the data of Zilliacus et al.[17] and argued that blood clotting and clot lysis develop in parallel. Levels of factor V approach the adult range by 12–15 weeks.[18,19] Substantial levels of factor VIII (23%) and vWF (37%) were detected at this developmental age.[19] Plasma concentration of fibrinogen approaches 100 mg/dl by 12–15 weeks.[15,19,20]

Development of ultrasound-guided periumbilical blood sampling (PUBS) opened the door to direct blood sampling in utero without disturbance to the fetus. Using samples from 285 healthy fetuses obtained by PUBS, Reverdiae-Moalic et al. were able to determine the development of plasma concentrations of 16 procoagulant and anticoagulant proteins from 19 to 38 weeks' gestation.[23] Their results showed measurable levels of all the proteins assayed from 19 weeks onwards and supported much of the work relating to earlier gestations. In essence, plasma concentrations of most coagulation proteins were maintained at a constant level throughout gestation until some time after 33 weeks, when a maturational increase occurred. From 19 weeks onwards, coagulation proteins circulate at 50–100% of the level achieved by 38 weeks. Exceptions to this general maintenance of a constant plasma concentration during midgestation include factors V, VII, VIII, and XII, and antithrombin, which show steady increases throughout the second and third trimesters.

Results obtained on healthy full-term infants after delivery are significantly higher than are those documented on healthy, full-term infants in utero.[1,2,23] The difference between in utero and postnatal results from infants of the same gestational age probably represents alterations induced by labor and early adaptations to extrauterine life. Awareness of differences in plasma concentrations of coagulation proteins related to birth status is important in the evaluation of published data on fetuses versus preterm infants. Likewise, the postnatal maturation of coagulation proteins in preterm infants is faster than that in undisturbed fetuses.[1,4,5]

The developmental expression of coagulation proteins in utero on cell surfaces, in liver and bone marrow tissue, and in plasma is depicted in Figure 23.1. Relative plasma concentrations of coagulation proteins in the fetus at term are shown in Table 23.1. Levels of vitamin K-dependent proteins are generally 30–50% of adult levels after term birth, although factor IX activity can be as low as 15% of adult levels in a healthy newborn. Plasma concentrations of contact factors are also low after term delivery. Levels of fibrinogen, factors V and VIII, and antiplasmin

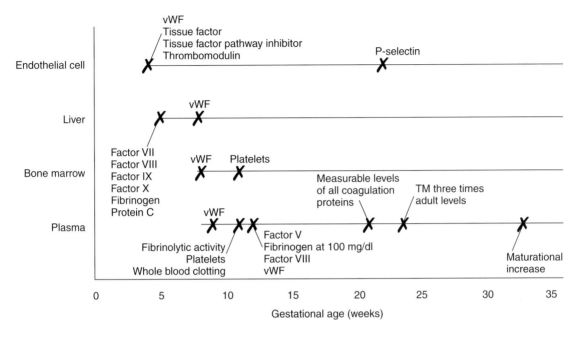

Figure 23.1 Developmental expression of the fetal hemostatic system. This graph depicts the temporal expression of fetal coagulation proteins and platelets in endothelial cells, hepatic cells, bone marrow, and plasma during gestation.

are within the normal adult range while concentrations of vWF and α2-macroglobulin are increased postnatally at term relative to adults. Certain proteins modulate activities of coagulation proteins in the neonate. Plasma concentration of C4b-binding protein is generally less than 10% of the adult level at birth.[23,24] Because the compartment of protein S bound to C4b-binding protein does not participate as a cofactor for activated protein C, free protein S (and consequently protein S activity) are increased relative to the level of total protein S. Similarly, levels of histidine-rich glycoprotein are often undetectable in the fetus.[25] Since this protein competes with fibrin for plasminogen binding, its deficiency contributes to increased fibrinolytic activity in the fetus and neonate.

EVIDENCE FOR FETAL CHARACTERISTICS OF COAGULATION PROTEINS

Most coagulation proteins in the fetus differ from the corresponding adult protein in plasma concentration, while molecular form and specific activity are equivalent. Proteins that exhibit unique fetal form and function include fibrinogen, plasminogen, and vWF.

Fibrinogen

The thrombin time is slightly prolonged in full-term infants at birth, and this prolongation persists for the first 3 weeks of postnatal life.[1] A unique fetal form of fibrinogen was first hypothesized by Burnstein *et al.*, who noted that fibrin clot formed in blood from newborn infants was more transparent and less resistant than clot from adult blood.[26] Subsequent investigators characterized fetal fibrinogen biochemically. Fetal fibrinogen has been reported to have greater negative charge in diethylaminoethyl–cellulose chromatography, prolonged clotting at alkaline pH, and increased chromatographic mobility of tryptic digest fingerprints.[27] The fetal molecule has an increased content of organically bound phosphorus to approximately twice that

Table 23.1 Coagulation screening tests and coagulation factor levels in fetuses, full-term newborns, and adults

Parameter	In utero fetuses			Postnatal Term newborns (n = 60)	Adults (n = 40)
	19–23 weeks' gestation (n = 20)	24–29 weeks' gestation (n = 22)	30–38 weeks' gestation (n = 22)		
Prothrombin time (s)	32.5 (19–45)	32.2 (19–44)†	22.6 (16–30)†	16.7 (12.0–23.5)*	13.5 (11.4–14.0)
Prothrombin time (INR)	6.4 (1.7–11.1)	6.2 (2.1–10.6)†	3.0 (1.5–5.0)*	1.7 (0.9–2.7)*	1.1 (0.8–1.2)
Activated partial thromboplastin time (s)	168.8 (83–250)	154.0 (87–210)†	104.8 (76–128)†	44.3 (35–52)*	33.0 (25–39)
Thrombin clotting time (TCT) (s)	34.2 (24–44)*	26.2 (24–28)	21.4 (17.0–23.3)	20.4 (15.2–25.0)†	14.0 (12–16)
Factor					
I (g/l, von Clauss)	0.85 (0.57–1.50)	1.12 (0.65–1.65)	1.35 (1.25–1.65)	1.68 (0.95–2.45)†	3.0 (1.78–4.50)
I Ag (g/l)	1.08 (0.75–1.50)	1.93 (1.56–2.40)	1.94 (1.30–2.40)	2.65 (1.68–3.60)†	3.5 (2.50–5.20)
IIc (%)	16.9 (10–24)	19.9 (11–30)*	27.9 (15–50)†	43.5 (27–64)†	98.7 (70–125)
VIIc (%)	27.4 (17–37)	33.8 (18–48)*	45.9 (31–62)	52.5 (28–78)†	101.3 (68–130)
IXc (%)	10.1 (6–14)	9.9 (5–15)	12.3 (5–24)†	31.8 (15–50)†	104.8 (70–142)
Xc (%)	20.5 (14–29)	24.9 (16–35)	28.0 (16–36)†	39.6 (21–65)†	99.2 (75–125)
Vc (%)	32.1 (21–44)	36.8 (25–50)	48.9 (23–70)†	89.9 (50–140)†	99.8 (65–140)
VIIIc (%)	34.5 (18–50)	35.5 (20–52)	50.1 (27–78)†	94.3 (38–150)	101.8 (55–170)
XIc (%)	13.2 (8–19)	12.1 (6–22)	14.8 (6–26)†	37.2 (13–62)†	100.2 (70–135)
XIIc (%)	14.9 (6–25)	22.7 (6–40)	25.8 (11–50)†	69.8 (25–105)†	101.4 (65–144)
Prekallikrein (%)	12.8 (8–19)	15.4 (8–26)	18.1 (8–28)†	35.4 (21–53)†	99.8 (65–135)
High molecular weight kininogen (%)	15.4 (10–22)	19.3 (10–26)	23.6 (12–34)†	38.9 (28–53)†	98.8 (68–135)
Antithrombin III (%)	20.2 (12–31)*	30.0 (20–39)	37.1 (24–55)†	59.4 (42–80)†	99.8 (65–130)
Heparin cofactor II (%)	10.3 (6–16)	12.9 (5.5–20)	21.1 (11–33)†	52.1 (19–99)†	101.4 (70–128)
Tissue factor pathway inhibitor (ng/ml)‡	21.0 (16.0–29.2)	20.6 (13.4–33.2)	20.7 (10.4–31.5)†	38.1 (22.7–55.8)†	73.0 (50.9–90.1)
Protein C Ag (%)	9.5 (6–14)	12.1 (8–16)	15.9 (8–30)†	32.5 (21–47)†	100.8 (68–125)
Protein C activity (%)	9.6 (7–13)	10.4 (8–13)	14.1 (8–18)*	28.2 (14–42)†	98.8 (68–129)
Total protein S (%)	15.1 (11–21)	17.4 (14–25)	21.0 (15–30)†	38.5 (22–55)†	99.6 (72–118)
Free protein S (%)	21.7 (13–32)	27.9 (19–40)	27.1 (18–40)†	49.3 (33–67)†	98.7 (72–128)
Ratio of free protein S to total protein S	0.82 (0.75–0.92)	0.83 (0.76–0.95)	0.79 (0.70–0.89)†	0.64 (0.59–0.98)†	0.41 (0.38–0.43)
C4b-BP (%)	1.8 (0–6)	6.1 (0–12.5)	9.3 (5–14)	18.6 (3–40)†	100.3 (70–124)

Values are the mean, followed in parentheses by the lower and upper boundaries including 95% of the population

Ag, antigenic value; c, coagulant activity; (s), seconds

*$p < 0.05$

†$p < 0.01$

‡Twenty samples were assayed for each group, but only 10 for 19- to 23-week-old fetuses

From Reverdiau-Moalic et al.[23]

of the adult molecule.[28] A shorter fibril length between branch points and thinner fibrils have been demonstrated for fetal fibrin.[29] Fetal fibrinogen consists of decreased N-terminal alanine residues in the A-α chain.[30] Finally, fetal fibrinogen has been determined to contain increased sialic acid.[31,32]

The relative contribution of each of these biochemical differences to clot formation has been debated. Fetal fibrinogen exhibits faster plasma elimination than adult fibrinogen.[33] Increased turnover may be a general characteristic of fetal coagulation proteins.

Plasminogen

Benevent et al. described a fetal plasminogen molecule with 23% specific activity of the active site compared with the adult molecule.[34] Fetal plasminogen was subsequently found to contain increased sialic acid, as does fetal fibrinogen.[35] Despite decreased and slower activation of fetal plasmin, clot lysis is more rapid in fetal plasma, owing to decreased inactivation of fetal plasmin by α2-antiplasmin.[36] An enhanced sensitivity of fetal plasminogen to activation by tissue plasminogen activator (tPA) at lower concentrations has been reported by Ries et al. in comparison with adult plasminogen, while no differences have been found for urokinase-plasminogen (UPA) activator.[36,37]

von Willebrand factor

vWF is made up of ultralarge multimers (UlvWF) in all fetal plasmas up to 35 weeks' gestation, and it changes to the adult plasma form by 8 weeks after birth.[38] The UlvWF multimers in fetal and neonatal plasma are very similar to those constitutively released from endothelial cells. A vWF protomer is present in 97% of fetal blood samples, 83% of cord blood samples, and 11% of neonatal heel stick samples, suggesting altered processing of the vWF up to the time of birth. Fetal vWF shows an enhanced capacity to support platelet deposition on subendothelium under high-shear flow conditions.[39] Fetal vWF contributes to the shorter bleeding time and increased

susceptibility to arterial thrombosis found in the neonate.

VITAMIN K-DEPENDENT PROTEINS

Vitamin K is an essential cofactor for the post-translational modification of certain γ-glutamic acid residues to form unique γ-carboxyglutamic acids known as Gla proteins.[40] The carboxylation process requires the enzyme γ-glutamyl carboxylase and takes place within the endoplasmic reticulum.[41] Vitamin K is recycled via vitamin K1 epoxide reductase. Elevations of vitamin K1 epoxide reflect inefficient hepatic reductase cycling, a potentially rate-limiting step in the fetus and neonate if hepatic function is immature or impaired. At least four classes of vitamin K-dependent proteins have been identified. The coagulation proteins, factors II, VII, IX and X, protein C, protein S, and protein Z, are all characterized by a 45 amino acid Gla domain that contains between nine and 12 Gla residues, which confer Gla-mediated, calcium-dependent anionic phospholipid binding to membranes where coagulation activations occur physiologically.[42–44] Recently, Gas6, the ligand for the receptor tyrosine kinases Axl and Sky has been identified as belonging to this category of Gla protein.[45,46] Gas6 is involved in cell growth and apoptosis. Osteocalcin and matrix Gla protein are involved in bone growth and calcification of cartilage.[47] The enzyme γ-glutamyl carboxylase is itself a Gla protein.[48] Finally, there is a family of broadly expressed transmembrane Gla proteins whose structure is consistent with potential cell surface receptors capable of mediating cytoplasmic signaling.[49] Whereas once vitamin K was thought to play a biological role solely in the function of certain coagulation proteins, vitamin K-dependent proteins are now recognized to be involved in many critical physiological processes. The myriad possible links of vitamin K-dependent proteins to embryogenesis and fetal development are in the early stages of exploration.

Vitamin K-dependent coagulation proteins achieve a basal plasma level by approximately mid-gestation, a level that is maintained until an increase around the time of birth, followed by gradually increasing levels throughout childhood. Karpatkin *et al.* documented expression of fetal rabbit hepatic mRNA for prothrombin equal to or greater than expression in adult liver, while plasma concentrations of prothrombin remained low.[50] Ineffective protein synthesis, decreased intracellular protein stability, decreased protein secretion from the cell, or the production of unstable proteins with accelerated plasma elimination are possible explanations of this phenomenon.

Vitamin K-dependent proteins undergo complex post-translational modification, including glycosylation, γ-carboxylation, sulfation, and β-hydroxylation. Vitamin K inhibition by warfarin has been shown to decrease protein antigen concentrations of dependent proteins in the plasma, as well as resulting in dysfunctional molecules, suggesting a role of vitamin K in the regulation of protein synthesis.[51–53] Experiments using HepG2 cells in culture demonstrated that prothrombin secretion from the cell increased up to 100% and total prothrombin synthesis increased by 50% in the presence of excessive vitamin K1.[54] Secretion of prothrombin decreased by 19% following warfarin exposure in this model. However, the total amount of prothrombin mRNA was unchanged by either vitamin K1 or warfarin exposure. This and other data suggest that secretion of prothrombin and other vitamin K-dependent proteins from the hepatocyte is linked to conformational changes that occur with γ-carboxylation and is decreased in vitamin K deficiency states.[54,55]

The placenta maintains a steep gradient of vitamin K during gestation with fetal levels one-tenth or less that of maternal levels.[56,57] The gradient appears to increase towards the end of gestation.[57] Shapiro *et al.* reported evidence of non-carboxylated prothrombin in 2.7% of cord bloods from otherwise healthy full-term infants.[58] Similar rates for high concentrations of non-carboxylated vitamin K-dependent proteins at birth have been reported by Bovill *et al.* who used a monoclonal antibody to non-carboxylated prothrombin and protein C in 496 neonates across a wide range of gestational ages

and reported evidence of undercarboxylation of prothrombin in 7% of cases and protein C in 27% of cases.[59] The prevalence of deficient carboxylation increased with increasing gestational age, consistent with evidence of the increasing placental–fetal vitamin K gradient. It has been speculated that high concentrations of vitamin K promote mutagenesis of DNA *in vitro*, and low levels of vitamin K are maintained during fetal development to diminish mutagenic risk in rapidly proliferating cells.[60–62] It is possible that diminished availability of hepatic vitamin K is an important physiological determinant of plasma protein expression in the ontogeny of the vitamin K-dependent proteins.

Administration of certain anticonvulsants or antibiotics to the pregnant woman increases the risk of vitamin K deficiency in the fetus and neonate. Anticonvulsant therapy (including phenytoin, phenobarbital, valproic acid, and carbamazepine) has been shown to decrease fetal and neonatal levels of vitamin K1 and to increase the frequency of non-carboxylated prothrombin.[63] Vitamin K-deficient bleeding has occurred in infants of mothers on anticonvulsants within the first 24 hours of life. Antenatal maternal supplementation with vitamin K1 (10 mg/day by mouth) from 36 weeks of pregnancy onwards prevents neonatal vitamin K deficiency.[64] Of course, maternal oral anticoagulation with warfarin causes fetal and neonatal vitamin K deficiency and should be replaced by low molecular weight heparin therapy when indicated.

CELLULAR ACTIVITIES

Most coagulation proteins are synthesized and secreted from liver and endothelial cells, while platelet and endothelial cell surfaces contribute physiologically relevant surfaces for coagulation activations. Because of their relative inaccessibility, cellular proteins and processes have become the last frontier of neonatal hemostasis research.

Tissue factor is a transmembrane protein that serves a central role in thrombin generation. Following exposure to blood by endothelial cell damage or expression on activated mononuclear phagocytic cells or endothelial cells, tissue factor forms complexes with factors VII and VIIa to activate factor X. *In situ* hybridization and immunohistochemical studies have demonstrated strong and widespread expression of tissue factor in ectodermal and endodermal cells, with high levels of morphogenic activity during early organogenesis.[65] High levels of tissue factor expression were detected in neuroepithelial cells as well as in tissues that do not express this protein later in adulthood, including skeletal muscle and the pancreas.[65] However, lack of evidence for factor VII during early embryology suggested that tissue factor serves as an ontological role in tissue proliferation and differentiation rather than in coagulation.

Mouse 'knock-out' models using manipulated gene deletions or disruptions have been helpful in assessing the physiological relevance of various coagulation proteins in fetal growth and development. Because thrombin causes cell proliferation, a potential relationship between thrombogenesis and embryogenesis has been hypothesized. Early mouse knock-out models of tissue factor deficiency showed complete lethality by 10.5 days.[66–68] Early organogenesis in the mouse models was normal. The animals died from hemorrhage, with leakage of red cells from abnormal embryonic vasculature. The role of fetal tissue factor in angiogenesis and embryogenesis as opposed to thrombogenesis has not yet been fully resolved. Regardless of the role of tissue factor in cellular proliferation and differentiation, it is evident that fetal hemostasis is necessary to prevent spontaneous hemorrhage. Fetal mice with homozygous mutations resulting in complete lack of prothrombin or factor V suffer excess fetal wastage at 10.5 days of embryogenesis, and the few fetuses that survive to term die of hemorrhage shortly after birth.[69,70]

Evidence of increased tissue factor activity from cord blood leukocytes was first reported in 1975.[71] Employing a model of whole blood flow through human term umbilical veins, Grabowski *et al.* determined increased tissue factor activity from neonatal endothelial cells.[72]

In addition, Streif *et al.* showed accelerated thrombin generation in the plasma of preterm infants related to increased tissue factor activity *in vivo*.[73] The tissue factor pathway of coagulation activation is likely to play an important role in thrombin generation in the near-term fetus and neonate.

The tissue factor pathway inhibitor (TFPI) is synthesized and secreted from endothelial cells. Immunohistochemical techniques have demonstrated that TFPI is widely expressed in human tissues from 8 to 24 weeks' gestation.[74] Plasma levels of TFPI are decreased in newborn infants.[75,76] Mouse knock-out models of TFPI also show excess lethality at 10.5 embryonic days.[77] Tissue histology suggests consumptive coagulopathy and diffuse fibrin deposition in TFPI-deficient embryonic mice. Although many endothelial cell-associated proteins show early, diffuse, and intense developmental expression, the fetal endothelial cell adhesive protein, P-selectin, was not detected in human fetal tissue before 22 weeks.[78]

Fibrinolytic components, tPA, uPA and plasminogen activating factor (PAI)-1 are all synthesized in and secreted from endothelial cells. In contrast to the increased expression of tissue factor and TFPI, tPA and uPA levels have been reported to be slightly decreased in fetal plasma, while fetal PAI-1 activity is significantly decreased.[25] Fibrinolytic proteins also exhibit a role in embryogenesis. After the 10th week of gestation, immunohistochemical techniques can demonstrate uPA and PAI-1 in osteoblasts and chondrocytes in areas of endochondral ossification and in perivascular chondrocytes of the epiphyseal secondary ossification centers.[15] uPA and PAI-1 are progressively expressed proximal to distal bones, implicating fibrinolytic enzymes in the desmal and enchondral ossification processes in the osseocartilaginous compartment.[15]

Thrombomodulin (TM) is an endothelial proteoglycan that serves as a surface receptor for thrombin in the activation of the coagulation regulatory protein, protein C. Immunoreactive TM can be detected in plasma. Circulating levels of TM have been determined to be increased in the fetus, with a peak level of 165 ng/ml achieved between 23 and 26 weeks' gestation.[79] Plasma concentrations of TM decrease progressively during the last trimester of pregnancy and throughout childhood until they reach their adult normal median value of 56 ng/ml by later childhood or adolescence.[79,80]

PLATELETS

Platelets have been consistently detected in fetuses from 11 weeks' gestation.[16] Somewhat large platelets have been observed at 10–12 weeks' gestation, with essentially normal mean platelet volume thereafter depending on measurement technique.[16,81–84] The platelet count is within the adult normal range by 20 weeks' gestation, even though mean cell numbers are significantly lower than in healthy adults.[16,81,82] It is known that the bleeding time, which measures global platelet–vessel interaction, is shorter in the full-term neonate than in the adult and within adult normal limits in the preterm infant.[7] Similar results have been reported recently with the use of the whole blood platelet function analyzer (PFA-100).[8]

Hepatocytes are the primary site of thrombopoietin in the fetus.[85] Increased levels of thrombopoietin relative to maternal values have been determined in fetuses who require periumbilical blood sampling.[86,87]

The relatively higher hematocrit of neonatal whole blood contributes to increased blood clotting both by increasing the concentration of platelets directed to the vessel wall by the dynamics of laminar flow, as well as by offering a larger surface for the formation of fibrin clots. vWF, which facilitates adhesion of platelets to collagen, reaches normal adult levels by 20 weeks' gestation and is increased in both plasma concentration as well as in the proportion of larger (stickier) UlvWF multimers after full-term birth. Fetal platelet receptors are mature as early as 12–16 weeks' gestation, except for epinephrine receptors, which exhibit decreased receptor coupling.[84,88,89] Neonatal platelet function, as measured by aggregation in response to a number of physiological agonists, is diminished.[90–94] Recent evidence suggests diminished calcium channel transport and impaired signal transduction as an etiology of delayed change in platelet shape and delayed granular release in response to activators.[95–97] In spite of this, *in vivo* platelet function appears to be very adequate in the well full-term neonate, who manifests remarkably few petechiae and bruises after the strenuous process of vaginal delivery.

Neonatal alloimmune thrombocytopenia (NAIT), caused by maternal production of antiplatelet antibodies against fetal platelet antigens of paternal origin, occurs in one delivery in 1000.[98] Affected babies are generally asymptomatic unless the platelet count is less than 10,000 cells/µl. However, intracranial hemorrhage has been documented *in utero* in infants with NAIT. In contrast, *in utero* hemorrhage secondary to defects of bone marrow megakaryocytes is rare.

CONCLUSION

In general, individual components of the coagulation system can be detected very early in gestation, mature late in fetal development, and increase postnatally throughout much of the first year of life. The best evidence for unique fetal forms of coagulation proteins are found in fibrinogen, plasminogen, and vWF. Decreased concentrations and activities of coagulation proteins account for the mild prolongations of global screening tests detected in healthy full-term infants. Exceptions to the generally low plasma levels of coagulation proteins include vWF, factors VIII and V and fibrinogen. Together with hematocrit, platelet number and platelet adhesiveness, these four coagulation proteins which are all within or above the normal adult range at full-term gestation, make a major contribution to hemostatic potential in the neonate and probably contribute to hypercoagulability seen clinically in sick infants.

Despite apparent deficiencies of procoagulant, regulatory, and fibrinolytic activities, the hemostatic system of the well full-term infant is balanced and intact. However, the neonatal hemostatic system lacks reserve capacity adequate to cope with massive stresses of low blood flow, acidosis, and sepsis, which often challenge the sick preterm infant.

REFERENCES

1. Hathaway WE, Bonnar J. *Hemostatic Disorders of the Pregnant Woman and Newborn Infant*. New York: Elsevier Science, 1987:57–75.

2. Andrew M, Paes B, Johnston M. Development of the haemostatic system in the neonate and young infant. *Am J Pediatr Hematol Oncol* 1990;**12**: 95–104.

3. Aronis S *et al*. Indications of coagulation and/or fibrinolytic system activation in healthy and sick very-low-birth-weight neonates. *Biol Neonate* 1998;**74**:337–44.

4. Barnard DR, Simmons MA, Hathaway WE. Coagulation studies in extremely premature infants. *Pediatr Res* 1979;**13**:1330–5.

5. Andrew M, Paes B, Johnston M *et al*. Development of the human coagulation system in the healthy premature infant. *Blood* 1988;**72**: 1651–7.

6. Markarian M, Githens JH, Jackson JJ *et al*. Fibrinolytic activity in premature infants. Relationship of the enzyme system to the respiratory distress syndrome. *Am J Dis Child* 1967;**113**: 312–21.

7. Feusner JH. Normal and abnormal bleeding times in neonates and young children utilizing a fully standardized template technic. *Am J Clin Pathol* 1980;**74**:73–7.

8. Israels SJ, Cheang T, McMillan-Ward EM, Cheang M. Evaluation of primary hemostasis in neonates with a new in vitro platelet function analyzer. *J Pediatr* 2000;**138**:116–19.

9. Gitlin D, Biasucci A. Development of gamma G, gamma A, gamma M, beta IC-beta IA, C1 esterase inhibitor, ceruloplasmin, transferrin, hemopexin, haptoglobin, fibrinogen, plasminogen, alpha 2-macroglobulin, and prealbumin in the human conceptus. *J Clin Invest* 1969;**48**: 1433–46.

10. Travis PA, Bovill EG, Hamill B, Tindle B. Detection of factor VIII von Willebrand Factor in endothelial cells in first-trimester fetuses. *Arch Pathol Lab Med* 1988;**112**:40–2.

11. Tuddenham EGD, Shearn SAM, Peake IR *et al*. Tissue localization and synthesis of factor-VIII-related antigen in the human foetus. *Br J Haematol* 1974;**26**:669–77.

12. Kawamoto S, Matsumoto Y, Miuno K *et al*. Expression profiles of active genes in human and mouse livers. *Gene* 1996;**174**:151–8.

13. Malhotra K, Luehrsen KR, Costello LL *et al*. Identification of differentially expressed mRNAs in human liver across gestation. *Nucleic Acids Res* 1999;**27**:839–47.

14. Hassan HJ, Leonardi A, Chelucci C *et al*. Blood coagulation factors in human embryonic-fetal development: preferential expression of the FVII/tissue factor pathway. *Blood* 1990;**76**:1158–64.

15. Hackel C, Radig K, Rose I, Roessner A. The urokinase plasminogen activator (u-PA) and its inhibitor (PAI-1) in embryo-fetal bone formation in the human: an immunohistochemical study. *Anat Ambryol (Berl)* 1995;**192**:363–8.

16. Bleyer WA, Hakami N, Shepard TH. The development of hemostasis in the human fetus and newborn infant. *J Pediatr* 1971;**79**:838–53.

17. Zilliacus H, Ottelin AM, Mattison T. Blood clotting and fibrinolysis in human foetuses. *Biol Neonate* 1966;**10**:108–12.

18. Ekelund H, Hedner U, Astedt B. Fibrinolysis in human foetuses. *Acta Paediatr Scand* 1970;**59**: 369–76.

19. Heikinheimo R. Coagulation studies with fetal blood. *Biol Neonate* 1964;**7**:319–27.

20. Holmberg L, Henriksson P, Ekelund H, Åstedt B. Coagulation in the human fetus. *J Pediatr* 1974;**85**:860–4.

21. Creter D, Goldman JA, Djaldetti M. The fibrinolytic pathway in the human fetus. *Biol Neonate* 1977;**32**:94–6.

22. Terwiel J, Veltkamp JJ, Bertina RM, Muller HP. Coagulation factors in the human fetus of about 20 weeks of gestational age. *Br J Haematol* 1980;**45**:641–50.

23. Reverdiau-Moalic P, Delahousse B, Body G *et al*. Evolution of blood coagulation activators and inhibitors in the healthy human fetus. *Blood* 1996;**88**:900–6.

24. Moalic P, Gruel Y, Body G *et al*. Levels and plasma distribution of free and C4b-BP-bound protein S in human fetuses and full-term newborns. *Thromb Res* 1988;**49**:471–80.

25. Reverdiau-Moalic P, Gruel Y, Delahousse B *et al*. Comparative study of the fibrinolytic system in human fetuses and in pregnant women. *Thromb Res* 1991;**61**:489–99.

26. Burnstein M, Lewis S, Walter P. Sur l'existence du fibriogène foetal. *Sang* 1954;**25**:102–7.

27. Witt I, Müller H, Künzer W. Evidence for the existence of foetal fibrinogen. *Thromb Diath Haemorrh* 1969;**22**:101–9.

28. Witt I, Müller H. Phosphorus and hexose content of human foetal fibrinogen. *Biochim Biophys Acta* 1970;**221**:402–4.

29. Müller M, Burchard W. Fibrinogen–fibrin transformation. Part III. Particularities for foetal fibrinogen. *Thromb Res* 1981;**24**:339–46.

30. Hasegawa N, Sasaki S. A deficiency in A alpha chain's *N*-terminal alanine residue as a major cause of the slow coagulation of fetal fibrinogen. *Thromb Res* 1989;**54**:595–602.

31. Francis JL, Armstrong DJ. Sialic acid and enzymatic desialation of cord blood fibrinogen. *Haemostasis* 1982;**11**:223–8.

32. Galanakis DK, Martinez J, McDevitt C, Miller F. Human fetal fibrinogen: its characteristics of delayed fibrin formation, high sialic acid and AP peptide content are more marked in pre-term than in term samples. *Ann NY Acad Sci* 1983;**408**:640–3.

33. Karitsky D, Kleine N, Pringsheim W, Kunzer W. Fibrinogen turnover in the premature infant with and without idiopathic respiratory distress syndrome. *Acta Paediatr Scand* 1971;**60**:465–70.

34. Benavent A, Estelles A, Aznar J *et al.* Dysfunctional plasminogen in full term newborn: study of active site of plasmin. *Thromb Haemost* 1984;**51**:67–70.

35. Ries M. Molecular and functional properties of fetal plasminogen and its possible influence on clot lysis in the neonatal period. *Semin Thromb Hemost* 1997;**23**:247–52.

36. Ries M, Klinge J, Rauch R *et al.* In vitro fibrinolysis after adding low doses of plasminogen activator and plasmin generation with and without oxidative inactivation of plasmin inhibitors in newborns and adults. *J Pediatr Hematol Oncol* 1996;**18**:346–51.

37. Ries M, Zenker M, Gaffney PJ. Differences between neonates and adults in the urokinase-plasminogen activator (u-PA) pathway of the fibrinolytic system. *Thromb Res* 2000;**100**:341–51.

38. Katz JA, Moake JL, McPherson PD *et al.* Relationship between human development and disappearance of unusually large von Willebrand factor multimers from plasma. *Blood* 1989;**73**:1851–8.

39. Shenkman B, Linder N, Savion N *et al.* Increased neonatal platelet deposition in subendothelium under flow conditions: the role of plasma von Willebrand factor. *Pediatr Res* 1999;**45**:270–5.

40. Stenflo J. Vitamin K and the biosynthesis of prothrombin. IV. Isolation of peptides containing prosthetic groups from normal prothrombin and the corresponding peptides from dicoumarol-induced prothrombin. *J Biol Chem* 1974;**249**:5527–35.

41. Vermeer C. The vitamin K-dependent carboxylation reaction. *Mol Cell Biochem* 1984;**61**:17–35.

42. Bristol JA, Ratcliffe JV, Roth DA *et al.* Biosynthesis of prothrombin: intracellular localization of the vitamin K-dependent carboxylase and the sites of gamma-carboxylation. *Blood* 1996;**88**:2585–93.

43. Kurachi K, Davie EW. Isolation and characterization of a cDNA coding for human factor IX. *Proc Natl Acad Sci USA* 1982;**79**:6461–4.

44. Jorgensen MJ, Cantor AB, Furie BC, Furie B. Recognition site directing vitamin K-dependent gamma-carboxylation resides on the propeptide of factor IX. *Cell* 1987;**48**:185–91.

45. Varnum BC, Young C, Elliot G *et al.* Axl receptor tyrosine kinase stimulated by the vitamin K-dependent protein encoded by growth-arrest-specific gene 6. *Nature* 1995;**373**:623–6.

46. Ohashi K, Nagata K, Toshima J *et al.* Stimulation of sky receptor tyrosine kinase by the product of growth arrest-specific gene 6. *J Biol Chem* 1995;**270**:22681–4.

47. Price PA, Poser JW, Raman N. Primary structure of the gamma-carboxyglutamic acid-containing protein from bovine bone. *Proc Natl Acad Sci USA* 1976;**73**:3374–5.

48. Berkner KL, Pudota BN. Vitamin K-dependent carboxylation of the carboxylase. *Proc Natl Acad Sci USA* 1998;**95**:466–71.

49. Kulman JD, Harris JE, Xie L, Davie EW. Identification of two novel transmembrane γ-carboxyglutamic acid proteins expressed broadly in fetal and adult tissues. *Proc Natl Acad Sci USA* 2001;**98**:1370–5.

50. Karpatkin M, Lee M, Cohen L *et al.* Synthesis of coagulation proteins in the fetus and neonate. *J Pediatr Hematol Oncol* 2000;**22**:276–80.

51. Vigano S, Mannucci PM, Solinas S *et al.* Decrease in protein C antigen and formation of an abnormal protein soon after starting oral anticoagulant therapy. *Br J Haematol* 1984;**57**:213–20.

52. Takahashi H, Hanano M, Hayashi S *et al.* Plasma levels of protein C and vitamin K-dependent coagulation factors in patients on long-term oral anticoagulant therapy. *Tohoku J Exp Med* 1986;**149**:351–7.

53. Weiss P, Soff GA, Halkin H, Seligsohn U. Decline of proteins C and S and factors II, VII, IX and X during initiation of warfarin therapy. *Thromb Res* 1987;**45**:783–90.

54. Jamison CS, Burkey BF, Degen SJ. The effects of vitamin K1 and warfarin on prothrombin

expression in human hepatoblastoma (HepG2) cells. *Thromb Haemost* 1992;**68**:40–7.

55. Wallin R, Stanton C, Hutson SM. Intracellular maturation of the gamma-carboxyglutamic acid region in prothrombin coincides with release of the propeptide. *Biochem J* 1993:**291**:723–7.

56. Shearer MJ, Rahim S, Barkhan P, Stimmler L. Plasma vitamin K1 in mothers and their newborn babies. *Lancet* 1982;**2**:460–3.

57. Mandelbrot L, Guillaumont M, Leclercq M *et al.* Placental transfer of vitamin K1 and its implications in fetal hemostasis. *Thromb Haemost* 1988;**60**:39–43.

58. Shapiro AD, Jacobson LJ, Armon ME *et al.* Vitamin K deficiency in the newborn infant: prevalence and perinatal risk factors. *J Pediatr* 1986;**109**:75–80.

59. Bovill EG, Soll RF, Lynch M *et al.* Vitamin K1 metabolism and the production of des-carboxy prothrombin and protein C in the term and premature neonate. *Blood* 1993;**81**:77–83.

60. Israels LG, Friesen E, Jansen AH, Israels ED. Vitamin K1 increases sister chromatid exchange in vitro in human leukocytes and in vivo in fetal sheep cells: a possible role for 'vitamin K deficiency' in the fetus. *Pediatr Res* 1987;**22**:405–8.

61. Israels LG, Israels ED. Observations on vitamin K deficiency in the fetus and newborn: has nature made a mistake? *Semin Thromb Hemost* 1995;**21**:357–63.

62. Webster WS, Vaghef H, Ryan B *et al.* Measurement of DNA damage by the comet assay in rat embryos grown in media containing high concentrations of vitamin K(1). *Toxicol In Vitro* 2000;**14**:95–9.

63. Cornelissen M, Steegers-Theunissen R, Kollee L *et al.* Increased incidence of neonatal vitamin K deficiency resulting from maternal anticonvulsant therapy. *Am J Obstet Gynecol* 1993;**168**:923–8.

64. Cornelissen M, Steegers-Theunissen R, Kollee L *et al.* Supplementation of vitamin K in pregnant women receiving anticonvulsant therapy prevents neonatal vitamin K deficiency. *Am J Obstet Gynecol* 1993;**168**:884–8.

65. Luther T, Flossel C, Mackman N *et al.* Tissue factor expression during human and mouse development. *Am J Pathol* 1996;**149**:101–13.

66. Bugge TH, Xiao Q, Konbrinck KW *et al.* Fatal embryonic bleeding events in mice lacking tissue factor the cell-associated initiator of blood coagulation. *Proc Natl Acad Sci USA* 1996;**93**:6258–63.

67. Carmeliet P, Mackman N, Moons L *et al.* Role of tissue factor in embryonic blood vessel development. *Nature* 1996;**383**:73–5.

68. Toomey JR, Kratzer KE, Lasky NM *et al.* Targeted disruption of the murine tissue factor gene results in embryonic lethality. *Blood* 1996;**88**:1583–7.

69. Xue J, Wu Q, Westfield LA *et al.* Incomplete embryonic lethality and fatal neonatal hemorrhage caused by prothrombin deficiency in mice. *Proc Natl Acad Sci USA* 1998;**95**:7603–7.

70. Cui J, O'Shea KS, Purkayastha A *et al.* Fatal haemorrhage and incomplete block to embryogenesis in mice lacking coagulation factor V. *Nature* 1996;**384**:66–8.

71. Rivers RP, Hathaway WE. Studies on tissue factor activity and production by leukocytes of human umbilical cord and adult origin. *Pediatr Res* 1975;**9**:167–71.

72. Grabowski EF, Carter CA, Tsukurov O *et al.* Comparison of human umbilical vein and adult saphenous vein endothelial cells: implications for newborn hemostasis and for models of endothelial cell function. *J Pediatr Hematol Oncol* 2000;**22**:266–8.

73. Streif W, Paes B, Berry L *et al.* Influence of exogenous factor VIIa on thrombin generation in plasma of full-term and pre-term newborns. *Blood Coagul Fibrinolysis* 2000;**11**:349–57.

74. Edstrom CS, Calhoun DA, Christensen RD. Expression of tissue factor pathway inhibitor in human fetal and placental tissues. *Early Hum Dev* 2000;**59**:77–84.

75. Warr TA, Warn-Cramer BJ, Rao LV, Rapaport SI. Human plasma extrinsic pathway inhibitor activity: I. Standardization of assay and evaluation of physiologic variables. *Blood* 1989;**74**:201–6.

76. Weissbach G, Harenberg J, Wendisch J *et al.* Tissue factor pathway inhibitor in infants and children. *Thromb Res* 1994;**73**:441–6.

77. Huang ZF, Higuchi D, Lasky N, Broze GJ Jr. Tissue factor pathway inhibitor gene disruption produces intrauterine lethality in mice. *Blood* 1997;**90**:944–51.

78. Lorant DE, Li W, Tabatabaei N, Garver MK, Albertine KH. P-selectin expression by endothelial cells is decreased in neonatal rats and human premature infants. *Blood* 1999;**94**:600–9.

79. Menashi S, Aurousseau MH, Gozin D *et al.* High levels of circulating thrombomodulin in human foetuses and children. *Thromb Haemost* 1999;**81**:906–9.

80. Orbe I, Paramo JA, Pinacho A *et al*. Plasma thrombomodulin is increased in cord blood of healthy newborns. *Thromb Haemost* 1995;**73**:326.

81. Fruhling L, Roger S, Jobard P. L'hématologie normale (tissues et organes hématopoietiques sang circulant) de l'embryon, du foetus et du nouveau-né humains. *Sang* 1949;**20**:313–24.

82. Holmberg L, Gustavii B, Jonsson A. A prenatal study of fetal platelet count and size with application to fetus at risk for Wiskott–Aldrich syndrome. *J Pediatr* 1983;**102**:773–6.

83. Patrick CH, Lazarchick J, Stubbs T, Pittard WB. Mean platelet volume and platelet distribution width in the neonate. *Am J Pediatr Hematol Oncol* 1987;**9**:130–2.

84. Meher-Homji NJ, Montemagno R, Thilaganathan B, Nicolaides KH. Platelet size and glycoprotein Ib and IIIa expression in normal fetal and maternal blood. *Am J Obstet Gynecol* 1994;**171**:791–6.

85. Nomura S, Ogami K, Kawamura K *et al*. Cellular localization of thrombopoietin mRNA in the liver by in situ hybridization. *Exp Hematol* 1997;**25**:565–72.

86. Jilma-Stahlawetz P, Homoncik M, Jilma B *et al*. High levels of reticulated platelets and thrombopoietin characterize fetal thrombopoiesis. *Br J Haematol* 2001;**112**:466–8.

87. Murray NA, Watts TL, Roberts IA. Endogenous thrombopoietin levels and effect of recombinant human thrombopoietin on megakaryocyte precursors in term and preterm babies. *Pediatr Res* 1998;**43**:148–51.

88. Jones CR, McCabe R, Hamilton CA, Reid JL. Maternal and fetal platelet responses and adrenoreceptor binding characteristics. *Thromb Haemost* 1985;**53**:95–8.

89. Gruel Y, Boizard B, Daffos F *et al*. Determination of platelet antigens and glycoproteins in the human fetus. *Blood* 1986;**68**:488–92.

90. Mull MM, Hathaway WE. Altered platelet function in newborns. *Pediatr Res* 1970;**4**:229–37.

91. Pandolfi M, Astedt B, Cronberg L, Nilsson IM. Failure of fetal platelets to aggregate in response to adrenaline and collagen. *Proc Soc Exp Biol Med* 1972;**141**:1081–3.

92. Matsumoto T, Kihira M, Ito M, Sugiyama Y. Effects of prostacyclin on fetal platelet function. *Biol Res Pregnancy Perinatol* 1984;**5**:11–15.

93. Ahlsten G, Ewald U, Tuvemo T. Arachidonic acid-induced aggregation of platelets from human cord blood compared with platelets from adults. *Biol Neonate* 1985;**47**:199–204.

94. Nicolini U, Guarneri D, Gianotti GA *et al*. Maternal and fetal platelet activation in normal pregnancy. *Obstet Gynecol* 1994;**83**:65–9.

95. Gelman B, Setty BN, Chen D *et al*. Impaired mobilization of intracellular calcium in neonatal platelets. *Pediatr Res* 1996;**39**:692–6.

96. Niida K, Ejiri K, Suga K. Effect of intracellular free calcium mobilization in aggregation of umbilical cord blood platelets. *Acta Med Okayama* 1996;**50**:47–52.

97. Israels SJ, Cheang T, Robertson C *et al*. Impaired signal transduction in neonatal platelets. *Pediatr Res* 1999;**45**:687–91.

98. Bussel JB. Alloimmune thrombocytopenia in the fetus and newborn. *Semin Thromb Hemost* 2001;**27**:245–52.

24

Thrombophilia and neonatal thrombosis

Ulrike Nowak-Göttl and Andrea Kosch

INTRODUCTION

Venous thromboembolism, an obstruction of the circulation by clots that have formed locally in the veins or have been released from a thrombus elsewhere, is being increasingly recognized in infancy and childhood.[1–3] On the one hand, numerous clinical and environmental conditions (such as the use of central lines,[2–9] cardiac malformations,[9] renal diseases,[10] peripartal asphyxia, fetal diabetes, dehydration and septicaemia[11,12]) have resulted in increased thrombin generation with subsequent fibrin or thrombus formation in infancy and childhood. On the other hand, various genetic prothrombotic defects of proteins that regulate blood coagulation, particularly those that affect the physiological anticoagulant systems, have been well established as risk factors of thrombotic diseases in adults.[13–18]

Besides the high thrombotic risk reported in patients with homozygous factor V G1691A mutation, homozygous protein C deficiency, homozygous protein S deficiency and homozygous homocysteinuria caused by cystathionine-β-synthase deficiency,[17] a high risk of early thrombotic onset is observed in patients with heterozygous antithrombin deficiency, protein C deficiency of the so-called dominant type, and heterozygous protein S deficiency. In contrast, an intermediate or low risk of developing early thromboembolism is observed in adult patients with the heterozygous factor V G1691A mutation, the heterozygous prothrombin G20210A variant,[18] heterozygous recessive protein C deficiency, heterozygous defects of the heparin-binding site of the antithrombin molecule,[19] and moderate hyperhomocysteinaemia caused by homozygous methylene tetrahydrofolate reductase (MTHFR) deficiency C677T. Based on the great structural homology between lipoprotein (a) and plasminogen and on *in vitro* studies reporting that lipoprotein (a) inhibits fibrinolysis,[21] many prospective and case-control studies have identified elevated levels of lipoprotein (a) concentrations as a risk factor for premature myocardial infarction and stroke.[22] In addition, Soulat *et al.* very recently demonstrated that binding of lipoprotein (a) to lysine residues and cell surfaces is directly related to circulating levels of both plasminogen and lipoprotein (a).[23] In the latter model, it is suggested that both glycoproteins interact as competitive ligands for biological surfaces *in vivo*. As in premature myocardial infarction and stroke in adults, increased concentrations have been shown to enhance significantly the risk not only of thromboembolic events in children but also of deep venous thrombosis in children and adults.[24,25] In addition to the risk factors already mentioned, there is only scanty and conflicting information about the role of inherited or acquired deficiency of heparin cofactor II or factor XII or elevated levels of von Willebrand factor antigen or factor VIIIC.

Since the recent discovery of activated protein C resistance as a highly prevalent hereditary risk factor of thromboembolism,[15] evidence has been accumulating that thrombophilia is a multifactorial disorder and that the association of multiple haemostatic prothrombotic defects or the combination of established prothrombotic risk factors with acquired environmental or clinical conditions greatly increases the risk of thrombosis not only in adults but also in infants and children.[19,20,24–28]

DEVELOPMENTAL HAEMOSTASIS

It has been shown in several *in vivo* and *in vitro* studies that components of the haemostatic system (i.e. vascular endothelium, procoagulant and fibrinolytic factors) differ between infants and adults.[28–35] Different coagulation factors show different postnatal patterns of maturation. In the newborn, plasma concentrations of the vitamin K-dependent coagulation factors (factors II, VII, IX and X), contact factors (factors XII and XI and prekallikrein) and high molecular weight kininogen are approximately 50% of adult values.[28,29] These levels rapidly increase in the first weeks of life, and adult values for coagulation proteins are achieved in most components by 6 months of age.[29] In addition, the vitamin K-dependent natural inhibitors protein C and protein S are low in the neonatal period. However, despite reduced total protein S antigen levels in neonatal plasma, there is a relatively high level of active protein S, owing to nearly undetectable levels of C4b-binding protein; this may minimize the risk of vascular accidents.[31] Furthermore, the capacity of neonatal plasma to generate thrombin, which is clearly dependent on plasma concentrations of antithrombin and protein C, is reduced to approximately 50% of that of adult plasma.[32,33] This situation may act as a protection from thrombotic events during infancy and childhood.

Whereas some components of the procoagulant coagulation system may contribute to a reduced risk of thromboembolism during infancy and childhood, there is no evidence that plasma concentrations of the fibrinolytic proteins provide protection from vascular accidents in the young. Some plasma levels of fibrinolytic proteins are lower than in adults.[30] It is mainly the decreased plasma levels of plasminogen as well as a lower activity of neonatal plasminogen, along with increased concentrations of tissue type plasminogen activator inhibitors (PAI) that are responsible for the hypofibrinolytic state. They also explain the prolonged thrombus lysis times observed in neonates in response to urokinase, streptokinase and tissue type plasminogen activator (t-PA) (in high concentrations only) administration.[34] A second fibrinolytic shut down is described in girls during puberty, who show significantly higher PAI-1 activity, reduced t-PA antigen levels, and significantly reduced fibrinolytic capacity after venous occlusion, owing mainly to the higher PAI-1 activities.[35]

In summary, because of the special properties of the haemostatic system during infancy and childhood, symptomatic thrombotic manifestations in carriers of prothrombolic risk factors, acquired or inherited, occur in less than 5% of children compared with approximately 40% of adults. Among the entire childhood population, neonates are at the greatest risk of thromboembolic complications, and the incidence of vascular accidents decreases significantly after the first year of life, with a second peak during puberty and adolescence.

THROMBOTIC MANIFESTATIONS AND LOCATIONS IN THE NEWBORN BABY

Besides the involvement of inherited or acquired thrombophilic risk factors in fetal wastage, prematurity or intrauterine growth retardation caused by placental infarction (Fig. 24.1)[36–41] and peripartal thromboembolic stroke (Fig. 24.2),[42–45] common venous thromboembolisms in the newborn period are cerebral venous thrombosis (Fig. 24.3),[46] renal venous thrombosis,[47–49] portal vein thrombosis and mesenteric vein thrombosis.[7,8] Arterial vascular occlusions have been reported mainly as ischaemic stroke,[50–54] and occlusions in the aorta, the femoral artery and the subclavian artery.[2,3]

In addition, the Canadian and German thrombosis registries recently demonstrated high rates of catheter-related thrombosis in neonates and infants.[1-3] In the catheterized population, central venous lines lead to thrombus formation and thrombus growth near the catheter implantation site in axillary veins, jugular veins, subclavian

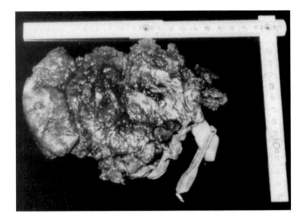

Figure 24.1 Placental thrombosis leading to premature birth at 28 weeks' gestation.

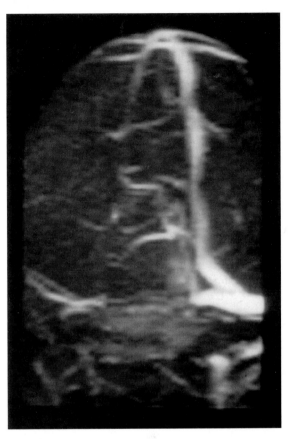

Figure 24.3 Spontaneous cerebral venous thrombosis (in the transverse sinus) in an infant with increased levels of lipoprotein (a).

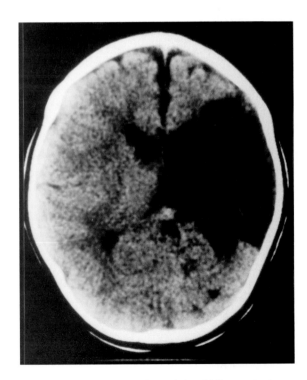

Figure 24.2 Infarction of the left middle cerebral artery acquired during birth in a newborn baby.

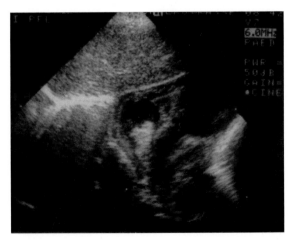

Figure 24.4 Intracardiac thrombus formation in a neonate heterozygous for the factor V G1691A gene mutation.

veins, superior vena cava, femoral veins, inferior vena cava and renal veins, especially when prothrombotic risk factors are involved. In addition, intracardiac thrombosis have been reported (Fig. 24.4). A further rare and life-threatening thrombotic disorder, 'purpura fulminans' (characterized by initial microvascular thrombosis in the dermis followed by perivascular haemorrhage) is observed within hours after birth in neonates with disseminated intravascular coagulation in response to septicaemia and in babies carrying homozygous protein C deficiency, homozygous protein S deficiency or the homozygous factor V G1691A mutation.

CLINICAL PRESENTATION AT DIAGNOSIS AND UNDERLYING BASIC DISEASES

Clinical symptoms of deep venous thrombosis include collateral vessel circulation and oedema and cyanosis of the dependent limbs, head, neck or chest (Fig. 24.5). An abdominal mass, thrombocytopenia or haematuria may give evidence of renal venous thrombosis.[47–49] Acute catheter-related thrombosis can include 'blockage' of a central venous line along with swelling, pain and discoloration of the involved limb; thrombosis related to a central venous line often presents with collateral circulation.[2]

Arterial thromboses present clinically with acute impairment of arterial blood flow, with cold, pale limbs, diminished or absent pulses, diminished peripheral perfusion or reduced skin temperature. Seizures, hemiparesis and coma are leading symptoms of vascular accidents within the central nervous system in the newborn baby and young infant.[46,47,53,54] In addition, respiratory failure, dyspnoea and tachypnoea give evidence of pulmonary embolism.

Clinical conditions associated with symptomatic thromboembolism in infancy (Table 24.1) include the use of central lines,[2,3,5–8] cardiac diseases and polycythaemia,[5,9] renal diseases such as congenital nephrotic syndrome and neonatal haemolytic–uraemic syndrome,[10] peripartal asphyxia, having a diabetic mother, dehydration, septicaemia,[11,12] necrotizing enterocolitis, acute respiratory distress syndrome, and extracorporeal membrane oxygenation. In addition, heparin-induced thrombocytopenia, thromboembolic events due to homocysteinuria, and 'spontaneous' thrombosis are diagnosed in neonates and infants.

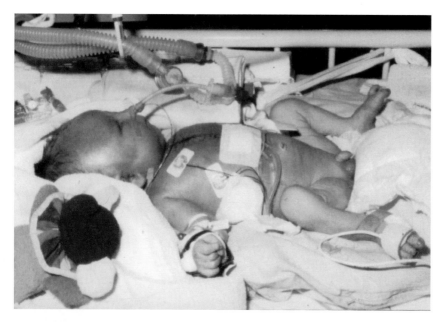

Figure 24.5 Six-month-old male infant with catheter-related thrombosis of the superior vena cava following a hemi-Fontan operation. The infant suffers additionally from increased levels of lipoprotein (a) and hyperhomocysteinaemia because of homozygosity for MTHFR C677T.

Table 24.1 Clinical conditions associated with thromboembolism during infancy

Umbilical catheters (arterial or venous)
Central venous lines
Cardiac diseases
Polycythaemia
Renal diseases
Peripartal or birth asphyxia
Having a diabetic mother
Dehydration
Septicaemia
Necrotizing enterocolitis
Respiratory distress syndrome
Extracorporeal membrane oxygenation
Heparin-induced thrombocytopenia
Metabolic disorders

IMAGING METHODS

Duplex ultrasound, venography, computed tomography and magnetic resonance imaging can be used to diagnose venous thrombosis.[2–4,24] However, venography is recommended for confirming suspected thrombosis in the upper venous system (e.g. the axillary veins, the superior vena cava). Magnetic resonance imaging and magnetic resonance angiography are recommended for confirming the diagnosis of thromboembolic ischaemic stroke.[25,46,53,54] Magnetic resonance angiography is a suitable method for diagnosing pulmonary embolism in neonates and infants.

PROTHROMBOTIC DEFECTS IN NEONATES AND YOUNG INFANTS

At present, various data suggest that symptomatic thromboembolism is a multicausal disease:[19,20] the younger the patient, the more risk factors are required to precipitate thrombosis.

Besides the underlying triggering factors mentioned above, other risk factors play a potential role in the aetiology of symptomatic venous thrombosis[24,56–60] and ischaemic cerebrovascular accidents[9,44,50–54] in the paediatric population. These risk factors include transient maternal antiphospholipid antibodies; inherited deficiency states of protein C, protein S and antithrombin; the factor V G1691A mutation; the prothrombin G20210A variant; increased fasting homocysteine; and increased lipoprotein (a) concentrations (Tables 24.2, 24.3

Table 24.2 Prothrombotic risk factors in Caucasian paediatric patients suffering from venous thrombosis

Risk factors	Controls (n = 370)	Patients (n = 261)	Odds ratio (95% CI)
Protein C deficiency	3 (0.8%)	24 (9.2%)	12.4 (3.7–41.6)
Protein S deficiency	3 (0.8%)	15 (5.7%)	7.5 (2.1–26.0)
Factor V 1691GA/AA	15 (4.1%)	83 (31.8%)	11.0 (6.2–19.7)
1691GA	14 (3.8%)	77 (29.5%)	10.6 (5.9–19.3)
1691AA	1 (0.3%)	6 (2.3%)	8.7 (1.0–72.6)
Prothrombin 20210GA	4 (1.1%)	11 (4.2%)	4.1 (1.3–12.8)
Antithrombin deficiency	0	9 (3.4%)	—
Liproprotein (a) > 30 mg/dl	19 (10.3%)	78 (42.0%)	7.2 (3.7–14.5)

Summary of results of case control studies in Caucasian paediatric patients recruited from various catchment areas in Germany. Data from Nowak-Göttl et al.[24] and Junker et al.[59]

Table 24.3 Distribution of established genetic prothrombotic risk factors in childhood patients with renal vein thrombosis, portal vein thrombosis and hepatic vascular occlusion

Risk factors	Renal vein thrombosis (n = 31)	Portal vein thrombosis (n = 24)	Hepatic vein thrombosis (n = 10)	Total (n = 65)	Controls (n = 100)	Odds ratio (95% CI)
Factor V 1691GA	9 (29.0%)	4 (16.6%)	—			
Factor V 1691AA	—	—	1 (10%)			
Factor V 1691GA/AA				14 (21.5%)	5 (5.0%)	5.2 (6.77–15.3)
MTHFR 677TT and elevated fasting homocysteine concentration	2 (6.5%)	1 (4.1%)	1 (10.0%)	4 (6.2%)	1 (1.0%)	6.5 (0.7–59.0)
Protein C deficiency	2 (6.5%)	1 (4.1%)	—	3 (4.6%)	—	—
Antithrombin deficiency	1 (3.2%)	1 (4.1%)	—	2 (3.1%)	—	—
Prothrombin 20210GA	—	—	—	—	1 (1.0%)	—
Total	14 (45.2%)	7 (29.2%)	2 (20.0%)	23 (35.4%)	7 (7.0%)	7.3 (2.89–18.27)

Summary of results from a case control study in Caucasian paediatric patients recruited in Germany. Data from Heller et al.[12]

Table 24.4 Prothrombotic risk factors in Caucasian children suffering from neonatal ischaemic stroke

Risk factors	Controls (n = 182)	Patients (n = 91)	Odds ratio (95% CI)
Protein C deficiency	—	6 (6.6%)	—
Factor V 1691GA	10 (5.5%)	17 (18.7%)	3.95 (1.72–9.0)
Prothrombin 20210GA	4 (2.2%)	4 (4.4%)	2.0 (0.5–8.3)
MTHFR 677TT	20 (10.9%)	15 (16.5%)	1.59 (0.77–3.29)
Lipoprotein (a) > 30 mg/dl	10 (5.5%)	20 (22.0%)	4.84 (2.16–10.86)

Summary of results from a case control study in Caucasian paediatric patients recruited in Germany. Data from Günther et al.[54]

and 24.4). The data presented in these tables may not be mirrored in other countries because of differences in the ethnic population background; the number of patients and controls investigated may also affect results in other studies.

Laboratory evaluation

Based on the data obtained from case control studies and matched-pair analysis, at least the symptomatic patient should be screened in a specialized coagulation unit. Activated protein C resistance, protein C activity and protein C antigen levels, free protein S antigen levels, antithrombin activity, antithrombin antigen levels, lipoprotein (a) levels and fasting homocysteine levels should be investigated, and DNA-based assays (factor V G1691A mutation, prothrombin G20210A variant and MTHFR C677T genotype should also be performed). However, potential variations are unavoidable, owing to different ethnic population backgrounds. In addition, rare prothrombotic defects (such as dysfibrinogenaemia, hypoplasminogenaemia, dysplasminogenaemia, heparin cofactor II deficiency, increased levels of histidine-rich glycoprotein, as well as other further genetic polymorphisms) should be kept in mind.[13] Besides being tested for prothrombotic defects, all symptomatic babies with thrombosis should be screened for transient antiphospholipid or anticardiolipin antibodies and the presence of lupus anticoagulants.[47]

Interpretation of laboratory results

To prevent results of protein-based assays from being affected by the acute thrombotic onset or oral anticoagulation, blood samples should be obtained at least 3–6 months after the thrombotic episode and at least 14–30 days after withdrawal of oral anticoagulant medication. In contrast, since DNA-based assays are not influenced by the acute thrombotic event screening for factor V G1691A, prothrombin G20210A and MTHFR C677T can be performed immediately at the onset of the vascular accident.

For all plasma-based assays a clotting abnormality should be documented as a defect only if the plasma level of a protein is outside the limits of its normal range in at least two different samples.[28,46] A type I deficiency state can be diagnosed when the functional plasma activity and immunological antigen concentration of a protein are below the lower age-related limit (Table 24.5). A type II deficiency is present when repeatedly low functional activity levels are combined with normal antigen concentrations. As in adults, the diagnosis of protein S deficiency is based on reduced free protein S antigen levels combined with decreased or normal total protein S antigen concentrations.[14]

OUTCOME IN NEONATES AND INFANTS WITH THROMBOSIS

Renal venous thromboses and vena caval occlusion occurring in neonates and infants

Table 24.5 Age-dependent normal reference values from 385 healthy Caucasian newborns and infants compared with older children

Parameter	Newborn. (n = 55) median (range)	3 months (n = 50) median (range)	6 Months (n = 60) median (range)	1–5 Years (n = 60) median (range)
Protein C activity	35 (14–55)	55 (25–82)	60 (38–95)	75 (45–102)
Protein C antigen levels	30 (12–50)	50 (22–75)	55 (40–100)	70 (45–98)
Fr. Protein S antigen levels	38 (15–55)	55 (35–92)	77 (45–115)	78 (62–120)
Antithrombin	52 (30–85)	90 (55–120)	98 (65–126)	101 (85–140)
Plasminogen	50 (35–70)	68 (45–95)	87 (65–100)	98 (63–123)

Data from Ehrenforth et al.[28]

frequently persist and lead to considerable long-term morbidity with a high incidence of irreversible organ damage (i.e. residual structural abnormalities, impairment of renal function and hypertension).[48,49,61] The Canadian registry reported on the follow-up of 405 paediatric patients for a mean of 2.8 years.[62,63] In this large series of patients the mortality rate was 2.2%, with recurrent thrombosis occurring in 8.1% of patients investigated and a postphlebitic syndrome being in 12.4%. These results confirm that venous thromboembolism has serious consequences for paediatric patients. In addition, a recent prospective study on recurrent vascular occlusion after a first episode of spontaneous venous thromboembolism (i.e. thrombosis in the absence of further secondary causes) indicated that a subgroup of paediatric patients suffering from combined prothrombotic risk factors (the factor V G1691A mutation, the prothrombin G20210A variant, increased lipoprotein (a) concentrations, antithrombin deficiency, protein C deficiency or protein S deficiency) carries a high risk of recurrent thrombosis.[64] In this consecutively recruited cohort of 301 paediatric patients followed up for a median of 7 years, recurrent thrombosis occurred in 64 patients within a median time of 3.5 years after withdrawal of anticoagulation; there was a significantly shorter cumulative thrombosis-free survival in subjects with combined defects.[64] These findings in children

challenge the widely adopted short course of anticoagulation in patients with symptomatic deep venous thrombosis.

TREATMENT IN CHILDHOOD THROMBOSIS

The management of newborns and infants with symptomatic thrombosis comprises acute thrombosis treatment and thromboprophylaxis. Life-threatening organ or limb dysfunction as a result of vascular occlusion is the most important indication for anticoagulation, thrombolysis or surgical intervention in neonates and infants. However, the lack of strong evidence for the benefits of antithrombotic therapy and the observation that thrombosis in neonates may resolve spontaneously do not justify routine anticoagulant and thrombolytic therapy or surgical intervention in asymptomatic patients. Thus, therapeutic options mentioned in this chapter are for use in symptomatic babies and infants. Before anticoagulant or thrombolytic therapy is performed in a symptomatic paediatric patient, intracranial haemorrhage or haemorrhagic infarction should be excluded with suitable imaging methods (cranial ultrasound or computed tomography).

Besides specific treatment of acute thromboembolism with anticoagulant or thrombolytic therapy, infants with acute purpura fulminans caused by homozygous protein C deficiency, protein S deficiency or activated protein C resistance should receive fresh frozen plasma or, if available, protein C concentrate.[55,65,66] However, detailed patient management is seriously hampered by the lack of appropriate clinical trials. Thus, until data are available for the treatment of symptomatic children, the following recommendations based on small-scale studies in paediatric patients and guidelines adapted from adult patient protocols are provided.

The Münster protocol for standard heparin administration is shown in Table 24.6. As in adults, routine heparin administration requires normal antithrombin levels. The therapeutic goal for achieving adequate anticoagulation in paediatric patients without an undue increase in the bleeding risk is a 1.5–2-fold activated partial thromboplastin time prolongation compared with the starting value.

A protocol for the use of low molecular weight heparin based on data published by Massicotte et al.[67] and by Dix et al.[68] and on the authors' experience in paediatric patients is given in Table 24.7.

Table 24.6 Systemic unfractionated heparin doses and administration for paediatric patients adjusted for body weight (Münster protocol)

A. Loading dose: 50–100 units/kg unfractionated heparin intravenously over 10 minutes
B. Maintenance: 20–30 units/kg per hour unfractionated heparin
C. Adjustment: aPTT 55–90 seconds (normal range 25–38 seconds) or 4 hour antifactor Xa level 0.4–0.8

aPTT (seconds)	Bolus (units/kg)	Stop infusion	Rate change (%)
< 55	0	—	+10%
56–90	0	—	0
91–120	0	—	–10%
> 120	0	1.5 hours	–15%

aPTT/antifactor Xa level control: 4 hours after loading dose and after increase or reduction of dosage
Cave HIT type II: complete blood cell count daily required; dose reduction in patients with reduced hepatic or renal function

aPTT, activated partial thromboplastin time; HIT, heparin induced thrombocytopenia.

Table 24.7 Low molecular weight heparin doses and administration for paediatric patients (Münster protocol)

	Infants	4–hour antifactor Xa level
Prophylactic	1.5 mg/kg once daily	0.2–0.4 units/ml Monitoring after dose finding not usually required
Therapeutic	1.5 mg/kg twice daily	0.4–0.8 units/ml Monitoring required

Information based on enoxaparin, which contains 110 antifactor Xa units/mg; maximum single dose 2.0 mg/kg
Data based on Massicotte et al.,[67] Dix et al.[68] and the authors' data

Table 24.8 Recommendations for thrombolytic therapy

	Urokinase	Streptokinase	Recombinant tissue-type plasminogen activator
Bolus	4400 units/kg over 10–20 minutes	3500–4000 units/kg over 30 minutes	0.1–0.2 mg/kg over 10 minutes
Maintenance	4400 units/kg per hour	1000–1500 units/kg per hour	*0.8–2.4 mg/kg per 24 hours
Duration	12–24 hours	12–72 hours	6 days maximum

*Bleeding risk is increased at dosages > 2.5 mg/kg per 24 hours; dose reduction is required in patients with reduced hepatic or renal function
Information from Kirk et al.,[69] Nowak-Göttl et al.,[70] Wever et al.,[71] Farnoux et al.,[72] Weiner et al.,[73] Nowak-Göttl et al.[74] and Manco-Johnson et al.[75]

Although thrombolytic agents are used in paediatric patients, no randomized prospective trials have been reported so far.[69–75] Table 24.8 summarizes widely used dosages for urokinase, streptokinase and recombinant tissue-type plasminogen activator. However, dose modifications, different combination ratios and different parallel heparin administrations may pertain.

Besides low molecular weight heparin, vitamin K antagonists, mainly warfarin, are widely administered for long-term anticoagulation in paediatric patients.[55,63] Table 24.9 shows the simplified Münster protocol for warfarin administration, which is in agreement with data recently published by the Canadian group.[55,63] As in adults, when warfarin therapy is started in paediatric patients after an acute thromboembolism, an adequate overlap with heparin is mandatory to avoid further enhanced coagulation activation, which might lead to vascular re-occlusion or warfarin necrosis (Fig. 24.6).

Duration of anticoagulant treatment

Data from adult patients have shown that patients with a first venous thromboembolism are at high risk for many years of recurrent vascular accidents, especially when transient

Table 24.9 Oral anticoagulation with warfarin in paediatric patients

Loading dose:
Normal INR 1.0–1.3: 0.2 mg/kg warfarin orally
Reduced hepatic function and Fontan-OP: 0.1 mg/kg

Loading dose, days 2–4

INR	Dose
1.1–1.3	Repeat initial dose
1.4–3.0	50% of initial dose
3.1–3.5	25% of initial dose
> 3.5	Stop until INR < 3.5, then restart at half of previous dose

Maintenance

INR	Dose
1.1–1.9	Increase dosage by 20%
2.0–3.0	No change
3.1–3.5	Reduce dosage by 10%
> 3.5	Stop until INR < 3.5, then restart at 20% less than previous dose

INR, international normalized ratio
Target INR: 2.0–3.0

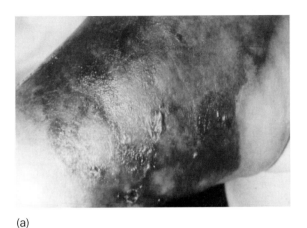
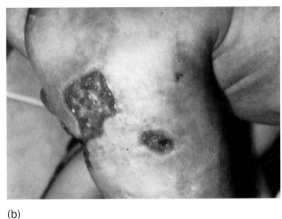

(a) (b)

Figure 24.6 Warfarin necrosis before (a) and after (b) therapy with protein C concentrate. (From Dr K Kurnik, University Children's Hospital, Munich, Germany.)

acquired risk factors not contributory or the patient carries more than one genetic prothrombotic risk factor.[64] The high recurrence rates reported by Monagle et al.[62] and by Streif et al.[63] for patients monitored in the Canadian registry, in addition to the authors' data for paediatric patients with spontaneous thrombosis who carry combined prothrombotic risk factors,[64] challenge the adopted short course of anticoagulation in patients with symptomatic venous vascular accidents. Thus, until prospective randomized data on long-term anticoagulation in paediatric patients are available, it may be helpful to manage paediatric patients on an individual basis according to the following recommendations.

In symptomatic neonates and infants with deep vein thrombosis, pulmonary embolism, or arterial vascular accidents associated with clinical underlying conditions (see Table 24.1) with or without additional prothrombotic defects, secondary anticoagulation should be individualized. If secondary anticoagulation is not used, the thrombus should be closely monitored with suitable imaging methods, and if the thrombus is found to be extending, anticoagulant treatment should be initiated immediately. From the authors' multicenter experience, secondary anticoagulant treatment should be continued for at least 3 months in cases in which the acquired

clinical condition persists (Nowak–Göttl, unpublished data).

Symptomatic neonates and infants with spontaneous thrombosis (i.e. without identifiable underlying prothrombotic triggering factors) who carry one homozygous or one heterozygous prothrombotic defect should receive oral anticoagulation or low dose heparin, usually administered for 3–6 months after the acute thrombotic onset. In these patients, anticoagulant therapy may be given in subsequent situations known to provoke thrombosis.

In homozygous symptomatic children or in patients carrying combined heterozygous prothrombotic risk factors with spontaneous thrombosis or with a history of life-threatening recurrent thrombosis, long-term anticoagulant therapy is considered on an individual patient basis.[64]

In each case, an assessment must be made with respect to the relative benefit conferred by long-term anticoagulant therapy in preventing future thromboembolism versus the potential haemorrhagic side effects, costs and inconvenience for the paediatric patient.

ACKNOWLEDGEMENT

The authors thank Susan Griesbach for help in editing this manuscript.

REFERENCES

1. Andrew M. Developmental hemostasis: relevance to thromboembolic complications in pediatric patients. *Thromb Haemost* 1995;**74**: 415–25.
2. Schmidt B, Andrew M. Neonatal thrombosis: report of a prospective Canadian and international registry. *Pediatrics* 1995;**95**:936–4.
3. Nowak-Göttl U, von Kries R, Göbel U. Neonatal symptomatic thromboembolism in Germany: two year survey. *Arch Dis Child* 1997;**76**:F163–7.
4. Nowak-Göttl U, Dübbers A, Kececioglu D, *et al.* Factor V Leiden, protein C and lipoprotein (a) in catheter related thrombosis in childhood: a prospective study. *J Pediatr* 1997;**131**:608–12.
5. Vitiello R, McCrindle BW, Nykanen D, *et al.* Complications associated with pediatric cardiac catheterization. *J Am Col Cardiol* 1998;**32**:1433–40.
6. Salonvaara M, Riikonen P, Kekomaki R, *et al.* Clinical symptomatic central venous catheter-related deep venous thrombosis in newborns. *Acta Paediatr* 1999;**88**:642–6.
7. Boo NY, Wong NC, Zulkifli SS, *et al.* Risk factors associated with umbilical vascular catheter-associated thrombosis in newborn infants. *J Pediatr Child Health* 1999;**35**:460–5.
8. Schwartz DS, Gettner PA, Konstantino MM, *et al.* Umbilical venous catheterization and the risk of portal vein thrombosis. *J Pediatr* 1997;**131**:760–2.
9. Sträter R, Vielhaber H, Kassenböhmer R, *et al.* Genetic risk factors of thrombophilia in ischaemic childhood stroke of cardiac origin. A prospective ESPED survey. *Eur J Pediatr* 1999;**158**: S122–5.
10. Schlegel N. Thromboembolic risks and complications in nephrotic children. *Semin Thromb Haemost* 1997;**23**:271–80.
11. Hagstrom JN, Walter J, Bluebond-Langner R, *et al.* Prevalence of the factor V Leiden mutation in children and neonates with thromboembolic disease. *J Pediatr* 1998;**133**:777–81.
12. Heller C, Schobess R, Kurnik K, *et al.* Abdominal venous thrombosis in neonates and infants: role of prothrombotic risk factors: a multicentre case-control study. *Br J Haematol* 2000;**111**:534–9.
13. Lane DA, Mannucci PM, Bauer KA, *et al.* Inherited thrombophilia: Part 1. *Thromb Haemost* 1996;**76**:651–62.
14. Lane DA, Mannucci PM, Bauer KA, *et al.* Inherited thrombophilia: Part 2. *Thromb Haemost* 1996;**76**:824–34.
15. Dahlbäck B, Carlsson M, Svensson PJ. Familial thrombophilia due to a previously unrecognized mechanism characterized by poor anticoagulant response to activated protein C: prediction of a cofactor to activated protein C. *Proc Natl Acad Sci USA* 1993;**90**:1004–8.
16. Bertina RM, Koeleman BPC, Koster T, *et al.* Mutation in blood coagulation factor V associated with resistance to activated protein C. *Nature* 1994;**369**:64–7.
17. Mudd SH, Skovby F, Levy HL, *et al.* The natural history of homocystinuria due to cystathionine-β-synthase deficiency. *Am J Hum Genet* 1985;**37**: 1–31.
18. Poort SR, Rosendaal FR, Reitsma PH, Bertina RM. A common genetic variation in the 3'-untranslated region of the prothrombin gene is associated with elevated plasma prothrombin levels and an increase in venous thrombosis. *Blood* 1996;**88**:3698–703.
19. Seligsohn U, Zivelin A. Thrombophilia as a multigenetic disorder. *Thromb Haemost* 1997;**78**: 297–301.
20. Salomon O, Steinberg DM, Zivelin A, *et al.* Single and combined prothrombotic factors in patients with idiopathic venous thromboembolism. Prevalence and risk assessment. *Arterioscler Thromb Vasc Biol* 1999;**19**:511–18.
21. Uterman G. The mysteries of lipoprotein (a). *Science* 1989;**246**:904–10.
22. Berg K, Dahlen G, Frick MH. Lp(a) lipoprotein and pre-beta 1 lipoprotein in patients with coronary heart disease. *Clin Genet* 1974;**6**:230–5.
23. Soulat T, Loyau S, Baudouin V, *et al.* Effect of individual plasma lipoprotein (a) variations *in vivo* on its competition with plasminogen for fibrin and cell binding: an *in vitro* study using plasma from children with idiopathic nephrotic syndrome. *Arterioscler Thromb Vasc Biol* 2000;**20**: 575–84.
24. Nowak-Göttl U, Junker R, Hartmeier M, *et al.* Increased lipoprotein (a) is an important risk factor for venous thrombosis in childhood. *Circulation* 1999;**100**:743–8.
25. Nowak-Göttl U, Sträter R, Heinecke A, *et al.* Lipoprotein (a) and genetic polymorphisms of clotting factor V, prothrombin and methylenetetrahydrofolate reductase are risk factors of ischaemic stroke in childhood. *Blood* 1999;**94**: 3678–82.
26. Formstone CJ, Hallam PF, Tuddenham EGD, *et al.* Severe perinatal thrombosis in double and triple heterozygous offspring of a family segregating two independent protein S mutations and a protein C mutation. *Blood* 1996;**87**:3731–7.

27. Brenner B, Zivelin A, Lanir N, *et al.* Venous thromboembolism associated with double heterozygosity for R506Q mutation of factor V and for T298M mutation of protein C in a large family of a previously described homozygous protein C deficient newborn with massive thrombosis. *Blood* 1996;**88**:877–80.

28. Ehrenforth S, Junker R, Koch HG, *et al.* Multicentre evaluation of combined prothrombotic defects with thrombophilia in childhood. *Eur J Pediatr* 1999;**158**:S97–104.

29. Andrew M, Paes B, Johnston M. Development of the hemostatic system in the neonate and young infant. *Am J Pediatr Hematol Oncol* 1990;**12**:95–104.

30. Ries M, Klinge J, Rauch R. Age-related reference values for activation markers of the coagulation and fibrinolytic systems in children. *Thromb Res* 1997;**85**:341–4.

31. Schwarz HP, Muntean W, Watzke H, *et al.* Low total protein S antigen but higher protein S activity due to decreased c4b-binding protein in neonates. *Blood* 1988;**71**:562–5.

32. Cvirn G, Gallistl S, Muntean W. Effects of antithrombin and protein C on thrombin generation in newborn and adult plasma. *Thromb Res* 1999;**93**:183–90.

33. Andrew M, Schmidt B, Mitchell L, *et al.* Thrombin generation in newborn plasma is critically dependent on the concentration of prothrombin. *Thromb Haemost* 1990;**63**:27–30.

34. Ries M, Klinge J, Rauch R, *et al.* In vitro fibrinolysis after adding low doses of plasminogen activators and plasmin generation with and without oxidative inactivation of plasmin inhibitors in newborns and adults. *J Ped Hematol Oncol* 1996;**18**:346–51.

35. Siegbahn A, Ruusuvaara L. Age dependence of blood fibrinolytic components and the effects of low-dose oral contraceptives on coagulation and fibrinolysis in teenagers. *Thromb Haemost* 1988;**60**:361–4.

36. Salafia CM, Vintzileos AM, Silberman L, *et al.* Placental pathology of idiopathic intrauterine growth retardation at term. *Am J Perinatol* 1992;**9**:179–84.

37. Brenner B, Sarig G, Wiener Z, *et al.* Thrombophilic polymorphisms are common in women with foetal loss without apparent cause. *Thromb Haemost* 1999;**82**:6–9.

38. Dizon-Townson DS, Meline L, Nelson LM, *et al.* Fetal carriers of the factor V Leiden are prone to miscarriage and placental infarction. *Am J Obstet Gynecol* 1997;**177**:402–5.

39. Berg K, Roland B, Sande H. High Lp(a) lipoprotein level in maternal serum may interfere with placental circulation and cause foetal growth retardation. *Clin Genet* 1994;**46**:52–6.

40. Göpel W, Kim D, Gortner L. Prothrombotic mutations as a risk factor for preterm birth. *Lancet* 1999;**353**:1411–12.

41. Verspyck E, Le Camp-Duchez V, Gravier A, *et al.* Small for gestational age infant in association with maternal prothrombin gene variant (nt 20210A). *Eur J Obstet Gynecol Reprod Biol* 1999;**83**:143–4.

42. Vries de LS, Eken P, Groenendaal F, *et al.* Antenatal onset of haemorrhagic and/or ischaemic lesions in preterm infants: prevalence and associated obstetric variables. *Arch Dis Child* 1998;**78**:F51–6.

43. Kraus FT, Acheen VI. Fetal thrombotic vasculopathy in the placenta: cerebral thrombi and infarcts, coagulopathies, and cerebral palsy. *Hum Pathol* 1999;**30**:759–69.

44. Debus O, Koch HG, Kurlemann G, *et al.* Factor V Leiden and genetic defects of thrombophilia in childhood porencephaly. *Arch Dis Child* 1998;**78**: F121–4.

45. Govaets P, Matthys E, Zecic A, *et al.* Perinatal cortical infarction within middle cerebral artery trunks. *Arch Dis Child* 2000;**82**:F59–63.

46. Vielhaber H, Ehrenforth S, Koch HG, *et al.* Cerebral venous thrombosis in infancy and childhood: role of genetic and acquired risk factors of thrombophilia. *Eur J Pediatr* 1998;**157**:555–60.

47. Nuss R, Hays T, Manco-Johnson M. Childhood thrombosis. *Pediatrics* 1995;**96**:291–4.

48. Mocan H, Beattie TJ, Murphy AV. Renal venous thrombosis in infancy: long-term follow-up. *Pediatr Nephrol* 1991;**5**:45–9.

49. Bökenkamp A, von Kries R, Nowak-Göttl U, *et al.* Neonatal renal venous thrombosis in Germany between 1992 and 1994: epidemiology, treatment and outcome. *Eur J Pediatr* 2000;**159**:44–8.

50. Riikonen RS, Vahtera EM, Kekomäki RM. Physiological anticoagulants and activated protein C resistance in childhood stroke. *Acta Paediatr* 1996;**85**:242–4.

51. Zenz W, Bodo Z, Plotho J, *et al.* Factor V Leiden and prothrombin gene G20210A variant in children with stroke. *Thromb Haemost* 1998;**80**:763–6.

52 Van Beynum IM, Smeitink JA, den Heijer M, *et al.* Hyperhomocysteinemia: a risk for ischaemic stroke in children. *Circulation* 1999;**99**:2070–2.

53. Kenet G, Sadetzki S, Murad H, *et al.* Factor V Leiden and antiphospholipid antibodies are

significant risk factors for ischaemic stroke in children. *Stroke* 2000;**31**:1283–8.

54. Günther G, Junker R, Sträter R, *et al.* Symptomatic ischaemic stroke in full-term neonates: role of acquired and genetic prothrombotic risk factors. *Stroke* 2000;**31**:246–51.

55. Andrew M, Michelson AD, Bovill E, *et al.* Guidelines for antithrombotic therapy in pediatric patients. *J Pediatr* 1998;**132**:575–88.

56. Manco-Johnson M, Abshire T, Jacobson L, Marlar R. Severe neonatal protein C deficiency: prevalence and thrombotic risk. *J Pediatr* 1991;**119**: 793–8.

57. Manco-Johnson MJ, Nuss R, Key N, *et al.* Lupus anticoagulant and protein S deficiency in children with postvaricella purpura fulminans or thrombosis. *J Pediatr* 1996;**128**:319–23.

58. Laeson SE, Butler D, Enayat MS, Williams MD. Congenital thrombophilia and thrombosis: a study in a single centre. *Arch Dis Child* 1999;**81**: 176–8.

59. Junker R, Koch HG, Auberger K, *et al.* Prothrombin G20210A gene mutation and further prothrombotic risk factors in childhood thrombophilia. *Arterioscler Thromb Vasc Biol* 1999;**19**:2568–72.

60. Bonduel M, Hepner M, Sciuccati G, *et al.* Prothrombotic abnormalities in children with venous thromboembolism. *J Pediatr Hematol Oncol* 2000;**22**:66–72.

61. Häuseler M, Duyue D, Merz U, *et al.* The clinical outcome after inferior vena cava thrombosis in early infancy. *Eur J Pediatr* 1999;**158**:416–20.

62. Monagle P, Adams M, Mahoney M, *et al.* Outcome of pediatric thromboembolic disease: a report from the Canadian childhood thrombophilia registry. *Ped Res* 2000;**47**:763–6.

63. Streif W, Andrew M, Marzinotto V, *et al.* Analysis of warfarin therapy in paediatric patients: a prospective cohort study of 319 patients. *Blood* 1999;**94**:3007–14.

64. Nowak-Göttl U, Junker R, Kreuz W, *et al.* Risk of recurrent thrombosis in children with combined prothrombotic risk factors. *Blood* 2001;**15**:858–62.

65. Marlar RA, Montgommery R, Broeckmans AW. Diagnosis and treatment of homozygous protein C deficiency. *J Pediatr* 1989;**114**:528–34.

66. Dreyfus M, Magny JF, Bridey F, *et al.* Treatment of homozygous protein C deficiency and neonatal purpura fulminans with purified protein C concentrate. *N Engl J Med* 1991;**325**:1565–8.

67. Massicotte P, Adams M, Marzinotto V, *et al.* Low molecular weight heparin in pediatric patients with thrombotic disease: a dose finding study. *J Pediatr* 1996;**128**:313–18.

68. Dix D, Andrew M, Marzinotto V, *et al.* The use of low molecular weight heparin in pediatric patients: a prospective cohort study. *J Pediatr* 2000;**136**:439–45.

69. Kirk CR, Qureshi SA. Streptokinase in the management of arterial thrombosis in infancy. *Int J Cardiol* 1989;**25**:15–20.

70. Nowak-Göttl U, Schwabe D, Schneider W, *et al.* Thrombolysis with recombinant tissue-type plasminogen activator in renal venous thrombosis in infancy. *Lancet* 1992;**340**:1005 (letter).

71. Wever ML, Liem KD, Geven WB, Tanke RB. Urokinase therapy in neonates with catheter related central venous thrombosis. *Thromb Haemost* 1995;**73**:180–5.

72. Farnoux C, Camard O, Pinquier D, *et al.* Recombinant tissue-type plasminogen activator therapy of thrombosis in 16 neonates. *J Pediatr* 1998;**133**:137–40.

73. Weiner GM, Castle VP, DiPietro MA, Faix RG. Successful treatment of neonatal arterial thrombosis with recombinant tissue plasminogen activator. *J Pediatr* 1998;**133**:133–6.

74. Nowak-Göttl U, Auberger K, Halimeh S, *et al.* Thrombolysis in newborns and infants. *Thromb Haemost* 1999;**82**:S112–16.

75. Manco-Johnson MJ, Nuss R, Krupski W, *et al.* Combined thrombolytic and anticoagulant therapy for venous thrombosis in children. *J Pediatr* 2000;**136**:446–53.

25

Bleeding disorders in neonates

Gili Kenet

INTRODUCTION

The clinical and laboratory diagnosis of congenital and acquired bleeding disorders is different in neonates from the diagnosis in older children or adults. In an adult, a tentative diagnosis can usually be established from the bleeding history, an assessment of the extent of hemorrhage against the background of any provoking challenges (e.g. trauma, surgery), a careful physical examination, and an initial set of hemostatic tests.

Most severe forms of hemostatic disorders can present in the neonatal period, but since physiologically decreased levels of plasma proteins may overlap with pathological values, a diagnosis may be difficult to establish.[1–5]

Hemorrhagic disorders can be classified as either congenital or acquired. Alternatively, they can be classified according to the mechanism of the defect. Neither the thrombocytopenias, which are the most frequently encountered acquired disorders, nor the functional platelet disorders are discussed in this chapter.

GENERAL INFORMATION AND DEVELOPMENTAL HEMOSTASIS

The hemostatic system during infancy undergoes dynamic physiological changes. Coagulation factors are synthesized by the fetus and begin to appear at 10 weeks' gestational age. The physiological concentrations of coagulation proteins gradually increase and are lower in premature infants than in full-term babies or healthy children.[1–5] In the neonate, plasma concentrations of vitamin K-dependant coagulation factors (factors II, VII, IX and X) and contact factors (factors XI and XII, prekallikrein and high molecular weight kininogen) are about 50% of adult values.[4,5] Furthermore, the capacity of neonates to generate thrombin (which is dependent on plasma concentrations of procoagulants) is reduced.[6–8] These facts, which would theoretically increase the risk of severe bleeding, are balanced by the protective effects of physiological deficiencies of the inhibitors of coagulation, as well as by the decreased capacity of the fibrinolytic system in infants.[4,9] Activation of platelets,[10,11] and coagulation proteins[12] and release of tissue plasminogen activator[13] usually occur during the birth process and probably represent a developmental, non-pathological phenomenon. Nevertheless, any complications of delivery that result in birth asphyxia may play an important role in the pathogenesis of consumptive coagulopathy and promote the risk of significant bleeding.

CLINICAL PRESENTATION

The clinical presentation of bleeding disorders is characterized by one or more of:

- bleeding into the scalp, with the consequent formation of cephalhematomas;

Table 25.1 The clinical presentation of bleeding disorders and the association between bleeding symptoms and specific coagulation defects

Bleeding manifestation	Coagulation defect
Intracranial hemorrhage	Severe hemophilia (A or B)
	Severe factor VII deficiency
	Severe factor XIII deficiency
	Vitamin K deficiency bleeding
Facial purpura	Platelet dysfunction
	Glanzmann's thrombasthenia
	Severe thrombocytopenia
Oral mucosal bleeding	Severe thrombocytopenia
	Severe von Willebrand's disease
Cephalhematoma	Severe factor deficiencies
	Vitamin K deficiency bleeding
Intramuscular bleeding	Severe factor deficiencies
	Vitamin K deficiency bleeding
Injury-related bleeding (e.g. from needle pricks)	Any coagulation defect
Umbilical stump bleeding	Factor XIII deficiency
	Fibrinogen deficiency

- injury-related bleeding after invasive procedures or intramuscular injections and at sites of peripheral venepunctures;
- bleeding after circumcision; and
- bleeding into the skin, manifesting itself as petechiae, purpura and ecchymoses.

Defects of primary hemostasis (such as thrombocytopenia, platelet function disorders and von Willebrand disease) are usually associated with superficial bleeding in the skin and mucous membranes whereas clotting factor deficiencies cause deeper bleeding. The associations between bleeding symptoms and specific coagulation defects are shown in Table 25.1.

Persistent oozing from the umbilical stump is typical for infants with defective production or function of fibrinogen and for infants with factor XIII deficiency. A small proportion of infants with severe coagulation factor deficiencies present with intracranial hemorrhage as the first manifestation of their bleeding tendency.[14–17]

Facial purpura following birth is usually associated with severe platelet dysfunction or thrombocytopenia. Oral mucous membrane bleeding is common for thrombocytopenic infants, however gum bleeding and epistaxis hardly ever present in neonates. Joint hemarthroses, typical for severe hemophilias, rarely occur before ambulation.

Bleeding isolated to a single organ or system is more likely to occur as a result of a local cause rather than a hemostatic abnormality. Hemoptysis, hematemesis, gastrointestinal tract bleeding and hematuria are rarely presenting symptoms of a bleeding disorder (in contrast, hematuria in neonates may be the presenting symptom of renal vein thrombosis). Nevertheless, hemostatic abnormalities may exacerbate those symptoms in sick children with acquired deficits, such as disseminated intravascular coagulation, liver failure or vitamin K deficiency.

LABORATORY SCREENING TESTS

The initial set of tests, providing important information on the possible causes of hemorrhagic disorders, includes a platelet count, a prothrombin time (PT) and an activated thromboplastin time (aPTT). Fibrinogen levels, thrombin clotting time (TCT) and sometimes bleeding time (BT) may be added in some cases; these tests are followed by specific factor assays as required. Diagnostic problems of special concern are the need to adapt all coagulation assays for small amounts of blood and the age-related interpretation required for the test results.

The prolonged aPTT in neonates reflects decreased plasma concentrations of the contact factors, whereas the prolonged PT reflects decreased plasma levels of vitamin K-dependant factors.[2–5] Plasma concentrations of fibrinogen may be skewed upwards; even so, TCT may be prolonged, owing to a normally present 'fetal'

fibrinogen.[18] BT, the test that measures platelets and vessel wall interaction, is shorter in healthy neonates than in adults, probably because of increased concentrations and enhanced function of von Willebrand factor and its large multimers,[2–4,19,20] increased hematocrit, and the presence of large red cells.

The interpretation of the results of coagulation factor assays requires special consideration. In the neonate, the lower normal boundary for the assays of factors II, X and XI may overlap with values typical for heterozygous deficiency,[2,3] making it difficult to diagnose this condition. The levels of other factors, such as factors VIII, V and XIII, correlate well with the 'normal' boundaries; thus the diagnoses of hemophilia A, factor V deficiency and factor XIII deficiency can easily be established.

In general, when the initial laboratory test results reveal abnormalities compared with normal age-related values, a stepwise diagnostic approach should be followed in order to characterize specific defects. The interpretation of abnormal laboratory screening tests of the bleeding neonate is presented in Table 25.2.

Table 25.2 Interpretation of abnormal laboratory screening tests in bleeding neonates

Test	Coagulation defect
Only PT prolonged	Factor VII deficiency
Only aPTT prolonged	Factor VIII, factor IX, and/or factor XI deficiency
	Severe von Willebrand's disease
PT and aPTT prolonged	Factor X, factor V, and/or factor II deficiency
	Fibrinogen deficiency
	Combined factor V and factor VIII deficiency
	Vitamin K deficiency bleeding
Only TCT prolonged	Fibrinogen disorders
	Heparin
	Fibrin degradation products
Fibrinogen decreased	Afibrinogenemia or hypofibrinogenemia
All tests normal	Factor XIII deficiency
	Platelet function defects

A prolonged PTT as a sole laboratory abnormality can stem either from a deficiency of factor VIII, IX, XI or XII (although infants with factor XII deficiency do not bleed) or from the presence of an inhibitor. Factor-specific coagulation inhibitors do not appear in neonates before exposure to blood-borne products; however in cases when a non-specific inhibitor (e.g. heparin) is suspected, mixture studies with normal plasma yield the answer. A prolonged PT reflects factor VII deficiency (or an inhibitor). When PT and PTT are prolonged, combined deficiencies of coagulation factors or disorders of fibrinogen, prothrombin, factor V or factor X are suspected. A prolonged thrombin time may result from afibrinogenemia, hypofibrinogenemia, dysfibrinogenemia or the presence of heparin.

In patients with disseminated intravascular coagulation, an abnormal PT and PTT may be observed, owing to consumptive coagulopathy; a prolonged TCT (caused by inhibition of fibrin polymerization in the presence of high fibrin degradation products) and low fibrinogen levels may also be seen.

In the bleeding neonate with no laboratory abnormality, factor XIII activity should be assessed by direct measurement or using a simple test, based on dissolving a fibrin clot in 5M urea. A blood film, enabling detection of some platelet disorders, and the use of BT may provide information for further diagnosis in such cases.

CONGENITAL FACTOR DEFICIENCIES

Prenatal diagnosis of most severe congenital factor deficiencies is currently possible in families with a history of inherited coagulation factor deficiency. Fetal DNA, obtained through amniocentesis or chorionic villus biopsy, can be tested for the presence of known mutations or analyzed to compare linkage and sequences against the sick proband and his or her parents. Early diagnosis allows for termination of pregnancy or early intervention and therapy, as indicated. The clinical presentation of a severe factor deficiency is spontaneous bleeding or excessive bleeding following minor trauma in an otherwise healthy infant. Intracranial hemor-

rhage may be the presenting symptom.[14–17] The correct diagnostic assays and appropriate management vary according to the underlying basic disorder. Therapeutic options for treatment of the various bleeding disorders in neonates are summarized in Table 25.3.

HEMOPHILIA A

This X-linked recessive deficiency of factor VIII is the most common congenital factor deficiency that presents in neonates. The prevalence of hemophilia is estimated at one in 5000–10,000 males. A detailed epidemiological survey in the USA yielded a prevalence of one in 10,000 males for hemophilia A, whereas the combined prevalence of both hemophilias (A and B) was estimated as one in 5000 live male births.[21] Severe hemophiliacs account for 43–70% of the diagnosed patients. The risk of intracranial hemorrhage in severe hemophilia A or B during infancy is 2–8%.[14,16] In cases where hemophilia of the fetus has been diagnosed *in utero*, the use of instrumental delivery (e.g. vacuum, forceps) should be avoided to reduce the risk of bleeding after birth.

The lower normal limit of factor VIII level at birth is 0.50 units per ml;[2] this is consistent with severe deficiency correlates with a level of < 0.01 units/ml, moderate deficiency with a level of 0.01–0.05 units/ml and mild deficiency with a level of > 0.06 units/ml.

The gene for factor VIII is located on the long arm of chromosome X (Xq28) and contains 26 exons.[22] The specific configuration of this gene makes it prone to a unique rearrangement and inversion, disrupting intron 22. This mutational event accounts for about 45% of all severe hemophilia A patients.[23] Among the remaining 55% of severe hemophilia A patients, gene deletions and specific point mutations have been identified.[24]

Treatment of bleeding manifestations in hemophilia consists of replacement with factor concentrates (see Table 25.3). A bolus intravenous injection of 0.1 units/kg usually raises the plasma factor VIII concentration by approximately 0.2 units/ml. The optimal dosing and frequency of administration are dependent on

Table 25.3 Disease- and product-related therapy of bleeding disorders in neonates

Product	Disease
Vitamin K	Vitamin K deficiency bleeding, prophylaxis after birth
Fresh frozen plasma	Vitamin K deficiency bleeding
	Deficiency of factor II, V, VI, IX*, X, XI, and/or XIII
Cryoprecipitate	Hemophilia A,* von Willebrand's disease*
	Afibrinogenemia, hypofibrinogenemia, or dysfibrinogenemia
	Factor XIII deficiency
Prothrombin complex concentrate	Deficiency of factor II, VII, IX or X
	Vitamin K deficiency bleeding
Factor concentrates:	
Factor VIII	Hemophilia A
von Willebrand factor	von Willebrand's disease
Factor IX	Hemophilia B
Factor XI	Factor XI deficiency
Factor VII, recombinant activated factor VII	Factor VII deficiency
Fibrinogen	Afibrinogenemia, hypofibrinogenemia, or dysfibrinogenemia
Fibrogamin	Factor XIII deficiency

*Only when factor concentrates not available

the severity of bleeding, as well as on individual response, reflecting factor plasma recovery and clearance. Phase I clinical trials for ultimate hemophilia cure by gene therapy, are currently in progress.[25,26]

OTHER GENETIC DISORDERS ASSOCIATED WITH REDUCED FACTOR VIII LEVELS

von Willebrand's disease

von Willebrand's disease is caused by a quantitative reduction or a qualitative abnormality von Willebrand factor. von Willebrand factor is a large, multimeric protein that circulates in the plasma and can also be secreted from granules of endothelial cells or platelets. Unlike other coagulation proteins, it has a role in primary hemostasis by mediating platelet adhesion to sites of vascular injury. It also serves as a carrier protein for plasma factor VIII.[22] von Willebrand's disease affects males and females with a prevalence of 0.8–1.3%.[27,28] Despite the high prevalence of the disease, patients with severe von Willebrand's disease are very rare.[29]

Most forms of von Willebrand's disease cannot be diagnosed in neonates since physiological concentrations of von Willebrand factor and the proportion of high molecular weight multimers of von Willebrand factor are increased.[5,20] Severe von Willebrand's disease is associated with reduced factor VIII activity since circulating plasma factor VIII is bound to von Willebrand factor.[22] Thus, type 3 von

Willebrand's disease (the severe form, with a complete factor deficiency) can be diagnosed in neonates, whereas the diagnoses of mild or qualitative deficiencies (type 1 or 2 von Willebrand's disease respectively) are troublesome and require repeated testing for confirmation in later infancy.

The von Willebrand factor gene, containing 51 introns, was identified on the short arm of chromosome 12. A pseudogene, representing the middle half of von Willebrand factor gene has been mapped to chromosome 22.[30] Large deletions within the gene were found in patients with type 3 disease;[31] other molecular defects correlate to different types and subtypes of von Willebrand's disease.[32]

For the treatment of severe von Willebrand's disease, factor concentrates of factor VIII enriched with von Willebrand factor are used (e.g. Haemate P (Centeon), 8y (BPL), Innobrand (LFB) – see also Table 25.3). Desmopressin, frequently administered to improve hemostasis in some cases of mild hemophilia or von Willebrand's disease, is generally avoided in neonates, because of its side effects of water retention and hyponatremia.[33]

Combined deficiency of factors V and VIII

Combined deficiency of factors V and VIII is a rare recessive disorder that was reported in about 100 families clustered in southern Europe or the Middle East. It can be diagnosed in infants, with simultaneous reductions of activity for both factors down to 10–15% of the normal ranges. Mutations in ERGIC-53, a protein required for efficient transport of factor V and factor VIII, have been identified, yet some patients possess mutations in another gene.[34,35] Treatment consists of factor VIII concentrates combined with fresh frozen plasma, required to raise factor V levels.

HEMOPHILIA B

Congenital factor IX deficiency accounts for 20–25% of all hemophilia cases. Like hemophilia A, the disease is inherited as an X-linked recessive disorder. The prevalence of hemophilia B in the USA is estimated as one in 35,000 males.[21] The severe and moderate forms of hemophilia B can be diagnosed in neonates; however, since the lower normal limit for factor IX at birth is about 0.15 units/ml, the diagnosis of mild hemophilia B requires repeated testing and is confirmed at later infancy.[2,3,36] The factor IX gene, which contain eight exons, is located on the long arm of chromosome X. A number of deletions and point mutations have been identified in this gene.[37,38]

Preliminary data from gene therapy studies for hemophilia B patients seem to be encouraging.[39] Bleeding manifestations are treated with specific factor IX concentrates (0.1 units/kg FIX concentrate raises plasma levels by approximately 0.1 units/ml).

FACTOR XI DEFICIENCY

Factor XI contributes to fibrin clot formation via thrombin generation. It also promotes the activation of thrombin activatable fibrinolysis inhibitor.[40] Patients with factor XI deficiency suffer variable bleeding abnormalities, especially when tissues with high fibrinolytic activity (e.g. the urinary tract, nose, oral cavity, tonsils) are injured.[41] Factor XI deficiency results from mutations of the factor XI gene located on chromosome 4. Severe deficiency is established in adults as well as children when factor levels are below 0.02 units/ml. The disease is common in Ashkenazi Jews (among whom two predominant mutations have been identified); it is present to a lesser degree in other Jewish populations and it occurs sporadically in non-Jewish populations.[42,43]

Homozygous (or compound heterozygous) factor XI deficiency is inherited as an autosomal-recessive trait; it causes severely reduced plasma factor XI concentrations. It can present in neonates following hemostatic challenges such as circumcision.[36] Since physiologic factor XI levels may be low after birth, infants with borderline factor XI levels should be retested before any elective surgical procedures.

For treatment of bleeding episodes or during surgery, either fresh frozen plasma or factor XI concentrate is sometimes required (depending on the site of the procedure and the baseline plasma level of factor XI – trough levels of factor XI of about 30% of normal or even lower are sufficient). Antifibrinolytic therapy may be used as well.[44]

FACTOR VII DEFICIENCY

Factor VII deficiency is a rare autosomal-recessive disorder with an estimated incidence of one per 500,000 in the general population.[45] Severe homozygous factor VII deficiency (plasma levels less than 0.03 units/ml) can present with intracranial hemorrhage after birth.[17,46] Milder deficiencies are usually diagnosed at an older age, owing to lower normal limits of the vitamin K-dependent factor VII at birth as well as more subtle bleeding manifestations.

The factor VII gene, which comprises nine exons, is located at chromosome 13q34. More than 30 different mutations, four short deletions and eight polymorphisms have been identified within this gene. Some of them influence factor VII activity and correlate to the variable hemorrhagic diathesis in factor VII deficient patients.[47] The minimum level of factor VII required to achieve hemostasis is not certain; however, it is generally believed that plasma levels of 15–25% of normal are sufficient. To maintain these levels in bleeding factor VII-deficient infants, fresh frozen plasma, prothrombin complex concentrates that contain factor VII, plasma-derived factor VII concentrate, or recombinant activated factor VII is used, at short intervals, since the product has a very short half-life.[44]

FACTOR XIII DEFICIENCY

A common presentation of factor XIII deficiency (a rare disorder) is delayed bleeding from the umbilical stump. One-third of children with severe, homozygous factor XIII deficiency suffer spontaneous intracranial hemorrhage.[15] Wound dehiscence, impaired healing, and scar formation are typical manifestations at older ages. Once suspected, the diagnosis is confirmed by obtaining a low plasma factor XIII activity or by performing clot stability tests (clots that lack factor XIII stabilizing effect dissolve in 5M urea).

The molecular basis for factor XIII deficiency has been investigated in recent years. Mutations of factor XIII have been described in two genes that encode the A and B subunits of factor XIII. These genes are located on chromosomes 6p24–25 and 1q31–32, respectively.[48]

Bleeding symptoms can easily be treated, since the half-life of factor XIII is long and hemostasis is maintained at low plasma factor XIII levels.[49] Therapeutic options are the use of fresh frozen plasma, cryoprecipitate, or specific factor XIII concentrate.[50]

DISORDERS OF FIBRINOGEN

Afibrinogenemia, severe hypofibrinogenemia, and dysfibrinogenemia may present in neonates with a clinical picture similar to that of factor XIII deficiency.[15,36] Low plasma fibrinogen levels and a prolonged age-related TCT establish the laboratory diagnosis. Cryoprecipitate, usually containing fibrinogen at 200–300 mg per bag, is often used for treatment of bleeding related to these defects. Fibrinogen concentrates are also available. The half-life of fibrinogen is about 3 days.[51]

OTHER RARE FACTOR DISORDERS

Deficiencies of factor XII, prekallikrein, and high molecular weight kininogen are of no clinical significance in neonates. Rare autosomal-recessive homozygous severe factor V deficiency (diagnosed by plasma concentrations > 0.1 units/ml) as well as homozygous severe factor II or factor X deficiency (plasma concentrations lower than 0.2 units/ml and 0.1 units/ml, respectively) can cause hemorrhagic symptoms. The exact prevalence of these disorders is unknown. All infants suffering these disorders demonstrate abnormal coagulation screening tests, with prolonged PT and PTT. Whereas factor V deficiency is easily diagnosed in neonates, borderline-low levels of factor II or factor X (both vitamin K-dependent factors) may overlap with neonatal physiological levels, making the diagnosis difficult. Therapy consists of administration of fresh frozen plasma (for factor V deficiency) or prothrombin complex concentrates. The latter, which contains factors II, VII, IX, and X, confers a risk of thrombosis but solves the issue of therapy-related volume overload. Specific factor concentrates are not available.[44]

VITAMIN K DEFICIENCY

Charles Townsend was the first to describe the classical form of vitamin K deficiency, known as hemorrhagic disease of the newborn (HDN). Thirty-one out of 50 neonates reported by him in 1894 died of HDN.[52] The term is still used as a synonym for vitamin K deficiency bleeding (VKDB). Neonatal stores of vitamin K and the plasma levels of vitamin K-dependent factors are low, and only a small fraction of maternal administered vitamin K reaches the fetus.[53,54] On the other hand, warfarin derivatives, some antibiotics, tuberculostatics and anticonvulsant drugs, when given to pregnant women, can enter the fetal circulation and further decrease the action of vitamin K.[55] Low intake of breast milk (which has particularly poor vitamin K concentrations) in the first days of life and the sterile neonatal gut also confer a risk of VKDB.[56–58]

Classic HDN mostly presents on days 2–5 postnatally. Estimates of its frequency vary between 0.25 and 1.5% (quoted in old reviews)[59] to up to four per 1000 in more recent papers.[60] Bleeding symptoms include gastrointestinal bleeding, ecchymoses, umbilical bleeding, and bleeding at needle prick sites. Intracranial hemorrhage was also reported, with an incidence as high as 65–100% in the early reports. The incidence of intracranial hemorrhage and the mortality in infants with VKDB have declined markedly following the increase in vitamin K prophylaxis.[60] A rare, early form of VKDB presents in the first 24 hours of life with cephalhematomas, internal bleeding or intracranial

hemorrhage. This form is usually associated with maternal drug intake, although occasionally no predisposing factor is found.[61] The delayed form, occuring between week 2 and week 8 of postnatal life in breastfed infants, may also present with intracranial hemorrhage. This form can be associated with various conditions that affect vitamin K supplementation and absorption (e.g. hepatitis, cystic fibrosis, diarrhea) or conditions such as long-term administration of antibiotics or parenteral nutrition, which affect the natural flora of the gut and decrease vitamin K absorption.[60,61]

In all infants with VKDB, laboratory assays of PT and PTT are prolonged, and direct measures of plasma vitamin K-dependent factors yield low levels. Since vitamin K is responsible for the carboxylation of these factors, infants that lack vitamin K produce decarboxylated forms of vitamin K-dependent factors (protein induced by vitamin K absence), which can provide indirect evidence for vitamin K deficiency.[60]

Most studies support generalized vitamin K prophylaxis. Although a possible association between neonatal vitamin K administration and an increased risk of childhood cancer was reported in 1990,[62,63] further studies have failed to prove this risk.[64,65] The recommended prophylactic dose is either a single intramuscular dose of 0.5–1 mg or an oral dose of 2–4 mg at birth.[65,66] Multiple-dose oral prophylaxis may be acceptable as well.[61] Symptomatic patients should be treated with extra doses of vitamin K. In the case of life-threatening bleeding or intracranial hemorrhage, fresh frozen plasma, prothrombin complex concentrate and even recombinant activated factor VII may be considered.

Hereditary combined deficiency of vitamin K-dependent factors

Hereditary combined deficiency of vitamin K-dependent factors is a very rare autosomal recessive disorder. It can manifest itself by a mild or severe bleeding tendency, the latter being similar to that seen in HDN. A mis-sense mutation in the γ-glutamyl carboxylase gene has been identified in one case; this mutation results in combined deficiency of all vitamin K-dependent blood factors.[66]

REFERENCES

1. Reverdiau-Moalic P, Delahousse B, Bardos GBP, et al. Evolution of blood coagulation activators and inhibitors in the helthy human fetus. *Blood* 1996;**88**:900–6.

2. Andrew M, Payes B, Milner R, et al. Development of the human coagulation system in the full-term infant. *Blood* 1987;**70**:165–72.

3. Andrew M, Payes B, Milner R, et al. Development of the human coagulation system in the healthy premature infant. *Blood* 1988;**72**:1651–7.

4. Andrew M, Payes B, Johnston M. Development of the hemostatic system in the neonate and young infant. *Am J Pediatr Hematol Oncol* 1990;**12**:95–104.

5. Andrew M, Vegh P, Johnston M, et al. Maturation of the hemostatic system during childhood. *Blood* 1992;**80**:1998–2005.

6. Cvirm G, Gallistl S, Muntean W. Effects of antithrombin and protein C on thrombin generation in newborn and adult plasma. *Thromb Res* 1999;**93**:183–90.

7. Andrew M, Schmidt B, Mitchell L, et al. Thrombin generation in newborn plasma is critically dependant on the concentration of prothrombin. *Thromb Haemost* 1990;**63**:27–30.

8. Andrew M, Mitchell L, Vegh P, Ofosu F. Thrombin regulation in children differs from adults in the absence and presence of heparin. *Thromb Haemost* 1994;**72**:836–42.

9. Summaria L. Comparison of human normal, full-term, fetal and adult plasminogen by physical and chemical analyses. *Haemostasis* 1989;**19**:266–73.

10. Israels S, Daniels M, McMillan E. Deficient collagen-induced activation in the newborn platelet. *Pediatr Res* 1990;**27**:337–43.

11. Suarez CR, Gonzalez J, Menendez C, et al. Neonatal and maternal platelet activation at time of birth. *Am J Hematol* 1988;**29**:18–21.

12. Suarez CR, Menendez CE, Welenga JM, Fareed J. Neonatal and maternal hemostasis. Value of molecular markers in the assessment of hemostatic status. *Semin Thromb Hemost* 1984;**10**:280–4.

13. Runnebaum IB, Maurer SM, Daly L, Bonnar J. Inhibitors and activators of fibrinolysis during and after childbirth in maternal and cord blood. *J Perinat Med* 1989;**17**:113–19.

14. Yoffe G, Buchanan GR. Intracranial hemorrhage in newborn and young infants with hemophilia. *J Pediatr* 1988;**113**:333–6.

15. Abbondanzo SL, Gootenbeg JE, Lofts R, McPherson R. Intracranial hemorrhage in congenital deficiency of factor XIII. *Am J Pediatr Hematol Oncol* 1988;**10**:65–8.

16. Struwe FE. Intracranial hemorrhage and occlusive hydrocephalus in hereditary bleeding disorders. *Dev Med Child Neurol* 1970;**12**:165–72.

17. Mariani G, Mazzucconi MG. Factor VII congenital deficiency. *Hemostasis* 1983;**13**:169–77.

18. Witt I, Muller H, Kunter LJ. Evidence for the existence of fetal fibrinogen. *Thromb Diatherm Haemorrhage* 1969;**22**:101–9.

19. Katz JA, Moake JL, McPherson PD, et al. Relationship between human development and disappearance of unusually large von Willebrand factor multimers from plasma. *Blood* 1989;**73**:1851–8.

20. Weinstein M, Blanchard R, Moake J, et al. Fetal and neonatal von Willebrand factor (vWf) is unusually large and similar to the vWF found in patients with thrombotic thrombocytopenia purpura. *Br J Haematol* 1989;**72**:68–72.

21. Soucie JM, Evatt B, Jackson D. Occurrence of hemophilia in the United States. The Hemophilia Surveillance System Project Investigators. *Am J Hematol* 1998;**59**:288–94.

22. Kaufman RJ. Biological regulation of factor VIII activity. *Annu Rev Med* 1992;**43**:325–39.

23. Antonarakis SE, Rossiter JP, Young M, et al. Factor VIII gene inversions in severe hemophilia A: results of an international consortium study. *Blood* 1995;**86**:2206–12.

24. Tuddenham EDG, Schwaab R, Seehafer J, et al. Hemophilia A: database of nucleotide substitutions, deletions, insertions and rearrangements of the factor VIII gene, second edition. *Nucleic Acids Res* 1994;**22**:3511–33.

25. Jolly D. In vivo delivery of factor VIII retroviral vectors for treatment of hemophilia A. Corporate Symposium, Progress Toward Hemophilia Gene Therapy. Program of the Second Annual Meeting of the American Society of Gene Therapy. Washington DC;1999:52.

26. Selden R. Nonviral ex vivo gene transfer. National Hemophilia Foundation, the Third Workshop on Gene Therapies for Hemophilia. Washigton DC; 2000.

27. Rodeghiero F, Castaman G, Dini E. Epidemiological investigation of the prevalence of von Willebrand's disease. *Blood* 1987;**69**:454–9.

28. Werner EJ, Emmett H, Tucker D, et al. Prevalence of von Willebrand disease in children; a multicentric study. *J Pediatr* 1993;**123**:893–8.

29. Mannucci PM, Bloom AL, Larrieu MJ, et al. Atherosclerosis and von Willebrand factor. I.

Prevalence of severe von Willebrand's disease in western Europe and Israel. *Br J Haematol* 1984;**57**:163–9.

30. Mancuso DJ, Tuley EA, Westfield LA, *et al.* Human von Willebrand factor gene and pseudogene: structural analysis and differentiation by polymerase chain reaction. *Biochemistry* 1991;**30**:253–69.

31. Ngo KY, Glotz VT, Koziol JA, *et al.* Homozygous and heterozygous deletions of the von Willebrand factor gene in patients and carriers of severe von Willebrand disease. *Proc Natl Acad Sci USA* 1988;**85**:2753–7.

32. Ginsburg D, Sadler JE. von Willebrand disease: a database of point mutations, insertions and deletions. *Thromb Haemost* 1993;**69**:177–84.

33. Sheperd LL, Hutchinson RJ, Worden EK, *et al.* Hyponatremia and seizures after intravenous administration of desmopressin acetate for surgical hemostasis. *J Pediatr* 1989;**114**:470–2.

34. Nichols WC, Seligsohn U, Zivelin A, *et al.* Mutations in the ER–Golgi intermediate compartment protein ERGIC-53 cause combined deficiency of coagulation factors V and VIII. *Cell* 1999;**12**:714–17.

35. Nichols WC, Terry VH, Wheatley MA, *et al.* ERGIC-53 gene stucture and mutation analysis in 19 combined factors V and VIII deficiency families. *Blood* 1999;**93**:2261–6.

36. Andrew M. The relevance of developmental hemostasis to hemorrhagic disorders of newborns. *Semin Perinatol* 1997;**21**:70–85.

37. Koerbert DD, Bottema CDK, Ketterling RP, *et al.* Mutations causing hemophilia B: direct estimate of the underlying rates of spontaneous germ-like transitions, transversions, and deletions in a human gene. *Am J Hum Genet* 1990;**47**:202–17.

38. Giannelli F, Anagnostopoulos T, Green PM. Mutation rates in humans. II. Sporadic mutation-specific rates and rate of detrimental human mutations inferred from hemophilia B. *Am J Hum Genet* 1996;**65**:1580–7.

39. Kay MA, Manno CS, Rangi MV, *et al.* Evidence for gene transfer and expression of factor IX in haemophilia B patients treated with AAV vector. *Nat Genet* 2000;**24**:257–61.

40. Bouma BN, Mosnier LO, Meijers JCM, *et al.* Factor XI dependent and independent activation of thrombin activatable fibrinolysis inhibitor in plasma associated with clot formation. *Thromb Haemost* 1999;**82**:1703–8.

41. Bouma BN, Meijers JCM. Role of blood coagulation factor XI in downregulation of fibrinolysis. *Curr Opin Hematol* 2000;**7**:266–72.

42. Peretz H, Mulai A, Usher S, *et al.* The two common mutations causing factor XI deficiency in Jews stem from distinct founders: one of ancient Middle Eastern origin and another of more recent European origin. *Blood* 1997;**90**;2654–9.

43. Goldstein DB, Reich DE, Bradman N, *et al.* Age estimates of two common mutations causing factor XI deficiency: recent genetic drift is not necessary for elevated disease incidence among Ashkenazi Jews. *Am J Hum Genet* 1999;**64**:1071–5.

44. Seligsohn U, White GC. Inherited deficiencies of coagulation factors II, V, VII, XI and XIII and the conbined deficiencies of factors V and VIII and of the vitamin K-dependent factors. In: Beutler E, Lichtman MA, Coller B, Kipps TJ, Seligsohn U, eds. *Williams' Hematology*, 6th edn. New York: McGraw-Hill; 2001:1617–38.

45. Triplett D, Brandt J, McGann Batard M, *et al.* Hereditary factor VII deficiency: heterogeneity defined by combined functional and immuno-chemical analysis. *Blood* 1985;**66**:1284–7.

46. Herrmann FH, Wulff K, Auberger K, *et al.* Molecular biology and clinical manifestation of hereditary factor VII deficiency. *Semin Thromb Hemost* 2000;**26**:393–400.

47. Hunault M, Bauer KA. Recombinant factor VIIa for the treatment of congential factor VII deficiency. *Semin Thromb Hemost* 2000;**26**:400–5.

48. Mikkola H, Palotie A. Gene deficiency. *Semin Thromb Hemost* 2000;**22**:393–8.

49. Mikkola H, Muszbek L, Laiho E, *et al.* Molecular mechanism of a mild phenotype in factor XIII deficiency, a splicing mutation permitting partial correct splicing of factor XIII A subunit mRNA. *Blood* 1997;**89**:1279–87.

50. Karges HE, Metzner HJ. Therapeutic factor XIII preparations and perspective for recombinant factor XIII. *Semin Thromb Hemost* 1996;**22**:427–36.

51. Brettlet D, Levine P. Clinical manifestations and therapy of inherited coagulation factor deficiencies. In: Colman RW, Hirsh J, Marder VJ, Salzman EW, eds. *Hemostasis and Thrombosis: Basic Principles and Clinical Practice*, 3rd edn. Philadelphia: JB Lippincott; 1999:169–83.

52. Townsend CW. The haemorrhagic disease of the newborn. *Arch Pediatr* 1894;**11**:559–65.

53. Hiraike H, Kimura M, Itokawa Y. Distribution of K vitamins (phyloquinone and menaquinones) in human placenta and maternal and umbilical cord plasma. *Am J Obstet Gynecol* 1988;**158**:564–9.

54. Hamulyak K, de Boer-van den Berg MAG. The placental transport of (3H) vitamin K1 in rats. *Br J Haematol* 1987;**65**:335–8.

55. Birger A. Antenatal drug affecting vitamin K status of the fetus and the newborn. *Semin Thromb Hemost* 1995;**21**:364–70.

56. Shinzawa T, Mura T, Tsunei M, Shiraki Z. Vitamin K absorption capacity and its association with vitamin K deficiency. *Am J Dis Child* 1989;**143**:686–9.

57. Von Kries R, Becker A, Gobel U. Vitamin K in the newborn: influence of nutritional factors on carboxy-prothrombin detectability and factor II and VII clotting activity. *Eur J Pediatr* 1987;**146**:123–7.

58. Sutherland JM, Glueck HI. Hemorrhagic disease of the newborn: breast feeding as a necessary factor in the pathogenesis. *Am J Dis Child* 1967;**113**:524–33.

59. American Academy of Pediatrics: Committee on Nutrition. Vitamin K compounds and water soluble analogues: use in therapy and prophylaxis in pediatrics. *Pediatrics* 1961;**28**:501–7.

60. Sutor A. Vitamin K deficiency bleeding in infants and children. *Semin Thromb Hemost* 1995;**21**: 317–29.

61. Monagle P, Andrew M. Hemorrhagic and thromboembolic complications during infancy and childhood. In: Colman RW, Hirsh J, Marder VJ, Salzman EW, George JN, eds. *Hemostasis and Thrombosis: Basic Principles and Clinical Practice*, 4th ed. Philadelphia: JB Lippincott; 2001: 1053–70.

62. Golding J, Paterson M, Kinlen L. Factors associated with childhood cancer in a national cohort study. *Br J Cancer* 1990;**62**:304–8.

63. Golding J, Birmingham K, Greenwood R, Mott M. Intramuscular vitamin K and childhood cancer. *BMJ* 1992;**305**:341–6.

64. Sutor AH, von Kries R, Cornelissen EAM, *et al.* Vitamin K deficiency bleeding (VKDB) in infancy. ISTH pediatric/perinatal sub-committee. International Society on Thrombosis and Haemostasis. *Thromb Haemost* 1999;**81**:456–61.

65. Brousson MA, Klein MC. Controversies surrounding the administration of vitamin K to newborns: a review. *CMAJ* 1996;**154**:307–15.

66. Brenner B, Sanchez-Vega B, Wu SM, *et al.* A missense mutation in gamma-glutamyl carboxylase gene causes combined deficiency of all vitamin K-dependent blood coagulation factors. *Blood* 1998;**92**:4554–9.

Index